Your
Best
Medicine

Your
Best
Medicine

From Conventional and Complementary Medicine—Expert-Endorsed
Therapeutic Solutions to Relieve Symptoms and Speed Healing

**Mark A. Goldstein, MD, Myrna Chandler Goldstein, MA,
and Larry P. Credit, OMD**

RODALE

Rodale books may be purchased for business or promotional use or for special sales. For more information, please write to: Special Markets Department, Rodale Inc., 733 Third Avenue, New York, NY 10017

Printed in the United States of America
Rodale Inc. makes every effort to use acid-free ♾, recycled paper ♻.

Book design by Christopher Rhoads

Library of Congress Cataloging-in-Publication Data

Goldstein, Mark A. (Mark Allan)
    Your best medicine : from conventional and complementary medicine—expert-endorsed therapeutic solutions to relieve symptoms and speed healing / Mark A. Goldstein, Myrna Chandler Goldstein, and Larry P. Credit.
        p.   cm.
    Includes bibliographical references and index.
    ISBN-13 978–1–59486–826–9 hardcover
    ISBN-10 1–59486–826–3 hardcover
    ISBN-13 978–1–59486–849–8 paperback
    ISBN-10 1–59486–849–2 paperback
    1. Middle-aged persons—Health and hygiene.   2. Medicine, Popular.   3. Alternative medicine.
I. Goldstein, Myrna Chandler   II. Credit, Larry P.   III. Title.
RA777.5.G65 2008
613'.0434—dc22   2008010300

Distributed to the trade by Macmillan

8   10   9   hardcover

2   4   6   8   10   9   7   5   3   1   paperback

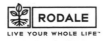

LIVE YOUR WHOLE LIFE™

We inspire and enable people to improve their lives and the world around them

For more of our products visit **rodalestore.com** or call 800-848-4735

To our children, Brett, Samantha, and Sarah, whose work in law enforcement, medicine, and public health will help improve the lives of countless members of society.

In loving memory of our parents, Samuel, Jean, Craig, and Sarah, whose lives were shortened by heart disease and cancer.

—*Mark A. Goldstein and Myrna Chandler Goldstein*

To my family, friends, and patients—with thanks for your continued support and guidance.

—*Larry P. Credit*

Contents

Part 3: References

Introduction: How to Use This Book

Every week consumers like you hear or read reports of medical advances that may leave them wondering what truly is the "best" in diagnosis and treatment. Just a few examples:

- An article in a recent issue of the *New England Journal of Medicine* compared the ability of computed tomographic colonography (CTC) and traditional colonoscopy to detect advanced colon polyps that could lead to colon cancer. The two screening techniques were equally accurate—but the CTC is much more comfortable for patients, which means that it may be a better option.

- A study published in the *Archives of General Psychiatry* attempted to discern the best treatment for adolescents with depression. It turned out to be not one treatment but, rather, a combination of drug therapy (with fluoxetine, or Prozac) and cognitive behavioral therapy.

- For an article in the journal *Nature*, researchers at Massachusetts General Hospital described how capsaicin—the active ingredient in chili peppers—helps relieve pain, including after surgery. Their report cites scientific evidence to demonstrate that capsaicin, which has a long history as a complementary treatment, actually works.

In writing this book, one of our goals has been to sort through evolving and sometimes conflicting health information, to help identify what truly is "best" in terms of effectiveness, accessibility, safety, and cost. We've taken the broadest view of the options, presenting conventional and complementary treatments for 81 common health concerns. To compile this information, we have drawn on prestigious medical journals such as the *New England Journal of Medicine*, the *Journal of the American Medical Association*, and *Lancet* as well as reliable clinical resources such as UptoDate (www.uptodate.com) and the *BMJ Clinical Evidence Handbook*. Two of us have also drawn on our collective clinical experience—Dr. Goldstein as an allopathic or conventionally trained physician who is a division chief at Massachusetts General Hospital in Boston and Dr. Credit as an oriental medicine doctor (OMD) who maintains a private practice at Sancta Maria Hospital in Cambridge, Massachusetts.

We should note at the outset that compared to conventional treatments, which must undergo extensive testing prior to going on the market, complementary treatments seldom are subject to the same level of clinical evaluation. This doesn't mean they don't work; in fact, many have hundreds if not thousands of years of anecdotal evidence to demonstrate their therapeutic properties. It does mean you (and your doctor) should carefully weigh all of your options when deciding on a treatment plan. Take care not to assume that a complementary treatment is safer, and therefore better, simply because it's "natural."

Getting Around

If you've scanned the table of contents, you already know that we've organized our book into two parts, each of which serves a distinct purpose. Part 1 reviews the principles of good health maintenance, such as when to get key medical screenings and how to recognize life-threatening medical emergencies. It also offers brief descriptions of the various conventional and complementary therapies, which will provide a framework for the information in Part 2.

The condition entries in Part 2 account for the lion's share of the book. With a handful of exceptions, each entry offers the following:

- A general overview of the condition, including its causes and risk factors
- A list of signs and symptoms
- Conventional treatments
- Complementary treatments
- Lifestyle recommendations
- Preventive measures

We've structured the entries in this way in order for you, the reader, to have quick and easy access to the information you need, as soon as you need it. Let's say you're returning home from a visit to your doctor, who told you that you have high blood pressure. Just turn to the appropriate page in this book, and there you'll find out why you're a candidate for high blood pressure and—perhaps more important—what you can do about it. After reviewing your options, you may want to follow up with your doctor to find out if you really need a beta-blocker to rein in your blood pressure, or if you first could try a combination of diet, nutritional supplements, herbs, and relaxation techniques.

If you want to learn more about high blood pressure, you can flip to the resources at the back of the book for a listing of organizations that can provide further information and support. We've also included a listing of professional associations for the various complementary therapies, many of which can help direct you to qualified practitioners in your area. We realize that while finding a conventionally trained physician (an MD or DO) is rather easy, the same may not be true for complementary practitioners—acupuncturists and reflexologists, for example. Certainly, convenience should be a consideration when you're deciding whether to try a particular complementary therapy.

Before You Proceed

We've done our best to make this book as up-to-date, authoritative, and complete as possible. In turn, we encourage you to use it wisely and responsibly. To this end, we offer the following caveats.

• Please exercise your best judgment in deciding when to seek your physician's advice and when to try self-care. For example, you probably can handle a bout of garden-variety constipation on your own. But if it persists, or it's exceptionally painful, or it's accompanied by blood in the stool, then it requires medical intervention. Some symptoms or conditions, like chest pain, should be checked out by a physician as soon as possible. Pay attention to your body's internal and external cues; then you'll learn to recognize when something unusual is going on, and you'll be able to respond accordingly. When in doubt, call your doctor. As the saying goes, it's better to be safe than sorry.

• Do not discontinue any conventional treatment, or replace it with a complementary treatment, without first consulting your physician. If you are taking a medication, for example, reducing the dosage—or going off the drug completely—can have serious health implications. So can adding an herbal or nutritional supplement, which could undermine a medication's intended effects. We believe that conventional and complementary therapies can coexist in a treatment plan; in cases of chronic illness, in particular, an integrated approach to care may offer the best chance for alleviating symptoms and improving quality of life. But you and your doctor should work together to determine the best course of treatment.

• As thorough and accurate as we've attempted to be in our reporting, we really can't advise you on your particular condition without knowing you and your health history. With this book, our purpose is to inform and educate, so you (and your doctor) can make intelligent decisions about your health care. If you believe that you should consult your doctor on a particular matter, by all means do. Caution and common sense can make all the difference in your treatment outcomes.

We hope that you find our book to be a helpful guide on your journey to complete healing and optimal health.

—Mark A. Goldstein, MD, Myrna Chandler Goldstein, and Larry P. Credit, OMD

The Basics of Good Health

WHILE THE FOCUS OF THIS BOOK is on understanding and treating specific medical conditions, everyone knows that good health care involves much more than addressing problems as they arise. If you are to enjoy and fully engage in all aspects of your life, you need to be proactive about your own care at all times—even when you're feeling well.

Part 1 provides the information and tools necessary to be an effective steward of your health, with chapters that offer the following:

• An overview of conventional and complementary therapies, and how they can be used together in an integrative approach to care

• Routine medical tests that can help to detect disease in its earliest stage, when it is most treatable

• The signs and symptoms of potentially life-threatening health crises, with important instructions on what to do in a medical emergency

These chapters can help establish the framework for safeguarding your health—and for taking action in the event that you do become sick. Prevention and preparation may be the best medicine of all.

Integrative Medicine:
The Best of All Worlds

In this book, you're going to find treatments from both conventional medicine and complementary disciplines. Combining the two in a treatment plan has come to be known as an integrative approach to care.

For many years, conventional and complementary medicine operated in separate universes, with little common ground except their mutual objective of helping patients to heal from illness or—in the case of chronic conditions—to minimize symptoms. Why are they coming together now? Mostly because health care consumers like you have demanded it. They recognized that conventional and complementary therapies alike have benefits as well as risks—and that combining the two can optimize healing while, in many cases, reducing costs.

In this chapter, we'll provide brief overviews of conventional and complementary medicine in turn. This information will provide a foundation for the condition-specific "prescriptions" in Part 2.

What Is Conventional Medicine?

Until relatively recently, the words "complementary medicine" seldom were spoken in a medical setting. For the most part, the care and treatment provided by doctors fell within the conventional realm.

Conventional medicine—sometimes called allopathic medicine or mainstream medicine—has been practiced by generations of traditionally trained physicians. Those who wish to pursue a career in medicine must complete 4 years of study (beyond a bachelor's degree), followed by an internship, a residency, and possibly a fellowship. Generally, students who attend one of the nation's 125 medical schools are taught to use medications, surgery, and other conventional modalities to treat medical conditions. They may not learn about complementary disciplines, unless they choose to do so. (Many schools are offering training on the relationship between body and mind, so doctors-to-be can recognize when treatment may need to involve a mental health practitioner.)

Among the key differences between conventional and complementary medicine is that conventional modalities must undergo a certain level of scientific scrutiny before they become available to the general public. Every day, medical researchers in laboratories throughout the United States are conducting thousands of studies in a continual effort to develop new diagnostic procedures, medications, and surgical techniques. To a certain extent, these endeavors are overseen and regulated by the federal government.

In recent years, many medical doctors have embraced evidence-based medicine—that is, the use of the best evidence from research studies to guide their clinical decisions. Thanks to the Internet, they now have quick and easy access to these findings, which allows them to provide their patients with the most up-to-date medical care possible.

Conventional medicine also places an emphasis on prevention. From a very young age, children are given vaccines to help protect against a host of different illnesses. Likewise, adults are encouraged to get certain shots—such as the one that prevents influenza—and to undergo regular screenings designed to detect various illnesses in their earliest and most treatable forms.

But conventional medicine isn't without challenges, particularly with regard to cost and access to care. There's a serious shortage of medical doctors—especially those who specialize in certain areas of medicine—in rural communities. Further, more than 46 million Americans have no health insurance, while another 40 million have inadequate coverage. These people all too often neglect preventive care, and they may put off treatment for their health problems until they require emergency intervention.

Perhaps not surprisingly, those with greater financial resources tend to receive better medical care in the conventional medical system. The recent emergence of "boutique practices" promises to widen the gap even more, with some doctors limiting their practices to a preset number of patients. Patients, in turn, pay thousands of dollars above their normal health insurance premiums for improved access to their doctors.

Despite the problems within a conventional medical system, it is a good idea to have a traditionally trained physician as your primary care provider. To some degree, whom you choose may be determined by your health plan, as some plans require their members to utilize certain physicians or practices. Beyond that, you want a doctor who's board-certified, meaning that he or she has met the training requirements and passed the certification exam of a medical organization such as the American Board of Internal Medicine. These exams are designed to assess competency in various medical specialties.

Also be sure to ask whether a doctor has hospital admitting privileges. This means that if you ever require hospitalization, your doctor can admit you to the appropriate facility.

These days, it's relatively easy to check out a doctor's training and credentials online through the Web sites of organizations such as the American Medical Association (www.ama-assn.org). Still, many people find their primary care providers by word of mouth—through family members, friends, and colleagues who are happy with the quality of care that a particular doctor provides. At the end of the day, perhaps what matters most is finding someone with whom you feel comfortable and in whom you have the confidence to entrust your care.

What Is Complementary Medicine?

Complementary medicine—also known as alternative or holistic medicine—is an umbrella term for a number of healing disciplines, some of which date back thousands of years. A typical complementary treatment plan takes into account all of the elements that influence a person's health—including the physical, mental, emotional, spiritual, and social, and sometimes the environmental. Complementary therapies also tend to be quite sensitive to the mind-body connection—that is, how a person's mental and emotional state can influence physical health and vice versa. A complementary practitioner will actively involve a patient in his or her own care by teaching the person to use remedies and techniques that not only support healing but also prevent future illness.

Where conventional medicine tends to focus on alleviating the symptoms of a disease, complementary therapies attempt to identify and treat the root cause. These perspectives may seem at odds, but as practitioners and patients are coming to realize, combining conventional and complementary modalities—that is, an integrative approach to care—often can be more effective than using either alone.

One of the enduring criticisms of complementary medicine is that very few of the treatments have been subject to the same rigorous scientific scrutiny as conventional medicine. Indeed, though certain complementary disciplines have thousands of years of anecdotal evidence to support their therapeutic powers, the scientific literature remains rather scant. Gradually that is changing, due in large part to the creation of the National Center for Complementary and Alternative Medicine in 1999. This government-funded institution—under the auspices of the National Institutes of Health—is training researchers, financing clinical trials, and disseminating authoritative information about various complementary therapies to physicians and laypeople alike.

Within complementary medicine, the philosophies and practices of the disciplines can vary greatly. If you're thinking about adding one of these therapies to your health care regimen, it's important for you to consider your personal preferences and comfort level when weighing your options. For example, acupuncture, massage, and therapeutic touch are all effective treatments for headaches, but they're very different in what they entail. Choosing the one that's best for you requires some research, and perhaps a bit of trial and error.

More and more insurance companies are expanding their coverage to include complementary therapies, so before you make a decision, you may want to check the provisions of your own health plan. Other factors that you should take into account: how far you'll be traveling to a qualified practitioner, how often you'll require in-office visits and treatments, and whether you can use the treatments at home, on your own.

Depending on the discipline, finding a qualified practitioner can take some legwork. To simplify the process, we've provided a listing of professional organizations beginning on page 563. Often the Web sites for these organizations have tools that allow you to search for practitioners by location. We've included a guide to practitioners' credentials (see page 567), which may help you assess whether someone has the appropriate training and certifications to practice a particular therapy.

What follows are brief descriptions of the complementary disciplines that you're most likely to encounter in this book. You'll find more detailed remedies in the condition entries of Part 2.

Acupressure

Based on the principles of acupuncture and traditional Chinese medicine, acupressure is the application of pressure to specific points on the body via deep circular movements of the thumbs, fingers, elbows, or palms. This pressure is said to release *chi*, or healing energy, which circulates throughout the body along specific pathways called meridians. By clearing blockages in the energy flow, acupressure improves the body's ability to heal itself.

Acupuncture

The main difference between acupuncture and acupressure is that the former uses hair-thin, sterile, disposable needles rather than firm pressure to release *chi*. Studies have shown that acupuncture treatment is able to stimulate various physical reactions, including changes in brain activity, blood pressure, blood chemistry, heart rate, endocrine function, and immune system response.

Alexander Technique

Developed by the Australian actor Frederick Matthias Alexander, who suffered from chronic hoarseness when performing, the Alexander Technique (AT) identifies poor postural habits and replaces them with improved body mechanics. An AT instructor teaches basic exercises that improve balance, posture, and coordination and help relieve posture-related problems such as back pain.

Aquatic Therapy

Also known as water therapy, aquatic therapy involves performing gentle, rhythmic movements and exercises in a warm (92° to 99°F), shallow pool. Participants may be seated or standing during their therapy sessions, and they may walk or float in the water. Since many aquatic therapy facilities have an additional pool that's set to a cooler temperature, a therapy session may include time in both pools.

Aromatherapy

Aromatherapy is the use of aromatic essential oils from herbs and flowers for therapeutic purposes. Aromatherapists believe that the perfume from the essential oils stimulates the release of neurotransmitters in the brain. These neurotransmitters, in turn, stimulate or calm the body and relieve pain. Moreover, certain essential oils may have antibacterial, anti-inflammatory, or astringent properties when applied directly to the skin. Each essential oil has unique therapeutic benefits.

Ayurveda

Developed in India more than 5,000 years ago, Ayurveda is a holistic (whole-body) discipline that tailors treatment to a person's body type (*prakriti*) and energy type (*dosha*). Each of the three energy types—*vata*, *pitta*, and *kapha*—corresponds to particular body types. Although everyone has a combination of the three *doshas*, one (sometimes two) tends to be most prevalent.

Once an Ayurvedic practitioner has determined your dominant *dosha*, he will make recommendations that collectively will bring the three energy types into balance. A typical Ayurvedic treatment plan will combine a number of approaches, including nutritional therapy, herbal remedies, physical exercise, massage, and meditation.

Biofeedback

In biofeedback, an electric monitoring device is placed on the surface of the skin to record data on vital functions such as heart rate, blood pressure, muscle tension, brain wave activity, and skin temperature. These data are transmitted to a biofeedback machine, which "translates" them into sounds (beeps), visual images (flashes), or dial readings. By paying attention to these signals, you become more aware of stress-related physical changes and better able to control them—usually through relaxation techniques such as deep breathing, meditation, and/or visualization. The goal of biofeedback training is to learn how to achieve and maintain a relaxed state even when you are not using a biofeedback machine.

Bodywork

Bodywork is a general term for a number of therapeutic approaches that use hands-on techniques to manipulate and balance the musculoskeletal system. These approaches relieve pain, facilitate healing, increase energy, and promote relaxation and well-being. Examples of bodywork techniques include acupressure, craniosacral therapy, reflexology, Rolfing, shiatsu, therapeutic touch, and trigger point therapy.

Chiropractic

Based on the premise that good health requires a strong, agile, and aligned spine, chiropractic medicine involves spinal manipulation and adjustment. This moves the backbone into its proper position, thereby facilitating the correct functioning of the nervous system and the well-being of the entire body. A chiropractic session also may include nutritional counseling.

Craniosacral Therapy

Craniosacral therapy is the gentle manipulation of the craniosacral system, which includes the brain, spinal cord, cerebrospinal fluid, dural membrane, cranial bones, and sacrum. The pressure applied to these parts is no more than the weight of a nickel. By reducing stress and correcting systemic imbalances, craniosacral therapy may stimulate the body's innate healing powers.

Diet

Proper nutrition is vital to the healing process, and to optimal health. In general, we advocate a well-balanced diet that's high in fiber and low in unhealthy fats, with an abundance of whole grains, fresh fruits and vegetables, and lean proteins. Try to avoid hydrogenated fats, fried foods, and processed foods containing artificial colors and other chemicals. For certain medical conditions in Part 2, we recommend eating some foods that help heal the body while avoiding other foods that can contribute to or aggravate the problem.

Feldenkrais Method

Similar to the Alexander Technique, the Feldenkrais Method teaches you to become more aware of your movement patterns and to correct unhealthy habits by relearning proper body mechanics. Sessions may be one-on-one or group instruction. In a private session, the instructor manually guides you through the various movements, a technique called Functional Integration. Group sessions involve a technique called Awareness Through Movement, in which the instructor provides verbal cues to the movement sequences. The goal of the Feldenkrais Method is to reduce pain, increase mobility, and enhance well-being.

Flower Essences

First developed by the English physician Dr. Edward Bach in the 1930s, flower essences are liquid extracts of various flowers and plants that help to stabilize emotions, which in turn cultivates physical healing. Unlike the essential oils of aromatherapy, flower essences are highly diluted, and the fragrance does not contribute to their therapeutic properties. The essences may be mixed into a beverage; placed under the tongue; or applied directly to the temples, wrists, elbows, or knees or behind the ears. Because each essence has unique soothing or healing properties, practitioners tailor their recommendations to a person's personality and emotional state.

Herbal Medicine

Herbal remedies are among the most popular and accessible of the complementary therapies. Each herb has its own set of therapeutic properties, and often it's necessary to use a particular part of the plant—perhaps the roots, stems, leaves, or flowers—to obtain an optimal dose of the medicinal constituent(s). Herbal remedies are available as pills, teas, tinctures, creams, and ointments. Herbalists may recommend multiple herbs to treat a particular condition.

Although herbs are available over-the-counter, they are potent substances that can interact with medications and cause side effects. For this reason, we strongly advise talking with your doctor or a qualified herbalist before adding any herbal remedy to your self-care regimen.

Homeopathy

Homeopathy is a healing system based on the principle that substances capable of producing symptoms of sickness in healthy people can have a healing effect when given in very minute quantities to sick people who exhibit the same symptoms. Homeopathic remedies—which are derived from plants, animals, and minerals—work in part by encouraging symptoms to run an accelerated course through the body, thereby speeding the healing process.

Although high-dose homeopathic remedies are available from homeopaths and other trained practitioners, you can find lower-dose products in health food stores, some drugstores, and online. Most remedies are tiny pills that dissolve when placed under the tongue.

Hydrotherapy

Hydrotherapy is the use of water in any of its various forms—liquid, solid, or vapor—to relieve discomfort and promote healing. As a therapeutic discipline, hydrotherapy dates all the way back to ancient Greece and Rome. Today, it's most likely to entail steam baths, saunas, hot tubs, whirlpools, and/or applications of hot and cold packs or ice. All of these treatments have different physiological effects, which makes hydrotherapy a versatile remedy capable of soothing sore or inflamed muscles, reducing fever, rehabilitating injured limbs, relieving headache, and promoting relaxation.

Hypnotherapy

In a hypnotherapy session, the therapist guides the patient into a trancelike state, characterized by extreme suggestibility, heightened imagination, and relaxation. The therapist then uses posthypnotic suggestion to alter the patient's perceptions and behaviors. Hypnotherapy may be beneficial for improving a person's emotional state or helping to overcome addictive behaviors such as smoking and overeating.

Naturopathy

Naturopathy is a holistic healing system that utilizes an array of natural therapies, such as nutritional therapy, herbal medicine, exercise, acupuncture, massage, and hydrotherapy. Together, these therapies strengthen and support the body's innate ability to heal itself.

Nutritional Supplements

Even if you're eating a relatively healthy diet, you may not be getting sufficient amounts of all the vitamins, minerals, and other nutrients that your body needs to carry out its most basic functions. One reason is that nutrient-depleted soils tend to produce nutrient-deficient foods. Storing, cooking, and otherwise processing foods can further deplete their nutrient supplies. Add to this the nutrient-robbing properties of certain medical conditions as well as certain medications (both prescription and over-the-counter), and your body may be at risk for nutritional shortfalls.

Supplements can help cover your nutritional bases when, for whatever reason, your diet may be coming up short. In this book, we recommend supplements both for general nutritional support and for targeted treatment of conditions that may cause or result from a vitamin or mineral deficiency. In nearly every condition entry in Part 2, you will find recommendations for specific supplements.

Just as for herbal remedies, we do strongly advise talking with your doctor before adding nutritional supplements to your self-care regimen. Though they are natural and generally safe, they can cause harm—especially when taken in too-large amounts or when used in combination with certain herbs or medications.

Polarity Therapy

Polarity therapy builds on the principle that energy flows freely in nature, and that stagnation of this energy is the fundamental cause of disease. The goal of treatment is to balance the energy field within the body, thus helping to restore the body to a healthy state.

A polarity therapy session usually begins with a series of finger or hand placements, which are designed to locate areas of energy stagnation while fostering relaxation. These are followed by light touches and subtle manipulations that help release any blocked energy. Polarity therapy also may include nutritional counseling, exercise, and verbal interactions.

Qigong

Much like acupressure and acupuncture, qigong facilitates the flow of *chi*, or energy, along specific pathways throughout the body. It does this through a series of gentle movements, postures, meditations, and breathing patterns. By encouraging the flow of *chi*, qigong supports healing while increasing stamina, flexibility, and relaxation.

Reflexology

In reflexology, certain points on the feet, hands, and ears correlate to specific parts of the body. As a reflexologist stimulates these points (using pressure and massage techniques), he or she can direct blood, energy, nutrients, and nerve impulses to the corresponding parts, thereby stimulating the healing process.

Reiki

Reiki—a 2,500-year-old Tibetan Buddhist practice—is based on the belief that a universal life force flows around us and connects us to one another. This force can be channeled through the hands of a trained practitioner to help restore the flow of a person's innate healing energy. The practitioner may use a light touch, or he may simply place his hands over the affected area. This releases old energy while directing new energy to cells, stimulating the body's systems and normalizing its functions.

Relaxation/Meditation

In this book, we often recommend meditation and/or other relaxation techniques to counteract the harmful effects of stress and to support healing. In some cases, we have provided specific exercises that you can try on your own. In general, though, whenever you see a reference to "relaxation/meditation," feel free to use any technique that helps calm you and helps reduce your heart rate and blood pressure. Among your choices: biofeedback, deep breathing, hypnosis, meditation, tai chi, and yoga.

Rolfing

Developed by Ida Rolf, PhD, Rolfing involves deep manipulation and massage of the connective tissues in order to relieve physical and emotional tension. Practitioners, called Rolfers, may use their fingers, thumbs, forearms, and elbows to physically alter the body's posture and structure. This fosters proper postural alignment, increases mobility, and reduces pain throughout the body.

Shiatsu

Shiatsu, a Japanese term meaning "finger pressure," is a hands-on therapy in which practitioners use their fingers, palms, and thumbs to identify irregularities within the body and to correct those irregularities by applying pressure to specific points—the same points used in acupressure and acupuncture. (In fact, you may hear shiatsu described as "needle-free acupuncture.") In this way, shiatsu unblocks and facilitates energy flow, which in turn relieves muscular tension, improves lymph circulation, and fosters the body's natural healing powers.

Tai Chi

Similar to qigong, tai chi—also a traditional Chinese discipline—consists of a series of slow, gentle movements that require a significant amount of concentration as well as synchronized breathing. The movements help unite body and mind, build inner strength, and stimulate energy flow throughout the body.

Therapeutic Massage

Therapeutic massage involves kneading or otherwise manipulating muscles and soft tissues to alleviate pain, muscle spasms, and stress and to promote relaxation. Swedish massage is the most common technique; others include deep-tissue massage, neuromuscular massage, and sports massage.

Therapeutic Touch

A practitioner trained in therapeutic touch is able to redirect energy flow simply by moving his or her hands over a client's body, without actually touching the person. In this way, therapeutic touch has much in common with Reiki. By properly channeling energy, or *chi*, therapeutic touch can relieve pain, promote relaxation, and restore balance to the body.

Traditional Chinese Medicine

Traditional Chinese medicine (TCM) embraces a range of therapeutic disciplines, all developed in China over thousands of years. Acupressure, acupuncture, herbal medicine, qigong, and tai chi are components of TCM.

Trager Approach

Developed by Milton Trager, MD, the Trager Approach uses a series of gentle, rhythmic movements and touch to create deep relaxation and increased mobility. There are no rigid procedures in this discipline; rather, the practitioner tailors the movements to each individual, helping to relax tight muscles without pain.

Trigger Point Therapy

Also known as myotherapy and neuromuscular therapy, trigger point therapy targets so-called trigger points—tender spots on the muscle tissue that radiate pain to other areas of the body. Applying pressure to these areas helps to relieve tension, relax muscle spasms, improve circulation, and break the cycle of pain.

Yoga

From its roots as a Hindu system for achieving a heightened state of spiritual insight, yoga has evolved into a popular discipline for stress reduction, relaxation, and gentle physical activity. A yoga session combines physical postures, breathing exercises, and meditation to release the emotions, clear the mind, and energize the body—ultimately fostering the healing process and general wellness. Hatha yoga is the most common form.

Keeping an Eye on Your Health

If you have a family history of heart disease, cancer, or another serious medical condition, you may be convinced that you're destined to become sick, too. In fact, though you may be at increased risk for a particular illness, you can take steps to safeguard your health or, at least, to detect any problem at its earliest and most treatable stage.

Your first line of defense is to make appropriate lifestyle changes. If you aren't already doing so, now is the time to improve your eating habits, get regular exercise and adequate sleep, quit smoking, and moderate your alcohol consumption—all central to a healthy lifestyle. It also is important to keep tabs on your health status through medical exams and tests.

In this chapter, we'll provide an overview of the routine screenings that many physicians recommend for their patients. We suggest reviewing this list with your doctor; depending on your family history and other risk factors, he or she may want to increase the frequency of certain screenings.

Learning about the various exams and tests is one way in which you can play a more proactive role in your health and health care. We can't overemphasize how vital this is. With doctors' office visits getting shorter and shorter, it's up to you to make the most of the appointment time you have. By educating yourself about regular screenings, among other aspects of your health care, you can make informed decisions in collaboration with your doctor—and give yourself a leg up on maintaining the best health possible.

Body Measurements

In order to determine your body mass index (BMI)—a measure of body fat—your doctor should check your height and weight at least once a year. He or she can use these measurements to calculate your BMI. If you wish to do so on your own, visit the following Web site: www.nhlbisupport.com/bmi/. Here you'll find a BMI calculator provided by the National Heart, Lung, and Blood Institute, a division of the National Institutes of Health. In general, a BMI of less than 18.5 is considered underweight; between 18.5 and 24.9, normal weight; between 25 and 29.9, overweight; and 30 or higher, obese.

Blood Pressure

It's likely that your doctor checks your blood pressure at least at your annual physical exam, and perhaps more often—especially if you have high blood pressure. A typical screening involves wrapping an inflatable cuff around your upper arm, then using a device to monitor the force applied to the arterial walls as blood pumps throughout your body. These days, many drugstores and department stores have their own blood pressure screening stations for customers. In addition, many stores carry monitoring devices that allow you to check your blood pressure at home. If you buy one of these devices, just be sure to follow the instructions carefully.

Laboratory Tests

Routine blood analysis. Also called a complete blood count or CBC, a routine blood analysis uses a small blood sample to establish levels of various types of cells, including red blood cells, white blood cells, and platelets. It also measures the total amount of hemoglobin, the component of red blood cells that is responsible for transporting oxygen to the body's cells; hematocrit, or the proportion of blood that's comprised of red blood cells; and the size of red blood cells. Your doctor will determine when and how often you require a routine blood analysis.

Blood chemistry. This test measures levels of various chemical substances in the blood—such as sodium, potassium, calcium, and phosphorus, as well as liver enzymes—as a means of determining how well organs such as the liver and kidneys are functioning. As with the routine blood analysis, your doctor will decide when and how often you need a blood chemistry test.

Cholesterol test. This simple blood test assesses total cholesterol as well as high-density lipoproteins (HDL, or "good" cholesterol), low-density lipoproteins (LDL, or "bad" cholesterol), and triglycerides. Generally, if your cholesterol levels are consistently normal, you may need a cholesterol test only once every 5 years. Your doctor may recommend more frequent screenings if you have high cholesterol.

Fasting blood sugar test. For this test, you'll fast for 12 hours, after which you'll give a small blood sample to check your blood sugar (glucose) level. This is not a routine test; generally, doctors use it only to confirm a diabetes diagnosis. (The American College of Obstetricians and Gynecologists, or ACOG, does recommend a fasting blood sugar test every 3 years for women at midlife or older.)

Thyroid-stimulating hormone test. Your doctor will recommend this test if he or she suspects that your thyroid gland is overactive or underactive. It involves drawing a small amount of blood to check the level of thyroid-stimulating hormone, or TSH. Since women are more likely than men to have thyroid problems, they're more likely to require this test. Although it's usually performed only when clinically indicated, ACOG recommends screening every 5 years for women at midlife or older.

HIV test. This test uses a blood sample to detect HIV antibodies, an indicator that HIV has entered the body.

Pap test (cervical cancer screening). Performed on women, the Pap test examines a sample of cervical cells for the presence of cervical cancer, precancerous cell changes, or human papillomavirus (a common cause of cervical cancer). Women over age 30 whose Pap tests are normal should undergo this screening every 2 or 3 years. For women in the same age range whose tests show abnormal results, once-a-year screening is recommended. Once a woman reaches age 65 and she has no recent history of abnormal test results, her doctor may recommend discontinuing the Pap test.

Prostate-specific antigen test. Performed on men, this test uses a blood sample to measure the amount of prostate-specific antigen (PSA) released by the prostate. High PSA can be an indicator of prostate enlargement, prostate cancer, or another related condition. Your doctor will decide how frequently you should have this test, based on your individual risk.

Urinalysis. Urinalysis is a physical and/or chemical examination of the urine to check for the presence of abnormal metabolites (metabolism by-products), which can be an indicator of diabetes, kidney disease, urinary tract infection, or another problem. This test should be performed only when clinically indicated.

Clinical Examinations

Clinical breast examination. This physical exam of a woman's breasts and armpits is meant to detect any lumps or enlarged lymph nodes, which may indicate the presence of cancer. ACOG recommends an annual clinical breast exam as part of a woman's routine ob-gyn exam, in addition to monthly self-exams.

Pelvic examination. For this procedure, the doctor first checks a woman's external genitals for sores, cysts, warts, swelling, or other signs of trouble. Then using an instrument called a speculum, the doctor inspects the inside of the vagina and the cervix for any abnormalities. ACOG recommends an annual pelvic exam.

Digital rectal examination (DRE). This exam involves the insertion of a gloved, lubricated finger into the rectum; in some cases, the examining physician will use the other hand to apply pressure to the abdomen or pelvic area. The DRE can help detect various potential problems, including abnormalities of the prostate gland in men; abnormalities of the uterus and ovaries in women; and hemorrhoids or growths in the rectum. It also can help identify the cause of symptoms such as rectal bleeding and pelvic pain. All men and women over age 50 should have a yearly DRE.

Testicular examination. In this procedure, the doctor performs a complete physical exam of a man's groin and genitals—including the penis, scrotum, and testicles—to detect any lumps, swelling, shrinking, or other abnormalities. Men should get a testicular exam once a year. This exam also is helpful to identify the cause of any groin or genital pain, among other symptoms.

Skin examination. This exam involves

checking the skin from head to toe for any lesions, mole changes, or other possible signs of skin cancer. Generally, doctors perform a skin exam as part of a patient's annual exam. If you're at high risk for skin cancer, your doctor may recommend more frequent screenings.

Diagnostic Imaging

Mammogram. A mammogram uses low-dose radiation to produce an image of the breast, which the doctor then examines for tumors, cysts, or other abnormalities. To improve the quality of the image and avoid blurring, the breast is compressed by a mammography machine while the x-ray is being taken. Both ACOG and the US Preventive Services Task Force recommend mammograms every 1 or 2 years for women between ages 40 and 49. For women 50 and older, ACOG suggests once-a-year screenings.

Chest x-ray. A chest x-ray uses low-dose radiation to produce an image of the heart, lungs, and chest. Doctors may order chest x-rays to help diagnose (or rule out) heart disorders, lung cancer, emphysema, and other medical conditions. These screenings are administered only when they're deemed clinically necessary.

Bone density measurement. A number of different tests are available to assess bone density, or bone mass. Usually, these tests measure bone in the spine, hip, or wrist—the most common sites for fractures due to low bone density (osteopenia) or osteoporosis (porous bones). Your doctor will determine how often you require bone density screening, based on your risk. According to the National Osteoporosis Foundation, all women over age 65—the group at highest risk for low bone density—should get screenings. Women at high risk for osteoporotic fractures should begin screenings at age 60, though there is no consensus on how often to screen.

Colon Cancer Screening

Beginning at age 50, all men and women should undergo colon cancer screenings. The frequency of these screenings often depends on a person's individual risk factors. The following are the most common methods of colon cancer screening.

Fecal occult blood test. For this test, two or three stool samples are collected at home and then sent to a laboratory. There a clinician places the samples on special testing materials that indicate whether blood is present in the stool. The general recommendation is to perform this test annually, in conjunction with other screenings.

Flexible sigmoidoscopy. In a sigmoidoscopy, a thin, flexible tube called a sigmoidoscope is inserted through the anus into the rectum and the lower portion of the colon. Once in place, the sigmoidoscope allows the doctor to check for signs of colon polyps or colorectal cancer. Generally, people over age 50 should get a sigmoidoscopy once every 5 years.

Double contrast barium enema. This procedure—which combines a liquid barium enema with x-rays—helps detect colon polyps and colorectal cancer. Usually it's performed in conjunction with the flexible sigmoidoscopy.

Colonoscopy. This test uses a colonoscope—a thin, flexible instrument attached to a small video camera—to view the entire colon. In addition to detecting ulcers, polyps, tumors, and areas of inflammation and bleeding, a colonoscopy permits the collection of tissue samples and the removal of abnormal growths such as polyps. The general recommendation for a colonoscopy is once every 10 years, or more often if you're at high risk for colorectal cancer.

One study compared the effectiveness of optical colonoscopy (OC) against that of another technology, computed tomographic colonography (CTC), in detecting advanced colon lesions. ACTC is different from an OC in that it uses a CT scanner and computer software to generate images of the colon for a physician to review. Both tools had similar detection rates, which suggests that CTC—which is more comfortable than OC—could serve as a primary screening test. However, if the CTC identifies colon polyps, then the OC still would be necessary for polyp removal.

Other Tests

Electrocardiogram. Perhaps best known as an ECG or EKG, an electrocardiogram involves attaching electrode patches to the chest, arms, and legs in order to record the electrical impulses of the heart. An ECG can diagnose abnormal heart rhythms (arrhythmia), heart muscle damage, heart enlargement, and other cardiac problems. Doctors will order this test only when it's clinically necessary.

Dental checkup. You should see your dentist at least twice a year for a routine cleaning and exam. During the exam portion of your visit, your dentist will check your teeth, gums, and mouth for signs of tooth decay, gum disease, oral cancer, and other problems. He or she also may take dental x-rays.

Eye examination. A complete eye examination should include an external exam followed by specific tests for visual acuity, pupil function, muscle motility, visual fields, and intraocular pressure, as well as an ophthalmoscopy (examination of the inside of the eye). According to the American Academy of Ophthalmology, people between ages 40 and 65 should get eye exams every 2 to 4 years.

Hearing test. A hearing test can identify any hearing loss, as well as the type and degree of impairment. The American Speech-Language-Hearing Association advises those over age 50 to get a hearing test every 3 years.

Signs and Symptoms of Life-Threatening Conditions

In Part 2 of this book, we'll turn our attention to medical conditions that generally fall into one of two categories. Either they're mild problems that tend to respond well to home care or they're chronic illnesses for which treatment emphasizes long-term symptom management.

At some point in your life, however, you or a loved one may face a medical crisis that requires immediate care. In this chapter, we'll briefly explore the most critical of these medical emergencies—how to recognize them and how to treat them until professional help arrives. In situations like these, your most important action is to call 911 or your emergency services number as quickly as possible. Every minute matters to survival.

Cardiac Arrest

A person is said to be in cardiac arrest when his or her heartbeat and cardiac function stop, preventing oxygen-rich blood from circulating through the body. Cardiac arrest occurs quite suddenly. Among its most common symptoms are:

- Loss of consciousness
- No breathing
- Loss of pulse and blood pressure
- Collapse

If you suspect that someone has experienced cardiac arrest, you should call 911 or the local emergency services number right away. Then you can begin cardiopulmonary resuscitation (CPR), which will keep blood flowing to the heart and brain until professional help arrives. See page 20 for a brief overview of CPR.

Heart Attack

A heart attack is characterized by the sudden interruption of bloodflow to the heart, often because of a blockage in a coronary artery that feeds the heart muscle. While the classic symptom of a heart attack is severe, sharp chest pain, a person may experience only mild pain or discomfort at first. In fact, women tend not to have chest pain at all; their symptoms can be much more subtle. The following lists illustrate how heart attacks can manifest differently in women and men.

Cardiopulmonary Resuscitation

Cardiopulmonary resuscitation—or CPR, as it is more commonly known—is a lifesaving technique that's called upon in medical emergencies such as cardiac arrest and heart attack. It uses chest compressions to help move oxygen-rich blood through the body, and especially to the heart and brain—just as a healthy heart would do on its own. CPR is an emergency intervention that can help sustain life until further medical treatment restores a normal heart rhythm.

Though we'll outline the basics of CPR here, we strongly urge you to obtain appropriate training through the American Heart Association, the American Red Cross, your local hospital, or another qualified training organization. It's the best way to learn proper technique, so you can administer CPR effectively and safely.

In the meantime, you might want to familiarize yourself with the following instructions, just in case you find yourself in a situation where CPR is necessary. They're based on newly revised recommendations from the American Heart Association, released in 2008. You can find more information about this "hands-only" version of CPR at http://handsonlycpr.eisenberginc.com.

Check for Responsiveness

1. If a person appears unconscious, tap or shake his shoulder and loudly ask, "Are you okay?"

2. If he does not respond, call 911 or your local emergency services number, or direct someone else to do it for you. Then continue with the steps below.

Begin Chest Compressions

1. If the person isn't already on his back, roll him into position and kneel beside him.

2. Place the heel of one hand over the center of the person's chest, between his nipples. Place the other hand on top and clasp your fingers. Lean in so that your shoulders are directly above your hands, with your elbows straight and locked.

3. Using your body weight, push straight down on the person's chest, compressing the chest about 2 inches. Do about 100 compressions per minute, lifting your hands slightly after each one to allow the chest to recoil.

4. Continue the compressions until emergency personnel arrive. If other bystanders are on the scene, take turns administering CPR. Try to keep disruptions to a minimum.

If an automatic external defibrillator (AED) is available, you should use it. However, you will need to continue with CPR before and after AED treatment until emergency personnel arrive to relieve you.

Women's Symptoms

- Shortness of breath, perhaps without chest pain of any kind

- Flulike symptoms, especially nausea, clamminess, and cold sweats

- Unexplained weakness, fatigue, and/or dizziness

- Pain in the chest, upper back, shoulder, neck, or jaw

- Anxiety and/or loss of appetite

Men's Symptoms

- Chest pain—often described as a heavy, squeezing, or crushing sensation

- Discomfort or pain in the stomach, back, neck, jaw, or one or both arms

- Vague upper abdominal discomfort, coupled with nausea

- Shortness of breath

- Lightheadedness, fainting, or cold sweats

- Profound weakness

- Confusion

Time is of the essence when dealing with a heart attack. If you suspect one—whether in yourself or in someone else—call 911 or your local emergency services number without delay. Today, treatments are available that dramatically increase the odds of surviving a heart attack. To be effective, though, they must be given as quickly as possible.

Keep in mind that you should not administer CPR to someone who is having a heart attack as long as he or she remains conscious. Simply stay with the person and monitor the situation until professional help arrives.

Stroke

During a stroke, brain cells begin to die because of a lack of bloodflow—and therefore oxygen—to the brain. Symptoms of a stroke may include the following:

- Sudden numbness or weakness on one side of the body

- Sudden confusion and difficulty understanding or speaking

- Sudden disturbances in vision

- Sudden trouble with balance or walking

- Sudden severe headache, with no known cause

As is the case with cardiac arrest and heart attack, a stroke requires immediate intervention. If you suspect that someone is having a stroke, call 911 or your local emergency services number right away. Then monitor the person until professional help arrives.

Once the person arrives at the emergency room, hospital personnel may choose to administer drugs that increase the odds of survival while reducing the chances of long-term health effects. The sooner the person receives these drugs, the more effective they are.

Choking

In a choking emergency, something—most likely food—is blocking the airway to the lungs. A person who is choking may display any or all of the following symptoms.

- Wheezing or coughing

- An inability to speak

- Skin that is pale or bluish in color

- Perspiration

- Collapse

To help someone who is choking, you need to clear the person's airway. You can do this by administering the Heimlich maneuver. For instructions, see page 22.

Hypothermia

In its most severe form, hypothermia—which involves a significant drop in internal body temperature—may lead to brain damage, cardiac arrest, or death. The symptoms of hypothermia change as the condition progresses. Here's what to watch for at each stage.

Mild Hypothermia (Internal Body Temperature between 90° and 95°F)

- Bouts of shivering

- Grogginess and confusion
- Rapid breathing and heart rate
- Waxy pallor

Moderate Hypothermia (Internal Body Temperature between 82° and 89°F)

- Violent shivering
- Inability to think and concentrate
- Loss of balance and coordination

The Heimlich Maneuver

The Heimlich maneuver is an emergency technique for preventing suffocation when a person's airway becomes blocked by a piece of food or another object. You can administer the Heimlich to others as well as to yourself, if no one else is around to assist you. Here's what to do.

Using the Heimlich Maneuver on Others

If someone around you is choking, you can use either back blows or abdominal thrusts—or a combination of the two—to expel the object from the person's airway. Actually, the American Red Cross recommends five back blows followed by five abdominal thrusts—referred to as the "five and five"—for someone who's choking but conscious and seated or standing upright. If the person is lying down, sitting abdominal thrusts are the better option.

Back Blows

Use back blows only if the person who's choking is seated or standing upright. They should be your first choice in a choking emergency.

1. Stand behind the person.

2. Place one of your hands on the person's chest, and use the heel of your other hand to give five quick blows between the shoulder blades. This may be enough to expel the foreign object. If the person is able to breathe, cough, and speak, then you know that her airway is open.

Abdominal Thrusts

If back blows fail to clear the person's airway, then switch to abdominal thrusts.

1. Still standing behind the person, wrap your arms around her waist.

2. Make a fist with one hand and clasp it with your other hand. Your fist should be below the person's breastbone, just above her navel.

- Slow, shallow breathing

- Slow, weak pulse

- Blue pallor

- Inappropriate undressing (called paradoxical undressing)

Severe Hypothermia (Internal Body Temperature below 82°F)

- No shivering

- Loss of consciousness

- Little or no breathing

- Weak, irregular, or nonexistent pulse

- Blue pallor

Because the symptoms of hypothermia can mimic other health concerns—such as low blood sugar, hormonal imbalances, medication side effects, and malnutrition—it's best to seek medical attention without delay. Of course, you might reasonably suspect hypothermia if you know that the person has

3. Give five quick upward thrusts. This forces air up through the person's airway.

4. Continue alternating between five back blows and five abdominal thursts until the person expels the foreign object and is able to breathe, cough, and speak.

Sitting Abdominal Thrusts
If the person who's choking is lying down, this version of the Heimlich maneuver is most effective.

1. Roll the person onto her back. Straddle the person's hips or kneel to one side.

2. Position the heel of one hand below the breastbone, just above the navel. Place your other hand on top of the first and clasp your fingers.

3. Keeping your elbows straight but not locked, thrust upward. Continue until the person expels the foreign material and is able to breathe, cough, and speak.

Using the Heimlich Maneuver on Yourself
If you are choking and no one is around to help you, you can clear your own airway with this variation of the Heimlich.

1. Find a blunt, stable object that is just below chest height—perhaps the back of a chair, the edge of a sink, or the headboard of a bed.

2. Place the soft area of your abdomen, just below your breastbone, against the object. Relax the area as much as possible.

3. Without attempting to breathe, thrust your abdomen against the object. This creates pressure under the diaphragm. Continue until you successfully clear your airway.

been outdoors for an extended period, or otherwise exposed to cold temperatures. In cases of mild hypothermia, first-aid measures include moving the person to a warm (not hot) room and covering him with a blanket until help arrives. More severe hypothermia requires more active rewarming, which may include warm intravenous fluids and heated oxygen. These can be administered only in a hospital setting.

Part 2

The Best Medicine for 81 Common Health Concerns

NO MATTER WHAT YOUR health concern, there's a good chance that you'll find effective solutions here. The entries that follow—arranged alphabetically—provide in-depth profiles of 81 specific medical conditions, with conventional and complementary treatments for each. You'll also get vital information about:

- Causes and risk factors
- Signs and symptoms
- Self-testing options, when appropriate
- Lifestyle recommendations and preventive measures

Before you start exploring the individual entries, we do want to say a word about the herbal and nutritional supplements that we've chosen to present here. For the vast number of people with a given condition, the recommended herbs and supplements will enhance treatment without any adverse effects. Still, it's important to remember that herbs and nutrients can be powerful substances. To ensure proper dosing, and to guard against possible interactions with any medications you may be taking, we advise you to consult your doctor before adding herbal or nutritional supplements to your self-care regimen.

Age Spots

Age spots—also called liver spots or lentigines—are flat, darkened patches of skin that are larger than freckles, up to an inch in size. Most often, they appear on the shoulders, face, forehead, and forearms, and on the backs of hands.

As you grow older, your chances of developing age spots increase. In fact, these brown lesions are one of the most common signs of aging, especially in fair-skinned people.

Causes and Risk Factors

Age spots are caused by increased amounts of a brown color, or pigment, called lipofuscin. As skin ages, it thins, and the number of cells with pigment declines. In response, the remaining cells with pigment get bigger and tend to group together. It is believed that exposure to sunlight hastens this process. This is why age spots most often occur on areas of the body not protected from the sun. Aging skin is more fragile and vulnerable to the sun's ultraviolet (UV) rays.

Signs and Symptoms

Age spots simply appear on the skin. Unlike moles and warts, which protrude beyond the surface of the skin, age spots tend to be flat and dark brown in color. They may vary widely in size and shape. Although there is no pain or itching associated with age spots, some people find them unsightly. On occasion, spots like these may signal the development of a more serious skin condition such as skin cancer. So if you develop age spots, you might want to have a health care professional examine them.

Conventional Treatments

Age spots do not normally require treatment. As long as they are not masking a serious problem, such as skin cancer, they may be left alone. Still, if you find them unsightly, there are several conventional options that you may wish to consider.

Cryotherapy

Cryotherapy involves freezing the age spot with liquid nitrogen. During application, there is a stinging sensation. After the procedure, you will need to keep the area clean. Within a month or so, the age spot should turn white, but you may be left with a permanent white spot or scar.

Hydroquinone

Hydroquinone, a bleaching agent that is sold in creams, gels, lotions, and solutions, may fade age spots. Examples of products containing hydroquinone are Eldopaque and Esoterica, both of which are available without a prescription. These remove the dark pigment. Unfortunately, hydroquinone tends to be irritating, so products containing this substance should not be used for more than 3 consecutive months.

Laser Therapy

Laser therapy removes the pigment from an age spot. The treatment involves targeting the spot with an intense beam of light. In a matter of seconds, the laser shatters the pigment into small pieces, which then are carried away by the body's immune system. Often one treatment is enough for an age spot to disappear; sometimes a few office visits are necessary.

Generally, laser therapy doesn't require anesthesia, and it doesn't permanently damage the skin. The laser feels like snaps from a rubber band. After treatment, the area will appear red, and there may be light crusting, tenderness, and pinpoint bleeding. Within a week, though, healing should be complete.

Complementary Treatments

The best way to treat age spots is to prevent them. Eating foods rich in antioxidants and taking nutritional supplements can help protect your skin.

Diet

Among the antioxidants, carotenes—natural compounds found in red, yellow, and orange fruits and vegetables—are especially beneficial for preventing age spots. Carotenes strengthen skin cells while warding off damaging free radicals. They also keep skin looking vibrant. Aim for at least five servings of vegetables and four servings of fruits—especially carotene-rich choices, such as cantaloupe, carrots, and tomatoes—in your daily diet. Carotenes also are found in dark green, leafy vegetables, but the dark green color overpowers the reddish tones.

Nutritional Supplements

Sun exposure can cause the pigment of the skin to clump together, causing age spots. The following supplements help to support and strengthen the skin, preventing age spots from forming.

- Vitamin A: 10,000 IU daily. Keeps skin smooth, prevents skin aging, and improves the body's ability to heal itself. Also important for cell growth.

- B-complex vitamins: Take as directed on the label. Promote healthy, clear skin and reduce dry skin.

- Vitamin C with bioflavonoids: 2,000 milligrams daily, in divided doses (1,000 milligrams at breakfast and 1,000 milligrams before bed). May help stop skin pigment from clumping together. *Note:* Vitamin C and selenium interfere with each other's absorption, so it's best not to take these two supplements at the same time.

- Vitamin E: 400 IU daily as natural d-alpha tocopherols, taken with selenium (below) at lunch or dinner. Helps prevent premature aging and age spots. Vitamin E and selenium are better absorbed when taken together.

- Selenium: 300 micrograms daily. Works well with vitamin E.

- Zinc: 30 milligrams daily. Necessary for a strong immune system and healthy skin.

Lifestyle Recommendations

Conceal age spots. If age spots are unsightly to you, try covering them with a concealing makeup product. Be sure to choose a product made from natural ingredients. The chemicals in commercially available beauty products are not regulated by the FDA. These chemicals are toxic, and they may contribute to the buildup of free radicals, which are damaging to the skin.

Fade your age spots. Cover your age spots with the pulp from a lemon once a day, and repeat for several consecutive days. The citric acid in the pulp will cause the spots to lighten gradually. Try to leave the pulp in place for 3 to 5 minutes, so the citric acid can be absorbed into the skin. The pulp will dry quickly and become pastelike.

Preventive Measures

Limit sun exposure. The sun's ultraviolet rays, which cause the damage that leads to age spots, are strongest from 10:00 a.m. to 4:00 p.m. During those hours, you may want to limit the time you spend outside.

Avoid products that increase sensitivity. Limit your use of perfumes and aftershave lotions. These products have the ability to increase the skin's sensitivity to sunlight. Certain prescription and over-the-counter medications have the same effect, so be sure to read drug labels carefully and ask your doctor or pharmacist whether you need extra protection from the sun.

Use sunscreen. Throughout the year, use a good-quality sunscreen that blocks both ultraviolet-A (UVA) and ultraviolet-B (UVB) rays and has an SPF of at least 30. Apply sunscreen at least 30 minutes before heading outdoors, and repeat every 2 hours, as sunscreen loses its effectiveness over time. You may need to reapply sunscreen even more frequently if you are swimming or perspiring.

Wear protective clothing. If you plan to spend more than 30 minutes outside, consider wearing a shirt with long sleeves, pants, and a hat. This will give your skin extra protection from the sun.

Alzheimer's Disease

Alzheimer's disease is the most common form of dementia—a disorder in which the loss of intellectual and social abilities is so marked that it interferes with daily functioning. While the disease may begin with confusion and memory problems—a condition known as mild cognitive impairment—a person with Alzheimer's disease gradually becomes unable to learn, reason, remember, and imagine. Changes in personality may precede the changes in cognition.

Once diagnosed with Alzheimer's, patients live an average of 8 years, though some survive up to 20 years. Many die from other causes—infection being the most common—before the disease progresses to its final stages.

It has been estimated that about 4.5 million American adults have Alzheimer's. Most are over age 65. There is a rare form of the condition, known as familial or early-onset Alzheimer's, that occurs between ages 30 and 60.

Causes and Risk Factors

The exact cause of Alzheimer's disease remains unknown. What is known is that in people with Alzheimer's, certain neurons (nerve cells) in their brains are dying off. A normal brain has about 100 billion neurons. The transmission of electrical and chemical signals from one neuron to another is what enables us to think, feel, and remember. This transmission is facilitated by chemicals known as neurotransmitters. In the early stages of Alzheimer's disease, the number of neurons declines, as does the production of neurotransmitters. This creates a signaling problem in the brain.

It also has been determined that the brains of people with Alzheimer's contain abnormal clumps (plaques) and irregular knots of brain cells (tangles). Composed of a normally harmless protein known as beta-amyloid, plaques are believed to form between neurons even before neurons die and cognitive symptoms appear. Meanwhile, in order to work properly, the internal support structure of neurons requires the correct functioning of a protein called tau. In people with Alzheimer's, the threads of this protein become twisted. As a result, researchers theorize, neurons are damaged and eventually die. In some people with Alzheimer's, the brain shows signs of inflammation. This may occur as immune cells (microglia) respond to the development of beta-amyloid plaques between neurons. Researchers postulate that the microglia view the plaques as foreign substances and attempt to damage or destroy them, triggering inflammation. The microglia also may prompt other substances to cause inflammation.

Your risk for Alzheimer's increases as you age. You may be at slightly higher risk if one of your first-degree relatives—a parent, sister, or brother—has the disease. High blood pressure and high cholesterol also may be risk factors. As for familial or early-onset Alzheimer's, researchers have identified three genetic mutations that set the stage for the disease.

Signs and Symptoms

Alzheimer's disease usually begins with mild memory loss and confusion. In time, it evolves into increasing and persistent forgetfulness, such as the failure to remember a recent event or simple directions. There may be problems with abstract thinking, such as dealing with numbers, and difficulty finding the correct word to express thoughts. People with Alzheimer's often lose their sense of time and have a tendency to wander. They may experience a diminished ability to complete even some of the most basic daily activities, such as food preparation and personal hygiene. There may be a loss of judgment, such as forgetting to turn off the stove. There also may be personality changes, such as anxiety, aggression, depression, and inappropriate behavior.

In the more advanced stages of Alzheimer's, people lose the ability to care for themselves. They tend to have problems with eating and remaining continent. As a result, they are at increased risk for secondary health issues, such as pneumonia, infections,

A Quick Guide to Symptoms

- ☐ **Memory impairment and confusion**
- ☐ **Persistent forgetfulness**
- ☐ **Sleeplessness, agitation, and anxiety**
- ☐ **Problems with abstract thinking**
- ☐ **Difficulty with communication**
- ☐ **Loss of sense of time**
- ☐ **Tendency to wander and pace**
- ☐ **Diminished ability to complete basic daily tasks**
- ☐ **Loss of judgment**
- ☐ **Personality changes**
- ☐ **In the end stages of the illness, a loss of speech, appetite, and bladder and bowel control, and a complete dependence on others**

and falls. Most people with Alzheimer's eventually die from one of these complications.

Conventional Treatments

At present, there is no cure for Alzheimer's, and the current treatments do not reverse the course of the disease. At best, they slow its progression and alleviate its symptoms.

Medications

Cholinesterase inhibitors. Cholinesterase inhibitors work to increase the level of acetylcholine, a neurotransmitter in the brain. Approximately half of those who are prescribed these medications show improvement in their symptoms. Examples are rivastigmine

It is important to note that the early symptoms of Alzheimer's disease can be mimicked by other health issues, including medication side effects, mild strokes, depression, fatigue, and thyroid problems. A physician can order tests to determine whether a person actually has Alzheimer's.

(Exelon), galantamine (Reminyl), tacrine (Cognex), and donepezil (Aricept).

Memantine (Namenda). Used to treat moderate to severe Alzheimer's, this medication protects brain cells from damage caused by the chemical messenger glutamate. In so doing, it slows the loss of daily living skills.

Other medications. Doctors may recommend other medications to treat the behavioral problems—including anxiety, depression, agitation, sleeplessness, and wandering—associated with Alzheimer's. For example, atypical antipsychotic medications, such as risperidone (Risperdal), may be prescribed for agitation and psychosis. Mood stabilizers, such as carbamazepine (Tegretol), are helpful for agitation. Anxiety, depression, agitation, and psychosis may be treated with selective serotonin reuptake inhibitors, such as fluoxetine (Prozac), sertraline (Zoloft), and paroxetine (Paxil).

Complementary Treatments

Presently, there is no proven way to prevent Alzheimer's disease. By maintaining proper nutrition, staying physically and mentally active, and practicing healthy lifestyle habits, you may be able to reduce your risk or slow the progression of the disease.

Diet

The brain can function only as well as it is fed, which means that a diet of nutrient-rich foods may help slow or prevent Alzheimer's. Be sure to include lots of fresh, antioxidant-rich fruits and vegetables, as well as whole grains. Beta-carotene and vitamin C, both abundant in fruits and vegetables, appear to improve cognitive performance. Aim for at least five servings of vegetables, four servings of fruits, and six servings of whole grains each day.

Berries, broccoli, flaxseeds, and linseeds contain lignans, one of the major classes of plant chemicals known as phytoestrogens. A Dutch study, published in the May 2005 issue of the *Journal of Nutrition*, measured cognitive function in 394 premenopausal women. It found that the women with high lignan intakes performed better on a mini-mental state examination (MMSE) than those with lower intakes.

Other preliminary research suggests that monounsaturated fats, such as olive oil, may protect against memory loss and age-related cognitive decline (ARCD). This condition can be a precursor to Alzheimer's.

Take care to avoid fried foods, hydrogenated fats, and processed foods containing artificial colors and chemicals.

Herbal Medicine

A number of studies have shown that the antioxidant herb *Ginkgo biloba* improves mental clarity and memory, in addition to overall circulation to the brain. The typical recommended dose is 120 milligrams, twice daily, of an extract standardized to 24 percent flavone glycosides and 6 percent terpene lactones. The flavone glycosides give ginkgo its antioxidant benefits, while terpene lactones increase circulation and have a protective effect on nerve cells. *Note:* If you're taking a prescription blood-thinning medication, be sure to consult your doctor before using ginkgo supplements.

Nutritional Supplements

A number of nutrients are important for improving brain function and reducing—in some cases, reversing—memory loss.

- Multivitamin: Take as directed on the label. The supplement should contain calcium, copper, magnesium, and zinc, which together help the brain retain memory.

- B-complex vitamins: Take as directed on the label. The B vitamins increase circulation to the brain and work to prevent and reverse memory loss.

- Vitamin B_{12}: Administered by injection, which enhances absorption. Can significantly improve memory.

- Vitamin C: 1,000 milligrams daily, in divided doses (500 milligrams at breakfast and 500 milligrams before bed). Helps reduce memory loss. *Note:* Vitamin C and selenium interfere with each other's absorption, so be sure to take these supplements separately.

- Vitamin E: 400 IU daily, taken with selenium (below) at lunch or dinner. Helps reduce memory loss. Vitamin E is better absorbed when taken with selenium.

- L-carnitine: 1,500 milligrams daily. Improves memory and can delay the progression of Alzheimer's.

- Selenium: 400 micrograms daily, in divided doses (200 micrograms each). May protect the brain against the toxic effects of mercury.

- Zinc: 30 milligrams daily. Along with selenium, may protect the brain against the toxic effects of mercury.

Preventive Measures

As mentioned above, there is no proven way to prevent Alzheimer's disease. However, some preliminary evidence suggests that statins—medications used to lower cholesterol—also may lower Alzheimer's risk.

In addition, since autopsies on people who died from Alzheimer's have revealed high levels of aluminum, it may be helpful to avoid cooking with aluminum pots and pans. Foods, especially acidic foods such as tomato products, absorb the aluminum from the cookware. Also pay attention to foods and beverages packaged in aluminum. And read labels on personal care items, as many products—including deodorants, shampoo, antacids, and buffered aspirin—can contain aluminum. Bear in mind that as of this writing, there is no solid evidence that aluminum exposure causes Alzheimer's disease.

Avoid conditions that can lead to Alzheimer's. A Finnish study involving close to 1,500 participants showed that elevated cholesterol and blood pressure are even more closely linked to Alzheimer's than the APOE-4 gene, the genetic risk factor for the disease. Other

Caring for a Person with Alzheimer's

Dealing with Alzheimer's is challenging both for people with the disease and for their caregivers. If you're caring for a loved one with Alzheimer's, the following suggestions may help make the best of the situation.

Deal realistically with Alzheimer's issues. As time passes, a person with Alzheimer's will need additional assistance with activities of daily living. Allow him or her more time to complete these tasks, and try to remain flexible. It is helpful to focus on how the task can best be accomplished now, rather than how it was done in the past.

Before a person with Alzheimer's requires considerable help with daily activities, start to think about where you can get the needed support. Will family members be able to provide assistance? Will it be necessary for your loved one to move to an assisted living or skilled nursing facility? Will there be sufficient financial resources to cover the costs—which may be quite sizeable? It is never too soon to begin planning.

Limit alcohol. Since alcohol consumption can increase confusion, it isn't appropriate for someone with Alzheimer's.

Encourage physical activity. Exercise tends to ease some of the symptoms associated with Alzheimer's, such as depression and anxiety. It can help prevent falls, reduce wandering, and improve sleep and overall quality of life. Exercise also builds overall strength and cardiovascular health.

Improve safety inside the home. To help reduce the chances of a fall, keep furniture in the same place rather than rearranging it, remove throw rugs, and eliminate as much clutter as possible. In particular, make sure that areas around the bed are tidy and that there is a clear path to the bathroom and soft lighting throughout the night. Place locks on any cabinets that contain potentially dangerous products, such as toxic substances and medications. Install grab rails in bathrooms and set the hot water heater to no higher than 120°F. To help prevent electrical shock, remove electrical appliances from the bathroom.

Keep communication simple. Use short, familiar words and sentences. Don't yell; rather, adopt a quiet tone. Don't argue, as it will only increase agitation in a person with Alzheimer's.

Maintain good sleep habits. Encourage your loved one to go to bed and awaken at the same time each day. Avoid unsettling activities, such as changing clothing or personal hygiene, close to bedtime. Develop a prebedtime relaxation ritual, such as playing soothing music or providing a back rub. If you are unable to keep the person from taking daytime naps, limit nap time and encourage him or her to rest on a recliner or a couch. This will help associate the bedroom with nighttime sleeping. Make sure that the bedroom is cool and comfortable, but have extra blankets available.

research suggests that those who have blood sugar levels indicative of prediabetes are 70 percent more likely to develop Alzheimer's than if their blood sugar levels were normal.

Eat well. Improve your diet, and you may well preserve your brain. The results of a Finnish study presented at the 10th International Conference on Alzheimer's Disease and Related Disorders showed higher test scores for coordination, decision-making, memory, and reasoning among those who ate a diet rich in antioxidants and omega-3 oils

Prepare for sundowning. *Sundowning* is a term that refers to increased agitation and wandering during the early evening hours in those with Alzheimer's. While you can't eliminate it, you can adopt effective coping strategies. These include turning on the lights before the evening hours and trying to keep your loved one focused on a particular task.

Prevent nighttime problems. The negative behaviors associated with Alzheimer's tend to worsen at night. Reduce the amount of caffeine consumed during the day, and especially after lunch, so that your loved one may fall asleep more easily. As mentioned above, exercising helps promote sound sleep, as does limiting daytime napping. To reduce the possibility of disorientation during the night, keep the bedroom softly lit.

Provide a degree of structure. People with Alzheimer's tend to become agitated fairly easily. By creating structure in the daily schedule, you will reduce the level of agitation. Try to avoid large groups, noise, and activities that are too difficult to complete. Create a serene environment with soft background music, and avoid excessive stimulation. Limit the number of houseguests or visitors, and keep visits short.

Rely on memory aids. Set aside a place in the kitchen to list the day's activities as well as important phone numbers. In addition, post instructions on how to complete everyday tasks, such as warming food in the microwave and preparing a cup of coffee.

Try to limit wandering. It is very common for people with Alzheimer's to wander—and it is potentially dangerous. If you can determine what's causing your loved one to wander, you may be able to take steps to prevent it.

Keep your home's front and back doors locked. Avoid storing keys, shoes, umbrellas, and coats by the door; these are associated with leaving, and they may confuse a person with Alzheimer's. Whenever leaving home, have your loved one carry a pocket card that says "Call Home" and list the phone number. Consider purchasing a bracelet that notes the person's name and phone number, and indicates "Memory Impaired." These are available through membership in the Alzheimer's Association, which also sponsors a 24-hour hotline as part of its Safe Return program. (See Resources for Specific Disorders on page 541.)

Join a support group. People with Alzheimer's, as well as their families and caregivers, can benefit from meeting with others who are coping with the disease. To find a support group in your area, ask your physician or local hospital for a referral. (Also see Resources for Specific Disorders on page 541.)

compared with those whose diets included lots of saturated fat. The people with high saturated fat intakes doubled their risk of mild cognitive impairment.

Stay active. *Lancet Neurology* published a study in which people in their forties and fifties who exercised for 20 to 30 minutes at least twice a week cut their risk for Alzheimer's and dementia by 50 percent. The reduction in risk was almost 60 percent in those genetically predisposed to the disease.

Stimulate your brain. People who engage their minds throughout their lives, especially as they get older, build up a defense against Alzheimer's. In particular, those with higher education appear to have better protection against the disease. One study that compared rural, uneducated populations in Taiwan with more educated populations in the United States and Japan found that the Taiwanese developed dementia 10 to 20 years earlier.

Other research suggests that older adults from blue-collar backgrounds benefit the most from practicing mentally stimulating puzzles and games. In a study at York University in Toronto, published in the February 2007 issue of *Neuropsychologia*, older adults who were bilingual since their youth showed signs of cognitive decline 4 years later than those who spoke only one language.

Maintain a strong social circle. An active social life can help you age better, according to the Rush University Alzheimer's Disease Center. The larger your social network, the better.

Stop oxidative stress. The catechin resveratrol that's found in red wine may help reduce oxidative stress, which kills brain cells. Patients with Alzheimer's have high levels of oxidative stress.

In a recent study involving laboratory mice, conducted by the National Institute on Aging and Harvard Medical School, high doses of resveratrol appeared to offset the consequences of an unhealthy, high-fat diet. But in order for an average 150-pound human to obtain the dose fed to the mice, he or she would need to drink 750 to 1,500 bottles of red wine a day. Resveratrol is available as a standardized extract, but no dose has been established as yet.

Anemia

Anemia is characterized by a deficiency of red blood cells and/or hemoglobin, the component of red blood cells that transports oxygen from the lungs to the rest of the body. In people with anemia, the body makes too few red blood cells, loses too many of them, or destroys them before they are replaced.

The most abundant cells in the human body, red blood cells form in the bone marrow. In adults, only the marrow of the ribs, spine, and pelvis produces red blood cells. For every cubic millimeter of blood, men have about 5.2 million red blood cells, and women, about 4.7 million. When these cells are in low supply, the blood isn't as effective in carrying oxygen to tissues.

As mentioned above, it's the hemoglobin inside each red blood cell that actually is responsible for shuttling oxygen throughout the body. Each red blood cell contains between 200 and 300 hemoglobin molecules. Each of these molecules, in turn, contains protein and iron.

Anemia is far more widespread than most people realize. Considered the most common blood disorder, it is believed to affect at least 3.4 million Americans to some degree. Since many people are unaware that they have anemia and remain untreated, the actual number probably is higher.

Causes and Risk Factors

Anemia is not a single disease. Rather, it is like a fever—an indication that something is wrong. Because malfunctions can occur at any stage of the manufacturing, recycling, and regulating of red blood cells, anemia may have several causes. In adults, the three most common forms of the disorder are iron deficiency anemia, megaloblastic anemia, and anemia of chronic disease.

In iron deficiency anemia, the body has depleted the excess iron that it stored in the bone marrow, liver, and spleen. As a result, it lacks the iron it requires to produce hemoglobin, which in turn is necessary to make red blood cells. Generally, iron deficiency anemia is not caused by a lack of iron in the diet. Rather, in adult men and women, it most often occurs because of internal bleeding from another underlying health condition, which may be as benign as hemorrhoids or as serious as colon cancer. *Helicobacter pylori*, a bacterium that causes peptic ulcers, may trigger iron deficiency anemia by impairing iron absorption. Women who still are menstruating may lose iron as they bleed. People who suffer from a condition known as pica—in which they eat unusual substances such as clay, cardboard, and dirt—also are at increased risk for iron deficiency.

Megaloblastic anemia most often occurs

because of a deficiency of folic acid (folate), vitamin B_{12} (cobalamin), or both. (When it is a result of the failure to absorb vitamin B_{12}, it is called pernicious anemia.) In this form of anemia, the red blood cells are abnormally large and have shorter than normal life spans.

Poor diet, sometimes coupled with alcoholism, is the usual cause of folate deficiency. But folate deficiency can also be a by-product of other conditions that impair the absorptive ability of the small intestine, including parasitic diseases such as giardiasis, short bowel syndrome, inflammatory bowel disease, and celiac disease. Some medical conditions, such as cancer, psoriasis, hyperthyroidism, and hemolytic anemia, create a high demand for folate and so may lead to a deficiency. Certain medications also may interfere with folate absorption, thereby causing megaloblastic anemia. These drugs include phenytoin (Dilantin), methotrexate (Rheumatrex), trimethoprim (Proloprim, Trimpex), and triamterene (Dyrenium).

While vitamin B_{12} deficiency may occur after gastrointestinal surgery, it more often is the result of impaired absorption of the vitamin. This may be due to a number of factors, such as celiac disease or overgrowth of bacteria in the intestine.

In general, anemia of chronic disease (ACD) is caused by ongoing inflammation from a persistent medical problem. Among the conditions that can lead to ACD are lymphoma, Hodgkin's disease, inflammatory bowel disease, rheumatoid arthritis, and long-term infection. These disorders stimulate the immune system to produce substances that interfere with the transport of iron and the production of red blood cells. Further, they shorten the life span of red blood cells. For a number of medical conditions, the presence of ACD is associated with a poorer prognosis.

Although the risk of anemia tends to decline with age, it is still a prevalent medical concern, especially among those who have a chronic disease that causes inflammation or bleeding.

Signs and Symptoms

Not everyone with anemia experiences symptoms. In its mild form, the most likely symptoms are weakness and fatigue. Moderate to severe anemia may have more obvious symptoms such as lightheadedness, headache, shortness of breath, rapid heartbeat, ringing in the ears, restless legs syndrome, irritability, mental confusion, pale skin, and reduced pinkness of the lips, gums, eyelid linings, nail beds, and palms. In addition to these symptoms, megaloblastic anemia can be accompanied by an abnormally smooth and tender tongue and neurological problems, such as numbness and tingling in the hands and feet, loss of balance, and staggering.

The most serious cases of anemia may affect the heart. In high-output heart failure, the heart must work harder to supply a sufficient amount of oxygen to the brain and other organs. If the heart becomes unable to keep up with the demand, it may lead to symptoms of heart failure, such as difficulty breathing and leg swelling. If there has been a narrowing of the blood vessels that supply blood to the heart, or if there is coronary artery disease, a person may experience angina or chest pain as a result of inadequate bloodflow.

Conventional Treatments

Once your doctor has determined the cause of your anemia, he or she can recommend an appropriate course of treatment. Here's what you might expect, depending on the type of anemia you have.

Iron Deficiency Anemia

Treatment for iron deficiency anemia usually begins with dietary changes. (For recommendations, see the Diet section on page 40.) If they don't bring about improvement, then the next step is iron supplements. But they must be used with caution, as supplements may cause gastrointestinal problems, especially constipation, and aggravate existing gastrointestinal disorders. Further, excess iron may increase the risk of heart disease, diabetes, and some cancers. So it's important for your doctor to monitor your anemia throughout treatment, and to discontinue supplementation once your iron levels return to normal.

There are different types of iron supplements on the market, among them ferrous salts, usually ferrous sulfate (Ferosol, Fer-In-Sol, Mol-Iron, and others). Others include ferrous fumarate (Femiron, Feostat, Fumerin, Hemocyte, Ircon, and others), ferrous gluconate (Ferfon, Ferralet, Simron), and polysaccharide-iron complex (Niferex, Nu-Iron). There also is a prolonged-release ferrous sulfate (Slow Fe) that may be better absorbed and have fewer side effects.

In some instances, supplemental iron is injected or administered intravenously. Injectable iron may cause pain at the injection site, while intravenous iron may result in pain in the vein, flushing, and a metallic taste in the mouth. Other possible side effects of both treatments include blood clots, fever, joint aches, headache, and rash. Oral iron and injectable iron should never be used at the same time.

A Quick Guide to Symptoms

- ☐ Weakness and fatigue
- ☐ Lightheadedness or headache
- ☐ Shortness of breath
- ☐ Rapid heartbeat
- ☐ Ringing in the ears
- ☐ Restless legs syndrome
- ☐ Mental confusion
- ☐ Irritability
- ☐ Pale skin
- ☐ Reduced pinkness of the lips, gums, eyelid linings, nail beds, and palms
- ☐ Signs of heart failure, such as difficulty breathing and leg swelling

About Iron Supplements

If your doctor recommends iron supplements for your anemia, always take them with an 8-ounce glass of water. Though pairing your supplements with ascorbic acid (vitamin C) can improve iron absorption, the ascorbic acid could worsen any side effects.

While you are taking iron supplements, expect your stools to be dark. In fact, if they are *not* dark, you should contact your doctor. This means that your body is not absorbing the iron.

Avoid consuming bran or using bran supplements in combination with your iron supplements. Iron is lost through the stool, so bran may sweep the iron right along with it. Similarly, taking antacids around the same time as your iron supplements will reduce the effectiveness of the supplements. Iron also may reduce the usefulness of other medications, such as the antibiotics tetracycline, penicillamine, and ciprofloxacin, and the anti-Parkinson's drugs methyldopa, levodopa, and carbidopa. Allow at least a 2-hour window between these medications and your iron supplements.

Remember to store your iron supplements in a cool location. The bathroom medicine cabinet probably is too warm.

Megaloblastic Anemia

For megaloblastic anemia caused by a vitamin B_{12} deficiency, the usual prescription is vitamin B_{12} injections and oral folic acid supplements. These reverse the production of overly large red blood cells and produce a rapid rise in hemoglobin levels. During recovery, the red blood cells may use up your body's potassium supply, so your doctor may advise you to take potassium supplements as well.

If you have a folate deficiency, you may be advised to take daily oral doses of folic acid.

Anemia of Chronic Disease

If anemia of chronic disease is mild, your doctor will concentrate on treating the underlying medical condition rather than the anemia itself. For example, if anemia is a result of chronic renal failure, then your doctor will prescribe medication to treat renal failure.

However, if anemia is severe, medication or a transfusion may be necessary. Some patients with moderate anemia of chronic disease may benefit from recombinant human erythropoietin (rHuEPO). This is a genetically engineered form of erythropoietin, a substance required for red blood cell production. In people with ACD, erythropoietin levels are low.

Complementary Treatments

The presence of anemia indicates an underlying medical problem that must be identified through testing. Once you have an accurate diagnosis, complementary therapies may help to treat or alleviate the condition.

Diet

Eat foods that are rich in iron, folic acid, and vitamin B_{12}. Good sources of iron include oysters, clams, beans (especially black beans, kidney beans, and soybeans), peas, iron-fortified cereals, whole-grain breads and pastas, foods containing corn flour, dark green, leafy vegetables (especially spinach), okra, asparagus, broccoli, dried fruit, nuts, seeds, and rhubarb. Folic acid is abundant in fresh fruits (especially citrus fruits), vegetables (especially dark green, leafy vegetables such as spinach), fortified cereals, pumpkin, and all kinds of beans. Large amounts of B_{12} are available in meat, fish, and dairy products. Note that beef and chicken livers have higher concentrations of B_{12} than the meat itself.

Because animal products are the primary dietary source of vitamin B_{12}, strict vegetarians are at higher risk for B_{12} deficiency. If you're vegetarian, be sure to eat lots of tempeh, tofu, and miso, which contain some B_{12}.

Blackstrap molasses—sold in supermarkets and health food stores—is rich in iron and B vitamins. You might try taking a tablespoon daily. Brewer's yeast, a good source of B vitamins and other essential nutrients, is another good dietary addition. So are fruits and vegetables rich in vitamin C, which enhances iron absorption. Try keeping a record of what you eat. You may find that many of the foods in your usual diet are lacking in iron, folic acid, or vitamin B_{12}, or are interfering with the absorption of iron. For example, beverages that contain caffeine interfere with the absorption of iron, so you should not drink them with meals. Black tea contains compounds called tannins that have

a similar effect, so it is a good idea to limit your consumption of black tea, whether caffeinated or decaffeinated.

Herbal Medicine

Dandelion and nettle. Both dandelion and nettle are good sources of iron. Dandelion is best as a fresh juice, but as an alcohol-based tincture, the bitter properties may be more soluble. Take 1 teaspoon of fresh juice or 5 to 10 milliliters of tincture with water twice a day.

For nettle, look for a freeze-dried standardized extract of the leaf. Take a 250-milligram capsule three times a day with meals. In tincture form, take 1 to 4 milliliters three times a day. As a tea, pour 1 cup of boiling water over 1 to 3 teaspoons of the dried herb and steep for 10 minutes. Strain the leaves and drink. The recommended dose is 3 cups of tea per day.

Parsley, chives, and watercress. All three are excellent sources of iron. Try adding them to salads, soups, or sandwiches.

Nutritional Supplements

A number of essential nutrients are necessary for red blood cell formation and production, as well as for iron absorption.

- Multivitamin/mineral: Take as directed on the label. The supplement should contain vitamin A and natural beta-carotene. Note that the safe upper limit for vitamin A is 10,000 IU daily, and for natural beta-carotene, 15,000 IU daily.

- B-complex vitamins: Take as directed on the label. The B vitamins work best when they're taken together. Additional B_{12} may be necessary if you have megaloblastic anemia or if you don't eat meat or dairy. Take a 1,000-microgram tablet sublingually (under the tongue).

- Vitamin C: 2,000 milligrams daily, in divided doses of 1,000 milligrams. May be beneficial for iron deficiency anemia, as it aids in iron absorption. The multivitamin will provide some vitamin C, but a separate supplement is necessary to make up the difference.

- Vitamin E: 400 IU daily. Assists in extending the life span of red blood cells.

- Zinc: 30 milligrams daily. Required for the production of red blood cells.

Traditional Chinese Medicine

Traditional Chinese medicine (TCM) has been very effective in treating various types of anemia. In TCM, anemia generally is regarded as a result of deficient blood and deficient spleen *chi* (vital energy). The usual recommendation is to follow a diet containing iron-rich foods and to use herbal remedies such as dong quai, which strengthens (fortifies) the blood. Dong quai is rich in vitamin B_{12}, which helps stimulate red blood cell production and, in turn, improves energy and reduces fatigue. The recommended daily dose of dong quai is 400 to 800 milligrams, taken as two or three divided doses, of a standardized extract containing 0.8 percent to 1.1 percent ligustilide. In tincture form, the dose is ½ to ¼ teaspoon of liquid extract three times a day.

Although dong quai is available over-the-counter, it is best to consult a TCM practitioner for specific guidance. (For further information, see Professional Organizations for Complementary Therapies on page 563.)

Lifestyle Recommendations

Using cast-iron pans will increase the iron content of your meals, as food absorbs iron from the pans during the cooking process.

Preventive Measures

The best way to prevent iron deficiency anemia is to eat a sound diet, as outlined above. Anemia resulting from other causes may not be preventable, but it usually is treatable.

Angina

The characteristic chest pain of angina is caused by ischemia—a lack of bloodflow and, hence, a lack of oxygen supply to the heart muscle, or myocardium. Angina may manifest simply as chest pain, or as heaviness, tightness, squeezing, pressure, or a burning sensation in the chest, back, arms, neck, throat, or jaw.

Angina (sometimes referred to as angina pectoris) is a common problem in midlife and beyond. An estimated 6.4 million Americans have the condition, with about 400,000 new cases being diagnosed each year.

Of the four main types of angina, the two most common are stable and unstable angina. Stable angina, also known as common angina, is predictable chest pain. It is caused by factors that increase the heart's demand for oxygen, such as exercise, cold weather, emotional turmoil, and large meals. A high proportion of stable angina attacks take place between 6:00 a.m. and noon. An attack generally lasts no more than 2 to 5 minutes. This type of angina tends to respond well to rest and medication, and it causes no permanent damage to the heart.

Unstable angina, on the other hand, is not predictable. The pain may occur while you are resting, sleeping, or participating in less than strenuous activities. It may increase in intensity and persist for more than 20 minutes at a time. Unstable angina may be a warning sign of an impending heart attack, which is why it must be handled as a medical emergency. The good news is that when unstable angina is treated with aggressive medical therapy, up to 80 percent of patients will stabilize within 48 hours.

The less common types of angina are variant angina, also known as Prinzmetal's angina, and microvascular angina. Variant angina is triggered by a spasm of a coronary artery. It's most likely to occur while you are resting, between the hours of midnight and 8:00 a.m. The majority of people who experience this type of angina have narrowed arteries from plaque deposits. Treatment provides immediate pain relief.

Microvascular angina also causes chest pain, but without any evidence of coronary artery blockage. Instead, the pain—which can occur during exercise or rest—is caused by poorly functioning blood vessels.

Causes and Risk Factors

The lack of sufficient oxygen flow to the heart may be associated with a number of medical problems. The most widespread cause is coronary artery disease, a condition in which the walls of the arteries that carry blood to the heart are narrowed by fatty deposits, and thus have a reduced capacity to carry blood. Other, less common causes of angina include abnormal heart valves, abnormal heart rhythm, coronary artery spasm (temporary narrowing of the artery), anemia, polycythemia (too many red blood cells, resulting in thickening of the blood), and hyperthyroidism.

Signs and Symptoms

The symptoms of angina may vary in intensity from mild to moderate to severe. Severe symptoms do not necessarily mean that you are about to have a heart attack, and mild symptoms do not always mean that your problem is insignificant. People with angina often describe feeling as though there were something heavy pressing on their chests. Sometimes the pain is intense; sometimes it's more of a burning sensation. The pain may extend to the neck, jaw, shoulder, arm, or back. Some people experience palpitations, fatigue, or shortness of breath. The skin may be more sensitive to heat.

A Quick Guide to Symptoms

☐ **Mild to moderate to severe chest pain**
☐ **A feeling of something heavy pressing on the chest**
☐ **Intense chest pain or a burning sensation**
☐ **Pain radiating to the neck, jaw, shoulder, arm, or back**
☐ **Palpitations**
☐ **Fatigue**
☐ **Shortness of breath**

Conventional Treatments

To manage angina effectively, conventional medicine tends to focus on lifestyle changes and medication. In severe cases, surgery may be necessary.

Lifestyle Changes

For angina associated with coronary artery disease, treatment often begins with lifestyle changes. Your doctor likely will review aspects of your lifestyle that may require modification. For example, he or she may recommend improving your diet, starting an exercise program, losing weight, quitting smoking, reducing your alcohol consumption, and keeping stress in check.

Medications

Anticoagulants. If you have angina, you may be advised to take low-dose aspirin or another anticlotting medication. Aspirin inhibits the action of blood platelets, which is how it helps keep blood from clotting. It's important to note that the prolonged use of aspirin may increase your risk of gastrointestinal ulcers and bleeding. Other medications that inhibit blood platelets include clopidogrel (Plavix) and ticlopidine (Ticlid).

Beta-blockers. Beta-blockers are drugs that reduce heart rate and lower blood pressure. Although they do not stop angina attacks, they may reduce the frequency of attacks and the need for nitrate medications (see below). Examples of beta-blockers are propranolol (Inderal), atenolol (Tenormin), and carvedilol (Coreg). Possible side effects of beta-blockers include a moderate decline in HDL ("good") cholesterol, along with fatigue and lethargy. Among those who use these medicines, there have been reports of vivid dreams, nightmares, memory loss, cold extremities, and depression. Some people have a diminished capacity for exercise, decreased heart function, sexual dysfunction, and gastrointestinal upset.

Calcium-channel blockers. These medications reduce heart rate and dilate blood vessels, thereby increasing the supply of oxygen while decreasing the demand for it. Examples of calcium-channel blockers are verapamil (Calan, Isoptin), nifedipine (Adalat, Procardia), nicardipine (Cardene), diltiazem (Cardizem, Tiazac), and amlodipine (Norvasc). Withdrawal from calcium-channel blockers should be gradual. If you are taking a calcium-channel blocker, do not mix it with grapefruit juice, as this may intensify its effects.

Nitrates. These are the most frequently prescribed drugs for angina. They relax the blood vessels, allowing more blood to flow and reducing the workload of the heart. The most popular of the nitrates is nitroglycerin. It is administered as a pill that you place under your tongue, or between your upper lip and gum, and allow to dissolve. It also is available in a metered-dose spray.

The basic dosage regimen for nitroglycerin is as follows.

• One dose at the first signs of an angina attack

• A second dose 5 minutes after the onset of pain, if pain persists

• A third dose 10 minutes after the onset of pain, if pain persists

If you are experiencing chest pain, you must get to an emergency room without delay. Call 911 or your local emergency medical services number, or ask someone to call for you.

If pain doesn't subside within 15 minutes of onset, then you must seek emergency medical assistance.

Since nitroglycerin is very volatile, it can easily lose its potency. Do not purchase more than 100 tablets at one time. Store them in a cool, dry place in their original container, but discard the cotton filler and close the cap tightly. Always carry nitroglycerin tablets with you. Ask your pharmacist to suggest a suitable container.

In addition to prescribing nitroglycerin for acute episodes of angina, your doctor may recommend a long-acting nitrate medication. This drug is available as a topical ointment, patches, and oral tablets. The ointment should be placed, not rubbed, on the chest, stomach, or thigh. Before it's reapplied, the previous application must be removed. The patch should be affixed each morning to a hairless, injury-free area on the back, chest, upper arm, stomach, or thigh. To avoid skin irritation, change the application site each time. Be sure to wash your hands after handling a patch or the ointment.

Since the long-acting forms of nitrate medication may lose their effectiveness over time, many health care providers suggest nitrate-free periods. However, abruptly stopping a nitrate medication may trigger an angina attack, so withdrawal always should be gradual.

Potential short-term side effects of nitrate medications include dizziness, headache, flushing, blurred vision, nausea, rapid heartbeat, and sweating. There are no known long-term side effects. If you experience low blood pressure or dizziness, it may help to lie down and elevate your legs.

Ranolazine (Ranexa). Approved for the treatment of chronic angina, ranolazine (Ranexa) may be given to patients who have not responded to other medications.

Other medications. If your blood cholesterol is too high, your doctor may prescribe a cholesterol-lowering medication. Likewise, for elevated blood pressure, a blood pressure medication may be recommended.

Surgery

If lifestyle changes and medication do not relieve your angina symptoms, your doctor may recommend surgery. There are a number of procedures available.

Angioplasty. In a balloon angioplasty, the physician inserts a catheter with a tiny balloon at the end into an artery in the arm or groin. Where the artery is narrowed, the balloon is inflated, flattening deposits against the arterial wall. To keep the area open, a stent—a small metal tube—may be placed in the artery.

Coronary bypass surgery. In this procedure, the surgeon removes pieces of veins and arteries from the legs (and possibly the chest), and sews them into the arteries of the heart. This allows the blood to "bypass" the blocked arteries and flow through the replacement vessels. Although these surgeries tend to be very successful, they are major medical procedures, requiring at least a week of hospitalization and several weeks of recovery time.

Complementary Treatments

Complementary approaches to angina include lifestyle changes that reduce stress, strengthen the heart muscle, and increase arterial circulation. These treatments are most effective when used in conjunction with conventional medicine.

Acupuncture

Several studies of acupuncture have shown that it can be effective in reducing angina pain, while also promoting relaxation and reducing stress. To locate an acupuncturist in your area, visit the Web site of the National Certification Commission for Acupuncture and Oriental Medicine (NCCAOM) at www.nccaom.org.

Ayurveda

Originating in India more than 5,000 years ago, Ayurveda is a healing system that combines nutrition, herbal remedies, exercise, massage, and meditation. Ayurveda views the heart as the most important organ and the seat of human consciousness. Further, problems such as angina occur because the heart is not receiving proper attention—characterized not just by poor diet and a lack of physical activity, but also by a lack of emotional attachment and spirituality. In Ayurveda, the emotions play a major role in heart health and always factor into treatment.

Ayurveda has been successful in treating the frequency and severity of angina attacks. One helpful remedy is Abana, a combination of herbs and minerals based on your *prakriti,* or body type. Other recommendations may include diet and lifestyle changes, yoga, and meditation.

An Ayurvedic practitioner will make dietary and lifestyle recommendations based on your *dosha,* which is the cornerstone of Ayurvedic diagnosis and treatment. The objective is to restore balance to your dosha, so you can achieve better health. To find a qualified practitioner in your area, begin by visiting the Web site for the Ayurvedic Institute at www.ayurveda.com.

Bodywork

Two forms of bodywork—acupressure and shiatsu—may help alleviate the symptoms of angina. In these techniques, a practitioner applies controlled pressure to selected points along the heart and pericardium meridians—pathways through which the healing energy of the body flows. By strengthening and toning the meridians, these techniques may reduce the frequency and severity of angina attacks.

A practitioner of acupressure or shiatsu can show you how to use these techniques on your own, so when necessary, you can help relieve mild angina pain. To find a qualified practitioner in your area, visit either of the following Web sites: www.aobta.org (American Organization for Bodywork Therapies of Asia) or www.ncbtmb.org (National Certification Board for Therapeutic Massage and Bodywork).

Diet

A healthy diet rich in nutrients and fiber allows blood to flow more freely, reducing pressure on the heart muscle. Foods high in saturated fat and cholesterol, such as red meat and butter, as well as processed and refined foods—especially fried and sugary foods, and anything containing hydrogenated fats—should be avoided. Steer clear of salty foods, too; sodium causes the body to retain fluids, creating more work for your heart. If you do consume meat products, choose only those that are low in fat, such as skinless poultry.

Be sure to include in your diet foods that contain essential fatty acids, as they help reduce inflammation and blood clots, and regulate heart rhythm. Pink salmon and other cold-water fish, olive oil, and raw nuts are all good choices. Vitamin C—found in abundance in raw fruits and vegetables such as grapefruit, kiwifruit, oranges, peaches, bell peppers, and tomatoes—is vital for heart health. So, too, is magnesium, found in green, leafy vegetables such as spinach, parsley, kale, and mustard and turnip greens as well as raw almonds.

Because caffeine increases production of stress hormones, putting you at greater risk for heart problems, limit your consumption of coffee to 1 cup a day. Cut back on other caffeine-containing beverages and foods as well.

Herbal Medicine

Ginkgo biloba. Ginkgo is an antioxidant herb that supports circulation. It is sold both raw and in capsule form. The recommended daily dose is 120 milligrams, twice a day, of an extract standardized to 24 percent flavone glycosides and 6 percent terpene lactones. The flavone glycosides give ginkgo its antioxidant benefits, while terpene lactones increase circulation and have a protective effect on nerve cells. *Note:* If you're taking any blood-thinning medication, be sure to check with your doctor before trying ginkgo supplements.

Green tea. Green tea contains high levels of substances called polyphenols, which have powerful antioxidant properties. It also helps to lower cholesterol and blood pressure, and to keep arteries from clogging. Green tea may be taken as a tea or in capsules. By drinking 3 cups of green tea per day, you'd get 240 to 320 milligrams of polyphenols. In capsule form, a standardized extract of EGCG (a polyphenol) may provide 97 percent polyphenol content, which is the equivalent of drinking 4 cups of tea per day.

Hawthorn. Like green tea, hawthorn works to lower cholesterol and blood pressure. In addition, hawthorn helps to strengthen the heart muscle, improve circulation, and rid the body of unnecessary fluid and salt. Hawthorn is available in capsule or tincture form, standardized to 2.2 percent total bioflavonoid content. The recommended daily dose of hawthorn capsules varies widely, ranging from 100 to 300 milligrams, two or three times per day. Be aware that higher doses may significantly lower blood pressure, which may cause you to feel faint. For the tincture, the recommended dose is 4 to 5 milliliters, three times per day. It can take up to 2 months for hawthorn to have any noticeable effect on your health.

Nutritional Supplements

A number of nutritional supplements are very helpful for maintaining a healthy heart and reducing angina symptoms. These supplements can be taken together.

- Vitamin B_6: 50 milligrams daily, in divided doses of 25 milligrams. Improves the absorption of calcium, L-carnitine, and magnesium.

- Vitamin C: 1,000 milligrams daily, in divided doses of 500 milligrams. Converts cholesterol into bile, lowering LDL cholesterol; strengthens arterial walls; and stops the buildup of cholesterol.

- Vitamin E: 400 IU daily. Increases the oxygen supply to heart tissue and reduces excessive blood clotting.

- Calcium: 1,500 milligrams daily, in divided doses of 750 milligrams. Lowers total cholesterol while increasing HDL cholesterol.

- Coenzyme Q_{10}: 200 milligrams daily, in divided doses of 100 milligrams. Increases the oxygen supply to heart tissue.

- L-carnitine: 1,000 milligrams daily, in divided doses of 500 milligrams. Lowers total cholesterol while increasing HDL cholesterol.

- Magnesium: 800 milligrams daily, in divided doses of 400 milligrams. Regulates heartbeat, helps lower total cholesterol, and helps increase HDL cholesterol.

Relaxation/Meditation

Many complementary health care practitioners recommend various relaxation techniques to help reduce stress, control emotions, and lower blood pressure. In clinical trials, a combination of biofeedback, yoga, and meditation has been the most successful in reducing blood pressure.

Lying still and focusing on your breath can quiet the mind and relieve tension, too. Try this exercise for yourself: Lie flat on your back on the floor or your bed and place both hands on your abdomen. Slowly inhale through your nose, pushing your abdomen upward as if inflating a balloon. Then slowly exhale through your mouth, feeling your abdomen deflate as you do. Continue for 8 to 10 full cycles of inhalation and exhalation. Repeat as often as you're able throughout the day.

Lifestyle Recommendations

Stay active. If you have angina, you may be tempted to stop exercising, but don't give in. Instead, work with your doctor to develop an appropriate exercise plan. If you have not been getting regular exercise, you might start with something as brief as a 5-minute walk. Then gradually increase the duration of your walks as your fitness level improves.

By lowering your blood pressure and slowing your heart rate, exercise will improve bloodflow in your arteries. It also alleviates stress and supports weight loss. So over time, a sound exercise routine will help reduce angina symptoms.

Raise the head of your bed. To decrease the likelihood and/or frequency of angina attacks at bedtime, raise the head of your bed up to 4 inches by putting wooden blocks under the bed frame. This will lower the pressure on your arteries, reducing angina pain.

Stop smoking. Because it decreases the amount of oxygen in the blood, forcing the heart to work harder, the carbon monoxide produced by cigarette smoking only aggravates angina. Smoking also causes blood platelets to stick together, which may lead to an arterial blockage. And smoking interferes with certain prescription medications, making them less effective.

Preventive Measures

Maintain a desirable weight. If you are overweight, lose the extra pounds. Excess weight places additional strain on the cardiovascular system, increasing the risk of angina. Ask your doctor to refer you to a dietitian or a supervised weight-loss program.

Practice yoga. The gentle stretches of yoga have been shown to be very effective in strengthening all of the body's muscles, including the heart muscle. When muscles are stronger, circulation is more efficient, allowing for more effective pulling of oxygen from the blood. This may help prevent angina altogether, or at least help minimize acute attacks. Yoga classes are available at a reasonable cost in most communities, whether through yoga centers, private instructors, or adult education courses.

Anxiety Disorders

Anxiety disorders are not simple nervousness. Rather, they are characterized by an excessive and often unrealistic state of apprehension and fear, which may or may not be related to a specific situation. Derived from the Latin word *angere*, which means "to choke or strangle," anxiety has the potential to take over your life, leaving you unable to function in a normal manner. Of course, there are different degrees of anxiety, ranging from apprehension to paralyzing and profoundly debilitating fear. In extreme cases, people are unable to lead any semblance of a normal life.

Anxiety disorders take many different forms. Generalized anxiety disorder (GAD), which affects some 10 million Americans, is a constant state of worry about various situations. Panic disorder is characterized by periodic panic attacks. People with phobic disorder struggle with irrational fears. In obsessive-compulsive disorder (OCD), people have mental images that can trigger compulsive behaviors, such as repeated checking to make sure that the stove is turned off. Post-traumatic stress disorder (PTSD) is an extreme reaction to a traumatic event.

Anxiety disorders are the most common psychiatric conditions in the United States. As many as 25 million Americans have some form of anxiety-related medical problem—yet only about 25 percent of these people seek professional assistance. On the whole, anxiety disorders are two to three times more common in women than in men.

Anxiety disorders can exact a serious toll on the body. Anxiety can be accompanied by a rise in blood pressure, increased heart rate, rapid breathing, nausea, and other troubling and even dangerous physical symptoms. People with anxiety disorders are more likely than the general population to develop high blood pressure, irritable bowel syndrome, and chronic tension headaches. In studies, phobias and panic disorders have even been correlated with sudden death from heart-related problems.

Causes and Risk Factors

Researchers have identified a number of potential causes of anxiety disorders. There is a good deal of evidence that brain abnormalities—and specifically, imbalances of chemical messengers known as neurotransmitters—play a role in the process. Genetics also seems to be a factor. If you have a close relative with an anxiety disorder, there is about a 20 to 25 percent chance that you will experience one as well.

Family psychological dynamics are thought to contribute to anxiety disorders. Many people with anxiety disorders report having been raised in families that were simultaneously overprotective and unaffectionate, with parents who were quite controlling. There may be a history of childhood abuse.

Panic reactions have been seen in people who are hypersensitive to certain chemicals, such as those in perfumes. Some studies suggest that high levels of carbon dioxide, which can be found in crowded spaces, may trigger anxiety in susceptible adults.

Anxiety disorders may be related to depression. It has been reported that between 20 and 75 percent of people who are prone to panic attacks have experienced at least one major depression. Two of every three people with obsessive-compulsive disorder have depression, while more than one-quarter of people with panic disorder report suicidal thoughts.

People who suffer from alcoholism are at greater risk for anxiety disorders, especially social phobia. Conversely, people with anxiety disorders are at greater risk for alcoholism, smoking, and other forms of addictive behavior.

Signs and Symptoms

All anxiety disorders share a number of physical symptoms, including a rise in blood pressure, increased muscle tension, rapid breathing, and rapid heart rate. In addition, each disorder has its own unique symptoms, which we'll explore here.

Generalized Anxiety Disorder

The primary symptom of GAD is an overall state of tension that persists for more than 6

Medications and Anxiety

A number of medications—including some prescribed for diabetes, thyroid disorders, and high blood pressure—can cause anxiety symptoms. If you are investigating the possibility of an anxiety disorder, give your doctor a list of all the medications you are taking, along with the doses. Your anxiety might be caused by something you are taking for another medical problem. Also, the overuse of caffeine and the abuse of amphetamines may trigger symptoms that appear to be a panic attack.

months. Although there is no obvious stressor, people with GAD are unable to control their level of worrying. They have a constant sense of impending doom, which may impair their ability to go about their daily

A Quick Guide to Symptoms

- ☐ **Elevated blood pressure**
- ☐ **Increased muscle tension**
- ☐ **Rapid breathing or difficulty breathing**
- ☐ **Rapid heart rate**
- ☐ **Disturbed sleep patterns**
- ☐ **Nausea**
- ☐ **Upset stomach**
- ☐ **Dizziness**
- ☐ **Headache**

routines. In cases of GAD, three or more of the following symptoms usually are evident: muscle tension, restlessness, fatigue, disturbed sleep, irritability, and difficulty concentrating.

Panic Disorders

The 3 million to 6 million Americans with panic disorders experience periodic attacks of anxiety and terror that can last for 15 to 30 minutes, if not longer. The attacks, which are twice as common in women as in men, vary in frequency and severity from person to person. They may take place in response to a specific set of circumstances, for no apparent reason, or even during sleep. During an attack, people with panic disorder experience at least four of the following symptoms: shortness of breath, fear of dying, numbness, nausea, dizziness, rapid heartbeat, hyperventilation (overbreathing), hot flashes, chills, chest pain, sweating, shakiness, fear of losing control, a sense of choking, a feeling of unreality, and fear of going insane.

If you have two recurrent attacks followed by at least 1 month of worry that you will have another, your doctor likely will diagnose you with panic disorder. People with panic disorder tend to spend quite a bit of time worrying about when the next attack will occur. They also may avoid locations where attacks have occurred in the past. For example, if you experience an attack while in a supermarket, you may fear going food shopping.

Panic disorders, which often are accompanied by alcoholism or depression, can significantly restrict a person's daily routine. In about one-third of cases, people avoid leaving their own homes (a condition known as agoraphobia), fearful of having an attack. Early treatment of panic disorder can prevent the progression to agoraphobia.

Phobic Disorders

Phobias are extreme irrational fears of a specific object or set of circumstances. Examples of phobias include fear of highway driving, flying, heights, escalators, tunnels, dogs, spiders, crowds, bridges, and snakes. Whatever the phobia, the person is quite aware that it is groundless and absurd. Yet phobia disorders are common: More than 10 percent of the population has a phobia of some kind. If you are among them, you may find yourself working hard to avoid the object or situation that you fear. When you are face-to-face with it, you experience panicky feelings and other symptoms, such as rapid heartbeat and difficulty breathing.

One relatively common—although often undiagnosed—phobia is social phobia, or the fear of being evaluated, scrutinized, and humiliated by others. People with social phobia tend to be uncomfortable in social situations and have unrealistic ideas about the amount of attention others are paying to how they look and what they do and say. The most common form of social phobia is the fear of public speaking, but social phobia may range from a general fear of attending parties to a fear of using a public bathroom. Some people are even uncomfortable writing a check in front of another person or eating in a public place.

Obsessive-Compulsive Disorder

People with OCD have obsessive thoughts that tend to manifest as compulsive, repetitive actions. They also have a heightened sense of concern that if they fail to engage in their rituals, they will cause harm. Some common behaviors include excessive washing, repeated checking (to see if a door is closed, for example), hoarding, and counting. But obsessive thoughts can exist without ritualistic behaviors.

If you have OCD, you may recognize the senselessness of your thoughts and actions, yet be unable to stop them. Your thoughts and actions may use up a considerable amount of time.

Post-Traumatic Stress Disorder

PTSD is an extreme emotional response to experiencing or witnessing a life-threatening event, such as military combat or a violent personal assault. Over and over again, the crisis or incident replays in a person's mind. People with PTSD may have upsetting memories, flashbacks, and nightmares; they may be filled with anger and anxiety; they may struggle to concentrate. Other symptoms of PTSD include excessive avoidance of things and places that are reminders of the traumatic event, emotional withdrawal, self-destructive behavior, mood swings, personality changes, insomnia, and survivor's guilt.

Generalized Anxiety Disorder Self-Test

The following self-test will help determine whether you have generalized anxiety disorder (GAD). If you suspect that you do, it is important for you to consult your doctor, who will be able to make a formal diagnosis and recommend treatment.

For each question, check either "yes" or "no," as appropriate. When you have completed the test, count the number of questions to which you have answered "yes." If the total is four or more, you may have GAD.

1. Are you constantly worrying about things big and small? ☐ Yes ☐ No

2. Do you have difficulty controlling your worries and anxieties? ☐ Yes ☐ No

3. Do you have headaches and other pains for no obvious reason? ☐ Yes ☐ No

4. Do you sometimes feel like throwing up when you're worried? ☐ Yes ☐ No

5. Do you feel keyed up or on edge much of the time? ☐ Yes ☐ No

6. Do you have trouble relaxing? ☐ Yes ☐ No

7. Do you easily become angry or irritable? ☐ Yes ☐ No

8. Do you often have trouble concentrating on the task at hand? ☐ Yes ☐ No

9. Do you often have trouble falling asleep or staying asleep? ☐ Yes ☐ No

10. Does your worrying interfere with normal routine, such as work, school, or social activities? ☐ Yes ☐ No

Conventional Treatments

Conventional treatment for anxiety disorders used to begin with a prescription for an anti-anxiety drug from the group known as benzodiazepines, such as diazepam (Valium) or alprazolam (Xanax). Now, since many people with anxiety have an underlying depression, treatment more often involves an antidepressant in combination with cognitive-behavioral therapy (CBT). The medications of choice are the selective serotonin reuptake inhibitors (SSRIs), because they have fewer potential side effects and are nonaddictive. One well-designed study demonstrated that an 8-week course of the SSRI paroxetine (Paxil) was more effective in reducing anxiety and improving patient functioning than a placebo.

One drawback of the SSRIs is that they may take weeks to work. Normally, you will not notice an improvement for at least 2 to 4 weeks, and some medications may require up to 12 weeks. On occasion, anxiety will increase before it decreases. This is why about one-third of all patients stop using their antidepressants before completing the initial phase. As a result, doctors now begin treatment with both a benzodiazepine and an antidepressant. Once the benzodiazepine is phased out, the patient may remain on the antidepressant.

Medications

Azapirones. Azapirones are drugs that appear to be useful for generalized anxiety disorder. Probably the best known is buspirone (BuSpar). Regrettably, these medications take several days or even weeks to become fully effective, so they do not help with panic attacks. People who have recently taken a benzodiazepine may not respond as well to these medications as other people. Potential side effects include nausea, dizziness, and drowsiness. *Note:* Do not take an azapirone if you already are on a monoamine oxidase inhibitor (MAOI).

Benzodiazepines. As mentioned earlier, benzodiazepines once were the standard treatment for anxiety. Diazepam (Valium), lorazepam (Ativan), chlordiazepoxide (Librium), and halazepam (Paxipam) were prescribed for generalized anxiety disorder; clonazepam (Klonopin) and alprazolam (Xanax) were used for panic disorder and agoraphobia, as well as GAD. Unfortunately, benzodiazepines have a number of potential side effects, including daytime drowsiness and worsening of respiratory problems. They also stimulate eating, which can result in weight gain. Moreover, benzodiazepines may interact with other medications, such as cimetidine (Tagamet) and antihistamines, and may be deadly when combined with alcohol.

Over time, benzodiazepines lose their effectiveness, so to control their anxiety, patients use larger doses and may become dependent on the drugs. If you have been taking benzodiazepines for several months and you discontinue them all at once, you may experience withdrawal symptoms, including sleep problems, anxiety, upset stomach, and sweating. To reduce the risk of withdrawal symptoms, try to wean yourself off the medication gradually.

Beta-blockers. Beta-blockers, such as atenolol (Tenormin) and propranolol (Inderal), block the nerves that stimulate the heart to beat faster. Although they affect only physical anxiety symptoms, they can be beneficial for performance anxiety, which is a type of panic disorder.

Designer antidepressants. The so-called designer antidepressants, such as venlafaxine (Effexor) and nefazodone (Serzone), relieve anxiety by elevating levels of serotonin and other neurotransmitters. Mirtazapine (Remeron) may prove effective for GAD, panic disorder, OCD, and PTSD. It appears to work more quickly and have fewer sexual side effects than other medications. Since it may cause drowsiness, it has the potential to help those who suffer from insomnia. Mirtazapine also may cause blurred vision, weight gain, and slight elevations of cholesterol and triglyceride levels.

Monoamine oxidase inhibitors (MAOIs). Monoamine oxidase inhibitors, such as phenelzine (Nardil) and tranylcypromine (Parnate), are antidepressants that may be prescribed for panic disorders and OCD conditions that have not responded to other treatments. These drugs must be used with caution, however, as they're associated with serious side effects, including insomnia, drowsiness, weight gain, and sexual dysfunction. If a person who's taking an MAOI eats foods that are high in the amino acid tyramine—such as red wine, vermouth, canned figs, fava beans, dried meat, fish, and cheese—it may trigger sudden high blood pressure. MAOIs also may interact with over-the-counter medications such as decongestants and cough medications, and may cause a life-threatening reaction when combined with an SSRI (see below).

Selective serotonin reuptake inhibitors (SSRIs). Selective serotonin reuptake inhibitors, such as fluoxetine (Prozac), sertraline (Zoloft), paroxetine (Paxil), fluvoxamine (Luvox), escitalopram oxalate (Lexapro), and citalopram (Celexa), are the first line of treatment for obsessive-compulsive disorders. They work by increasing the concentration of serotonin, a chemical messenger in the brain. In about half of all patients, SSRIs reduce symptoms by 25 to 35 percent.

Sertraline and fluvoxamine have proven beneficial for panic disorders and agoraphobia, and they may be helpful in cases of social phobia. They must be combined with cognitive-behavioral therapy, however, or the social phobia may reappear. There is some indication that fluoxetine, sertraline, and paroxetine could help people with PTSD.

Among the potential negative side effects of SSRIs are nausea, agitation, insomnia, restlessness, weight gain, and sexual dysfunction.

Tricyclic antidepressants (TCAs). This group of drugs has been found effective for panic and obsessive-compulsive disorders. The most common TCA is imipramine (Tofranil, Janimine), which is used to treat panic disorders. Doxepin (Adapin, Sinequan) may help those who suffer from generalized anxiety disorder and depression. Clomipramine (Anafranil) is prescribed for panic disorders and OCD. TCAs have significant potential side effects, such as weight gain, sexual dysfunction, mental disturbance, sleep disturbance, and a sudden reduction in blood pressure upon standing.

Cognitive-Behavioral Therapy (CBT)

Cognitive-behavioral therapy builds on the premise that you can learn to objectively view the thoughts that cause anxiety, and so alter your response to them. This may be enough to stop the anxiety response, though most patients with anxiety disorders also require medication.

Generally, treatment begins with a daily diary in which you record every anxiety attack and the events and thoughts associated with them. As time passes, it is possible to identify the incorrect assumptions underlying the anxiety, which in turn leads to new ways of coping with the feared objects or situations. Treatment normally lasts 12 to 20 weeks.

Systematic desensitization. In this form of therapy, you gradually increase your exposure to the source of your fear, which enables you to master your anxiety through a series of controlled scenarios. Systematic desensitization appears to be particularly useful for agoraphobia, social phobias, simple phobias, and post-traumatic stress disorder.

Exposure and response treatment. Unlike systematic desensitization, which tends to take a relaxed approach, exposure and response treatment involves confronting an extreme form of the source of your fear from the outset. The theory is that with repeated exposure—either literally or mentally—to the feared object or situation, it should lose its effect over time.

Modeling treatment. During modeling treatment, which is for phobias, you watch an actor cope with an anxiety-producing situation or object. This is done in an attempt to teach you how to act in similar circumstances. Computer simulations have been used as well.

Breathing retraining and relaxation techniques. Cognitive-behavioral therapy usually includes training in techniques that can reduce the physical toll of anxiety. For example, if you know how to use controlled breathing during the early stages of a panic attack, you may be able to avoid a full-blown attack. Learning how to relax the various muscles throughout your body also may be helpful.

Surgery

On rare occasions, surgery may be recommended for patients who have severe forms of OCD or certain phobia syndromes, as well as for those who have not responded to any other treatments. In one procedure, called a cingulotomy, the cingulated gyrus—a bundle of nerves in the front of the brain—is disabled. Cingulotomy is considered a treatment of last resort. In cases where it is deemed necessary, it should be performed only by a highly skilled neurosurgeon at a top medical center.

Complementary Treatments

Acute anxiety triggers the so-called fight-or-flight response, in which the body releases hormones that increase heart rate and blood pressure, alter breathing patterns, and send a rush of blood sugar to the muscles—all in preparation for dealing with a stressful situation. Complementary approaches that help release subconscious emotions, aid in relaxation, cultivate a sense of well-being, and allow a person to gain control over fears can help defuse the fight-or-flight response and its physical effects.

Acupuncture

Acupuncture is useful for treating anxiety symptoms such as dizziness, rapid heart rate, fatigue, headache, increased blood pressure, muscular tension, nausea, rapid breathing, restlessness, and disturbed sleep. Traditional Chinese medicine regards anxiety as an imbalance in the body's energy flow (*chi*). The purpose of acupuncture is to restore balance to *chi*, thereby improving the function of both body and mind. To locate an acupuncturist in your area, visit the Web site of the National Certification Commission for Acupuncture and Oriental Medicine (NCCAOM) at www.nccaom.org.

Aromatherapy

For an acute anxiety attack that is causing hyperventilation, put 6 to 9 drops of essential oil of bergamot, sandalwood, or sweet marjoram on a cloth and inhale. These essential oils have known sedative qualities, as do chamomile, lavender, and valerian. Try placing 8 to 10 drops of one of these oils—or a combination of these oils, using 3 to 4 drops each—in warm bathwater and soaking for 20 minutes. For a nervous system that is fatigued from stress, soaking in a warm bath with oils of neroli, ylang-ylang, peppermint, and jasmine can be helpful.

Biofeedback

In biofeedback, an electric monitoring device provides data on vital bodily functions such as blood pressure and heart rate. During a biofeedback session, you will learn how to use various relaxation techniques—such as meditation and visualization—to alter or slow your body's signals. Because you're getting immediate feedback from the monitoring device, you are able to work on and improve your relaxation skills from the very first session. With practice, a healthier emotional state will become natural.

To locate a biofeedback practitioner in your area, visit the Web site for the Biofeedback Certification Institute of America: www.bcia.org.

Diet

As much as possible, avoid processed foods as well as foods that are high in saturated fat, hydrogenated fats, or sugar. It's best to curb your alcohol consumption, too. All of these foods contain chemicals that can create disturbances in your body functions, particularly the production of brain chemicals that affect mood. Instead, build your meals around fresh, nutrient-dense choices such as whole grains, fruits, and vegetables.

Try to eliminate or at least cut back on caffeine, as it can aggravate anxiety symptoms. For some people, as little as 200 milligrams of caffeine—about 2 cups of brewed coffee—can cause rapid heartbeat, sweating, and shakiness. Remember, too, that caffeine is not limited to regular coffee; it's also found in tea, chocolate, cocoa, and cola beverages. Even some over-the-counter medications contain caffeine.

Flower Essences

Flower essences have been shown to be beneficial for anyone experiencing emotional distress. Those essences that are particularly effective for anxiety are agrimony, elm, red chestnut, and rock rose.

Rescue Remedy, a combination of five flower essences, is a common complementary treatment for acute physical or emotional trauma. It also can be helpful for people suffering from anxiety, which taxes the nervous system. It's available as a liquid for emotional trauma and as a cream for physical injury.

Herbal Medicine

Bacopa. Bacopa is a popular Ayurvedic tincture made from the leaf of the plant. It has a tranquilizing effect, while also improving mental clarity. Bacopa has been shown to play a role in the physiological process of relaxation. Place 30 drops of the tincture in 8 ounces of water, hot or cold, and drink twice a day.

Chamomile and valerian. Like bacopa, chamomile and valerian have sedative qualities, and so can be helpful for reducing anxiety. Look for prepared teas that are labeled for reducing tension; they likely contain these two herbs.

Skullcap. Skullcap is known for its sedative qualities as well as for its ability to reduce anxiety. To prepare a tea using the dried herb, steep 1 or 2 teaspoons of the herb per cup of boiling water, and strain out the leaves before drinking. Drink 3 cups of the tea each day.

Skullcap also is available in tincture form. Place 2 to 4 milliliters in a cup of cold or warm water, or in any other beverage.

Nutritional Supplements

- B-complex vitamins: Take as directed on the label. Protect nerves and reduce anxiety.

- Vitamin C: 1,000 milligrams daily in divided doses of 500 milligrams. Supports the immune system, which is stressed by constant anxiety.

- Calcium: 1,000 milligrams daily. Aids the absorption of magnesium.

- Magnesium: 500 milligrams daily. Reduces nervous tension, relieves anxiety. Best taken with calcium at bedtime, as a sleep aid.

Relaxation/Meditation

Any form of meditation in which the mind is focused on a particular object, sound, mental image, breath, or activity is helpful in reversing the body's fight-or-flight response. Yoga and tai chi are considered meditation in motion; they help to relax muscles, quiet the mind, and create inner peace. You also can meditate while you are lying down or in a seated position. To create a temporary escape, close your eyes and imagine being in a place or doing an activity that you enjoy. The goal is to tell your mind to "be in the moment" instead of dwelling on worries. Experiment with different forms of meditation until you find one that you can easily commit to and practice daily.

Lifestyle Recommendations

Breathe. Focusing on the breathing process can slow your heart rate and take your mind off your anxiety. While lying flat on your back, place both hands on your abdomen. Slowly inhale through your nose, pushing your abdomen up as if inflating a balloon. Then exhale slowly through your mouth, and feel your abdomen deflate. Continue for 8 to 10 full cycles of inhalation and exhalation. Practice at least twice a day, once in the morning and once at night.

Don't smoke. Cigarettes increase blood pressure and contain nicotine, which is a stimulant. People dealing with anxiety disorders don't need the extra stimulation provided by smoking.

Use your senses to create a relaxing environment. By tapping into your senses of smell, sight, and hearing, you can create a therapeutic environment that is conducive to relaxation. You've already learned about the aromatherapy scents that can promote relaxation. Try filling your bathtub with warm water and adding a few drops of the oils noted under Aromatherapy on page 57. Then dim the lights and light a blue or green candle, as both of these colors have a relaxing, calming effect on the body. Finally, put on some relaxing music. Then climb in your tub, sit back, and enjoy. When you are finished, wrap yourself in a blue or green towel, and crawl into bed for a good night's sleep.

Get moving. Any form of exercise can help relieve mental and muscular tension. It also triggers the release of neurotransmitters that alleviate anxiety. Aim for at least 40 minutes of physical activity a day. Among your options are walking, running, skating, swimming, dancing, and other aerobic activities, any of which can help increase your sense of well-being.

Atherosclerosis

Also known as "hardening of the arteries," atherosclerosis is the buildup of plaque—a substance made of cholesterol, cellular waste products, and other materials—in the walls of the arteries. Over time, plaque makes the arteries stiffer than normal and either partially or completely blocks the flow of blood and oxygen. A narrowing of the artery is called a stenosis; a total blockage is an occlusion. The reduction in bloodflow is known as ischemia.

Atherosclerosis is the leading cause of death and disability in the United States. More than 5 million Americans have been diagnosed with it, while at least 5 million more are thought to have it but not know about it.

Atherosclerosis tends to occur near the branching points of the arteries. Most often, it affects medium-size arteries, such as those that feed the heart (coronary arteries), the brain (cerebral arteries), and the neck (carotid arteries), as well as those in the kidneys. It also can affect the aorta—the largest artery, which carries blood from the heart to the rest of the body.

Causes and Risk Factors

Atherosclerosis is thought to begin with an injury to the inner lining of an artery—perhaps caused by high blood pressure, a virus, nicotine, drugs, or an allergic reaction. In an attempt to repair the injury, white blood cells release a chemical that promotes plaque for-mation and acts as a soothing coating for the arterial wall. As the plaque continues to grow, it reduces bloodflow. If the surface of the plaque breaks off, it can cause a clot, impeding or stopping bloodflow and leading to a heart attack, stroke, or kidney failure.

The risk for atherosclerosis increases with age. Those who have high blood pressure, high cholesterol, diabetes, and/or a family history of atherosclerosis are more vulnerable to the disease, as are those who smoke. In a 3-year study of 10,914 middle-age adults, both active smoking and exposure to environmental tobacco were associated with the progression of atherosclerosis. The effect was most significant for those with diabetes and high blood pressure.

Signs and Symptoms

Particularly in its early stages, atherosclerosis produces no symptoms. However, as the level of blockage increases, it can lead to a number of symptoms, which tend to vary according to the affected artery. They include chest pain (angina), dizziness, calf pain during exercise, and transient ischemic attacks (TIAs, or "mini-strokes"). In men, atherosclerosis also may cause erectile dysfunction.

Conventional Treatments

The development of atherosclerosis is a lifelong, additive process. With early intervention, it's possible to slow and even stop the course of the disease.

Lifestyle Changes

In conventional medicine, the treatment of atherosclerosis often begins with lifestyle changes. Your doctor will review your habits and behaviors, with an eye toward possible modifications. Among the strategies that your doctor may suggest are eating a healthier diet, starting an exercise program, losing weight, quitting smoking, cutting back on your alcohol consumption, and reducing the amount of stress in your life.

Medications

To reduce the possibility of a blood clot, your doctor may recommend taking a daily low-dose aspirin. If you have chest pain (angina), you may need nitroglycerin, which helps open your arteries.

Other medications for treating atherosclerosis include beta-blockers, which slow the heart rate and decrease blood pressure. They also appear to lower the risk of fatal heart attacks. (To learn more about beta-blockers, see Angina on page 43.) Your physician also may prescribe an angiotensin-converting enzyme (ACE) inhibitor to facilitate blood-flow from the heart, thus reducing the heart's workload. Examples of ACE inhibitors are lisinopril (Prinivil and Zestril) and captopril.

Many people with atherosclerosis have elevated cholesterol. If you do, your doctor may advise you to take a cholesterol-lowering medication. These drugs include statins, nia-

A Quick Guide to Symptoms

- ☐ Chest pain (angina)
- ☐ Dizziness
- ☐ Calf pain during exercise
- ☐ Transient ischemic attacks (TIAs or "mini-strokes")
- ☐ Erectile dysfunction in men

cin, fibrates, and bile acid sequestrants. (These are described in detail in High Cholesterol, beginning on page 289.) Similarly, if you have high blood pressure, you may require medication to bring it under control. (To explore your options, see High Blood Pressure on page 278.)

Surgery

If lifestyle changes and medication do not improve your atherosclerosis, your doctor may recommend surgery. One option is a procedure known as balloon angioplasty, which involves inserting a catheter with a tiny balloon at the end into an artery in the arm or groin. The catheter is threaded through the artery until the balloon can be inflated in the areas that are narrowed by plaque. As the balloon inflates, it pushes the plaque against the artery wall, which opens up the artery. To keep it open, a stent—a small metal tube—may be put in place.

For some patients who are unable to undergo balloon angioplasty, an atherectomy may be necessary. As in angioplasty, a tube is inserted into the narrowed coronary artery. Then a high-speed drill at the end of the tube shaves the plaque from the artery wall. The shaved plaque is removed via the catheter.

Complementary Treatments

The best complementary approach to slowing or stopping the progression of atherosclerosis involves dietary modification, nutritional supplementation, herbal therapies, and stress reduction techniques.

Ayurveda

Ayurveda is an ancient healing discipline that originated in India more than 5,000 years ago. Ayurvedic practitioners consider the heart to be the most important organ and the seat of human consciousness. Any problems with the heart occur because it's not being given proper care and attention—not just through diet and exercise, but also through emotional attachment and spirituality. In Ayurveda, the emotions play a key role in heart health and are a factor in treatment. A typical Ayurvedic "prescription" may include diet, herbs, yoga, meditation, and lifestyle changes.

Because Ayurvedic practitioners tailor their recommendations to each person's *dosha*, or mind/body type, it's best to see a practitioner for a consultation. The Ayurvedic Institute may be able to direct you to the names of qualified professionals in your area. Visit the organization's Web site at www. ayurveda.com.

Diet

A healthy diet is critical to a healthy cardiovascular system. It should include lots of vegetables, fruits, whole grains, and nuts and seeds (walnuts, almonds, and sesame seeds). Avoid fried foods, sugar, and processed foods, all of which can compromise cardiovascular health. Also avoid foods rich in saturated fats and cholesterol, such as fatty meats, egg yolks, milk fat, and margarine. Replace whole-fat dairy products with their low-fat and nonfat counterparts.

By building your diet around fresh, whole plant foods, you naturally increase your intake of water-soluble fiber. This is the fiber that helps lower cholesterol and high blood pressure not only by reducing the absorption of fat but also by escorting fat from the intestines. Good sources of water-soluble fiber include fruits, legumes, and whole grains, especially oat and wheat bran.

Remember, too, to drink more water to help water-soluble fiber do its job. The minimum recommendation is eight 8-ounce glasses of water daily.

Any foods rich in essential fatty acids, beta-carotene, the B vitamins, vitamins C and E, magnesium, and the trace mineral selenium are beneficial for cardiovascular health. Essential fatty acids come from salmon and other cold-water fish, as well as flaxseed oil. Almost all fruits and vegetables contain beta-carotene, though in varying amounts. You can get your B vitamins from dark green, leafy vegetables, whole grains, avocados, beets, bananas, potatoes, low-fat or nonfat dairy products, nuts, beans, fish, and chicken. Good sources of vitamin C include almost all fruits and green vegetables, especially strawberries, cranberries, melons, oranges, mangoes, papayas, peppers, spinach, kale, broccoli, tomatoes, and potatoes. Vitamin E is available in vegetable oils, nuts, seeds, and wheat germ; green, leafy vegetables and whole grains provide smaller amounts. Magnesium is found in green, leafy vegetables such as spinach, parsley, broccoli, chard, kale, and mustard and turnip greens, as well as in raw almonds, wheat germ, potatoes, and tofu. As for selenium, good food sources include seafood, chicken, whole grain cereals, and garlic.

Antioxidant compounds known as anthocyanosides improve capillary circulation. The European species of blueberry, the bilberry, contains the most anthocyanosides of any food. Other excellent sources include blueberries, cherries, raspberries, red or purple grapes, and plums. An Israeli study, published in the August 2006 issue of *Atherosclerosis*, found that participants were able to reduce their risk of developing atherosclerosis by drinking 6 ounces of pomegranate juice every day for 3 months. Interestingly, the sugars in pomegranate juice did not elevate blood sugar levels in those participants who were diabetic. Instead, the sugars attached to certain antioxidants that help protect against atherosclerosis.

Herbal Medicine

Garlic. Beyond its antioxidant properties, garlic fights atherosclerosis not only by lowering cholesterol and blood pressure but also by improving the elasticity of blood vessel walls.

The recommended daily dose is two to three cloves of fresh garlic, or 500 milligrams in supplement form. If you have a choice, select fresh garlic over supplements; the supplements contain concentrated extracts, which may raise the risk of excessive bleeding.

Ginkgo biloba. Ginkgo is an antioxidant herb that supports healthy circulation. It is available both raw and in capsule form. The recommended daily dose is 120 milligrams, twice a day, of an extract standardized to 24 percent flavone glycosides and 6 percent terpene lactones. The flavone glycosides give ginkgo its antioxidant benefits, while terpene lactones improve circulation and have a protective effect on nerve cells. *Note:* If you're taking a prescription blood-thinning medication, be sure to check with your doctor before trying ginkgo supplements.

Green tea. Green tea contains high levels of substances called polyphenols, which have powerful antioxidant properties. It also helps to lower cholesterol and blood pressure and to keep arteries from clogging. Drinking 3 cups of green tea per day provides 240 to 320 milligrams of polyphenols. In capsule form, a standardized extract of EGCG (a polyphenol) may provide 97 percent polyphenol content, which is the equivalent of drinking 4 cups of tea per day.

Hawthorn. Like green tea, hawthorn helps to lower cholesterol and blood pressure. It also plays a role in strengthening the heart muscle, improving circulation, and ridding the body of unnecessary fluid and salt. Hawthorn is available in capsule or tincture form, standardized to 2.2 percent total bioflavonoid content. For the capsules, the recommended daily dose varies widely, from 100 to 300 milligrams, two or three times per day. Be aware that higher doses may significantly lower blood pressure, which may cause you to feel faint. For the tincture, the recommended dose is 4 to 5 milliliters, three times per day. Hawthorn does work slowly; it may take up to 2 months before you notice any effects.

Nutritional Supplements

The following nutritional supplements are very beneficial to maintaining a healthy heart.

- B-complex vitamins: Take as directed on the label. The B vitamins work best when they're taken together. B_6, B_{12}, and folic acid help reduce homocysteine, an amino acid that contributes to the artery-clogging process. In addition, B_6 improves the absorption of calcium, L-carnitine, and magnesium.

- Vitamin C: 1,000 milligrams daily, in divided doses of 500 milligrams. Converts cholesterol into bile, which lowers "bad" LDL cholesterol; strengthens the arterial walls; and stops cholesterol buildup in the arteries.

- Vitamin E: 400 IU daily. Prevents the oxidation of LDL cholesterol, protects and supports arterial walls and the heart muscle, improves circulation, and fortifies immune function. For the best absorption, pair your vitamin E capsules with selenium (see below). *Note:* Because vitamin E may thin the blood, consult your doctor before taking vitamin E if you already are using a blood-thinning medication.

- Calcium: 1,500 milligrams daily, in divided doses of 750 milligrams. Lowers total cholesterol while increasing "good" HDL cholesterol.

- Chromium: 200 micrograms daily. Helps prevent cholesterol buildup in the arteries.

- Coenzyme Q_{10}: 200 milligrams daily, in divided doses of 100 milligrams. Increases the oxygen supply to the heart tissues.

- L-carnitine: 1,000 milligrams daily, in divided doses of 500 milligrams. Lowers total cholesterol while increasing HDL cholesterol.

- Magnesium: 800 milligrams daily, in divided doses of 400 milligrams. May reduce angina symptoms. Also helps lower total cholesterol while increasing HDL cholesterol.

- Selenium: 400 micrograms daily, in divided doses of 200 micrograms. Thins the blood, helping to prevent heart disease and future heart attacks. *Note:* Consult your doctor before taking selenium if you already are on blood-thinning medication. For best absorption, do not take selenium at the same time as vitamin C.

Relaxation/Meditation

Conventional physicians and complementary health practitioners alike recommend relaxation techniques to help alleviate stress, defuse negative emotions, and lower blood pressure. Clinical trials have demonstrated that by combining biofeedback, yoga, and meditation, you can improve your ability to lower your blood pressure. Other effective relaxation techniques include qigong, tai chi, and visualization.

One 2006 study found that practicing mental relaxation or deep breathing can reduce both blood pressure and heart rate. To try deep breathing, first lie flat on your back either on a bed or on the floor. Place both hands on your abdomen. Slowly inhale through your nose, pushing your abdomen up as if inflating a balloon. Then slowly exhale through your mouth, feeling your abdomen deflate as you do. Continue deep breathing for 8 to 10 complete cycles of inhalation and exhalation. Repeat as often as needed throughout the day to keep stress in check.

Lifestyle Recommendations

Be active. By lowering blood pressure and slowing heart rate, exercise improves arterial bloodflow. It also may reduce plaque deposits, thereby reversing the atherosclerotic disease process. Of course, exercise is important for losing weight and managing stress, both cardiovascular risk factors.

If you have atherosclerosis, you may be tempted to avoid exercise. Instead, work with your doctor to develop an appropriate fitness program. If you have been relatively inactive, you should start with something as brief as a 5-minute walk, then gradually increase your duration over time. Aim for at least 20 minutes, three or four times a week.

Preventive Measures

Relax. Take steps to reduce the amount of stress in your life. As mentioned earlier, meditation, yoga, and other relaxation techniques can help offset the cardiovascular effects of stress.

Cut back on coffee consumption. Drinking coffee increases the body's production of stress hormones, which may place coffee drinkers at greater risk for cardiovascular problems. So far, studies have failed to establish a direct link between atherosclerosis and caffeine intake. Still, if you have other cardiovascular risk factors, you may want to limit your coffee intake to 2 cups a day.

Reduce your alcohol intake. Research into the effects of alcohol consumption on the heart has been mixed. Some studies have shown that red wine may be beneficial for the cardiovascular system, as the flavonoids in the wine help keep fatty deposits from forming in the arteries. On the other hand, alcohol can raise blood pressure and overtax the liver, causing cholesterol to build up in the arteries. While the jury is out, your best bet is to consume alcohol only in moderation. This means no more than one 5-ounce glass of wine daily for women, and no more than two 5-ounce glasses daily for men.

Stop smoking. Beyond the fact that smoking elevates blood pressure, the carbon monoxide produced by cigarette smoke lowers the amount of oxygen in the blood, forcing the heart to pump harder. Smoking also causes blood platelets to stick together, which can lead to arterial blockages. In some instances, smoking can interfere with prescription medications.

Back Pain

Back pain may affect the upper or lower back, and often the neck and legs as well. The pain may be accompanied by other symptoms, such as weakness, numbness, and tingling.

Generally, back pain is classified as either acute or chronic. Acute back pain tends to occur suddenly, and it lasts anywhere from a few days to as long as 3 months. It may subside for a while, only to return later on. When pain persists for more than 3 months, it is considered chronic back pain.

Back pain is extremely common, affecting more than 65 million Americans every year. Four in five of us adults will experience a bout of back pain at some point in our lives. Acute low back pain is the fifth most common reason for physician visits.

Causes and Risk Factors

Back pain has a number of potential causes, including injuries and accidents, muscle strains and spasms, infection, and disorders such as Paget's disease, Parkinson's disease, ankylosing spondylitis (an inflammatory disease of the spine), and osteoarthritis. In cases of acute back pain, however, the cause often remains unknown.

It's not unusual for back trouble to begin in the vertebrae—the 33 bone segments that make up the spinal column. If greater than normal pressure is exerted on one of the cushioning disks that separate the vertebrae, the disk may become herniated (ruptured), causing great pain. For someone with osteoporosis, a vertebral compression fracture could occur even with mild pressure, as in the case of a sneeze. In rare instances, a tumor may be responsible for compressing the spinal column.

Pain also may occur when the bony protrusions on the back of each vertebra deteriorate or become misaligned. Sometimes the spine undergoes painful arthritic changes, a condition known as spinal stenosis.

Pain in the lower back most often occurs because of a problem with the sciatic nerve, the major nerve that carries sensations between the lower back and legs. As many as 40 percent of Americans experience this type of pain, known as sciatica, during their lifetimes. Frequently the culprit is a herniated disk that pinches the nerve, producing pain that radiates into one or both legs. But sciatica can also be the result of an inflamed piriformis muscle (located in the buttocks), lumbosacral strain (muscle strain in the lower back), spinal stenosis, a ruptured disk, strained ligaments, endometriosis, uterine masses, prostatitis, arthritis, and weak abdominal and back muscles.

In some people, back pain may be an indicator of a problem with a nearby organ. For example, both kidney disease and pancreatitis can produce profound back pain. Likewise, conditions such as inflammatory bowel disease and rheumatoid arthritis can cause painful inflammation of the spine.

Even certain medications may have back pain as a side effect. For example, anticoagulants (blood thinners) are known to trigger bleeding and internal bruising that may trigger back pain.

A number of factors raise the risk of back pain—among them obesity, smoking, and a sedentary lifestyle. People who participate in strenuous sports or who do a good deal of heavy lifting are at even higher risk, as are those who have poor posture, who sit or stand in one position for long periods of time, or who improperly lift heavy items. Many people seem to have a genetic tendency for back pain; that is, they are born with spinal abnormalities that make them more vulnerable to problems. The risk of back pain also increases with age.

Signs and Symptoms

If you have back pain, you already know it. It may be dull and throbbing or sharp and piercing, as though someone just stabbed you with a knife. Back pain may occur only when you perform certain tasks or stand or sit in certain positions, or it may be relatively constant. Because the pain may radiate from the back into the legs, it can cause stiffness and restrict movement. It also may trigger tingling or numbness in the calf or foot. In some instances, back pain may interfere with bladder or bowel control.

A Quick Guide to Symptoms

☐ Persistent pain in your back, usually the lower back
☐ Pain may be dull and throbbing or sharp and piercing
☐ Pain may occur only when you're performing certain tasks, or when you're standing or sitting in a certain position
☐ Pain may radiate from your back into your legs
☐ Pain may trigger tingling or numbness in the calf or foot

Conventional Treatments

When acute back pain is not associated with an underlying medical problem, it tends to improve with minimal treatment, often within a few months. Bed rest, once the standard prescription, no longer is recommended. Now doctors advise patients to resume normal activity as soon as possible.

Immediate Pain Relief Measures

Unless acute back pain is the result of an obvious serious medical problem, your best

There are no self-tests for back pain, but if you have it, you know it. You may wish to keep a diary of your pain: When are your symptoms the worst? When do they seem better? This can help you and your doctor pinpoint the source of the problem.

first step may be one or a combination of the following treatments.

- Take an over-the-counter pain reliever such as acetaminophen, aspirin, or another non-steroidal anti-inflammatory drug (NSAID).

- Apply cold, then heat. For the cold treatments, you can use a gel pack or a bag of frozen vegetables, wrapped in a towel. Leave it in place for 20 minutes, and repeat every hour for the first 24 hours. Then switch to heat treatments, such as a heating pad or a warm towel. Apply for 20 minutes of every hour, and continue for as long as needed, up to several days.

- Apply an over-the-counter pain patch.

- Wear a supportive back brace for a short period of time.

- Get a good night's sleep. It might help to avoid caffeine from the afternoon on; to take a warm bath before bedtime; or to practice a relaxation technique such as deep breathing.

Electrical Nerve Stimulation

Transcutaneous electrical nerve stimulation (TENS) uses low-level electrical pulses to reduce back pain. In a typical course of treatment, the TENS unit administers 80 to 100 pulses per second for 45 minutes, three times per day. The sensations are barely felt.

In a similar procedure known as percutaneous electrical nerve stimulation (PENS), small needles deliver the pulses directly to acupuncture points. While this approach appears to provide some relief for many people with chronic back pain, it is not thought to be effective for sciatica. Interestingly, it tends to work better in men than in women.

Exercise

When dealing with acute back pain, it is important to find a balance between inactivity and overexertion. While you should avoid exercises that trigger pain, you do want to incorporate some level of activity into your daily schedule. Within 2 weeks of the onset of pain, most people should be able to begin walking, cycling on a stationary bike, swimming, or light jogging. It's best to steer clear of any exercise that places too much pressure on your back—for example, if it involves twisting or bending—as well as sports that are high-impact.

Exercise also is beneficial for people who are dealing with chronic back pain. In fact, those who engage in exercise tend to return to their normal routines faster than those who are sedentary. A review of randomized trials of various activities, including strengthening and stretching programs as well as physical therapy, found them to be reasonably equal in their effectiveness.

If you have chronic back pain, you may find the following to be particularly useful.

- **Aerobic activities that are low-impact.** These strengthen muscles in the back and abdomen, without straining the back. Examples include bicycling, swimming, and walking.

- **Exercises to strengthen the lower back.** Both partial situps and pelvic tilts can improve lower back strength. To perform partial situps, lie on your back with your knees slightly bent. Raise your head and shoulders off the floor for 2 seconds, then return to the starting position. Repeat 5 to 10 times. For a pelvic tilt, lie on your back with your arms stretched out to your sides. Your knees should be bent, with your feet shoulder-width apart and your heels on the floor. With your shoulders back, squeeze your buttocks and raise your pelvis, keeping your lower back on the floor. Hold for 1 second, then return to the starting position. Repeat 25 to 30 times.

Medications

COX-2 inhibitors. One group of medications found to be effective for relieving back pain is the COX-2 inhibitors, which include celecoxib (Celebrex) and meloxicam (Mobic). These drugs suppress the enzyme cyclooxygenase-2 (COX-2), which causes joint inflammation and pain, while preserving the COX-1 enzyme, which protects the stomach lining. Patients taking COX-2 inhibitors tend to have fewer gastrointestinal side effects than those taking NSAIDs. Nevertheless, many who use COX-2 inhibitors do experience gastrointestinal problems. Some report other side effects as well, such as headache, dizziness, and kidney problems.

People who are using anticoagulant drugs may be at greater risk for bleeding with COX-2s. In a small number of cases, higher doses of celecoxib have been associated with hallucinations, fluid buildup in the legs, high blood pressure, and excess potassium in the blood.

Because of safety concerns, one COX-2 inhibitor, rofecoxib (Vioxx), was taken off the market in 2004. Some researchers question the safety of all COX-2 medications.

Nonsteroidal anti-inflammatory drugs (NSAIDs). Doctors commonly advise their patients with back pain, especially those with chronic back pain, to take nonsteroidal anti-inflammatory drugs. These include aspirin, ibuprofen (Motrin, Advil), and naproxen (Aleve, Naprosyn). NSAIDs may be quite effective, though they may require a week or two to produce significant pain relief.

NSAIDs are known to cause gastrointestinal problems such as ulcers, stomach upset, and internal bleeding. These symptoms may occur even with intravenous administration of the medications. NSAIDs also may increase blood pressure, especially among those who already have high blood pressure. Other possible side effects include headaches, skin rash, ringing in the ears, dizziness, and depression. There is some evidence that NSAIDs may damage cartilage and/or cause kidney damage. The longer you take NSAIDs, the more likely they are to cause side effects, which is why you should use them with caution.

If your doctor determines that you are at risk for developing an ulcer from an NSAID, a number of medications may help prevent one. Among these are the proton-pump inhibitors, which include omeprazole (Prilosec), lansoprazole (Prevacid), rabeprazole (Aciphex), and pantoprazole (Protonix). In comparisons of people who took these medications with those who did not, the proton-pump inhibitors produced an 80 percent reduction in ulcer occurrence.

The drug misoprostol may be helpful in preventing (but not treating) NSAID-induced ulcers. The medication Arthrotec is a combination of misoprostol and the NSAID diclofenac. In one study, patients who took Arthrotec developed between 65 and 80 percent fewer ulcers than those who took NSAIDs alone.

Sometimes NSAIDs are combined with muscle relaxants such as cyclobenzaprine (Flexeril), diazepam (Valium), carisoprodol (Soma), or methocarbamol (Robaxin). Similarly, antidepressants known as tricyclics may be prescribed along with NSAIDs, even to people who are not depressed. This class of drugs includes amitriptyline (Elavil, Endep), desipramine (Norpramin), doxepin (Sinequan), imipramine (Tofranil), amoxapine (Asendin), nortriptyline (Pamelor, Aventyl), and maprotiline (Ludiomil). Although the tricyclic antidepressants have been successful in relieving pain, they may cause significant side effects, such as weight gain, sexual dysfunction, mental disturbance, sleep disturbance, and a sudden reduction in blood pressure upon standing that may lead to dizziness or fainting.

Other medications. For some patients with severe back pain, narcotics are an option. Narcotics fall into two categories: opiates and opioids. Opiates, such as morphine and codeine, are derived from natural opium; opioids—methadone is one example—are synthetic. Since these medications are potentially addictive, people who use them require close medical supervision. With this caveat, narcotics can be very successful in controlling chronic pain. Methadone, for instance, tends to lessen the intensity of pain, enabling people to participate in strength-building exercises, which are an important component of managing back pain.

Another choice for severe pain associated with nerve impingement, such as sciatica, is the injection of substances directly into the affected area. Perhaps the best known of these is the one-time injection of corticosteroid into the area around the spinal column. Other options include injections of local anesthetics, hypertonic saline (saltwater solution), hyaluronidase (an enzyme from mammalian testes), and botulinum toxin (Botox). Better known for reducing wrinkles, Botox temporarily paralyzes muscle tissues, and in doing so may relieve back pain for several months. But none of the injectable options offers a cure.

Surgery

The vast majority of back pain does not require surgery. Even severe pain caused by a herniated disk or spinal stenosis usually responds to more conservative treatments. Nevertheless, in those cases in which more conservative options fail to bring adequate relief and the pain becomes debilitating, surgery may be necessary. It also may be recommended when there is progressive weakening of the legs or evidence of a physical abnormality, such as a bone spur.

Be aware that all of the surgical procedures described below may cause complications, such as nerve and muscle damage, infection, and scarring. Also note that like any surgery, back surgery requires a period of recuperation afterward.

Discectomy. This procedure involves surgically removing the fragment of a spinal disk that is causing pressure and pain. One of the most common complications of a discectomy is the formation of scar tissue, which may lead to persistent pain.

Electrothermal surgery. In this procedure—formally known as an intradiskal electrothermal treatment (IDET)—the surgeon inserts a needle into the compromised disk, using x-rays for guidance. Electricity then heats and shrinks the injured disk tissue. Once healed, the disk is stronger, and often the pain is significantly reduced.

Laminectomy or laminotomy. Both of these procedures target the lamina, which is the back section of the vertebra. In a laminectomy, the entire lamina is removed; in a laminotomy, only a portion is removed. While these procedures tend to bring immediate pain relief, they are not always successful. Moreover, in more than half of all cases, the pain recurs to some degree.

Spinal fusion. Sometimes, when two or more vertebrae are positioned in such a way that they cause pain when they move, the surgeon may recommend fusing them together to eliminate the painful motion. A number of surgical methods are used for spinal fusion.

Complementary Treatments

Complementary medicine offers a number of approaches that have been successful in treating various types of back pain. Since complementary therapies can improve posture, relax tight muscles, address poor body mechanics, and alleviate pain, they should always be tried before scheduling surgery.

Acupuncture

An article published in *Annals of Internal Medicine* analyzed 33 acupuncture studies and concluded that acupuncture is a viable treatment for the relief of chronic back pain. To locate an acupuncturist in your area, visit the Web site of the National Certification Commission for Acupuncture and Oriental Medicine (NCCAOM) at www.nccaom.org.

Aquatic Therapy

Aquatic therapy is effective for relaxing tired, aching back muscles. People who cannot tolerate traditional exercise programs find the water to be the perfect medium for promoting pain relief, because it's buoyant. Health clubs, resorts, and gyms have back pain programs that are available to the general public. There are also physical therapy clinics that offer individual and group aquatic therapy classes specifically for low back pain. Treatments are generally provided by physical therapists, athletic trainers, and licensed aquatic therapists.

Aromatherapy

Peppermint oil relieves pain, eases muscle spasms, and reduces inflammation. The essential oils of eucalyptus, juniper, and rosemary also relieve muscle aches and pains. To promote muscular relaxation, try adding any of these oils to a warm bath. If you're using one oil at a time, you need only 2 or 3 drops in a tub full of water. Limit yourself to a total of 10 drops when combining oils.

You also might try massaging the sore area with one of the oils mentioned above. Just place 10 drops in 1 ounce of oil in a small bottle, and gently roll the bottle between your hands to combine. (If you do not want to purchase a special oil such as jojoba, grape seed, sunflower, or almond, common household oils such as canola or olive oil are fine.) Then use the oil to massage your back.

Bodywork

Various bodywork approaches have been shown to effectively relieve back pain, while also helping to address the underlying cause of the pain. These approaches include acupressure, craniosacral therapy, reflexology, Rolfing, shiatsu, therapeutic massage, and trigger point therapy.

Acupressure. Acupressure—the application of pressure at specific points—can eliminate obstructions in the flow of healing energy. This helps your back muscles and ligaments to relax, and your body to return to a healthier structure.

Craniosacral therapy. Through gentle manipulation of the craniosacral system, this therapy can reduce stress and correct systemic imbalances, allowing the body to heal itself and restore normal function.

Reflexology. Through application of pressure to specific areas of the hands and feet, reflexology can restore the natural flow of energy in the zones of the body. For the spine, the reflex area is located along the edge of each foot, from the big toe down to the heel, representing the area of the neck down to the base of the spine. Tenderness in this area means that circulation to the spine or back is blocked. You may even feel what seem to be tiny crystals when working on this area of the foot. If so, continue to apply gentle pressure, moving along the area until it feels smooth.

Rolfing. Rolfing involves deep manipulation of the connective tissue to restore the body's natural alignment.

Shiatsu. The deep finger pressure of shiatsu massage can help release obstructions in the muscles and vital energy system. Shiatsu can both stimulate and relax, bringing about relief from pain.

Therapeutic massage. Therapeutic massage helps relieve muscular tension and pain. It has an overall calming effect on the body and mind.

Trigger point therapy. Also known as myotherapy, trigger point therapy focuses on trigger points—tender, congested spots on muscle tissue that radiate pain to other areas of the body. Applying pressure to these areas helps alleviate tension, relax muscle spasms, improve circulation, and reduce pain.

Chiropractic

In chiropractic treatment, the chiropractor manipulates and adjusts the spine, placing the backbone in its proper position and thereby diminishing pain. The chiropractor may also integrate various massage therapy techniques to alleviate tension and spasm.

Diet

Maintain a healthy weight by eating lots of whole grains, fruits, and vegetables. This not only helps alleviate the pressure exerted by excess weight but also supports healing by properly nourishing the body. Aim for a minimum of six servings of whole grains, five servings of vegetables, and four servings of fruit each day.

Eliminate foods high in fat and sugar. Beyond their adverse effect on your weight, they rob your body of essential nutrients and interfere with their absorption.

But don't skip meals, particularly breakfast, in your quest to maintain a healthy weight. Strong muscles need food; weakened muscles create injured muscles. In the morning, 95 percent of your energy reserve is depleted. So be sure to eat breakfast to start your day off right.

Also, many people who are trying to lose weight eat the right kinds of food, but don't eat enough. Be sure to take in enough calories to fuel your muscles, so they're able to support your spine.

Energy Balancing

Stress and negative emotions can cause back muscles to tighten, resulting in muscle pain and tension. Energy balancing techniques such as polarity therapy, Reiki, and therapeutic touch can help to restore the flow of the body's natural healing energy, removing blockages and reducing pain and stress.

Polarity therapy. Polarity therapy is a gentle, noninvasive approach that allows the body's natural healing energy to return to balance, alleviating the energy blockages that reside in muscles, bones, and internal organs.

Reiki. Through the hand movements of a trained practitioner, Reiki releases old energy and allows new energy to flow into the body—revitalizing and strengthening each cell, stimulating the body's systems, and normalizing function.

Therapeutic touch. Therapeutic touch moves the body's energy, preventing it from stagnating and causing pain.

Herbal Medicine

Capsaicin. Extracted from the seeds of hot chili peppers, capsaicin reduces substance P, a naturally occurring compound that fosters inflammation and the delivery of pain impulses from the central nervous system. The over-the-counter creams Zostrix and Capzasin-P contain capsaicin in an easy-to-use form. Simply rub a small amount of cream on the affected area four times a day.

During the first few days of use, you may experience a localized sensation of warmth and stinging. This will pass, and pain relief will begin within 1 to 2 weeks.

Ginger. Ginger has a long-standing reputation for reducing the pain associated with inflammation. It is sold in tincture or powder form. Recommended doses are 2 milligrams of tincture, three times a day, or 3 grams of the dried powder, three times a day. Fresh ginger can be grated onto food or added when cooking. Use up to 3 tablespoons of raw ginger or 6 to 8 tablespoons of cooked ginger per day.

Note: If you are taking aspirin or using warfarin (Coumadin), consult your doctor before using therapeutic doses of ginger, since it can increase the potency of these medications and cause unexpected bleeding.

Movement Reeducation Therapies

The Alexander Technique, the Feldenkrais Method, and the Trager Approach are therapies that have successfully helped people with back pain to relearn proper body movements. This results in decreased pain, greater mobility, and improved posture.

Alexander Technique. You may benefit from a series of sessions with an Alexander Technique instructor, who will teach you how to avoid poor postural habits and replace them with healthy body mechanics.

Feldenkrais Method. Practitioners of the Feldenkrais Method train their clients to become more aware of movement patterns and practice proper body mechanics. This can relieve stiffness, inflammation, and pain.

Trager Approach. The Trager Approach uses movement reeducation to release tight muscles. As it is a passive treatment, it is especially useful for people with limited mobility. Over time, the body's nervous system is reeducated to respond in the proper manner to relieve pain and discomfort.

Nutritional Supplements

It is important to maintain proper levels of nutrients to support back health.

- Multivitamin/mineral: Take as directed on the label. Look for a supplement that contains vitamins A, B-complex, C, and E, as well as beta-carotene, calcium, copper, magnesium, selenium, and zinc. Such a supplement has anti-inflammatory properties and, more generally, ensures proper nutrient levels.

- Bromelain: 500 milligrams daily. An enzyme derived from pineapple, bromelain has anti-inflammatory properties.

- Essential fatty acids—omega-3 (flaxseed and fish oil) and omega-6 (borage, evening primrose, and black currant seed oils): Available in oil and capsule form; take as directed on the label. They increase the levels of anti-inflammatory agents in the body.

Personal Fitness Training

When a study published in *Annals of Internal Medicine* reviewed 61 trials involving more than 6,390 adults, it came to the conclusion that physical activity reduced acute and chronic back pain. Other studies have shown that exercises performed with the supervision of a knowledgeable professional, such as a personal trainer, yield better long-term results than exercises performed without professional supervision.

The best exercises for a painful back are those that strengthen and stabilize the core muscles—the muscles of the abdomen, pelvis, buttocks, and hips. These are the muscles that support the back. Appropriate exercises include strength training and Pilates.

To locate a certified personal trainer in your area, visit the Web site of the American

College of Sports Medicine at www.acsm.org. Click on "General Public" on the left side of the homepage, then on the link to "ProFinder."

Relaxation/Meditation

Since emotional stress often is a factor in low back pain, it can be helpful to reduce stress and increase relaxation. Therapies such as deep breathing, visualization, guided imagery, and meditation are useful for reducing stress.

John E. Sarno, MD, a physician and professor of rehabilitation medicine, has successfully worked with patients suffering from chronic back pain. He feels that chronic back pain is not a mechanical dysfunction, but rather is emotional in origin. To help reinforce the "pain as emotion" idea, Dr. Sarno discontinues all physical interventions during treatment, and instead instructs patients to practice positive affirmations to interrupt and eventually reverse the pain cycle.

Though it is not necessary to cease physical therapy when treating back pain, for best results, it is helpful to accept the mind-body connection and to work on healing the mind as well as the back.

Lifestyle Recommendations

Brace your back when sneezing. To avoid aggravating a back injury when sneezing, bend your knees and brace your back by holding on to a nearby support.

Maintain correct posture. To maintain healthy posture, keep your ears, shoulders, and hips in a straight line with your head and your stomach pulled in. Also, avoid excessive standing; standing for long periods of time places extra stress on your back.

For tasks such as washing your face or brushing your teeth, it is necessary to lean forward over the sink. If you have back pain, this position can be extremely difficult. To reduce the strain on your lower back, place one foot on a stool or box. If this is not possible, keep your feet shoulder-width apart, bend your knees slightly, and lean forward at the hips. Throughout this process, try to keep your back straight.

Take breaks on road trips. During longer drives, it is best to stop every hour and get out for a brief walk. Avoid lifting any heavy objects immediately after the drive, as your muscles and joints will be stiff and more vulnerable to injury. Depending on your personal preferences, you might consider using a contoured back pillow in your car.

Apply ice as needed. Ice reduces swelling and can alleviate the pain from back muscle strain. Fill a paper cup with water and freeze it. Then peel back the paper, and you're ready for an ice massage. Move the ice continuously over the painful area for 4 to 5 minutes. As an alternative, use a bag of frozen peas, which will conform to the shape of the painful area. After icing, you might switch to heat.

Relax before bedtime. If back pain compromises your ability to fall asleep, try some of these pampering strategies.

• Take a warm bath right before climbing into bed.

- Fill your room with the aroma of lavender. You can use the essential oil as a room spritzer or apply a few drops to a lamp ring and heat on a lightbulb.

- Listen to quiet music and release the tension of the day with deep abdominal breaths, slowly inhaling and exhaling.

Stretch carefully. When stretching, make sure that you feel the stretch in your muscles rather than in your joints. If you feel it in your joints, you are probably pulling the ligaments that connect the muscles to the joints. Ligaments are more likely to tear than stretch.

Push, don't pull. If at all possible, move a heavy object by pushing rather than pulling. When you push an object, you can use your legs and body weight, which takes the pressure off your lower back.

Take care in lifting heavy objects. If you *must* lift a heavy object, try to heed the following suggestions.

- To give a wider base of support, spread your feet apart.

- Stand close to the object you plan to lift.

- Do not arch your back.

- Bend at your knees.

- Lift with your leg muscles instead of your back muscles.

- While bending or lifting, do not twist from your waist.

Choose appropriate chairs. It is best to sit in chairs with straight backs or low-back support. Look for a chair that swivels and has arm rests. An adjustable chair back is preferable. When you are sitting, your knees should be higher than your hips; you might wish to place your feet on a low stool, if necessary.

Join a support group. If you have chronic back pain, you might consider joining a support group. You'll learn new ways to manage your pain in a more effective manner, and the psychological support of your fellow members may facilitate healing. To find a group in your area, ask your doctor or local hospital for a referral.

Preventive Measures

Get regular exercise. While regular exercise is an important component of any treatment plan for back pain, it also is a means of preventing back problems. By participating in regular exercise that incorporates stretching to increase flexibility, abdominal exercises to support your back, and cardiovascular activity such as walking, you will stretch and strengthen your back muscles as well as lubricate your joints, making them less vulnerable to injury. People who are active also are less likely to be obese, another risk factor for back pain. Aim for at least 40 minutes of physical activity per day.

Stop smoking. Probably because smoking impairs blood circulation, smokers are at higher risk for back problems. Further, smoking disrupts the delivery of vital nutrients to the spinal disks, leaving them more vulnerable to damage when under stress.

Cataracts

Cataracts form when protein in the lens of the eye clumps together. The once-transparent lens becomes cloudy and no longer allows light to pass through and focus on the retina. This leads to a gradual loss of clarity of vision, which over time may seriously interfere with sight and the activities of everyday living.

Because the light rays that are able to penetrate the lens tend to be scattered and distorted, cataracts affect vision in a number of different ways. There may be blurriness and difficulty seeing when lighting is dim. It may be harder to read signs, especially if there is insufficient contrast between the letters and the background. People with cataracts often have trouble driving at night, because of glare from the headlights of oncoming cars. Headlights and streetlights may appear to have halos. Initially, improved lighting and adjustments in eyeglass prescriptions may be of assistance. Eventually, surgery may be necessary.

Approximately 40 percent of Americans between ages 55 and 64 have some degree of opaqueness in the lenses of their eyes. In fact, after age 65, at least half of all Americans have some clouding of the lens, though there may be no noticeable impairment of vision.

Causes and Risk Factors

The most significant risk factor for cataracts is the aging process—the risk of cataracts increases with age. But other factors play a role as well. For example, women are at greater risk than men, and African Americans are at greater risk than whites. Family history also is important.

The presence of any of the following medical conditions may increase the likelihood of developing cataracts: diabetes, glaucoma (and glaucoma treatments), high blood pressure, and connective tissue diseases such as rheumatoid arthritis. Prolonged sun exposure, long-term corticosteroid use, excess abdominal fat, smoking, excess alcohol use, and radiation exposure also have been associated with an increased risk of cataracts. People who have had an eye injury or eye surgery are more vulnerable, too.

Signs and Symptoms

Cataracts tend to develop very slowly and are rarely noticeable in their early stages. There is no pain. Instead, symptoms center around diminished vision. People may experience blurred vision, double vision, or even ghost images. Their night vision may decline, and their perception of colors tends to fade.

People with cataracts may become more sensitive to light or perceive light from the sun or a lamp as too bright. Yet in order to see, they may require ever-increasing

A Quick Guide to Symptoms

- ☐ **Blurred vision**
- ☐ **Double vision**
- ☐ **Ghost images**
- ☐ **Increased sensitivity to light**
- ☐ **Diminished perception of colors**
- ☐ **Difficulty seeing at night**
- ☐ **Frequent changes in eyeglass prescriptions**

amounts of lighting. They also may need frequent changes in their eyeglass prescriptions and/or contact lenses. Those who were farsighted may notice a shift toward nearsightedness.

Conventional Treatments

During the early stages of cataracts, the easiest and best treatments entail modest lifestyle changes. Visit your eye-care professional annually, and obtain eyeglass prescriptions or contact lenses that adequately address your changing needs. When you read, make sure that you have proper lighting. In fact, it might be a good idea to improve the lighting throughout your home. Halogen lights and 100- to 150-watt incandescent bulbs are particularly good. If necessary, buy and use a magnifying glass. Wear sunglasses outside. Reduce or discontinue night driving. For many people, these

changes are sufficient to help them live with mild to moderate cataracts.

Surgery

At some point, a cataract may so impede vision that surgery becomes necessary. In cataract surgery, the clouded lens is removed and replaced with an artificial lens. In most cases, this is an outpatient procedure that's performed under local anesthesia and completed in less than an hour. You will probably be given medication to help you relax.

The most common procedure is called phacoemulsification, in which the surgeon breaks up the clouded lens by emulsifying it with ultrasound waves. The remaining fragments are removed with suction. The lens capsule, or outer layer of the lens, remains intact.

If the cataract is quite large, the surgeon may recommend an extracapsular cataract extraction. In this procedure, a slightly larger incision is made, and the hard center of the lens is removed. The softer outer layer is removed by suctioning, and the capsule shell is left intact.

Once the cataract is gone, an artificial lens is implanted in the empty lens capsule. This implant, which is called an intraocular lens (IOL), may be made from silicone, acrylic, or plastic. It becomes a permanent part of the eye and requires no care.

Shortly after the surgical procedure, you will be able to return home (though you won't be able to drive for a while). You may feel drowsy, so you should rest and relax for the next 24 hours. Don't lift any heavy objects, either. Your physician will probably want to check your eye the next day and again in a month to six weeks. Your vision will likely remain blurred for several weeks.

Expect some pain for a few days; you can treat it with an over-the-counter medication. If you experience vision loss, severe pain, light flashes, numerous floaters (tiny spots that appear to float in your field of vision), marked eye redness, or nausea, coughing, or vomiting, contact your doctor immediately.

While complications from cataract surgery are rare, they do occur. Two of the primary risks are infection and retinal detachment. (The retina is the "screen" at the back of the eye on which images focus.) During your surgical follow-up visits, your doctor will be looking for these problems. Generally, when complications are treated early, the eye heals well.

Cataract surgery has been known to cause glaucoma, a condition in which the pressure inside the eye rises. To reduce the possibility of this occurring, you should minimize physical activity—especially exercise—during the postoperative period. If you must retrieve something for which you'd normally bend over, kneel down to the level of the object instead. Sit down when you put on your shoes. Sleep on your back or on the side that hasn't been operated on. You may resume reading, walking, eating, and watching television the evening after you've had surgery.

Cataract surgery is very common. It is the most frequently performed surgery among Americans age 65 and older. In the United States, there are about 1.5 million cataract surgeries every year.

Complementary Treatments

When dealing with cataracts, complementary health care practitioners focus on stimulating bloodflow and strengthening the eyes. This is achieved primarily through improved nutrition and dietary supplements.

Diet

Studies show that antioxidant-rich foods, along with a healthy lifestyle, can reduce the risk of developing cataracts. Among the most

A Second Cataract

In about 15 to 20 percent of cases, the back of the lens capsule—the supporting part of the lens capsule, which is not removed during cataract surgery—becomes cloudy. This can occur months or years after the procedure. There is a quick treatment for this medical condition. It's called the neodymium: yttrium-aluminum-garnet (YAG) laser capsulotomy.

In a 5-minute procedure, the surgeon uses a laser beam to create a small opening in the clouded capsule, thereby allowing light to pass through. To ensure that the surgery has not raised eye pressure, you will probably be asked to remain at your doctor's office for an hour after the procedure.

beneficial antioxidants for eye health are lutein and zeaxanthin. Both are members of the carotenoid family, and they are the only carotenoids known to be present in the human eye—particularly the retina, the macula, and the lens. Good sources of lutein and zeaxanthin include corn, egg yolks, and green vegetables, particularly broccoli, kale, and spinach. They also are found in cabbage, collard greens, green beans, green peas, and lettuce. Aim for at least four or five servings of these foods each week; one serving a day is even better. Research suggests that people who eat lots of spinach are at lower risk for developing cataracts.

Also be sure to get plenty of vitamin C in your diet. The lens of the eye actually absorbs vitamin C, so the more you consume, the more the lens will contain. Good food sources of vitamin C include oranges, melons, tomatoes, strawberries, red and green peppers, and sweet potatoes.

Beyond these specifics, it's a good idea to adhere to the basic principles of healthy eating—building meals around whole grains, vegetables, and fruits while avoiding foods high in hydrogenated fats, such as solid shortening, margarine, and anything deep-fried. A good benchmark is four servings of fruit, five servings of vegetables, and six servings of whole grains per day.

Foot Reflexology

In foot reflexology, the eye points are located at the base of the second and third toes. By applying finger pressure to stimulate this area, you help to improve circulation to the eyes as well as throughout your body. Tenderness here means that circulation to the eyes is blocked.

When working this area, you may feel what seem to be tiny crystals underneath the skin. If so, continue to apply gentle pressure, moving along the area until it feels smooth.

Herbal Medicine

Ginkgo biloba and bilberry extract are two herbal remedies that have proven effective in maintaining eye health. Both aid in improving the delivery of oxygen to the eyes. And because they're antioxidants, scavenging for free radicals, they help to slow the progression of cataracts.

The recommended dose of ginkgo is 120 milligrams, twice a day, of an extract standardized to 24 percent of flavone glycosides and 6 percent terpene lactones. The flavone glycosides give ginkgo its antioxidant benefits; the terpene lactones increase circulation and have a protective effect on nerve cells. *Note:* If you are taking a blood-thinning medication such as aspirin, consult your doctor before using ginkgo.

The recommended dose of bilberry is one 100-milligram capsule, standardized to 25 percent anthocyanosides, three times a day.

Homeopathy

Homeopathy is a healing system in which substances that produce symptoms of illness in healthy people are believed to have a healing effect when given in very minute quantities to sick people who exhibit the same symptoms. For cataracts, one commonly recommended homeopathic remedy is *Cineraria*. A derivative of the plant known as dusty miller, it is applied as drops to the eyes—1 drop per eye, four or five times a day. This remedy has been used to treat corneal cloudiness. For optimal effectiveness, treatment must continue for several months.

Although high-dose homeopathic remedies are available from homeopaths and other trained practitioners, lower doses can be purchased in retail stores and online.

Nutritional Supplements

The best way to get the antioxidants that support eye health is through diet. If this is not possible, however, you may want to consider vitamin and mineral supplements. The nutrients below are helpful for maintaining eye health and, when taken in combination, may reduce your risk of developing cataracts.

- Vitamin A: 10,000 IU daily. Necessary for eye health; protects eyes from free radicals.

- B-complex vitamins: One capsule twice daily, with meals. The B vitamins help maintain eye health. They work best when taken together.

- Vitamin C: 1,000 milligrams daily, in divided doses (500 milligrams at breakfast and 500 milligrams before bed). Reduces the risk of developing cataracts. Because vitamin C and selenium interfere with each other's absorption, it's best to take these supplements separately.

- Vitamin E: 400 IU daily, taken at lunch or dinner. An antioxidant, vitamin E helps neutralize the free radicals that damage cell membranes.

- Copper: 2 milligrams daily. Plays a role in eye health.

- Lutein: 10 milligrams daily. An antioxidant that's present in the eye.

- Magnesium: 500 milligrams daily. Supports the absorption of vitamin C.

- Selenium: 200 micrograms daily, taken at lunch or dinner. Like vitamin E, selenium is an antioxidant. The two are better absorbed when taken together.

- Zinc: 30 milligrams daily. Zinc is another antioxidant, present in the retina of the eye. *Note:* Long-term use of zinc may impair the absorption of copper, potentially causing copper-induced anemia.

Lifestyle Recommendations

Certain prescription and over-the-counter medications may increase your risk of developing cataracts. They are photosensitizing—that is, they absorb light energy, which makes you more sensitive to sunlight. Moreover, the tissue of the eyes is chemically modified due to the photochemical reaction produced by the absorption of light. Among the drugs that have this effect are antihistamines, nonsteroidal anti-inflammatory drugs (including aspirin, ibuprofen, and drugs that contain them), birth control pills, antidepressants, oral diabetes medications, and sulfa drugs.

Even if it is medically necessary for you to use one or more of these medications on an ongoing basis, you may be able to limit your use. Ask your doctor. You should never stop or alter the dosage of any medication without your doctor's knowledge and approval.

Preventive Measures

Move your body for healthy eyes. Because it improves circulation, exercise enhances the delivery of nutrients to the eyes and facilitates the removal of waste products. The best form of exercise for the eyes is aerobic. Consider walking on a regular basis, gradually working up to daily 30-minute constitutionals.

Maintain proper weight. A high body mass index is a risk factor for cataract development. Excess abdominal weight, in particular, has a strong association with cataracts.

Stop smoking. The direct correlation between cataracts and smoking is well documented. In fact, it is believed that about 20 percent of cataract cases are related to smoking. Both men and women who smoke have significantly higher rates of cataracts than nonsmokers. Smoking is associated with high levels of the heavy metal cadmium in the lens. It also produces cyanide, a retinal toxin. If you smoke, quit. And do your best to avoid secondhand smoke.

Protect yourself from the sun. Most eye-care professionals agree that ongoing exposure to sunlight increases the risk of cataracts. When you head outdoors, it is a good idea to wear a protective hat and sunglasses that block out 100 percent of ultraviolet-A (UVA) and ultraviolet-B (UVB) rays and filter out at least 85 percent of blue-violet rays.

Be aware that certain medications, such as tetracycline, sulfa drugs, corticosteroids, and hydrocortisone, make the skin and the eyes more sensitive to light. Ask your doctor if any of your medications have this effect. If so, you need to be extra vigilant about protecting yourself from the sun.

Celiac Disease

Also known as celiac sprue, gluten-sensitive enteropathy, and nontropical sprue, celiac disease is a genetically transmitted autoimmune disorder. When someone with celiac disease eats foods containing the protein gluten (found in wheat, barley, and rye, and in oats from cross-contamination), an immune reaction occurs in the small intestine. Over time, the surface of the small intestine—with its hairlike projections known as villi—sustains damage. As a result, food cannot be absorbed properly (a problem known as malabsorption), and the nutrients vital to your body are eliminated in stool instead. This may lead to nutrient deficiencies in the nervous system, bones, brain, liver, and other organs, and may serve as a trigger for other illnesses. In addition, because of the damage to the villi, which contain the enzyme that helps to digest dairy products, many people with celiac disease are lactose intolerant.

Celiac disease is far more common than most of us may realize, affecting about one in 133 people by at least one estimate. Close relatives of those with celiac disease are at significantly higher risk themselves, with a one-in-22 chance of developing the condition. That said, only about 3 percent of cases of celiac disease have been diagnosed. This means that in the United States, more than 2.1 million Americans could have celiac disease and not know it.

People with celiac disease are at increased risk for other autoimmune disorders such as insulin-dependent (type 1) diabetes, thyroid disease, Sjögren's syndrome, and Addison's disease. Because of malabsorption, they are at higher risk for osteoporosis. Celiac disease has been linked to nervous system disorders such as seizures (epilepsy) and nerve damage. People who have celiac disease but continue to consume gluten are more likely to develop intestinal lymphoma and bowel cancer.

In Italy, researchers attempted to determine the prevalence of celiac disease in adults diagnosed with non-Hodgkin's lymphoma. Of 650 patients with lymphoma, six had antibody tests consistent with celiac disease. The researchers concluded that celiac disease is associated with an elevated risk of non-Hodgkin's lymphoma.

Causes and Risk Factors

Celiac disease has a strong genetic component. Though you may be born with the potential to develop the condition, experts believe that its onset requires some sort of environmental, physical, or emotional trigger, such as a particularly stressful situation or a bacterial or viral infection to which the immune system responds inappropriately. And you must be eating a diet that contains wheat, barley, rye, or oats.

Dermatitis Herpetiformis

Though sometimes confused with celiac disease, dermatitis herpetiformis is a separate illness. Just like celiac disease, dermatitis herpetiformis is an autoimmune disorder that is caused by gluten intolerance—only it affects the skin, producing severe, itchy blisters that tend to appear on the elbows, knees, and buttocks. While people with this disorder do not experience the digestive symptoms of celiac disease, they may still show signs of intestinal damage.

Celiac disease may have some connection to breastfeeding. Those who were breastfed for longer periods tend to develop celiac disease later in life, and their symptoms may be atypical. Moreover, when and how celiac disease manifests may have something to do with how old a person is when he or she starts eating gluten-containing foods and how much gluten the person is consuming.

Although anyone may develop celiac disease, people of European descent are at increased risk. Women are diagnosed more often than men.

Signs and Symptoms

The symptoms of celiac disease can vary widely from one person to the next. Most people experience some form of gastrointestinal distress such as abdominal pain and bloating, constipation, and/or diarrhea. Their symptoms may be similar to other conditions such as irritable bowel syndrome and Crohn's disease. They may notice weight loss and general weakness, and they may pass foul-smelling stools that float.

Other symptoms of celiac disease include stomach upset, joint pain, skin rashes, depression, irritability, gas, behavioral changes, pale sores inside the mouth (aphthous ulcers), chronic fatigue, migraines, rheumatoid conditions, muscle cramps, dental and bone disorders, and tingling in the legs and feet (neuropathy). In some cases, there are no obvious symptoms, even though there is damage to the small intestine.

If you suspect that you are experiencing symptoms of celiac disease, you should see your doctor. But until you receive an official diagnosis, do not eliminate gluten from your diet. If you do, there is no way to ensure the accuracy of your diagnostic tests.

Conventional Treatments

The most important treatment for celiac disease is to strictly avoid foods that contain gluten.

Dietary Modifications

Treatment for celiac disease involves the complete elimination of all gluten from the diet. This can be difficult, as gluten not only is found in obvious sources such as bread and pasta, it also may be hidden in sauces, soups, salad dressings, medications, supplements, and other products such as lipstick and postage stamps. There also is the problem of cross-contamination: In kitchens where there are gluten-containing ingredients, it is very easy for gluten to find its way into "gluten-free" foods.

You will need to read product labels very carefully. Frequently it may take a phone call to a manufacturer to find out if a specific product contains gluten. When in doubt about a product, avoid it.

It is very important that you adhere to a gluten-free diet. If you accidentally ingest gluten, there is a good chance that you will develop symptoms such as abdominal pain and/or diarrhea. Even if you don't have symptoms, the gluten will do damage to the lining of your small intestine.

On occasion, people following a gluten-free diet will not get better, because the damage to the small intestine is so severe. Their doctors may recommend another course of treatment, such as intravenous nutritional support.

Complementary Treatments

Complementary medicine strives to reduce or eliminate the symptoms associated with celiac disease, often with help from acupuncture, lifestyle modification, and dietary supplements.

A Quick Guide to Symptoms

- ☐ **Gastrointestinal problems such as abdominal pain and bloating, constipation, and/or diarrhea**
- ☐ **Weight loss**
- ☐ **General weakness or chronic fatigue**
- ☐ **Foul-smelling stools that float**
- ☐ **Joint pain or rheumatoid conditions**
- ☐ **Skin rashes**
- ☐ **Pale sores inside the mouth (aphthous ulcers)**
- ☐ **Depression, irritability, or behavior changes**
- ☐ **Gas**
- ☐ **Migraines**
- ☐ **Muscle cramps**
- ☐ **Dental and bone disorders**
- ☐ **Tingling in the legs and feet (neuropathy)**

Acupuncture

Acupuncture is very helpful for treating the pain associated with celiac disease. To locate a qualified acupuncturist in your area, visit the Web site of the National Certification Commission for Acupuncture and Oriental Medicine (NCCAOM) at www.nccaom.org.

Diet

A review of dietary studies, published in the *American Journal of Clinical Nutrition*, confirmed that the most effective treatment for celiac disease is a gluten-free diet. Among patients who strictly adhered to a gluten-free regimen, there was a rapid improvement in symptoms.

Of course, following a gluten-free diet means steering clear of the gluten-containing grains—barley, rye, and wheat—and any products made with them. Among the acceptable grains and flours are arrowroot, buckwheat, corn, flax, millet, quinoa, rice, soy, and tapioca.

On January 1, 2006, the Food Allergen Labeling and Consumer Protection Act (FALCPA) went into effect, requiring any food that contains one of the top eight food allergens (eggs, fish, milk, peanuts, shellfish, soy, tree nuts, and wheat) to declare this information on the food label. The new law also directs the FDA to develop and implement a policy for use of the term *gluten-free* on product labels by August 2008.

Naturopathy

Naturopathic medicine is very effective in the treatment of digestive disorders such as celiac disease. The first step in the naturopathic healing process is to determine the underlying cause of an illness. Once this is done, the naturopath assumes the role of educator, showing a client why and how to restructure his diet and lifestyle. In naturopathy, proper diet and nutritional supplements are fundamental to healing and strengthening the various systems of the body. In order for a naturopathic program to be most beneficial, a person must be willing to make a commitment to change, as it may be necessary to restructure lifelong habits.

To find a naturopathic practitioner in your area, visit the Web site for the American Association of Naturopathic Physicians at www.naturopathic.org.

Nutritional Supplements

Because of their impaired ability to absorb vitamins and minerals, people with celiac disease often run the risk of developing nutrient deficiencies. Taking a daily multivitamin/mineral supplement may help to maintain proper levels of vital nutrients within the body. A B-complex supplement also is recommended, as the B vitamins are not well absorbed in the presence of celiac disease. Beyond the B-complex, a sublingual (under the tongue) supplement of 1,000 micrograms of vitamin B_{12} each day is recommended to support proper digestion and nutrient absorption.

Lifestyle Recommendations

Be wary of beer. Beer, ale, and lagers contain gluten and so are off-limits for those with celiac disease. Because of the distillation process, spirits and wine are gluten-free.

Pay attention for cross-contamination. Cross-contamination can occur in many ways. Foods prepared on a common surface, shared utensils and toasters, flour sifters, foods cooked in the same oil, and shared condiments may easily be overlooked as potential gluten sources.

Take care when you eat out. A number of restaurants throughout the United States now offer gluten-free items on their menus. You might telephone or e-mail a particular restaurant in advance and ask if it's possible to accommodate your diet. Or list your food restrictions on an index card and ask your server to share the card with the chef. If you find a few restaurants that are particularly accommodating, be sure to patronize them often.

Take extra precautions. Remember that the following items may contain gluten: energy bars, communion wafers, prescription and over-the-counter medications, herbal and dietary supplements, and marinades.

Stay active. Regular exercise helps expedite the transit time of food through the digestive tract, reduces pressure inside the colon, and promotes normal functioning of the bowels. For improved bowel health, try to squeeze at least 30 minutes of exercise into every day, or at least as many days as possible. One of the best forms of exercise is walking. If you have been fairly sedentary, be sure to check with your doctor before beginning an exercise regimen.

Manage the stress in your life. When you are under stress, your digestive system can become a sort of "holding tank" for tension-causing emotions, contributing to digestive distress. Try to incorporate stress-reduction techniques into your daily routine. Among your options: biofeedback, deep breathing, hypnosis, massage, meditation, and yoga.

Join a support group. Following a gluten-free diet can be challenging. In a support group, you can learn about your illness, ask questions, share concerns, and see how others cope. If you aren't comfortable with a "live" group, you might try an online group instead. (For organizations that may sponsor support groups, see page 541 of Resources for Specific Disorders.)

Visit a registered dietitian. Many people with celiac disease benefit from one or two visits with a registered dietitian. You might ask your doctor or your local hospital to recommend someone who's particularly knowledgeable about your condition.

Preventive Measures

Right now, there is no way to prevent celiac disease. To reduce your chances of a symptom flare-up, it is very important to follow a gluten-free diet. Otherwise, the damage to your small intestine will not heal, and you will be much more likely to develop celiac-related health problems and complications.

Chronic Fatigue Syndrome

Chronic fatigue syndrome (CFS), also known as immune dysfunction syndrome, is a mysterious illness characterized by extreme fatigue, headaches, painful joints and muscles, and swollen lymph nodes. There are two forms of CFS: sudden onset and gradual onset. More than half of all people with CFS have the sudden-onset form of the illness. In these cases, CFS comes on quickly. The remaining cases are gradual onset, which takes longer to develop. Some experts have speculated that the sudden-onset form of the disease is caused by a virus or neurological abnormality, while the gradual form has psychological roots.

Causes and Risk Factors

While the cause of CFS remains unknown, experts have pointed to a number of contributing factors. They include environmental allergies, iron deficiency anemia, hypoglycemia (low blood sugar), mononucleosis and other infectious disorders, immune system dysfunction, changes in adrenal hormones (such as cortisol), and chronic low blood pressure. Most likely, there is a genetic connection; there may be a psychiatric or emotional component, too. Experts generally agree that the convergence of a number of these elements sets the stage for CFS.

Currently, chronic fatigue syndrome affects about 500,000 people in the United States, with women being diagnosed two to four times more often than men. African American women and Hispanic women are at higher risk than white women. CFS most often strikes between ages 40 and 50; it is less common in those younger than 29 or older than 60.

Signs and Symptoms

According to the Centers for Disease Control and Prevention, you must experience at least four of the following symptoms for at least 6 months in order to be diagnosed with chronic fatigue syndrome.

- Sore throat
- Unexplained muscle pain
- Short-term memory loss or severe inability to concentrate
- Swollen lymph nodes in the neck or armpits
- Pain in several joints, but without redness or swelling

- Profound weariness after exertion that continues for more than a day

- Intense or changing pattern of headaches

- Sleep that does not refresh

Other symptoms associated with CFS are alcohol intolerance, abdominal pain, chronic cough, diarrhea, constipation, dry eyes and mouth, bloating, chest pain, earache, jaw pain, irregular heartbeat, morning stiffness, night sweats, nausea, shortness of breath, tingling sensations, weight loss, depression, anxiety, panic attacks, and irritability. Symptoms tend to be worse in the early stages of the illness, improving over time.

That said, the course of CFS tends to vary significantly from person to person. Some recover within a year, while for others, symptoms linger much longer.

Conventional Treatments

Just as there is no single, precise test to diagnose CFS, there is no specific protocol for treating it. Still, your doctor may offer a number of suggestions to alleviate symptoms. He or she may advise you to slow down and to avoid unnecessary physical or emotional stressors, conserving your energy for essential activities.

As your symptoms improve, you should incorporate very mild physical activity into your life. After an extended period of inactivity, it is important to work your muscles and rebuild your strength.

A Quick Guide to Symptoms

☐ Sore throat
☐ Unexplained muscle pain
☐ Short-term memory loss or severe inability to concentrate
☐ Swollen lymph nodes in the neck or armpits
☐ Pain in several joints, but without redness or swelling
☐ Profound weariness after exertion that continues for more than a day
☐ Intense or changing pattern of headaches
☐ Sleep that does not refresh

Cognitive-Behavioral Therapy

Cognitive-behavioral therapy, which helps a person gain a sense of control over an illness, has been shown to be effective in many cases of CFS. Cognitive-behavioral therapists teach their patients to think about their fatigue differently and to manage their lives in a better way. A cognitive-behavioral therapy program for someone with CFS will probably include the following elements.

- Keeping an energy diary. You should record when your energy levels are better or worse, and what you are doing at the time. It should become evident that certain activities seem to boost energy while others deplete it.

- Adjusting your schedule. After you determine your energy highs and lows, you should plan any critical activities for your "up" times, and save less important tasks for your down times.

- Developing greater flexibility. Since your energy levels may be hard to predict in a consistent way, you need to become more adaptable and "go with the flow."

- Confronting negative thoughts. You will be taught to challenge any belief that you cannot overcome your illness.

- Learning to set limits. Break down a task into smaller, specific jobs. Then focus on doing one small job at a time.

- Prioritizing. You need to save your energy for your most important tasks. The less important ones can be delegated to someone else or set aside for another day.

- Coping with impaired concentration. Seek out the activities that you most enjoy, as they should be easier to complete. When you need instructions, ask that they be given as simple statements. Limit external distractions such as background music.

- Accepting your relapses. With CFS, relapses occur fairly frequently. Do not view them as a sign of failure.

- Beginning a graded exercise program. Research has shown that graded exercise can produce positive results for patients with CFS. In this sort of regimen, you gradually increase the intensity and duration of your exercise sessions. The idea is to build up your fitness in a measured or step-by-step manner. If your symptoms worsen, you can cut back on your physical activity until you feel better. Some experts believe that CFS symptoms such as fatigue, pain, and dizziness occur because of inactivity and will self-perpetuate unless a patient becomes more active.

Medications

Acetaminophen and pain relievers. If your CFS is causing a good deal of pain, your doctor probably will recommend a pain medication such as acetaminophen or a nonsteroidal anti-inflammatory drug (NSAID). If you take acetaminophen, you should know that exceeding the recommended dosage for an extended period will raise your risk of kidney and/or liver damage. An adult should not take more than 4,000 milligrams of acetaminophen per day. Anyone who drinks heavily, who takes blood-thinning medication, or who has liver disease must exercise extreme caution with acetaminophen.

NSAIDs, which include aspirin and ibuprofen, have potential side effects as well. For example, they frequently cause gastrointestinal problems such as stomach upset, ulcers, and internal bleeding—which can occur even with intravenous injection of a medication. NSAIDs also may raise blood pressure, especially among those who already have hypertension. Other potential side effects include headaches, skin rashes, ringing in the ears, dizziness, and possibly depression. There is some evidence that

NSAIDs may harm cartilage and/or cause kidney damage.

It's best to use NSAIDs with caution, as the longer you're on them, the more likely they are to cause side effects. If you have high blood pressure, a severe circulatory disorder, or kidney or liver problems, or if you are taking a diuretic or an oral diabetes medication, and your doctor prescribes an NSAID for an extended period, he or she needs to closely monitor you for the duration of your treatment. Also, if you happen to require surgery for any reason, be sure to stop taking your NSAID a week before the procedure. Since NSAIDs reduce blood clotting, they will increase your risk of excess bleeding.

COX-2 inhibitors are another class of medications that effectively relieve the pain associated with chronic fatigue syndrome. One example of a COX-2 inhibitor is celecoxib (Celebrex). These medications work by suppressing the enzyme cyclooxygenase-2 (COX-2), which causes joint inflammation and pain, while sparing the COX-1 enzyme, which protects the stomach lining. Patients taking COX-2 inhibitors tend to have fewer gastrointestinal concerns than those taking NSAIDs. Nevertheless, many still experience gastrointestinal problems. Other potential side effects of the COX-2 inhibitors include headache, dizziness, and kidney problems. Patients on anticoagulant drugs may be at greater risk for bleeding with a COX-2 inhibitor. In a small number of cases, larger doses of celecoxib and rofecoxib (Vioxx) have been associated with hallucinations, fluid buildup

NSAIDs and Ulcers

If your doctor determines that you are at risk for developing an ulcer from your ongoing use of a nonsteroidal anti-inflammatory drug (NSAID), or if you actually develop one, a number of medications can help treat it. Generally, a class of drugs known as proton-pump inhibitors is helpful in preventing ulcers among those who are at high risk. Examples of these drugs are omeprazole (Prilosec), lansoprazole (Prevacid), rabeprazole (Aciphex), and pantoprazole. When compared to no treatment, they reduce the rate of ulcers by up to 80 percent.

Misoprostol has been found valuable for preventing, but not treating, NSAID-induced ulcers. The medication Arthrotec is a combination of misoprostol and the NSAID diclofenac. In one study, patients who took Arthrotec developed between 65 and 80 percent fewer ulcers than those who took NSAIDs alone.

(edema), high blood pressure, and excess potassium in the blood.

Some researchers believe that all COX-2 inhibitors are unsafe. Rofecoxib was pulled from the market in 2004; another COX-2 inhibitor, valdecoxib (Bextra), suffered a similar fate in 2005.

Other medications. If you have allergy-like symptoms with your CFS, your doctor may prescribe an antihistamine, such as fexofenadine (Allegra) or loratadine (Claritin), and/or a decongestant, such as pseudoephedrine (found in Sudafed, Dimetapp, and many other products). If you have been dealing with a psychological symptom such as depression or anxiety, your doctor may recommend medication along with some form of talk therapy. The antidepressant medications known as tricyclics may be particularly effective in cases of CFS.

Complementary Treatments

The greatest success in the treatment of chronic fatigue has been through a combination of approaches, including those that follow. For you, the ideal treatment plan is one that's designed to meet your individual needs.

Acupuncture

By normalizing and supporting the immune system and increasing energy, acupuncture has been shown to be effective in the treatment of CFS. Often an acupuncture session will include moxibustion, a form of heat therapy. The procedure begins with the placement of a slice of gingerroot over the weakened area. Then a small amount of an herb (called moxa, mugwort, or *Artemisia vulgaris*) is placed over the gingerroot, and the herb is lit with an incense stick. The heat generated by the gingerroot and herb opens the pores; this allows the heat to penetrate internally, which increases circulation and stimulates organs.

To find an acupuncturist in your area, visit the Web site of the National Certification Commission for Acupuncture and Oriental Medicine (NCCAOM) at www.nccaom.org.

Aquatic Therapy

For anyone suffering from multiple symptoms of CFS, therapeutic exercises conducted in warm water can be beneficial. In particular, Watsu—a form of shiatsu massage performed in chest-high warm water—can alleviate pain and promote relaxation.

To find a certified Watsu practitioner in your area, visit the Web site of the National Certification Board for Therapeutic Massage and Bodywork at www.ncbtmb.com.

Craniosacral Therapy

Craniosacral therapy is an effective treatment for CFS as well as for anxiety, which contributes to fatigue. Through gentle manipulation of the craniosacral system, this therapy can reduce stress and correct systemic imbalances, allowing the body to heal itself and restoring normal function.

To find a qualified therapist in your area, visit the Web site of the International Association of Healthcare Practitioners at www. iahp.com.

Diet

Eating a nutritious diet full of whole grains, fruits, vegetables, nuts, and seeds is an excellent way to fight chronic fatigue. These foods are rich in the vitamins and minerals necessary to maintain optimal energy levels and a healthy immune system. Among the most beneficial nutrients for CFS are vitamin C, the B vitamins, magnesium, and essential fatty acids.

Vitamin C supports the adrenal glands, which regulate the production of stress hormones in the body. Good sources of vitamin C include almost all fruits and green vegetables, especially broccoli, cranberries, kale, mangoes, melons, oranges, papayas, potatoes, spinach, strawberries, and tomatoes.

In addition to supporting the immune system and the adrenal glands, the B vitamins are essential to a healthy nervous system. Good food sources of the Bs include avocados, bananas, beans, beets, chicken, dairy products, dark green, leafy vegetables, fish, nuts, oranges, potatoes, and whole grains. Many of these foods are complex carbohydrates, which means that they break down into glucose, an important fuel for the body.

The mineral magnesium helps form ATP, a molecule necessary for energy. Utilized by every cell in the body, magnesium is found in green, leafy vegetables such as broccoli, chard, kale, mustard greens, parsley, spinach, and turnip greens. Other food sources include corn, green beans, lima beans, pistachios, potatoes, pumpkin seeds, raw almonds, sesame seeds, squash, sunflower seeds, tofu, walnuts, wheat germ, yams, and fruits such as bananas, grapefruit, papayas, prunes, raisins, and pineapple juice.

Essential fatty acids (EFAs) help to fight fatigue and enhance immune function. In fact, the primary symptom of an essential fatty acid deficiency is fatigue, and people with CFS commonly run low on EFAs. Among the best food sources of these good fats are flaxseed oil and cold-water fish.

One particular type of essential acid, omega-3 (also known as linolenic acid), has three components: EPA (eicosapentaenoic acid), DHA (docosahexaenoic acid), and ALA (alpha-linolenic acid). EPA and DHA are found in fish oil, particularly from cold-water fish such as bluefish, herring, salmon, and tuna. Flaxseed oil is rich in ALA. Because your body converts ALA into EPA and DHA, taking flaxseed oil is another good way to reap the benefits of essential fatty acids.

Avoid foods and drinks that contain caffeine, which may remain in your system for

Hidden Sugars

Sugar is a common ingredient in our food supply. But because it goes by so many names, you may not recognize it on food labels. All of the following actually are forms of sugar: barley malt, brown rice syrup, cane juice, corn sweetener, corn syrup, date sugar, dextrin, dextrose, fructo-oligosaccharides, fructose, fruit juice concentrate, galactose, glucose, high-fructose corn syrup, lactose, malted barley, maltitol, maltodextrin, maltose, mannitol, maple syrup, microcrystalline cellulose, poly dextrose, raisin concentrate, raisin juice, raisin syrup, sorbitol, Sucanat, sucrose, turbinado sugar, and xylitol. All of these can contribute to weight gain and disrupt sleep patterns.

more than 10 hours and, as a result, may seriously disrupt your sleep. Moreover, caffeine robs your body of magnesium, and a magnesium deficiency can be a major contributor to fatigue.

Also avoid highly processed foods and other foods containing additives and chemicals, which will only aggravate CFS. So can high-fat foods, alcohol, and sweets.

Finally, instead of three large meals, try eating five or six small meals throughout the day. Large meals and overeating may disrupt sleep. Always eat breakfast; your body needs the fuel to get going. And never crash-diet, as it can cause or aggravate fatigue.

Exercise

You may think that exercise would aggravate your CFS symptoms. On the contrary, by engaging in physical activity on a regular basis, you may reduce your fatigue over time. According to studies, any form of gentle exercise that raises levels of brain chemicals known as endorphins can help alleviate anxiety and stress, as well as increase stamina and promote a general sense of well-being.

If you have been relatively inactive, gradually begin your exercise program with brief walks. These may be as short as 20 minutes per day. Work up to longer walks and additional activities, so you're active for at least 40 minutes every day. Get outside in the fresh air when you can.

Exercise may be particularly useful if you have a sedentary job or lead a sedentary lifestyle. In addition to walking, swimming, bicycling, stretching exercises, tai chi, yoga, and qigong may be helpful in reducing fatigue.

Just one caveat: Avoid exercise too close to your bedtime. It may impair your ability to get restful sleep.

Flower Essences

Flower essences are liquid extracts of various flowers and plants that are believed to stabilize emotions, thereby allowing the body to physically heal and remain well. Flower essences such as hornbeam and impatiens may alleviate some of the emotional distress associated with chronic fatigue. Hornbeam assists in relieving the feeling of utter exhaustion, while impatiens may help overcome nervousness, irritability, and tension.

Generally, several drops of either essence is recommended. The remedy is taken daily, often a number of times over the course of the day. Flower essences are gentle and non-addictive, and they have no side effects.

Herbal Medicine

Herbal remedies may help boost immune function, remove toxins from the body, increase energy, reduce anxiety and inflammation, and relieve insomnia—all benefits that counteract the effects of chronic fatigue syndrome.

Echinacea and goldenseal. Echinacea and goldenseal support the immune system and, when used together, may be very effective in fighting CFS. The herbs may be taken in capsule form, though they also are available as tinctures, including one that combines echinacea with goldenseal.

When using the combination tincture, follow the directions on the label. If you choose to alternate between the two herbs, start with 500 milligrams a day of echinacea standardized to at least 3.5 percent echinacosides. Then, after about 3 weeks, switch to goldenseal. Take one 125-milligram capsule, standardized to contain 8 to 10 percent alkaloids or 5 percent hydrastine, twice per day. By alternating the herbs in this way, you're less likely to develop a tolerance to them.

Note: Do not use goldenseal if you have heart disease, high blood pressure, diabetes, or glaucoma.

Garlic. Garlic boosts the immune system and helps fight fatigue. It also treats yeast infections, which appear to be quite common among women with CFS. Like echinacea, garlic enhances the activity of white blood cells and increases T-cell production to fight infections.

The recommended daily dose of fresh garlic is two or three cloves per day, while the dose in supplement form is 500 milligrams. If you have a choice, select fresh garlic over supplements, as the supplements contain concentrated extracts that may increase the risk of excessive bleeding.

Grape seed extract. Grape seed extract contains flavonoids called procyanidolic oligomers (PCOs) or proanthocyanidins (PACs). It's a valuable antioxidant that rids the body of damaging free radicals and helps protect muscle cells. Many who suffer from CFS experience constant muscular pain and tension, as well as depleted immune systems. The typical recommended dose is 100 milligrams, three times a day, of an extract standardized to 92 to 95 percent PCOs.

Green tea. A powerful antioxidant, green tea helps support the compromised immune systems of those with CFS. Prepared tea bags are readily available in grocery and health food stores, though you also can brew a tea from loose tea leaves. Steep 1 teaspoon of the leaves in 1 cup of boiling water for 2 to 3 minutes. Green tea can become bitter if steeped too long. Drinking 3 cups of tea per day will provide 240 to 320 milligrams of polyphenols, the therapeutic compounds in green tea.

A standardized extract of EGCG (a polyphenol) in capsule form will provide 97 percent polyphenol content. This is the equivalent of drinking 4 cups of tea per day.

Passionflower and valerian root. Passionflower and valerian root calm the central nervous system, thereby relieving the anxiety and insomnia that may accompany chronic fatigue. The herbs are available as prepared tea bags and tinctures, and in dried form.

For passionflower, look for a tincture containing no less than 0.8 percent total flavonoids. Take 1 to 4 milliliters in the evening to induce sleepiness. Or you can make a tea by pouring 1 cup of boiling water over 1 teaspoon of the dried herb and steeping for 10 to 15 minutes. Drink before bedtime.

Since valerian has a bitter taste and strong odor, you may prefer to take it in capsule form. Look for a product containing 0.8 percent valeric/valerenic acid, and take 400 to 450 milligrams 1 hour before bedtime.

As with echinacea and goldenseal, you can alternate between passionflower and valerian, using one for 2 weeks and then switching to the other. If you are taking any other sleep aid, be sure to check with your doctor before trying either herb.

Skullcap. Skullcap is helpful for insomnia. Generally, it is sold as a dried herb or a tincture. To make a tea, pour 1 cup of boiling water over 1 teaspoon of the dried herb, then steep for 20 to 25 minutes. Drink before bedtime. In tincture form, add 2 to 4 milliliters to water or juice and drink three times a day.

Naturopathy

Because naturopaths receive training in all facets of natural medicine, they can be especially knowledgeable about treating the symptoms of CFS. When creating a treatment plan, they will focus on reducing stress, identifying food allergies and sensitivities, and strengthening the immune system. They also can offer guidance on dietary changes, herbal and nutritional supplements, and exercise.

For CFS, naturopaths often will recommend hyperthermia hydrotherapy, on the belief that raising body temperature may stimulate the body's immune response. A 3-week intensive heat therapy program has proven effective for some people with chronic fatigue.

To find a naturopathic practitioner in your area, visit the Web site for the American Association of Naturopathic Physicians at www.naturopathic.org.

Nutritional Supplements

Many supplements can help alleviate CFS symptoms as well as replenish vitamins and minerals that may be deficient.

- Multivitamin/mineral: Take as directed on the label. Choose a supplement that provides calcium and potassium, as a shortage of either nutrient can aggravate fatigue. Steer clear of extra iron, however.

- B-complex vitamins: Take as directed on the label. The B vitamins are important for regulating energy and vitality, but they can run low due to stress or an unhealthy diet. They must be replenished, as your body does not store them.

- Vitamin B_{12}: 1,000 micrograms daily, as a sublingual (under the tongue) tablet. Because the body may not be absorbing enough vitamin B_{12}, this extra supplement is necessary. In fact, B_{12} injections may be more beneficial for CFS.

- Vitamin C: 1,000 milligrams daily, as divided doses of 500 milligrams. Supports adrenal function and strengthens the immune system.

- Vitamin E: 400 IU daily. Supports red blood cells, prevents anemia, and stimulates the immune system.

- Bromelain: 1,500 milligrams daily, as divided doses of 500 milligrams, taken between meals. A digestive enzyme, bromelain helps reduce inflammation.

- Coenzyme Q_{10}: 100 milligrams daily, in divided doses of 50 milligrams. An antioxidant involved in the production of ATP, the energy source for the body's cells.

- Evening primrose oil: 3,000 milligrams daily, in divided doses of 1,000 milligrams, each providing 240 milligrams of gamma-linolenic acid (GLA). Helps alleviate aches and pains.

- *Lactobacillus acidophilus*: 200 milligrams daily. Combats frequent yeast infections, which are common among women with CFS. Look for the words *live* or *active* cultures on the product label, with 1 billion to 2 billion organisms per capsule.

- L-carnitine: 1,000 milligrams daily, in divided doses of 500 milligrams. Necessary for the body to convert fatty acids into energy.

- Magnesium: 500 milligrams daily, at bedtime. As mentioned earlier, magnesium deficiency has been linked to chronic fatigue.

- Zinc: 30 milligrams daily. Combats fatigue while improving muscle strength and endurance.

Polarity Therapy

Polarity therapy is a gentle, noninvasive approach that alleviates CFS symptoms by allowing the body's natural healing energy to return to balance. In the body, as in all of nature, energy is characterized by the fundamental principles of attraction and repulsion. In order for energy to move, it needs two unobstructed, opposite fields—positive and negative—that create a polarity relationship. Polarity therapy has proven valuable in treating CFS, particularly in reducing stress and muscular tension. Internalized stress is a major source of energy blockages, which tend to reside in muscles, bones, and internal organs.

To find a practitioner trained in polarity therapy, visit the Web site of the American Polarity Therapy Association at www.polaritytherapy.org or the National Certification Board for Therapeutic Massage and Bodywork at www.ncbtmb.com.

Psychotherapy

Individual or group psychotherapy involving mind-body techniques—for example, hypnotherapy, visualization, and guided imagery—has proven beneficial for CFS patients coping with fatigue from anxiety or stress. Psychotherapy helps many patients assess their priorities and refocus their lives, creating a more manageable lifestyle and accelerating the recovery process.

Relaxation/Meditation

Stress may weaken the immune system, aggravating the symptoms of CFS or possibly triggering a relapse. Therefore, it is essential for people with CFS to find ways to reduce the stress in their lives. A regular routine of guided imagery, meditation, or deep-breathing exercises may promote relaxation, allowing the release of physical and emotional tension. If you don't have time to take a short nap during the day, set aside time to relax your body and mind. Even short breaks help relieve fatigue.

Therapeutic Massage

Therapeutic massage may alleviate CFS symptoms such as anxiety, stress, and muscular tension. It also helps promote a restful night's sleep and provide a general sense of well-being. To locate a massage therapist in your area, visit the Web site of the American Massage Therapy Association (www.massagetherapy.org) or of the National Certification Board for Therapeutic Massage and Bodywork (www.ncbtmb.org).

Trager Approach

The Trager Approach uses movement re-education to release tight muscles. Over time, the nervous system "learns" to respond in a proper manner to help alleviate pain and discomfort. For people with CFS, the Trager Approach can help reduce fatigue and muscle tension and promote a sense of deep relaxation. Because it is a passive treatment, it is especially useful for people with limited mobility.

To locate a Trager therapist in your area, visit the Web site of the United States Trager Association (www.trager-us.org) or of the National Certification Board for Therapeutic Massage and Bodywork (www.ncbtmb.org).

Yoga

A typical yoga session involves gentle stretches, postures, deep breathing, and meditation, which collectively can have an uplifting effect on the body and mind without draining energy. For someone with chronic fatigue, it is an excellent form of exercise. Many health clubs, community centers, and even churches offer yoga classes, usually at reasonable cost.

Lifestyle Recommendations

Avoid a quick fix from sweets. When you are tired, don't try to boost your energy by eating candy and other sweets. Instead, reach for complex carbohydrates such as nuts and fruits. Sweets reduce your blood levels of amino acids, which may worsen fatigue. Complex carbohydrates, on the other hand, elevate amino acids.

Spend some time in the sun. Just 15 minutes of sun exposure per day will ensure that you're getting an adequate amount of vitamin D. If it's cold outside, bundle up and breathe in some fresh air. This may lift your spirits and give you an energy boost.

Find time for you. Set aside 20 minutes each day to do something for yourself. It may be as simple as reading quietly, relaxing in a warm bath, or taking a walk in the fresh air. Whatever it is, it must be just for you.

Get adequate sleep. If you have trouble

falling asleep, try creating a better sleep environment. Begin your prebedtime ritual by drinking a cup of chamomile tea and taking a warm bath. To help relax your mind, listen to soothing music. Once you turn in, lie in bed and take deep, slow abdominal breaths. Let your belly become fully extended as you inhale, then slowly exhale through your mouth. Tell yourself that you are tired and ready to go to sleep. Keeping your bedroom cool, dark, and quiet may help, too.

No matter how well you sleep, try to awaken around the same time each day. It is okay to take a nap during the day, as long as it's brief and it's well before your normal bedtime. Otherwise, it could keep you awake at night.

Simplify your life. Too much stress and too little sleep can aggravate fatigue. So try to cut back on your personal responsibilities. Delegate what you can and prioritize the rest. This way, you may not feel so overwhelmed. Keeping lists may help you focus on what you need to do, without having to remember everything. As you complete tasks, you can cross them off, which gives you a satisfying sense of progress.

Pace yourself. As you feel better, you may be tempted to take on more responsibilities. But if you do too much too soon, your body may respond by feeling worse for several days.

Drink lots of fluids, especially water. Proper hydration helps prevent constipation, which may cause fatigue. Water flushes the system and removes toxins, a buildup of which may cause fatigue and muscular pain. Try to drink eight to ten 8-ounce glasses of water per day.

Stay involved. Remaining as mentally and socially engaged as possible is an important part of recovery from CFS. People who leave their jobs and remove themselves from all social activity tend to have worse outcomes than those who remain active.

Stop smoking. By inhibiting the delivery of oxygen to tissues, smoking robs the body of energy, which only worsens fatigue. If you smoke, quit. Try your best to avoid secondhand smoke, too.

Colon Polyps

Colon polyps are benign or precancerous growths that occur in the colon or rectum. They appear as bumps that vary greatly in size, from less than ¼ inch to several inches in diameter.

There are two main types of colon polyps. A biopsy is necessary to differentiate between them.

Hyperplastic polyps tend to be small and located in the rectum or left lower (sigmoid) section of the colon. They are benign and do not develop into cancer.

Adenomas—which account for about two-thirds of all colon polyps—are believed to be a precursor to almost all forms of colon cancer. Large adenomatous polyps are more likely to contain cancerous cells than smaller ones. A person who has an adenoma in his or her colon is about twice as likely to develop colon cancer as someone who doesn't.

Colon polyps are quite common. The average 50-year-old with no special risk factors for colon polyps has about a 25 percent chance of getting them.

Causes and Risk Factors

Though the cause of colon polyps remains unknown, it may have something to do with not getting enough dietary fiber. A lack of dietary calcium also seems to play a role. Other risk factors include eating lots of red meat and smoking cigarettes.

The odds of developing colon polyps increase with age, with the highest risk among those over age 50. There may be a genetic link as well; you're more likely to develop colon polyps if a first-degree relative has a history of colon polyps or colon cancer or if you've already had a polyp yourself. In rare instances, colon polyps/colon cancer syndromes run in families, and members of those families are more likely to develop polyps at a younger age.

Signs and Symptoms

In the vast majority of cases, colon polyps cause no symptoms. Sometimes there's painless bleeding from the rectum or blood in the stool. Other possible symptoms include anemia, rectal muscle spasms (which make you

A Quick Guide to Symptoms

- ☐ Painless rectal bleeding
- ☐ Blood in the stool
- ☐ Anemia
- ☐ Rectal muscle spasms
- ☐ Cramps or abdominal pain
- ☐ Intestinal obstructions

feel as though you're about to have a bowel movement), cramps, abdominal pain, and intestinal obstructions.

Conventional Treatments

Most colon polyps can be removed during a colonoscopy in a procedure known as a polypectomy. Smaller polyps are removed with an instrument known as a biopsy forceps, which snips off small pieces of tissue. Larger polyps usually are separated from the colon lining with a wire loop and/or burned at the base with an electric current. Since the colon lining is not sensitive to cutting or burning, there is no pain from either procedure. On rare occasions, a polyp may be too large to be removed during a colonoscopy, in which case surgery will be necessary.

If a polyp is benign, no further treatment is required. If it is cancerous, your doctor likely will recommend surgery. Generally, the surgeon will remove the section of the colon affected by the cancer, then stitch together the healthy ends of the colon. More serious cases may call for a colectomy, in which the entire colon or a significant section of it is removed.

When caught early, cancerous polyps may require no further treatment beyond surgery. Your doctor must make this determination.

Complementary Treatments
Diet

As mentioned earlier, people who don't get enough dietary fiber or who eat large amounts of red meat, fatty foods, and processed foods are more likely to develop colon polyps. If you have polyps or are at risk for a recurrence, try cutting back on red meat and other animal products and eating more fiber-rich plant

Anyone age 50 or older should be periodically screened for colon polyps.

foods—whole grains, fruits, and vegetables—instead. Aim for at least five servings of vegetables, four servings of fruit, and six servings of whole grains each day. This should get you to the American Dietetic Association's recommendation of 20 to 35 grams of fiber daily.

One caveat: If you haven't been eating a lot of fiber and you add too much fibrous food too quickly, you may trigger uncomfortable symptoms such as diarrhea, gas, bloating, cramping, or constipation. Increase your intake gradually. Be sure to drink enough fluids, too—at least eight 8-ounce glasses of water or noncaffeinated, nonalcoholic beverages each day.

Herbal Medicine

A natural anti-inflammatory, aloe vera juice may have a soothing effect on colon polyps. When buying aloe vera juice, look for a product with the label designation "IASC Certified," which means that it has been processed according to the standards of the International Aloe Science Council. The juice should be derived from the gel, not the latex, and contain 98 percent aloe vera. (Check the label for aloin or aloe-emodin compounds, both of which are substances in aloe latex. Aloe latex has a laxative effect.) The recommended dose is 1 tablespoon after each meal.

Nutritional Supplements

Certain supplements may be helpful in treating adenomatous colon polyps.

- Calcium: 1,500 milligrams daily; 1,200 milligrams daily for men over age 50. May help protect against a recurrence of adenomatous polyps. The lower dosage for men over age 50 is because of a possible connection between high doses of calcium and an increased risk of prostate cancer.

- Magnesium: 750 milligrams daily. Supports calcium absorption.

Lifestyle Recommendations

Be vigilant about screenings. If you've already had an adenomatous polyp, you are at higher risk for getting another one. So don't put off your next colonoscopy. Catching a polyp early allows for its removal while it's still small.

Take an aspirin. Preliminary studies show that a daily aspirin reduces the incidence of colon polyps. Aspirin therapy also may help keep polyps from developing into colon cancer.

Preventive Measures

One study identified several lifestyle factors that can help protect against colon polyps. They include taking aspirin (81 milligrams) or another nonsteroidal analgesic and getting more dietary fiber and vitamin D. In particular, taking a supplement of vitamin D (400 IU) plus calcium (500 milligrams) on a daily basis is a good preventive strategy, as is consuming dairy products.

Don't smoke. If you smoke, you are more likely to develop colon polyps, among other medical conditions.

Stay active. In studies, moderate to vigorous exercise for 60 minutes a day was shown to reduce the cell growth that leads to polyp formation.

Constipation

People vary widely in the frequency of their bowel movements; from three a day to three a week is considered normal. So not having a bowel movement every day doesn't necessarily mean that you're constipated.

Those with constipation struggle to move their bowels. Their stools are hard and don't pass easily. They may have fewer than three bowel movements per week.

As food passes through the colon, the water it contains is reabsorbed into the body. If too much water is reabsorbed, it leads to constipation. This occurs because the colon's contractions are too slow, and food remains in the colon for too long.

Constipation is the most common gastrointestinal complaint in the United States, particularly among older adults. As we age, just about all of us experience constipation at one point or another.

Constipation may lead to other medical problems. Straining to pass stool raises your risk for hemorrhoids (varicose veins in the rectum) and anal fissures (tears in the skin around the anus). You might even push a small amount of rectal lining outside the anus. This condition, known as rectal prolapse, may cause mucus to leak from the anus. In another condition called fecal impaction, the stool is too hard for the colon to move along, and fecal matter becomes stuck.

Causes and Risk Factors

Poor diet and lack of exercise are the most common causes of constipation. People who don't get enough dietary fiber or omega-3 fatty acids are especially prone to the condition, as are those who don't drink enough water. Other risk factors include changes in routine (such as during travel), medications (such as narcotics, calcium-channel blockers, and antacids that contain aluminum), abuse of laxatives, ignoring the urge to have a bowel movement, and conditions such as irritable bowel syndrome, diverticulosis, hypothyroidism, diabetes, and multiple sclerosis. Tumors, whether cancerous or benign, may narrow the intestine, contributing to constipation.

Chronic idiopathic constipation—also known as functional constipation—may be related to a number of nerve, muscle, and hormonal problems. One example is colonic inertia, a condition caused by a decline in muscle activity in the colon. In anorectal dysfunction (anismus), structural abnormalities in the anus or rectum prevent it from relaxing and allowing stool to exit.

More common in women than in men, functional constipation usually doesn't respond to standard treatment. Fortunately, it is rare.

Signs and Symptoms

People who are constipated have hard, dry stools, which may make bowel movements quite painful. Other symptoms include bloating, stomachache, a general sense of discomfort, and overall sluggishness. If you have hemorrhoids or anal fissures, constipation may cause rectal bleeding. You may notice bright red blood on the stool, in the toilet bowl, or on the toilet tissue.

Conventional Treatments

Generally, constipation is a temporary condition. You should seek medical attention if your constipation does not respond to ordinary measures, if you're experiencing a good deal of pain or any rectal bleeding, or if you notice any unexplained changes in your bowel patterns. Treatment will depend upon how long your symptoms have lasted and how serious they've been. In the vast majority of cases, dietary and lifestyle changes should bring about relief.

A Quick Guide to Symptoms

- ☐ Hard, dry stools
- ☐ Painful bowel movements
- ☐ Bloating
- ☐ Stomachache
- ☐ General discomfort
- ☐ Overall sluggishness

Medications

A bowel that has been sluggish for quite some time may need to be retrained. To accomplish this, your doctor may recommend short-term treatment with one of the following medications.

Laxatives. Bulk-forming laxatives such as Metamucil and Citrucel soften stool by absorbing water in the intestine. They also may interfere with the absorption of certain medications, so check with your doctor before using them.

Nonabsorbable saccharide/bulk laxatives such as lactulose and sorbitol work in much the same way as the bulk-forming laxatives, as do magnesium laxatives such as Milk of Magnesia and Citrate of Magnesia. Stimulant laxatives help move stool through the intestine by causing rhythmic muscle contractions. Examples of these are Correctol and Dulcolax.

If you have been using laxatives for some time, you should discontinue them gradually. This way the colon will have time to relearn to contract.

Lubricants. By literally greasing the stool, lubricants allow it to move through the intestine with greater ease. Mineral oil is one example of a lubricant. Taking mineral oil over a long period will inhibit the body's absorption of vitamins A, D, E, and K and also may cause rectal leakage.

Polyethylene glycol. Polyethylene glycol (Miralax), available over-the-counter, is recommended for occasional constipation. It's a powdered preparation that causes water to be retained in the stool, thereby facilitating bowel movements.

Stool softeners. Products such as Colace and Dialose moisten and soften stool. These are particularly useful following surgery.

Complementary Treatments

Some of the most effective remedies for constipation are the ones that you may try on your own. Dietary changes, exercise, and relaxation techniques not only help relieve symptoms but also may prevent a recurrence.

Acupuncture

For cases of acute constipation, acupuncture treatment is very effective and fast acting. A typical treatment session will involve stimulating points along the stomach, triple warmer, and large intestine meridians, which in turn stimulate the colon.

To locate an acupuncturist in your area, visit the Web site of the National Certification Commission for Acupuncture and Oriental Medicine (NCCAOM) at www.nccaom.org.

Aromatherapy

Because of their relaxing and stimulating properties, essential oils of orange and marjoram can be helpful for relieving constipation. You can prepare a therapeutic bath by adding 6 to 10 drops of either oil alone or 4 or 5 drops of each in combination. Orange oil assists in regulating the bowels, while marjoram improves digestion and promotes elimination. Since orange oil may increase the risk of sunburn and marjoram may cause drowsiness, it is best to plan your therapeutic bath for relatively close to bedtime.

Another option is to make your own massage oil and give yourself a gentle abdominal massage. Purchase a small plastic squirt bottle (not glass, which would be harder to manage) for storing the massage oil. A dark-colored bottle will protect the oil from light and increase its shelf life.

To prepare for your massage, fill the bottle with an oil such as canola, jojoba, or sesame. Place 4 or 5 drops each of marjoram and orange oils into the bottle and shake. Next, heat water in a small pan just to boiling, then remove it from the burner. Place the bottle in the heated water.

After you've warmed the massage oil, lie comfortably on your back. Place a small amount of the warmed oil in your hands and rub them together. Massage the oil over your abdomen, particularly along the colon area. Begin on the right side of your body, next to your hipbone. Gently stimulate the area with your fingertips until you reach the bottom of your ribs. Continue straight along to the left side of your body, downward toward your left hip. You have just stimulated your ascending, transverse, and descending colon.

Next, use both hands to massage the belly area, rhythmically and in a circular motion. This will relieve bloating and stimulate the bowels.

Biofeedback

Biofeedback uses an electric monitoring device to obtain data on vital body functions. During a biofeedback session, you will practice relaxation techniques to alter or slow these functions. If your constipation is the result of anorectal dysfunction, you may be a good candidate for biofeedback. With biofeedback, you are able to retrain the muscles that control the releasing of bowel movements.

To locate a biofeedback practitioner in your area, visit the Web site for the Biofeedback Certification Institute of America at www.bcia.org.

Diet

Increase your fiber intake by eating more high-fiber foods such as fruits, vegetables, and whole-grain products such as oatmeal. A good benchmark is four servings of fruit, five servings of vegetables, and six servings of whole grains each day. This should put you well within the range of 20 to 35 grams of fiber, which is the American Dietetic Association's recommended daily intake. High-fiber foods help create stool that is soft and bulky. Bran is a good fiber source, but it has a tendency to bind with minerals such as calcium and zinc, which may lead to deficiencies.

It's important to increase your fiber intake gradually. If you add too much fiber too quickly, you may experience uncomfortable symptoms such as diarrhea, gas, bloating, and cramping.

Limit or avoid foods that provide little or no fiber, such as meats, cheeses, and processed foods. And make sure that you're getting enough fluids—at least eight 8-ounce glasses of water or other noncaffeinated, nonalcoholic beverages per day. (Caffeine and alcohol may contribute to dehydration.)

Herbal Medicine

Chamomile. Drinking a cup of chamomile tea is soothing to the gastrointestinal tract, along with the rest of the body. You can find ready-made chamomile tea bags in supermarkets and health food stores.

Fennel. Fennel seeds help to prevent and relieve gas. They also are a good source of fiber, and they freshen your breath. Chew 1 tablespoon of seeds slowly and thoroughly.

Senna or *Cascara sagrada*. Both of these herbs are quick-acting, effective laxatives. Senna is quite potent and best taken as a tea. Pour 1 cup of boiling water over 1 teaspoon of dried senna leaves; let steep for 10 minutes, then strain and allow to cool. Drink 2 cups daily. *Cascara sagrada* is a gentle, nonaddictive herb that may be taken in tea form on an empty stomach before meals and at bedtime. Make the tea by adding 4 teaspoons of the herb

Make Your Own Natural Laxative

By crushing seeds and adding water, you can create your own natural laxative. Use 1 teaspoon of flaxseed, 2 teaspoons of psyllium seed, and 1 teaspoon of wheat, oat, or corn bran. Crush the seeds and bran in a coffee/seed grinder. Once they are reduced to a powder, stir them into an 8-ounce glass of water and drink.

Although it requires a day or two to begin working, this laxative will encourage your digestive system to work naturally. It helps soften stools, stimulate contractions, and facilitate the bowel movement process.

to 1 quart of boiling water. Let steep for 1 hour, then strain and allow to cool before drinking.

Nutritional Supplements

Certain nutritional supplements support proper digestion.

- Vitamin C: 1,000 milligrams daily. Helps heal the colon.

- Calcium: 1,000 milligrams daily. Supports muscle contractions in the colon.

- Magnesium: 500 milligrams daily as magnesium citrate or magnesium aspartate (not magnesium oxide) for easy absorption. Aids in the absorption of calcium.

- Omega-3 fatty acids: 1,000 milligrams daily. Necessary for proper digestion.

Polarity Therapy

Polarity therapy is especially useful for constipation and related symptoms such as low energy and emotional fatigue. It helps to relieve stagnation, as well as activate circulation and bodily systems, by focusing on what is known in traditional Chinese medicine as the fire element.

To help stimulate the fire element, a practitioner of polarity therapy might recommend squatting exercises. The squatting position stimulates the colon and moves matter downward. To try this exercise, your feet should be fairly close together and flat on the floor. Wrap your arms around the outside of your knees so that the inside crease of your elbows makes contact with your knees. Clasp your hands in front of you. Feel a stretch in your back between your shoulders. When you are comfortable, slowly rock forward, backward, and side to side. Hold this position for 3 minutes. Perform this exercise once in the morning and again at bedtime.

Another exercise that stimulates the fire element is the Woodchopper. Stand with your feet about 18 inches apart and clasp your hands above your head. Move your arms slightly behind your head, then swing them forward and down between your legs, as if chopping wood. As your arms swing between your legs, make a "ha" exhalation sound. Return to the starting position, letting the momentum carry you back up. Start by repeating this exercise 5 to 10 times each morning, then increase by intervals of five until you are able to perform the exercise 25 times at once.

Reflexology

In reflexology, the points for the colon and small intestine are located in the middle of the foot. Picture a square that begins just below the arch of your foot and ends just above the heel. The outer edges of this square are the colon, while the inside of the square is the intestine. Using your thumbs, apply gentle pressure along this entire area on each foot. It most likely will be very tender and sore. You may even notice what seem to be tiny crystals or bumps. If so, continue to apply gentle pressure, moving along the area until it feels smooth.

Lifestyle Recommendations

Stimulate your gallbladder. Each morning, take 1 tablespoon of cold-pressed extra virgin olive oil, followed by a small amount of fresh-squeezed lemon juice to eliminate the oily aftertaste. This combination jump-starts your gallbladder to begin breaking down fats, thereby aiding digestion.

Reduce stress. Many experts believe that stress slows the digestive process by evoking the so-called fight-or-flight response, which may stop your bowels from moving. According to anecdotal reports, relaxation techniques such as yoga and massage alleviate constipation as well as stress.

Preventive Measures

Pay attention to your bowel. Attempting to delay a bowel movement will result in stool that is harder and more difficult to pass, which increases pressure inside the colon.

Increase your fiber intake. Probably the best way to prevent constipation is to get more fiber in your daily diet. This will help reduce the pressure inside your colon. As mentioned earlier, the American Dietetic Association recommends between 20 and 35 grams of fiber each day. To avoid bloating, work up to this amount gradually.

Among the best food sources of fiber are apples, bananas, barley, blackberries, blueberries, carrots, cherries, cooked beans and peas, dates, figs, grapefruit, kiwifruit, nuts, oats, oranges, pears, prunes, raspberries, spinach, strawberries, sweet potatoes, and whole-grain products. Cruciferous vegetables such as bok choy, broccoli, brussels sprouts, cabbage, and cauliflower also are very good sources. Reduce or eliminate processed foods, which tend to be low in fiber.

Drink water. As you increase your fiber intake, don't forget to drink lots of fluids. Fiber absorbs water in the colon, creating soft, bulky stool that is easier to pass. If you don't replenish your water supply, you may become constipated. Try to drink at least eight 8-ounce glasses of water or other noncaffeinated, nonalcoholic beverages per day.

Move your body. Regular exercise helps move food through the digestive tract, reduces pressure inside the colon, and promotes normal functioning of the bowels. For improved bowel health, try to be active for at least 30 minutes a day, as many days of the week as possible. One of the best forms of exercise for constipation is walking. If you have been fairly sedentary, be sure to consult your doctor before beginning an exercise program.

Have a chuckle. Laughing is a great way to improve digestion. It not only relieves stress, it also has a relaxing effect on the intestines.

How to Get More Fiber in Your Diet

☐ **Unless absolutely necessary, don't peel fruits and vegetables.**
☐ **Whenever possible, eat vegetables raw.**
☐ **Add beans to salads, casseroles, stews, and soups.**
☐ **For breakfast, have a whole-grain cereal such as oatmeal and top it with berries or raisins.**

Coronary Artery Disease

Coronary artery disease, or CAD (sometimes called coronary heart disease), is caused by the gradual buildup of plaque deposits in the coronary arteries, a problem known as atherosclerosis. Over time, these deposits—which consist of fat, cholesterol, calcium, and other cellular sludge—narrow the coronary arteries. Less blood is able to flow to the heart, which may trigger chest pain, or angina. A sudden, complete blockage of an artery could lead to a heart attack.

CAD is the most common form of cardiovascular disease, affecting about 7 million Americans. It is also the leading cause of death in the United States. Every year, 500,000 Americans die from a heart attack caused by CAD.

Causes and Risk Factors

Recent studies suggest that inflammation plays an important role in coronary artery disease, as do other medical conditions such as high blood pressure (hypertension) and high blood levels of LDL cholesterol. Though people often are unaware that they have coronary artery disease—in its earliest stages, it may not produce symptoms—a number of factors are known to increase risk. These include a family history of heart disease, smoking, obesity, physical inactivity, diabetes, stress, and unexpressed anger.

Depression is a risk factor for the development of CAD in people who are otherwise healthy, as well as for adverse cardiovascular outcomes in those with known heart disease. In fact, depression is present in about 20 percent of outpatients and one-third of inpatients with CAD. What is not yet known is whether treating depression with medication will improve cardiovascular outcomes. Still, those with CAD should be considered at risk for depression.

While young people may develop coronary artery disease, it is much more common in those at midlife and older. Until then, men are more likely to have CAD than women. After menopause, a woman's risk increases to become roughly equal to a man's.

Signs and Symptoms

As mentioned earlier, coronary artery disease doesn't always produce symptoms. Even though the narrowed arteries are impeding the flow of blood—and therefore the delivery of vital nutrients and oxygen to the heart (a condition called ischemia)—a person may not notice any difference in his or her health. This is known as silent ischemia, and it is the most common manifestation of CAD.

When symptoms do occur, they may include shortness of breath, irregular heartbeat, and chest pain (angina). A heart attack caused by a blocked coronary artery is another symptom of CAD.

Conventional Treatments
Lifestyle Changes

Treating coronary artery disease often begins with lifestyle changes. Your doctor probably will review various lifestyle factors with you to determine whether they require modification. He or she may recommend improving your diet, starting an exercise program, losing weight, giving up smoking, cutting back on alcohol, and reducing the stress in your life (or learning to cope with stressors that you can't avoid).

Medications

Aspirin. To reduce the likelihood of a blood clot developing and lodging in a narrowed coronary artery, your doctor may advise you to take a low-dose aspirin daily. Aspirin helps to prevent blood platelets from sticking together and forming clots.

Beta-blockers and calcium-channel blockers. Among the prescription medications that help treat CAD are beta-blockers and calcium-channel blockers.

Beta-blockers, such as atenolol (Tenormin) and metoprolol (Lopressor), slow heart rate and lower blood pressure, so the heart doesn't need as much oxygen. These drugs have been shown to reduce the risk of dying from a heart attack, to prevent recurrent heart attacks, and to improve the odds of survival among patients who've had heart attacks.

Calcium-channel blockers, such as verapamil (Calan) and nifedipine (Procardia), relax the muscles surrounding the coronary arteries, so the arteries can open up.

Cholesterol-lowering medications. Many people with coronary artery disease have elevated cholesterol levels. If this is true for you, your doctor may prescribe a cholesterol-

The pain from a heart attack may be quite intense, and it lasts considerably longer than the pain of angina. But not all heart attacks cause chest pain, especially in women. They're more likely to experience pain in the jaw, neck, or back, as well as nausea, shortness of breath, weakness, or fatigue.

If you're experiencing these or any other symptoms of a heart attack, call 911 or your emergency medical number. It is vital to seek medical attention without delay.

lowering medication. There are several categories of these drugs (including statins, niacin, fibrates, and bile acid sequestrants), and they work in various ways. Besides lowering cholesterol, the statins have anti-inflammatory properties—and since CAD is an inflammatory process, it may respond particularly well to treatment with these drugs.

Nitrates. If you're experiencing chest pain (angina) from CAD, your doctor may recommend any of a class of medications called nitrates for use in emergencies. The best known of the nitrates is nitroglycerin, but these drugs are sold under a variety of generic and brand names. Some are meant to be swallowed; others dissolve under the tongue; and still others, in liquid form, are to be sprayed into the mouth. Nitrates work by opening the arteries and reducing the heart's need for oxygen.

Surgery

If lifestyle changes and medication do not relieve CAD symptoms, the next step may be surgery. Your doctor may recommend one of the following procedures.

Atherectomy. This procedure is an option for those patients who are not candidates for a balloon angioplasty (described next). In an atherectomy, a flexible hollow tube called a catheter is slowly threaded through a small incision underneath the arm or in the groin into the narrowed coronary artery. At the end of the tube is a tiny, high-speed drill, which shaves plaque from the arterial wall.

Balloon angioplasty and laser ablation. As in an atherectomy, a balloon angioplasty involves inserting a catheter into an artery and slowly threading it toward the heart. Once the catheter is in place in the narrowed area of the artery, a balloon at the tip of the tube is inflated. This compresses the plaque against the arterial wall, allowing blood to flow more freely.

In laser ablation, the cardiologist first uses a laser to burn away some of the arterial plaque. Then a balloon further opens the artery.

About 35 percent of people who undergo either of these procedures eventually develop more blockages in the treated area, a condition known as restenosis. To keep this from happening, the cardiologist may place a small metal rod, or stent, inside the artery to help keep it open. Among people who receive stents, the rate of restenosis is between 15 and 20 percent. The use of a polymer-based, paclitaxel-coated stent instead of a bare metal stent may lower the risk of restenosis even further.

Bypass surgery. In this procedure—the full name is coronary artery bypass graft surgery—the surgeon removes pieces of vein or artery from a patient's legs and/or chest and sews the pieces into the arteries of the heart. This allows blood to "bypass" the blocked arteries by flowing through the replacement vessels. Though these surgeries have an excellent success rate, they are major procedures, generally requiring at least 1 week of hospitalization and several weeks for recovery.

A newer procedure, called minimally invasive direct coronary artery bypass, may be performed on a beating heart without using a heart-lung machine. It also requires a smaller incision.

Transmyocardial laser revascularization. This procedure is particularly useful for patients who have angina that is not responsive to other treatment or who experience residual angina after bypass surgery. It may be performed by a cardiologist in a cardiac catheterization lab.

After numbing an area of the leg with anesthesia, the cardiologist inserts a catheter into a leg artery. Once the catheter reaches the heart, the laser makes 10 to 20 tiny channels in the heart muscle. Blood flows into these channels, giving the heart muscle the additional oxygen that it needs. The procedure may lead to the formation of additional vessels as well.

Complementary Treatments

The best complementary treatments for coronary artery disease are those that support a conventional treatment plan. A person with CAD always should be under a doctor's care.

Ayurveda

Ayurveda—a discipline with Indian roots dating back some 5,000 years—combines exercise, herbal remedies, massage, meditation, and nutrition in a holistic approach to healing. Ayurvedic practitioners view the heart as the most important organ and the seat of human consciousness. Health problems arise when we ignore the heart—not only through physical inactivity and poor diet but also through a lack of emotional attachment and spirituality. In Ayurveda, the emotions are key to the health of the heart and always are considered during treatment. An Ayurvedic treatment plan for coronary artery disease might include dietary and lifestyle changes, herbs, meditation, and yoga.

There is no professional organization that offers certification or membership to Ayurvedic practitioners. The Ayurvedic Institute may provide the names of practitioners in your area. Visit the institute's Web site at www.ayurveda.com.

Diet

Research shows that a diet heavy on fruits and vegetables—particularly leafy greens and vitamin C–rich produce—helps protect against coronary artery disease. According to an article in the March 2007 issue of the *American Journal of Clinical Nutrition*, some studies further suggest that these foods could reduce the risk of death from CAD. Try to eat at least four servings of fruits and five servings of vegetables, along with six servings of whole grains, each day.

Be sure to leave room in your diet for nuts and seeds such as walnuts, almonds, and sesame seeds, which help maintain a healthy heart. And don't forget the following foods and nutrients, all of which play roles in heart health.

- Fish oil from cold-water fish such as bluefish, herring, salmon, and tuna helps to lower blood pressure, cholesterol, and triglycerides. It also may prevent blood clots. Fish oil is rich in heart-friendly omega-3 fatty acids, which include EPA (eicosapentaenoic acid), DHA (docosahexaenoic acid), and ALA (alpha-linolenic acid). If you're not fond of fish or the aftertaste of fish oil supplements, you might try flaxseed oil instead. It's abundant in ALA, which the body converts to EPA and DHA.

- Beta-carotene is found in fruits and vegetables at the red-to-yellow end of the color spectrum. It's what gives these foods their vibrant hues.

- You can get a modest amount of vitamin C from virtually any fruit or vegetable. Among the very best sources are strawberries, cranberries, melons, oranges, mangoes, papayas, peppers, spinach, kale, broccoli, tomatoes, and potatoes.

- Vitamin E is found in vegetable oils, nuts, seeds, and wheat germ, with smaller amounts coming from leafy vegetables and whole grains.

- Food sources of the B vitamins include leafy dark green vegetables, whole grains, oranges, avocados, beets, bananas, potatoes, dairy products, nuts, beans, fish, and chicken.

- Magnesium—an important nutrient for heart health—comes from leafy green vegetables such as spinach, parsley, broccoli, chard, kale, and mustard and turnip greens, as well as raw almonds, wheat germ, potatoes, and tofu.

- Food sources of selenium include seafood, chicken, whole-grain cereals, and garlic.

- Anthocyanosides are compounds with antioxidant properties. They also help improve blood circulation in the capillaries. The European species of blueberry, called bilberry, contains the most anthocyanosides. Other good sources include blueberries, cherries, raspberries, red or purple grapes, and plums.

- Garlic, onions, cayenne pepper, ginger, turmeric, and alfalfa all reduce blood cholesterol, an important benefit for heart health. Garlic, onions, and cayenne pepper also help thin the blood, which keeps clots from forming.

- Foods derived from soybeans, such as tofu and soy milk, have been shown to help lower cholesterol as well.

Note: If you are taking a prescription medication—including any cholesterol-lowering drug—for a heart condition, talk with your doctor before making changes in your diet. This will reduce the likelihood of an interaction between the medication and any new foods or nutrients.

Herbal Medicine

Ginkgo biloba. Ginkgo is an antioxidant that supports circulation. It is sold raw or in capsule form. The recommended daily dose is

120 milligrams twice a day of extract standardized to 24 percent flavone glycosides and 6 percent terpene lactones. The flavone glycosides give ginkgo its antioxidant properties, while terpene lactones improve circulation. *Note:* If you are taking a prescription blood-thinning medication, be sure to consult your doctor before adding ginkgo supplements to your self-care regimen.

Green tea. Green tea contains high levels of substances called polyphenols, which have powerful antioxidant properties. It also helps to lower cholesterol and blood pressure, and to keep arteries from clogging.

Green tea may be taken as a tea or in capsules. Prepared tea bags are readily available in grocery and health food stores. To brew the tea from dried leaves, steep 1 teaspoon of the herb in 1 cup of boiling water for 2 to 3 minutes. (The tea can become bitter if it steeps too long.) Strain and allow to cool before drinking. Three cups of tea per day may provide 240 to 320 milligrams of polyphenols.

In capsule form, a standardized extract of EGCG (a polyphenol) provides 97 percent polyphenol content. This is the equivalent of drinking 4 cups of green tea per day.

Hawthorn. Hawthorn works to lower cholesterol and blood pressure. It also strengthens the heart muscle, improves circulation, and rids the body of unnecessary fluid and salt.

Hawthorn is available in capsule or tincture form, standardized to 2.2 percent total bioflavonoid content. The recommended daily dose of hawthorn capsules varies widely, ranging from 100 to 300 milligrams, two or three times per day. Be aware that higher doses may significantly lower blood pressure, which may cause you to faint. For the tincture, the recommended dose is 4 to 5 milliliters, three times per day.

It may take up to 2 months before you notice any effects from this herb.

Nutritional Supplements

All of the following nutritional supplements have proven benefits for heart health.

- B-complex vitamins: Take as directed on the label. Together the B vitamins help keep blood clots from forming and arteries from clogging.

- Vitamin B_6: 50 milligrams daily, in divided doses of 25 milligrams. Supports the absorption of calcium, magnesium, and vitamin C.

- Vitamin C: 1,000 milligrams daily, in divided doses of 500 milligrams. Essential for heart health. Vitamin C converts cholesterol into bile, strengthens the arterial walls, and stops cholesterol buildup.

- Calcium: 1,500 milligrams daily, in divided doses of 750 milligrams. Lowers total cholesterol while increasing HDL cholesterol.

- Chromium: 200 micrograms daily. Helps prevent cholesterol buildup; increases HDL cholesterol.

- Coenzyme Q_{10}: 200 milligrams daily, in divided doses of 100 milligrams. Supports the delivery of oxygen to the heart tissue. Also may help lower blood pressure and prevent oxidation of LDL cholesterol.

• Vitamin E: 400 IU daily; take with selenium (below) for optimal absorption. Stops the oxidation of LDL cholesterol, prevents damage to the arterial lining, improves circulation, and fortifies the immune system. *Note:* Because vitamin E may thin the blood, talk with your doctor before taking vitamin E if you are already on a blood-thinning medication.

• L-carnitine: 500 milligrams daily, in divided doses of 250 milligrams. Lowers total cholesterol while increasing HDL cholesterol.

• Magnesium: 800 milligrams daily, in divided doses of 400 milligrams. Helps to lower total cholesterol while increasing HDL cholesterol.

• Selenium: 400 micrograms daily, in divided doses of 200 micrograms. Helps prevent heart disease and future heart attacks by thinning the blood. For this reason, you should check with your doctor before taking selenium if you're already on a blood-thinning medication. Also, do not take selenium at the same time as vitamin C, as they interfere with each other's absorption.

Relaxation/Meditation

Many physicians recommend relaxation techniques to their patients with coronary artery disease to help alleviate stress as well as manage their blood pressure. In clinical trials, the combination of biofeedback, meditation, and yoga has proven effective in lowering blood pressure. For reducing stress, beneficial techniques include qigong, tai chi, visualization, and deep breathing exercises.

To try deep breathing, lie flat on your back on your bed or the floor. Place both hands on your abdomen. Slowly inhale through your nose, pushing your abdomen upward as though inflating a balloon. Then slowly exhale through your mouth, allowing your abdomen to "deflate" as you do. Repeat 8 to 10 times. Practice this exercise as often as necessary.

Lifestyle Recommendations

Exercise caution with coffee. To date, studies have not identified a definitive link between coffee consumption and heart disease risk. Still, there are points worth pondering. For example, caffeine can elevate stress hormones, which is not helpful if you're already under stress and dealing with high blood pressure. Caffeine also robs the body of essential nutrients, particularly calcium, magnesium, and the B vitamins, all of which are important for maintaining a healthy heart as you age. On the other hand, one study has shown that the caffeine in coffee may provide a beneficial boost for people with low blood pressure, or hypotension.

What does all of this mean? The current consensus is that moderate coffee consumption will not elevate your heart disease risk—

"moderate" being the operative word. This means no more than 2 cups of coffee a day. Be sure that the rest of your lifestyle supports a healthy heart through proper diet, regular exercise, adequate sleep, and plenty of relaxation.

Stay active. If you have coronary artery disease, you may be tempted to stop exercising. Don't. And if you haven't been exercising regularly, now is the time to start. Your doctor can help you develop a program that's appropriate for your health status and fitness level. You can ease into your exercise program with something as simple as a 5-minute walk, then gradually increase the length of your workouts over time until you're putting in at least 40 minutes a day.

Regular exercise, particularly aerobic activity, lowers blood pressure and heart rate, which in turn improves bloodflow through the arteries. Further, exercise can help you lose weight and manage stress, which together help manage and reduce CAD symptoms.

Stop smoking. The carbon monoxide produced by cigarette smoking decreases oxygen in the blood, forcing the heart to work harder. Smoking also causes blood platelets to stick together, which raises the risk of blood clots and blocked arteries. In some instances, smoking may interfere with prescription medication as well.

Crohn's Disease

Crohn's disease, also called ileitis or enteritis, is a form of inflammatory bowel disease that causes chronic inflammation in the gastrointestinal tract. Though it most often affects the area connecting the small and large intestines (the ileum and cecum, or the ileocecal region), it may occur anywhere in the GI tract, from the mouth to the anus. Crohn's disease frequently spreads deep into the layers of the affected tissues. A Crohn's flare-up may affect several areas of the GI tract at the same time.

Crohn's disease is somewhat common, and the incidence is on the rise. It is the second most prevalent inflammatory disorder after rheumatoid arthritis.

Since both are inflammatory bowel diseases, Crohn's often is confused with ulcerative colitis. Unlike Crohn's, however, ulcerative colitis affects only the innermost lining of the large intestine and rectum.

Causes and Risk Factors

Though the exact cause of Crohn's disease remains unknown, there are a number of possibilities. Some researchers believe that a virus or bacterium is to blame; the inflammation may be a direct result of the invading organism, or it may occur as the body attempts to fend off the virus or bacterium.

Since about 20 percent of those with Crohn's have a parent, sibling, or child with the disease, a genetic component is likely. Other potential culprits include a diet high in fat or refined foods, as well as environmental factors. Crohn's disease tends to be more common among those who live in cities and industrial nations.

Most people with Crohn's are diagnosed between ages 15 and 35, though the disease may appear at any age. It affects men and women about equally. White people are at highest risk, with those of Jewish and European descent four to five times more likely to have Crohn's compared to the general population.

Signs and Symptoms

Crohn's may develop slowly, or it may appear quite quickly. Its symptoms include chronic diarrhea, fatigue, abdominal pain and cramping, blood in the stool, diminished appetite, weight loss, and fever. Those with mild cases of Crohn's tend to experience abdominal discomfort and loose or more frequent stools, while those with more severe cases may have intense abdominal pain accompanied by

The symptoms of Crohn's disease tend to be worse in the autumn and winter and better in the summer. Why this is so isn't clear.

frequent, incapacitating bowel movements. Weight loss and fever also are common. While some people suffer continuously, others remain symptom-free for years or even decades.

People with Crohn's disease are at risk for a number of complications. For example, because the bowel may thicken and narrow, Crohn's may cause a bowel obstruction. Sometimes surgery is necessary to remove a diseased portion of the bowel. Other complications associated with Crohn's include ulcers, which can occur anywhere in the GI tract; GI fistulas, perforations that may be very deep; anemia; and malnutrition. If you have Crohn's disease, you also are at increased risk for colon cancer, arthritis, kidney stones, eye or skin inflammation, gallstones, and bile duct inflammation.

Conventional Treatments

Conventional treatments for Crohn's disease attempt to reduce inflammation in the GI tract. The goals are symptom relief and extended periods of remission.

Dietary Modifications

Though diet does not cause Crohn's, it may influence symptoms of the disease. Since many people with Crohn's disease are lactose-intolerant, you might try cutting back on dairy products or consuming only dairy products that are naturally low in lactose, such as Swiss and Cheddar cheeses. You also might try using Lactaid, an enzyme that breaks down lactose.

If Crohn's is affecting your small intestine, you probably have trouble digesting fat. So eating high-fat foods—such as mayonnaise, red meat, and ice cream—will only aggravate your diarrhea and other symptoms.

Carefully scrutinize the fibrous foods in your diet. If raw fruits and vegetables seem to bother you, you may need to steam, bake, or stew them before eating. You also might try juicing. It's an easy way to get nutrients into your body without further aggravating your GI tract. Plus, it allows you to try fruits and vegetables that you might not normally eat, or you aren't familiar with.

Some fruits and vegetables trigger symptoms, while others do not. In general, people with Crohn's disease tend to have more trouble with crunchy foods (raw apples and carrots) and foods in the cabbage family (cauliflower and broccoli).

Many people with Crohn's disease find that their symptoms worsen when they eat foods containing corn, gluten (found in

A Quick Guide to Symptoms

- ☐ **Chronic diarrhea**
- ☐ **Fatigue**
- ☐ **Abdominal pain and cramping**
- ☐ **Blood in the stool**
- ☐ **Diminished appetite**
- ☐ **Weight loss**
- ☐ **Fever**

wheat, oats, barley, or rye), soy, eggs, peanuts, and tomatoes. "Gassy" foods can cause problems, as can spicy foods, citrus fruits, fruits containing simple sugars (such as grapes, pineapples, and watermelon), dried fruits, and popcorn. Alcohol can aggravate symptoms, as can anything containing caffeine.

Try increasing your intake of lean proteins, especially oily fish such as salmon. You also might try eating five or six smaller meals throughout the day instead of two or three larger meals. And drink lots of water—at least eight 8-ounce glasses each day.

To reduce your risk of kidney stones—a common complication among people with Crohn's disease, particularly those who've had intestinal surgery—you should consider additional dietary modifications. Be sure to cut back on salt and increase your consumption of potassium-rich foods such as bananas, papayas, sweet potatoes, and canned salmon. Since many kidney stones are calcium oxalate, you should limit or avoid oxalate-rich foods such as beets, black tea, chocolate, nuts, parsley, spinach, and rhubarb.

Medications

If dietary changes do not bring sufficient relief from Crohn's symptoms, your doctor may prescribe medication. There are many medicines that help treat Crohn's, including anti-inflammatories, immune system suppressors, antibiotics, antidiarrheals, laxatives, pain relievers, iron supplements, and vitamin B$_{12}$ injections. It may take a little while to find the right combination for you, so don't become discouraged.

Antibiotics. Antibiotics, which help heal fistulas and abscesses, are a common treatment for Crohn's disease. In the past, metronidazole (Flagyl) was the antibiotic of choice. But because of side effects such as numbing and tingling in the hands and feet, muscle pain or weakness, nausea, headaches, dizziness, and loss of appetite, metronidazole has been replaced by ciprofloxacin (Cipro). It, too, has potential side effects, such as abdominal pain, irregular heartbeat, fainting, diarrhea, and fatigue.

Anti-inflammatories. An anti-inflammatory may be your doctor's first-choice drug treatment. Sulfasalazine (Azulfidine) has been around for many years, but it comes with some distressing side effects, such as nausea, vomiting, heartburn, and headache. Mesalamine (Asacol, Rowasa) and olsalazine (Dipentum) have fewer side effects. The chemical structure of mesalamine is similar to aspirin, so if you're allergic to aspirin, you shouldn't take mesalamine.

Corticosteroids are effective for Crohn's, but they can cause side effects such as puffy face, excessive facial hair, night sweats, insomnia, hyperactivity, high blood pressure, diabetes, osteoporosis, cataracts, and increased susceptibility to infection. Budesonide (Entocort EC) is a newer type of corticosteroid that seems to have fewer side effects.

Immune system suppressors. Some drugs reduce inflammation by suppressing the immune system. Among these are azathioprine (Imuran) and 6-mercaptopurine (Purinethol), which are widely prescribed for Crohn's—in particular, to heal the fistulas associated with Crohn's. Be aware that they work very slowly; it may take 4 months before you see any significant improvement in your symptoms.

Infliximab (Remicade) locates and removes tumor necrosis factor (TNF), a protein produced by the immune system, from the bloodstream. As a result, TNF is unable to cause inflammation in the intestines. The downside is that using infliximab increases your risk of serious infection.

Because some believe that Crohn's disease occurs because of a problem in the body's immune system, researchers are studying treatment with sargramostim, a substance that stimulates the intestinal immune system. There is some evidence that sargramostim may help reduce the severity of Crohn's symptoms and improve a patient's quality of life.

Methotrexate and cyclosporine. If you have not responded to other medications, your doctor may recommend methotrexate (Rheumatrex), a medication usually used to treat cancer. It may take 8 to 10 weeks to begin working. Short-term side effects include nausea, fatigue, and diarrhea; over time, it may scar the liver.

Cyclosporine (Neoral, Sandimmune) is another option for people with Crohn's who do not respond to other medications. It is helpful for healing fistulas, and it generally begins working in 1 to 2 weeks. Potential side effects include kidney damage, high blood pressure, and an increased risk of infection.

Other medications. If your diarrhea is mild to moderate, your doctor may suggest a fiber supplement such as psyllium powder (Metamucil) or methylcellulose (Citrucel). Loperamide (Imodium) may provide relief from more severe diarrhea.

If the inflammation in your intestines has caused constipation, you may need a laxative. But over-the-counter products are likely too strong for your system. Ask your doctor for advice.

For mild pain relief, your best option is acetaminophen (Tylenol). Do not take any nonsteroidal anti-inflammatory drugs such as aspirin, naproxen sodium (Aleve), or ibuprofen (Advil), as they probably will worsen your symptoms.

Crohn's can cause intestinal bleeding, which could leave you anemic. In this case, your doctor may recommend iron supplements.

Since the terminal ileum—the section of the small intestine where vitamin B_{12} is absorbed—often is inflamed with Crohn's disease, you may not be getting enough B_{12}, which is necessary for proper nerve function. Your doctor may decide to evaluate your B_{12} status.

Surgery

If your symptoms do not respond to medication, or if you develop certain complications, your doctor may recommend a surgical procedure called a resection or subtotal colectomy, in which the damaged section of the intestine is removed and the two healthy sections are reconnected. During this procedure, the surgeon may close any fistulas and drain any abscesses that he or she sees. Another common procedure in cases of Crohn's is a strictureplasty, which widens a section of the intestine that has become too narrow.

On occasion, people whose large intestines are affected by Crohn's are advised to have the entire colon removed. In this procedure, known as a proctocolectomy, the surgeon may create an opening, or stoma, in the lower right portion of the abdomen (a procedure called an ileostomy). This allows waste to leave the body through the stoma, where it's collected in a pouch. Whenever possible, surgeons will forgo the stoma, instead constructing a pouch from the end of the small intestine and attaching it to the anus. This procedure, an ileoanal anastomosis, permits the normal expulsion of waste. But bowel movements tend to be watery, since the colon—which normally absorbs the excess water—is gone.

About three-quarters of those with Crohn's disease eventually require some form of surgery. While it may bring relief, it isn't a cure. Crohn's frequently recurs, often near the section that was removed. About half of those who have a first surgery for Crohn's require a second surgical procedure; between 10 and 30 percent undergo a third procedure. Some Crohn's patients are more likely than others to experience recurrences. For example, those who smoke and those in whom the disease affected the lowest part of the small intestine (the ileum) and the colon are at greater risk, as are those who develop abscesses or fistulas and those who've had previous surgeries.

Some conditions related to Crohn's disease may require emergency surgery. These include severe intestinal bleeding, abscesses or fistulas that must be drained, small bowel obstructions, and perforations.

Complementary Treatments
Acupuncture

A 2004 German study found acupuncture and moxibustion (heat therapy) to be effective in treating Crohn's disease. In moxibustion, the practitioner places a slice of gingerroot over the weakened area, followed by a small amount of an herb (moxa, mugwort, or *Artemisia vulgaris*) over top of the gingerroot. Then the herb is lit with an incense stick. The heat generated by the gingerroot and herb opens the pores, allowing the heat to penetrate internally. This increases circulation and stimulates the weakened organs.

To locate an acupuncturist in your area, visit the Web site of the National Certification Commission for Acupuncture and Oriental Medicine (NCCAOM) at www.nccaom. org.

Herbal Medicine

Chamomile, licorice, and peppermint. Prepared as teas, all three of these herbs help soothe and relax the GI tract. You can purchase the herbs in ready-made tea bags or as loose leaves or for brewing similar to green tea.

Curcumin. Curcumin, a substance derived from turmeric (a key ingredient in curry powder), has both antioxidant and anti-inflammatory properties. In preliminary studies, curcumin has proven beneficial for people with Crohn's. The recommended dose is 400 milligrams three times a day, in capsule or tablet form. You also might try using curry powder as a seasoning in your cooking.

Green tea. Green tea is rich in substances called polyphenols, which have powerful antioxidant properties. Prepared tea bags are readily available in supermarkets and health food stores. If you wish, you can brew your own tea from loose tea leaves. Steep 1 teaspoon of the leaves in 1 cup of boiling water for 2 to 3 minutes. (Green tea can become bitter if it steeps too long.) Strain and allow to cool before drinking. Three cups of tea per day may provide 240 to 320 milligrams of polyphenols.

Nutritional Counseling

Once you're diagnosed with Crohn's disease, you might consider consulting a nutritional counselor. This practitioner can help design a diet that offers both variety and proper nutrition. He or she also can help identify any food hypersensitivities or intolerances that may be aggravating your Crohn's symptoms. Your doctor or local hospital can provide a referral.

Nutritional Supplements

People with Crohn's disease often have difficulty maintaining proper levels of key nutrients because of their inability to absorb vitamins and minerals, diminished appetite, chronic diarrhea, and/or side effects of prescription medications.

- Multivitamin/mineral supplement: Take as directed on the label. Look for a supplement that contains vitamins A, D, E, and K, folic acid, calcium, magnesium, and zinc.

- Vitamin B_{12}: 1,000-microgram tablet daily, taken sublingually (under the tongue). Necessary to ensure an adequate amount of B_{12}.

- Omega-3 fatty acids: 1 tablespoon of flaxseed oil daily *or* 4,000 milligrams of fish oil capsules daily. Prostaglandins formed from omega-3 fatty acids help regulate inflammation, pain, and swelling. These supplements are particularly effective in the GI tract.

Lifestyle Recommendations

Consider an elimination diet. Following an elimination diet can help identify the foods that trigger flare-ups of your Crohn's symptoms. For the first 10 days of the diet, eliminate all citrus fruits as well as any foods that contain corn, dairy, egg, or gluten. If your symptoms remain unchanged at the end of the 10 days, you probably aren't sensitive to any of these foods. If your symptoms improve and you notice that you're more energetic and in a better mood, your next step is to return the omitted foods to your diet—one at a time, every 3 or 4 days. This way, you can identify which food (or foods) is causing a reaction. Keeping a food journal during this time will help you track your symptoms.

Stay active. Regular exercise helps move food through your GI tract, reduces pressure inside your colon, and promotes normal functioning of your bowels. It also helps relieve stress, which can trigger Crohn's symptoms. Try to be active for at least 30 minutes a day, as many days as possible. One of the best activities is walking.

If you've been sedentary, be sure to consult your doctor before beginning an exercise regimen.

Manage the stress in your life. While stress does not cause Crohn's disease, it may trigger flare-ups and increase the severity of symptoms. When you are experiencing stress, the GI tract often becomes a holding area for tension-causing emotions, resulting in additional digestive difficulties. Try to incorporate stress-reduction techniques—such as deep breathing exercises, massage, meditation, and yoga—into your daily routine.

Stop smoking. Smoking is a risk factor for Crohn's disease and may aggravate symptoms.

Address related psychological issues. Living with Crohn's disease exacts a strong psychological toll. People with severe symptoms may fear leaving their homes as they worry about the accessibility of bathrooms. Even those with milder symptoms may curb their social activities. With Crohn's, it's very easy to become isolated, which is one reason that depression and anxiety are so common among Crohn's sufferers.

Consider joining a support group. Participating in a support group may enable you to better cope with Crohn's. It's comforting to be among people who understand what you're going through because they're going through it, too. You can learn from the information and advice they offer.

Deep Vein Thrombosis

In deep vein thrombosis (DVT), a thrombus—which is a mass of congealed blood, or a clot—forms in a vein. Normally clots will dissolve on their own, with the components being reabsorbed into the body. In DVT, the clot doesn't dissolve.

DVT most often occurs in the veins of the thighs and lower legs. In very rare cases, a clot will form in another area of the body, such as the armpit, upper arm, or abdomen.

Sometimes a clot will disrupt bloodflow and damage the vein. Or it will break apart into smaller but still congealed pieces, or separate from the vein and travel through the bloodstream. If a clot or a piece of a clot finds its way to the heart, brain, or lungs, it has the potential to cause serious damage. A blood clot in the heart can trigger a heart attack or stroke, while a clot in the brain can lead to a stroke. If a clot lodges in an artery in a lung, it can cause a pulmonary embolism.

DVT is far more common than many people realize. In fact, it is the second most common vascular problem in the United States

The word *thrombosis* means the presence of an abnormal blood clot. The clot itself is a *thrombus*.

(after varicose veins), affecting several hundred thousand Americans each year. While it most often occurs in people over age 60, it can happen at any age.

Causes and Risk Factors

Deep vein thrombosis most often results from prolonged physical inactivity. When you are less active, bloodflow through your veins declines. Muscle movement helps to propel blood from the extremities to the heart, while inactivity creates an ideal environment for formation of a clot.

People who are confined to bed because of illness, who have limited mobility (as in paralysis, for example), or who sit for relatively long periods—such as during car rides or plane trips—are more likely to develop DVT. So are those who've recently undergone surgery or suffered trauma, especially to the hip, knee, or gynecological organs. Some people have inherited thrombophilia, a condition that increases the likelihood of blood clots. This indicates a genetic tendency toward venous thromboembolism.

Certain types of cancer, such as pancreatic cancer, and hormone therapy (HT) may elevate blood levels of clotting substances, which can increase the likelihood of DVT. People with pacemakers and those with a central venous line for treating a medical condition are at greater risk, as are those with congestive heart failure or inflammatory bowel disease. Other risk factors include obesity, smoking, high blood pressure, and a previous bout of DVT.

Women are more likely than men to develop deep vein thrombosis, and risk increases with age. Genetics also plays a role;

if you have a genetic tendency toward DVT, it most likely will manifest before you turn 50.

Signs and Symptoms

About half of those with deep vein thrombosis experience no symptoms until the clot blocks a major vein. Then it can cause pain, tenderness, redness, and a change in skin color over the affected area. Sometimes these symptoms are accompanied by a fever. If the clot is in a leg vein, it can cause cramping, swelling, and warmth in the affected leg. If DVT leads to a pulmonary embolism, it can cause shortness of breath.

Conventional Treatments

The goals of treating deep vein thrombosis are to prevent the blood clot from increasing in size and to stop new clots from forming. It also is important to keep the clot from traveling to other parts of the body. Initially, your doctor may tell you to rest in bed and *not* massage your leg. This is to reduce the likelihood of the clot separating from the vein and entering the bloodstream.

Balloon Angioplasty and Stenting

If a vein is narrowed or damaged by DVT, this procedure can help reopen it. First a catheter is guided into the affected vein. Then a balloon attached to the end of the catheter is inflated, effectively pushing the vein back into shape. Often a small mesh cylinder called a stent is inserted through the catheter to prop open the vein.

A Quick Guide to Symptoms

☐ **Pain, tenderness, and redness in the affected area**

☐ **A change in skin color over the affected area**

☐ **If the clot is in the leg, cramping, swelling, and increased warmth in the affected leg**

☐ **Fever**

Catheter-Directed Thrombolysis

In this procedure, which usually is performed by an interventional radiologist, clot-busting drugs are injected directly into the clot. As in a balloon angioplasty, a catheter is inserted into the vein and threaded to the site of the clot. Once the catheter is in place, the medication is infused through the tube. Normally, the clot will dissolve in a few days. There is a risk of bleeding complications, such as bleeding in the brain.

Medications

If you are diagnosed with deep vein thrombosis, you will be placed on a blood-thinning medication or anticoagulant, such as heparin. Hospital patients may initially receive heparin as an intravenous infusion. There is a low-molecular-weight heparin that is suitable for home care. Either the patient or a family member can administer it as a skin injection.

Often heparin is combined with a second medication, warfarin (Coumadin), for 3 to

6 months. In some instances, warfarin must be taken for an indefinite period. While you are receiving drug treatment, your blood coagulation—that is, its clotting ability—will be checked frequently.

Blood-thinning medications have a number of potential side effects, including dizziness, fainting, stomach pain, headache, weakness, red or brown urine, bruising without injury, cuts that continue to bleed, coughing up blood, and unexpected bleeding from any body part. If you experience any of these side effects, you should contact your doctor without delay.

Since other medications may interfere with blood thinners, be sure to inform your doctor of any other medicines—prescription or over-the-counter—that you may be taking.

Complementary Treatments
Diet

Proper nutrition can help treat DVT and alleviate symptoms.

Post-Phlebitic Syndrome

It is not uncommon to continue experiencing symptoms of deep vein thrombosis even after a clot dissolves. This is known as post-phlebitic syndrome, and it may involve symptoms such as varicose veins, edema, skin pigmentation, induration (a feeling of hardness in the skin's surface), and ulceration. At present, there are no treatments for post-phlebitic syndrome.

- Bioflavonoids, which are common in fruits and vegetables, appear to improve circulation. One particular bioflavonoid, called rutin, is especially important because it supports vein health. It's found in citrus fruits and buckwheat.

- Fruits and vegetables—especially strawberries, cranberries, melons, oranges, mangoes, papayas, peppers, spinach, kale, broccoli, tomatoes, and potatoes—are good sources of vitamin C. A deficiency of vitamin C may make small capillaries more fragile and prone to breaking.

- The B-complex vitamins, found in brewer's yeast, help to strengthen blood vessels. You can sprinkle brewer's yeast on cereal or stir it into fresh juice.

- Fiber is crucial to vein health. It also helps prevent constipation, which can increase pressure on the vascular system. Be sure to eat plenty of whole grains—at least six servings a day—in addition to your fruits and vegetables.

- The enzyme bromelain, which comes from pineapple, may help prevent blood clots in people with varicose veins.

- Omega-3 essential fatty acids may reduce the risk of blood clots. Among the best food sources of omega-3's are cold-water fish such as salmon, bluefish, herring, mackerel, tuna, and cod, as well as almonds, peanuts, walnuts, and sunflower seeds. Flaxseed oil is another good source.

- Foods such as dark green, leafy vegetables, artichoke hearts, beets, carrots, and onions help keep your liver functioning as it should. This is important, as a liver operating less than optimally can stress the vascular system.

• Avoid processed foods and foods high in saturated fat. They don't support healthy circulation, nor do they properly nourish the body.

Herbal Medicine

To avoid interactions with prescription medications (particularly heparin), be sure to check with your doctor before trying any of the following herbal remedies.

Butcher's broom. Butcher's broom tones veins and reduces inflammation. In capsule form, the recommended dose is a standardized extract that provides 50 to 100 milligrams of ruscogenins per day.

Ginkgo biloba. Ginkgo supports vein health and increases bloodflow to the legs. Interestingly, ginkgo is rich in quercetin, a powerful flavonoid. The recommended dose is 40 milligrams of an extract standardized to 24 percent flavone glycosides and 6 percent terpene lactones, three times per day. The glycosides have antioxidant properties, while the terpene lactones improve circulation and protect nerve cells.

Gotu kola. Gotu kola improves circulation to the limbs and strengthens blood vessels. Preliminary double-blind, placebo-controlled studies—considered the gold standard of clinical research—have shown that gotu kola reduces swelling, pain, fatigue, and the sen-

Heparin—a blood-thinning medication that's a common treatment for deep vein thrombosis—may cause hyperkalemia, or high potassium levels. Many fruits contain potassium, so if you are taking heparin, be sure to ask your doctor about the amount of fruit you may consume.

sation of heaviness in the legs, as well as fluid leakage from veins. The recommended dose is 60 milligrams per day of an extract standardized to contain 100 percent total triterpenoids.

Gotu kola also is available as a tea and a tincture. Place 1 to 2 teaspoons of gotu kola leaves in 6 ounces of boiling water and let steep for 10 minutes. Strain and allow to cool before drinking. Repeat up to three times per day. If you choose the tincture, place 10 to 20 milliliters in a cup of water and drink. Repeat three times per day.

Green tea. Green tea contains proanthocyanidins, flavonoids that support the capillaries. You can find prepared green tea bags in supermarkets and health food stores. For vein health, drink a cup of the tea every day.

Nutritional Supplements

Various nutritional supplements strengthen blood vessels, support vein health, and improve circulation.

• Vitamin C: 1,000 milligrams daily, in divided doses of 500 milligrams. Improves circulation and strengthens vein walls.

- B-complex vitamins: Take as directed on the label. Strengthens blood vessels.
- Vitamin E: 400 IU daily. Improves circulation and reduces the risk of varicose veins.
- Fish oil: 3,000 milligrams daily, in divided doses of 1,000 milligrams. Prevents the formation of blood clots.
- Grape seed extract: 80 milligrams daily, in divided doses of 40 milligrams. Supports vein health.
- Pine bark extract: 80 milligrams daily, in divided doses of 40 milligrams. Supports vein health.
- Zinc: 30 milligrams daily. Helps maintain the proper concentration of vitamin E in the blood.

Lifestyle Recommendations

Avoid crossing your legs. Crossing your legs impairs bloodflow. If you just can't break the habit, then try crossing at the ankles rather than the knees.

Elevate your legs. When you are lying in bed or sitting down, prop up your legs. This encourages blood to make the return trip from the legs to the heart.

Wear support stockings. Studies show that below-the-knee compression stockings will help prevent swelling and reduce DVT complications.

Take precautions when traveling. If you are traveling by plane, wear compression stockings for your flight. While airborne, get up and take a walk at least once an hour. When seated, keep moving by flexing your ankles and stretching your legs. Steer clear of alcohol; drink lots of water instead.

If you're traveling by car, stop every hour or so and walk around for a few minutes. For long trips, ask your doctor if you might take an aspirin beforehand. It may help keep a clot from forming.

Just as sitting for long periods can aggravate DVT, so can standing. If you need to be on your feet, keep moving around.

Protect yourself after surgery. After a surgical procedure, you may be given compression boots to help prevent a blood clot. You also may be prescribed a blood-thinning medication. Be sure to read the directions for these medications, and take them exactly as your physician has indicated.

Preventive Measures

Stay active. Regular exercise is essential to preventing deep vein thrombosis. Walking a short distance several times a day will improve your circulation, endurance, and flexibility.

Maintain a healthy weight. People who are overweight or obese are at increased risk for DVT.

Quit smoking. Smoking is a significant risk factor for DVT.

Degenerative Disk Disease

Degenerative disk disease (DDD), also known as internal disk disruption and intervertebral disk disease, is the erosion of the disks in the spinal column. As we age, the normally soft, cushioning disks, which serve as shock absorbers between the vertebrae and prevent the vertebrae from hitting one another, become less flexible and less able to function effectively. Since they have diminishing amounts of blood and water, they lose some of their height. The disks become more vulnerable to tears, particularly in the outer layer, which has nerve cells. When this occurs, the gelatinous material inside the disk may bulge outward. The resulting herniated disk may put pressure on nerves. Adjacent vertebrae may rub against each other, which may pinch nerves and/or produce bone spurs (enlargements of normal bony structures).

Degenerative disk disease occurs most often in the cervical (upper) or lumbar (lower) spine and less often in the thoracic (middle) spine. If it affects the cervical spine, it may be called cervical disk disease.

DDD is extremely common. Though the statistics vary widely, there is a reasonable chance that you may have some evidence of disk degeneration by the time you reach midlife.

Causes and Risk Factors

While the very process of aging may cause degenerative disk disease, the condition also may result from trauma, infection, or injury to the disk. Working at a job that requires repeated heavy lifting or that involves vehicle vibration (being a truck driver, for example) can raise risk. Even leisure activities that place repetitive strain on the back may play a role in DDD.

Other risk factors for DDD include physical inactivity, obesity, diabetes, smoking, and heredity. People who have a genetic predisposition to the condition and/or who smoke are at highest risk. Women are believed to be more susceptible than men.

Signs and Symptoms

Many people who have degenerative disk disease experience no symptoms. Often they are completely unaware that there's a problem. When symptoms do appear, they may include midline back pain, which tends to be worse when sitting or standing and better when lying down. (This is because lying down reduces pressure on the degenerating disk.)

People with DDD may have trouble finding a comfortable sitting or standing position and so may keep shifting around. Their pain may worsen when bending or lifting heavy objects. In some instances, the pain may be severe and/or accompanied by a loss of bowel or bladder function. DDD also may cause referred pain in the buttocks, pelvis, or the back of the hips and thighs.

If you believe that you could have DDD, try keeping a diary of your symptoms—when they occur, what makes them worse, what makes them better, and so forth. This will help your doctor make an accurate diagnosis.

Conventional Treatments

If you are experiencing an acute flare-up of pain from degenerative disk disease, you might want to rest in bed for a day or two. Then try to resume your normal activities as soon as possible. Studies have shown that patients with lower back pain recover faster once they get back on their feet.

Medications

Nonsteroidal anti-inflammatory drugs. Doctors commonly advise their patients with degenerative disk disease—especially those in the midst of an acute flare-up—to take nonsteroidal anti-inflammatory drugs (NSAIDs). These include aspirin, ibuprofen (Motrin, Advil, and many other over-the-counter products), and naproxen (Aleve, Naprosyn).

Though NSAIDs are quite effective in alleviating pain and reducing soft-tissue swelling in and around the disk, they may cause gastrointestinal problems such as ulcers, stomach upset, and internal bleeding. These side effects may occur even when the medications are injected intravenously. NSAIDs also may increase blood pressure, especially among those who already have hypertension. Other potential side effects include headaches, skin rashes, ringing in the ears, dizziness, and depression. There is some evidence that NSAIDs may damage cartilage and/or the kidneys.

For these reasons, NSAIDs should be used with caution. The longer they are used, the more likely they are to cause side effects.

Once you begin taking an NSAID, a week or two may pass before you experience significant relief. If you have high blood pressure, a severe circulation disorder, or kidney or liver problems, or if you're already on diuretics or oral hypoglycemics, you need to be closely monitored while taking NSAIDs.

A Quick Guide to Symptoms

☐ **Midline back pain, which tends to be worse when sitting and standing and better when lying down**
☐ **Trouble finding a comfortable sitting or standing position**
☐ **Referred pain in the buttocks, pelvis, or the back of the hips and thighs**
☐ **Pain that worsens when bending or lifting heavy objects**

Also, since these drugs reduce blood clotting, you need to discontinue them a week before any scheduled surgical procedure.

Sometimes NSAIDs are prescribed in combination with muscle relaxants such as cyclobenzaprine (Flexeril), diazepam (Valium), carisoprodol (Soma), or methocarbamol (Robaxin).

Chymopapain and other injections. After the administration of a general or local anesthetic, the enzyme chymopapain is injected directly into the herniated disk. It dissolves the portion of the disk that is pressing against a nerve. Common side effects are back pain, stiffness, soreness, and muscle spasms in the lower back. Less common are dizziness, a burning sensation in the lower back, nausea, leg cramps, pain or mild weakness, reduced sensitivity to pain, and numbness or tingling in the legs or toes. There is a long list of rare side effects, the most serious of which are leg paralysis, severe allergic reaction, and death.

Some side effects of chymopapain may not appear until days or even weeks after treatment. If you believe that you may be having a reaction to the medication, consult your doctor. You should be especially vigilant if you have sudden, intense back pain or weakness or if you develop a skin rash, hives, or itching.

Another treatment option for severe pain caused by nerve impingement is the injection of different substances directly into the affected area. Perhaps the best known of these is a one-time injection of a corticosteroid into the area around the spinal column.

NSAIDs and Gastrointestinal Disorders

If your doctor determines that you are at risk for developing an ulcer as a result of taking a nonsteroidal anti-inflammatory drug (NSAID)—or if you actually develop one—a number of medications can help treat it. Generally, a class of drugs known as proton-pump inhibitors is useful in preventing ulcers in those who are at high risk. Examples are omeprazole (Prilosec), lansoprazole (Prevacid), rabeprazole (Aciphex), and pantoprazole (Protonix). When compared to no treatment, they reduce the rate of ulcers by up to 80 percent.

Misoprostol has been found valuable in preventing (but not treating) NSAID-induced ulcers. The medication Arthrotec is a combination of misoprostol and the NSAID diclofenac. In one study, patients who took Arthrotec developed between 65 and 80 percent fewer ulcers than those who took NSAIDs alone.

Although they provide temporary pain relief, none of the injectable treatments is a cure.

Physical Therapy

Early in your treatment for degenerative disk disease, you probably should arrange for a few visits with a physical therapist. He or she will design a series of exercises that will help you manage your condition. In some instances, if you practice your exercises regularly, you may not require any additional treatment.

When dealing with DDD, it is important to find a balance between inactivity and overexertion. While you should avoid actions and movements that trigger pain, try to incorporate some level of activity into your daily schedule. Don't include any exercise that places too much pressure on your spine or back.

The following exercises can be helpful for those dealing with DDD.

- Low-impact aerobic exercises. These strengthen muscles in the back and abdomen, without straining the back. Examples include bicycling, swimming, and walking.

- Exercises for lower back strength. These include partial situps and the pelvic tilt.

- Yoga and tai chi. These combine low-impact physical movements with meditation.

Surgery

The vast majority of cases of degenerative disk disease do not require surgery. Even the severe pain caused by a herniated disk or spinal stenosis usually responds to more conservative treatments. But sometimes these treatments fail to bring adequate relief, and the pain becomes debilitating. In addition, there may be progressive weakening in the legs or evidence of a physical abnormality, such as a bone spur. In these cases, surgery may be recommended.

There are several procedures for DDD. All can have complications such as nerve and muscle damage, infection, and scarring, and all require a period of recuperation.

Diskectomy. In a diskectomy, a diseased disk is surgically removed. One of the most common complications of this procedure is the formation of scar tissue, which may cause persistent pain.

Electrothermal surgery. In a procedure known as intradiskal electrothermal treatment, a needle is inserted into the disk under the guidance of x-rays. Electricity is used to heat and shrink the injured disk tissue. Once healed, the disk is stronger and desensitized. Following the procedure, you need to refrain from heavy lifting for a few weeks. It may bring about a significant reduction in pain.

Laminectomy. The lamina is a section of the bone over the spinal column. In a laminectomy, part of the lamina is removed. While the procedure tends to bring immediate pain relief, it is not always successful. Moreover, pain recurs in more than half of all cases. Nevertheless, in some studies, laminectomies with disk excision have produced excellent results in up to 90 percent of patients.

Spinal fusion. Spinal fusion rarely is used as a treatment for lower back pain due to DDD. But in cases in which the movement of the vertebrae places pressure on the nerves, it may be beneficial to fuse together the vertebrae.

Total disk replacement. In this relatively new procedure, an individual disk is replaced with an artificial one. Complete pain relief occurs for about 20 percent of patients, while 65 percent of patients report improvement in back pain.

Complementary Treatments

Several complementary therapies help relieve the pain associated with DDD by improving posture and poor body mechanics. Dietary and lifestyle changes also are addressed.

Acupuncture

Studies have shown that acupuncture with electrical stimulation may play a significant role in relieving the pain associated with degenerative disk disease. Many people who have been treated with acupuncture report considerable improvement in their general health. For help in locating an acupuncturist in your area, visit the Web site of the National Certification Commission for Acupuncture and Oriental Medicine (NCCAOM) at www.nccaom.org.

Aquatic Therapy

Aquatic therapy can be helpful in treating DDD. Many fitness facilities are equipped with heated pools. The warm water (92°F to 99°F) stimulates and then relaxes tired, aching back muscles. Patients with non-weight-bearing injuries and those who cannot tolerate traditional exercise programs find the buoyancy of water to be the perfect medium in which to work out.

Diet

Fill your diet with fruits, vegetables, and whole grains. Besides helping to maintain a healthy weight, these nutrient-rich foods support healing by properly nourishing your body. Aim for a minimum of four servings of fruits, five servings of vegetables, and six servings of whole grains each day.

Also avoid foods that are sugary or high in fat. They not only have an adverse effect on your weight, they also deprive your body of essential nutrients by interfering with their absorption.

Movement Reeducation Therapies

These disciplines—which include the Alexander Technique, the Feldenkrais Method, qigong, tai chi, and the Trager Approach—can benefit people with DDD by helping them to develop proper body mechanics. This may lead to reduced pain, improved posture, and greater mobility.

Alexander Technique. Over several sessions with an Alexander Technique instructor, you will learn how to identify and avoid poor postural habits and replace them with healthy ones. To learn more about this discipline and to locate a qualified instructor, visit the Web site of the American Society for the Alexander Technique at www.alexandertech.org.

Feldenkrais Method. Practitioners of the Feldenkrais Method teach students to become aware of their movement patterns and adopt proper body mechanics. This can relieve stiffness, inflammation, and pain. For help in finding a practitioner, visit www. feldenkrais.org.

Qigong and tai chi. These "moving meditations"—which date back to ancient times—use gentle, rhythmic postures and movements to facilitate the flow of energy throughout the body.

Many hospitals offer qigong and tai chi classes, as do YM/YWCAs, community colleges, and some churches. Check your local newspaper, or watch the bulletin board of your local library or community fitness center.

Trager Approach. The Trager Approach uses movement reeducation to release tight muscles. Over time, the body's nervous system "learns" to respond in the proper manner to relieve pain and discomfort. Trager is a passive treatment, meaning that the practitioner moves and holds the limbs without any resistance from the client. For this reason, it can be especially beneficial for people with limited mobility.

To find a Trager therapist in your area, visit the Web site for the United States Trager Association at www.trager-us.org.

Nutritional Supplements

Taking a high-quality multivitamin/mineral supplement can cover your nutritional bases for the essential vitamins and minerals, which are vital to optimal healing. Look for a supplement that has no additives or artificial colors or flavors. Take as directed on the label.

Therapeutic Massage

Studies have found therapeutic massage to be effective in reducing the pain of DDD by relaxing muscles and improving circulation. It also supports flexibility and allows for greater mobility, while offsetting the effects of stress. Therapeutic massage can be especially helpful when combined with movement reeducation therapies and exercise.

For help in locating a qualified massage therapist, visit the Web site of the National Certification Board of Therapeutic Massage and Bodywork at www.ncbtmb.com.

Lifestyle Recommendations

Be careful when lifting heavy objects. If you must lift, heed the following advice.

- Stand with your feet apart to get a wider base of support.
- Stand close to the object you plan to lift.
- Do not arch your back.
- Bend at your knees.
- While bending or lifting, do not twist from your waist.
- Lift with your leg muscles instead of your back muscles.

Practice proper posture. When sleeping, try to avoid lying on your stomach or your back with your legs fully extended. If you must sleep on your back, place a pillow under your knees. The best position for sleeping is on your side with a pillow under your neck and head and another between your knees. You also can use a full-length body pillow for this purpose.

When sitting or standing, keep your ears, shoulders, and hips in a straight line and your stomach pulled in. Avoid standing for long periods, as it places extra stress on your back. If you must be on your feet, prop one foot on any object (about 3 to 6 inches high) so that your knee is bent. This will take pressure off your lower back. Also, change your position often. If possible, stretch, bend, or lean against a wall.

For sitting, choose an appropriate chair—ideally, one with a straight back or with low-back support, a swivel, and arm rests. When you are seated, your knees should be higher than your hips. Prop your feet on a low stool, if necessary.

Try hot/cold therapy. For temporary pain relief, apply hot and cold packs in turn. The cold pack reduces pain and inflammation. Leave it on for 2 to 3 minutes, then switch to the hot pack for 5 minutes. The heat improves circulation and promotes relaxation.

Take care when driving. During long drives, stop every hour or so and take a brief walk. Also, immediately after the drive, avoid lifting any heavy objects.

Wear appropriate footwear. Proper footwear not only provides protection and support for your feet, it also serves as a cushion and shock absorber for the spine.

Join a support group. If you're suffering from chronic back pain, you may wish to join a support group. The psychological support can facilitate healing. Plus, you may learn ways to better manage your pain.

Preventive Measures

Don't smoke. The nicotine in cigarettes deprives disk cells of vital oxygen and nutrients.

Engage in regular exercise. While exercise is important to the treatment of DDD, it also helps to prevent the condition. Try to be active for at least 40 minutes each day. By participating in regular exercise, you will strengthen your back and make it less vulnerable to injury.

The best activities for your back are those that strengthen and stabilize the core muscles, such as strength training and Pilates. The core muscles—located in the abdomen, pelvis, hips, and buttocks—provide necessary support to your back.

Depression

We all have days when we feel unhappy and overwhelmed with problems. It would be abnormal to go through life in a perpetual state of gleefulness. But if negative feelings continue for at least 2 weeks and begin to interfere with work, family, and daily activities, you may be dealing with depression. Depression may impair your cognitive abilities as well as your mental and physical well-being. It may affect how you sleep and eat.

There are several forms of depression. The most common is major depression, in which you feel plagued with sorrow or grief and/or disinterested in everyday activities that you once enjoyed. You may be tired or have trouble sleeping, and you may gain or lose weight. Another form of depression is dysthymia, a low-intensity mood disorder that is not as intense as depression but can last for more than 2 years.

Some people cycle between periods of depression and periods of euphoria. This is called bipolar disorder (formerly manic depression), a condition that affects between 2 million and 3 million Americans. Others tend to experience depression in fall and winter but not in spring or summer. This condition, called seasonal affective disorder (SAD), affects about one in 20 adults—about 80 percent of whom are women. Those who live in colder climates, where there is limited sun in the late fall and winter, are more likely to develop SAD.

At any point in time, about 19 million Americans suffer from depression. During the course of their lives, about one in five Americans will have at least one period of depression. Yet about one-third of those who are depressed are unaware of it, while two-thirds of those who do know they are depressed fail to obtain the treatment they need. Their doctors may not recognize the illness, or they may not seek help for fear of being stigmatized socially or penalized by their insurance companies. Of course, the very nature of the illness makes it less likely that someone with depression will seek help.

Causes and Risk Factors

Depression affects people of all ages and all walks of life. Often it's triggered by a major life event such as the death of a close family member or the collapse of a marriage. Childhood abuse or other past trauma, chemical dependency, and surviving a catastrophe also can bring about a depressive episode.

A number of other factors can increase a person's chances of developing depression. Family history is important; if you have family members who've dealt with depression, you may be at higher risk. Women are twice as likely as men to be depressed, and their risk rises further during menopause, perhaps because of hormonal fluctuations. Similarly, people at midlife are vulnerable to depression, as they deal with various life adjustments and crises. Those who are highly creative are more likely than the general population to develop depression.

If you've already had one depressive episode, you have a 50-50 chance of a recurrence. Your risk jumps to 70 percent with two depressive episodes.

Certain medications can cause depression with long-term use. The list includes the following:

- Diazepam (Valium) and chlordiazepoxide (Librium), which are anti-anxiety drugs

- Interferon (Avonex, Rebetron), an anti-inflammatory

- Prednisone (Deltasone, Orasone), a corticosteroid

- Propranolol (Inderal), a heart and blood pressure medication

- Tamoxifen (Nolvadex), an anticancer drug

People with certain medical conditions are at greater risk for depression. For example, depression is a common symptom of an underactive thyroid, a condition known as hypothyroidism. Once the person begins treatment with thyroid hormones, the depression usually subsides. Similarly, about 30 percent of patients hospitalized for coronary artery disease have some form of depression, as do about half of all patients who've suffered heart attacks.

Depression also is common in people who've suffered strokes and in those with Alzheimer's or Parkinson's disease. And anyone who has ever dealt with chronic pain knows how easy it is to become profoundly depressed. Indeed, depression is routinely seen in people who are dealing with serious or chronic illness.

Signs and Symptoms

The most common symptom of depression is a depressed mood. You may be sad and tearful; you may feel that your situation is hopeless; you may have a sense of worthlessness. But not everyone with depression actually feels depressed. Instead, they may be irritable, annoyed, or agitated. Even if they don't feel sad, very little in life brings them pleasure or joy.

Depression may affect your memory and your ability to think clearly, making even the smallest decision seem too difficult. Depression also tends to interfere with sleep. You may awaken too early in the morning and be unable to fall back to sleep. Or you may spend a good deal of your day in bed; simply getting up requires a Herculean effort.

People who are depressed may neglect their appearance or disregard basic responsibilities, such as paying bills. On the job, they may be unable to keep up with their workload, and co-workers may notice changes in their behavior. It is not uncommon for people who are depressed to have more conflicts with spouses or family members.

Doctors will diagnose major depression in people who have at least five of the following symptoms: diminished energy, reduced self-esteem, a feeling of hopelessness, disturbed sleep, an inability to concentrate, impaired thinking, weight gain or loss, diminished sexual desire, restlessness or slowed movement, and thoughts of death or suicide. Major depression may occur along with another medical condition, such as anxiety disorder. Untreated, major depression may last for 6 to 18 months. Early treatment may prevent depression from becoming more severe, and continued treatment may prevent a recurrence.

A Quick Guide to Symptoms

- ☐ **Depressed mood**
- ☐ **A feeling of irritability, annoyance, or agitation**
- ☐ **Inability to find pleasure or joy in life**
- ☐ **Difficulty remembering and thinking clearly**
- ☐ **Disturbed sleep**
- ☐ **Neglect of appearance**
- ☐ **Disregard for basic responsibilities**
- ☐ **More conflicts with spouse or family members**
- ☐ **Diminished sex drive**
- ☐ **Reduced self-esteem**
- ☐ **A sense of hopelessness**
- ☐ **Weight gain or loss**
- ☐ **Thoughts of death or suicide**

Dysthymia has many of the same symptoms as major depression, but they tend to be less intense. They also last longer—at least 2 years. In fact, it is not unusual for dysthymia to persist for more than 5 years. In about three-quarters of cases, people with dysthymia have another medical condition.

As mentioned earlier, people with bipolar disorder experience manic symptoms in addition to depression. These include euphoria, irritability, grandiosity (a sense of importance out of proportion to reality), excessive talking, and disturbed sleep. Bipolar disorder may become much worse over time if it isn't treated properly.

Among people with seasonal affective disorder, the most common symptom is fatigue in the fall and winter. Their mood may change, with feelings of sadness. They also tend to eat more (especially carbohydrates) and sleep more than normal, which often leads to weight gain. A small number of those with SAD actually eat and sleep less.

Conventional Treatments

The best treatment for depression is a combination of medication and counseling. In recent years, however, insurers have begun limiting coverage for therapy and instead emphasize pharmacological treatment as a way to rein in costs. If a patient with depression seems in danger of harming himself or herself, the treating physician may recommend hospitalization.

Cognitive-Behavioral Therapy

The premise of cognitive-behavioral therapy is that you become what you think. Thus, if you continue to think negative, depressive thoughts, you're likely to remain depressed. Through sessions of CBT, you will learn to replace negative thoughts with positive ones. Your therapist may ask you to keep a journal of your thoughts and responses. Then, working together, the two of you will find alternatives to the negative thoughts.

CBT typically lasts for about 12 to 16 sessions. After these sessions, you will be able to practice the techniques by yourself. The combination of CBT and appropriate medication tends to be more effective than either treatment alone.

Electroconvulsive Therapy

Electroconvulsive therapy has improved dramatically since its earliest days, when it was known as shock therapy. Today, it's most often used as a treatment for severe depression, especially in cases that do not respond to medications. Generally, patients will receive 6 to 12 treatments over a period of about 4 weeks.

In a typical ECT session, a patient receives a muscle relaxant followed by a short-acting general anesthetic. Then a mild electric current is sent to the brain, causing a seizure that lasts for about 40 seconds. The entire treatment lasts only about 15 to 20 minutes, though recovering from the anesthesia adds time.

ECT does not require hospitalization. It does have a few potential side effects, including headache, nausea, muscle soreness, temporary confusion, memory lapses, and heart disturbances. ECT is successful in about 80 percent of cases.

If you think you may be depressed, you might want to complete a confidential diagnostic questionnaire. These forms are available online through a number of groups, such as the National Mental Health Association (www.depression-screening.org).

Medications

In prescribing medications for depression, a physician has two main objectives: relieving symptoms and keeping depressive episodes from returning. Depending upon each unique set of circumstances, a patient may require treatment for only a brief period, for an extended period, or for the rest of his or her life.

Keep in mind that if you don't see improvement with one medication, it doesn't mean that none of the antidepressants will work for you. Research has shown that after initial treatment with an SSRI failed to provide relief from depression, about one in four patients experienced improvement in their symptoms once they switched to another antidepressant.

Antianxiety drugs. It is not unusual for depression and anxiety to occur together.

Since antidepressants can take several weeks to begin working, your doctor may prescribe a short-term course of anti-anxiety medications. The most commonly prescribed of these medications, the benzodiazepines, work quickly—often in 30 to 90 minutes—to relieve anxiety. They have no effect on depression, however. Among the best known of the benzodiazepines are diazepam (Valium), alprazolam (Xanax), and chlordiazepoxide (Librium).

All of these drugs have potential side effects, such as sleepiness, dizziness, memory impairment, and reduced muscle coordination. It also is relatively easy to become addicted to them. When discontinuing these medications, do so gradually by slowly lowering the dosage. Then you're less likely to experience withdrawal symptoms such as insomnia, headache, trembling, nausea, irritability, and loss of appetite.

Anticonvulsants. Though generally used for seizure disorders, anticonvulsants such as valproate (Depakote) and carbamazepine (Tegretol) may be helpful for depression associated with bipolar disorder. Both have potential side effects. Valproate may cause digestive problems, sleepiness, increased appetite, and weight gain, while carbamazepine has been linked to headache, nausea, dizziness, sleepiness, skin rash, and confusion.

Anticonvulsants are known to cause liver problems in some people. For this reason, your doctor probably will want to do a blood test to check your liver function both before prescribing one of these drugs and during treatment.

Antipsychotic medications. Depression accompanied by hallucinations or delusions—a condition known as psychosis—may require treatment with an antipsychotic medication such as haloperidol (Haldol) or trifluoperazine (Stelazine). Though these medications generally are effective, they frequently cause side effects such as sleepiness, blurred vision, dry mouth, weight gain, constipation, and increased sun sensitivity.

Designer antidepressants. The so-called designer antidepressants relieve depression by elevating serotonin and inhibiting the uptake of norepinephrine, both of which are brain neurotransmitters. One of these drugs, venlafaxine (Effexor), may increase blood pressure. Another, mirtazapine (Remeron), may cause blurred vision, weight gain, and slight elevations of cholesterol and triglyceride levels. Because it may induce drowsiness, it may be helpful for those with insomnia.

Bupropion (Wellbutrin) has relatively few side effects, including a low incidence of sexual dysfunction. Still, in high doses, it has been linked to anorexia, bulimia, and an increased risk of seizures, usually in those with a history of seizures.

Lithium. Lithium, a well-known mood stabilizer, has been available in the United States since the 1970s. In 60 to 80 percent of people with bipolar disorder, it effectively controls mania and reduces sadness.

Some medications may raise blood levels of lithium by inhibiting its excretion by the kidneys. Among the medications known to have this effect are the nonsteroidal anti-inflammatory drugs such as ibuprofen (Advil, Motrin, and other over-the-counter products), naproxen (Aleve, Naprosyn), and ketoprofen (Orudis). Likewise, certain blood pressure medications may decrease blood levels of lithium. These medications include hydrochlorothiazide (Diuril, HydroDiuril) and angiotensin-converting enzyme inhibitors such as benazepril (Lotensin), captopril (Capoten), enalapril (Vasotec), fosinopril (Monopril), lisinopril (Prinivil, Zestril), moexipril (Univasc), perindopril (Aceon), quinapril (Accupril), ramipril (Altace), and trandolapril (Mavik). Your doctor likely will monitor your blood levels of lithium while you are taking the drug.

By itself, lithium can cause a number of unpleasant side effects, such as diarrhea, nausea, confusion, fatigue, hand tremors, thirst, and excessive urination.

Monoamine oxidase inhibitors. Monoamine oxidase inhibitors (MAOIs), such as phenelzine (Nardil) and tranylcypromine (Parnate), are effective antidepressants. They must be used with caution, however, since they can cause insomnia, drowsiness, weight gain, sexual dysfunction, and other side effects. Further, if someone who's taking an MAOI eats foods rich in the amino acid compound tyramine—such as red wine, vermouth, canned figs, fava beans, dried meat and fish, and cheese—the combination may trigger a sudden and dangerous rise in blood pressure.

MAOIs may interact with certain over-the-counter medications such as decongestants and cough medications. And if an MAOI is taken at the same time as an SSRI (see below), the combination can cause a fatal reaction. For this reason, MAOIs should never be used with other antidepressants. Still, this class of drugs may be helpful when other antidepressants have not been effective.

Mood stabilizers. Mood stabilizers are prescribed for people with bipolar disorder. They help control the swings between mania and depression by stimulating the release of the neurotransmitter glutamate.

Selective serotonin reuptake inhibitors. Commonly known as SSRIs, this class of drugs—which includes fluoxetine (Prozac), sertraline (Zoloft), paroxetine (Paxil), fluvoxamine (Luvox), escitalopram (Lexapro), and citalopram (Celexa)—works by raising the concentration of serotonin in the brain. These drugs need time to take effect—typically 2 to 4 weeks, longer in some people. Still, they've been very successful in treating depression.

SSRIs have some unpleasant side effects, including nausea, agitation, insomnia, restlessness, weight gain, and sexual dysfunction. Rarer, but potentially life-threatening, is a side effect known as serotonin syndrome. Usually it occurs when an SSRI interacts with another antidepressant, most commonly an MAOI, though it also can happen with a supplement that influences serotonin, such as the herb St. John's wort. Symptoms of serotonin syndrome include blood pressure and heart rhythm fluctuations, confusion, hallucinations, fever, seizures, and coma.

Tricyclic antidepressants. This class of drugs—which includes imipramine (Tofranil) and amitriptyline (Elavil, Endep)—has been in use since the 1950s. These drugs do have significant side effects, such as weight gain, sexual dysfunction, mental disturbances and sleep disturbances, and a sudden drop in blood pressure upon standing, which could lead to fainting. These drugs may be effective when other classes of antidepressants haven't produced the desired results.

Phototherapy

Phototherapy, or light therapy, is a common treatment for people with seasonal affective disorder. Since this type of depression is associated with a lack of sunlight, phototherapy involves exposure to very bright light from a specialized light box. The patient places the box on a table or desk and sits near it for 15 minutes to 2 hours every day. Some research suggests that phototherapy is most effective when done in the morning.

Talk Therapy

There are several forms of talk therapy, or psychotherapy. You might meet with a therapist on your own, or with a few family members present. There's also group therapy, in which several people—all unrelated—meet together for treatment.

Just as the forms of talk therapy vary, so do the training and credentials of the profes-sionals who offer it. A psychiatrist is a trained therapist who also is a medical doctor, and so is able to prescribe medication. Psychologists usually have doctorate degrees; they may provide counseling, but in general, they can't write prescriptions. Some social workers and psychiatric nurses are qualified therapists, as are some members of the clergy.

Talk with your doctor about the various options in talk therapy. Together, the two of you can decide which option is best for you.

Complementary Treatments

To treat depression, the best complementary approaches are those that stimulate the release of brain chemicals to relieve symptoms, raise your energy level, and improve your sense of well-being.

Acupuncture

Studies have shown that electroacupuncture may be as effective in relieving depression as the prescription drug amitriptyline, a tricyclic antidepressant. Acupuncture treatment prompts the release of serotonin, enkephalins, and endorphins, neurotransmitters that help improve mood and reduce pain.

Acupuncture works best when combined with movement therapies such as exercise, tai chi, and yoga. Together they facilitate the flow of stagnant energy, or *qi*.

To find an acupuncturist in your area, visit the Web site of the National Certification Commission for Acupuncture and Oriental Medicine (NCCAOM) at www.nccaom.org.

Aromatherapy

Certain essential oils have either sedating or stimulating effects on the nervous system. Depending on the characteristics of your depression, you may want to use calming oils such as chamomile, clary sage, jasmine, lavender, neroli, and ylang-ylang. If you're looking for something more energizing and uplifting, try rosemary or peppermint.

You may use these essential oils as inhalants by placing a few drops on the edge of your pillow at night, on a tissue, or in a bowl of steaming water, or by inhaling directly from the bottle. You also might try adding 10 drops of any one essential oil to 1 ounce of a carrier oil, such as sweet almond or jojoba oil, to create a massage blend. (A common household oil such as canola or olive oil works fine as well.) Put the oils in a small bottle and gently roll the bottle between your hands to warm it.

If you wish, you can combine the essential oils. Use no more than 10 drops total.

Color Therapy

Color can have a dramatic effect on your mood and behavior. Yellow and orange, which are energizing, and green, which is soothing and relaxing, may help ease depression's symptoms. Try to incorporate these colors into your environment—by wearing yellow, orange, or green clothing, for example, or eating and drinking from yellow, orange, or green plates and cups. Meditate with these colors around you. Take the time to let the colors do their healing.

Diet

Avoid refined foods and processed foods as much as possible. The same goes for trans-fatty acids, found in french fries, doughnuts, and some commercially baked goods. All of these foods contain unhealthy chemicals that may disrupt your body's functions, particularly the production of brain chemicals that influence your mood.

Replace these foods with healthier choices such as fruits, vegetables, soy foods, and starches such as pasta, rice, cereal grains, breads, and legumes. These are complex carbohydrates, which are necessary for energizing the body and creating a sense of well-being.

Flower Essences

Flower essences are liquid extracts of various flowers and plants. They help stabilize the emotions, thereby allowing the body to physically heal and remain well. Flower essences have been shown to be effective for anyone experiencing emotional distress. The best choices for depression are gentian, gorse, larch, and mustard. You can use any of these essences four drops at a time, up to four times a day. Place the drops under your tongue or mix them into a beverage. They also can be applied directly to the temples, behind the ears, or on the wrists, elbows, or knees.

Herbal Medicine

St. John's wort has a long-standing reputation as a treatment for depression. It is widely used in Europe as an antidepressant, and it's gaining popularity in the United States as well. But it's gotten mixed reviews in studies to date, producing either remarkable results or no effect at all. Most likely, the response simply varies from person to person. Because St. John's wort can interfere with certain prescription medications, be sure to talk with your doctor before you try it.

For clients with depression, some herbalists recommend a tea made from a combination of herbs such as St. John's wort, peppermint, and lavender. These herbs are readily available in health food stores. To make a tea, steep 1 teaspoon of dried lavender flowers, 1 teaspoon of dried peppermint leaves, and 2 teaspoons of dried St. John's wort in a cup of boiling water for 15 minutes. Strain the herbs and allow the tea to cool. Drink 1 cup, three times a day.

Hypnotherapy

The goal of hypnotherapy is to overcome old, unhealthy patterns of thinking, so you can function more positively and effectively, with less fear, pain, and/or distraction. Hypnotherapy is especially effective for alleviating stress and anxiety, both of which are symptoms of depression.

To locate a qualified hypnotherapist in your area, visit the Web site of the American Society of Clinical Hypnosis at www.asch.net or the National Guild of Hypnotists at www.ngh.net.

Nutritional Supplements

Certain nutritional supplements support the production and function of neurotransmitters in the brain, which help to relieve depression.

- Multivitamin/mineral supplement: Take as directed on the label. Helps to maintain proper nutrient levels.

- B-complex vitamins: Take as directed on the label. Improves energy, concentration, and mental function and reduces fatigue by helping to coordinate the activity of certain brain chemicals that transmit messages throughout the nervous system.

- 5-HTP: 150 milligrams daily, in divided doses of 50 milligrams. Works as an antidepressant. 5-HTP is a precursor to serotonin, the neurotransmitter that has a direct, positive effect on mood.

- SAMe (S-adenosyl-methionine): Start with 200 milligrams three times daily and work up to 400 milligrams three times daily; then, after several weeks, taper to 200 milligrams daily. SAMe is a quick-acting antidepressant; taken with the B-complex vitamins, it can help relieve severe depression.

Polarity Therapy

Polarity therapy can be extremely beneficial for people who suffer from depression. Treatment focuses on balancing the ether element, which is associated with the nervous system and regulates all communication within the body. Emotional disturbances occur when there is stagnation of energy in the ether element.

For help in locating a practitioner, visit the Web site of the American Polarity Therapy Association at www.polaritytherapy.org.

Reiki

Reiki is a gentle but powerful therapeutic discipline that works on four levels of a person's being: physical, emotional, psychological, and spiritual. It restores the flow of the body's natural healing energy and provides an outlet for the release of old emotional patterns. It also reduces stress and promotes relaxation.

In a Reiki session, a practitioner may use light touch or no touch at all, simply placing his or her hands above the affected area. This technique releases old energy while channeling new energy into the body's cells. This fresh energy, in turn, revitalizes and strengthens each cell, stimulating the body's systems and normalizing functions.

Many hospitals sponsor community programs to educate the public about Reiki. You also might find a practitioner by looking in the Yellow Pages under terms such as "Reiki," "Holistic Centers," or "Holistic Practitioners." To learn more about the discipline itself, you can visit the Web site for the Reiki Alliance at www.reikialliance.com.

Relaxation/Meditation

Excess stress and anxiety may cause blood sugar to rise drastically or drop precipitously, which can lead to mood swings. Further, people who are stressed or anxious may struggle to maintain a healthy lifestyle, especially eating nutritiously and exercising regularly. So make time in your daily routine to practice techniques that can help alleviate stress and anxiety, which in turn can relieve symptoms of depression and improve your general sense of well-being. Among the techniques that may be beneficial are biofeedback, yoga, meditation, qigong, tai chi, visualization, and deep breathing.

To try deep breathing, lie flat on your back on the bed or the floor. Place both hands on your abdomen. Slowly inhale through your nose, pushing your abdomen upward as though inflating a balloon. Then slowly exhale through your mouth, feeling your abdomen deflate. Repeat 8 to 10 times. Focusing on your breathing in this way can slow your heart rate and take your mind off any stress or anxiety.

Therapeutic Massage

Besides reducing levels of stress hormones, massage releases endorphins, the neurotransmitters that help improve mood. Regular massage treatments also ease muscular tension and help quiet the mind.

To find a certified massage therapist, visit the Web site of the National Certification Board of Therapeutic Massage and Bodywork at www.ncbtmb.com.

Lifestyle Recommendations

Stay active. Exercise can play a role in relieving mild to moderate depression by triggering the release of endorphins and other brain chemicals that boost mood. A long period of moderate physical activity can be just as beneficial as a short burst of intense exercise.

Avoid alcohol. Alcohol blocks the absorption of B vitamins, which are essential for proper cognitive function.

Diabetes

Diabetes, sometimes called diabetes mellitus, is a disease characterized by impaired production of the hormone insulin or by cells' resistance to the actions of insulin. Secreted by the pancreas, insulin affects the metabolism of blood sugar, or glucose, the basic fuel source for all cells. In people with diabetes, glucose accumulates in the bloodstream, a situation that has the potential to compromise health. A number of medical conditions are associated with diabetes, including vision loss (diabetes is the leading cause of adult blindness), kidney disease, and leg amputations.

People with diabetes face short-term health problems as well, some of which may be serious or even life-threatening. For example, if blood glucose levels climb too high, they can lead to diabetic ketoacidosis, which involves the buildup of dangerous substances known as ketones in the blood. High blood glucose can occur in people who are unaware that they have diabetes or who don't use their diabetes medications correctly. It also can affect people with diabetes who are on high-dose steroid medications, who have an infection such as a cold or flu, or who drink large amounts of alcohol. Even stress may cause blood glucose to rise.

Sometimes blood glucose can drop too low. This condition, known as hypoglycemia, can occur when someone with diabetes skips a meal, exercises more than usual, or takes an incorrect dose of diabetes medication.

Diabetes is very common in the United States, affecting some 17 million Americans—including about 15 percent of those over age 60. It's on the rise, too, with the incidence climbing by about 6 percent each year.

Causes and Risk Factors

Generally, diabetes is diagnosed as either type 1 or type 2. In type 1 diabetes, the body destroys the pancreatic cells that manufacture insulin. As a result, the pancreas makes little if any of the hormone on its own. Type 1 diabetes usually begins in childhood—hence its former name, juvenile-onset diabetes—though 25 percent of cases are diagnosed after age 35. It accounts for 5 to 10 percent of all diabetes diagnoses. Though the cause of type 1 diabetes remains unknown, genetic factors are believed to play a major role.

In type 2 diabetes—which is far more common than type 1, accounting for 90 to 95 percent of cases—the pancreas is able to produce insulin, but not as much as it should. Further, the body's cells are resistant to the hormone, keeping it from ushering glucose through the cell walls. Until recently, type 2 diabetes was thought of as primarily a disease of adulthood. Now it's turning up in children and adolescents, too.

A number of lifestyle factors can make a person more likely to develop type 2 diabetes, with overweight being the most significant. People who carry excess weight in the abdominal region are at higher risk. The more fatty cells the body has, the more resistant to insulin the cells may become.

Other factors that raise the risk of type 2 diabetes are aging and inactivity. People over age 45 are at increased risk, as are those who lead relatively sedentary lives. Physical activity uses up glucose, which not only makes cells more sensitive to insulin but also improves circulation and increases blood-flow.

Women who have a history of gestational diabetes and who deliver babies weighing more than 9 pounds are at risk for type 2 diabetes. Though gestational diabetes usually resolves after childbirth, women who develop this form of diabetes during pregnancy are 30 to 60 percent more likely to be diagnosed with type 2 diabetes later in life.

As with type 1 diabetes, type 2 has a strong association with genetics and family history. For 39 percent of patients diagnosed with type 2 diabetes, at least one parent also has the disease. Ethnic background plays a role, too: While type 1 diabetes is more common in white people, type 2 more often is found in African Americans, Latinos, and Native Americans (an alarming half of all adults in the Pima Tribe of Arizona have type 2 diabetes). Newly emigrated Asians are at high risk for type 2 diabetes, as they forgo the traditional Asian diet for an American diet. With weight gain and reduced physical activity, Asians tend to develop type 2 diabetes at lower weights than other ethnic groups.

Certain medical conditions can raise a person's risk for developing type 2 diabetes. These include pancreatitis (inflammation of the pancreas), polycystic ovary disease, hypertension, hepatitis C, and hyperthyroidism (an overactive thyroid). The incidence of diabetes is higher among people who've undergone pancreatic surgery as well as those who've been exposed to certain industrial chemicals. Some medications—including beta-blockers, corticosteroids, and phenytoin—may trigger diabetes, though it usually goes away once drug therapy stops.

Signs and Symptoms

The symptoms of type 1 diabetes tend to come on fairly quickly. For this reason, the disease tends to be diagnosed quite readily. With type 2 diabetes, symptoms develop more slowly. It's possible to have high blood glucose for years before a diagnosis is made.

For both types of diabetes, the two most common symptoms are increased thirst and frequent urination. This is because the excess glucose in your blood draws water from your tissues. As a result, you feel dehydrated, so you drink more fluids. Of course, this means you'll need to urinate more often.

Other diabetes symptoms include weight loss or weight gain, blurred vision, flulike symptoms, frequent infections, and gums that are red, swollen, and tender. Women

A Quick Guide to Symptoms

- ☐ Increased thirst
- ☐ Frequent urination
- ☐ Weight loss or weight gain
- ☐ Blurred vision
- ☐ Flulike symptoms
- ☐ Frequent infections
- ☐ Gums that are red, swollen, and tender

may develop vaginal yeast infections or fungal infections under the breasts or in the groin area. Men may experience erectile dysfunction.

There are kits on the market that allow you to self-test for diabetes. If you use such a kit and the test results suggest the presence of diabetes, or you simply suspect diabetes based on your symptoms, you need to see your doctor as soon as possible for proper testing and diagnosis.

Diabetes complications cause their own set of symptoms. For example, if your glucose drops below 60 milligrams per deciliter of blood (mg/dL), you may experience sweating, shakiness, hunger, dizziness, weakness, and nausea. Blood glucose below 40 mg/dL can lead to slurred speech, drowsiness, or confusion. If blood glucose drops too low, it can cause loss of consciousness and even what's known as a diabetic coma, a condition that's potentially life-threatening.

Too-high blood glucose—300 mg/dL or above—can cause excessive thirst, increased urination, weakness, confusion, leg cramps, and convulsions. As with low blood glucose, a diabetic coma may occur if glucose levels don't return to normal.

The symptoms of diabetic ketoacidosis resemble the flu: loss of appetite, nausea, vomiting, stomach pain, and fever. Your breathing may be abnormally deep and rapid, with frequent sighing, and your breath may smell sweet and fruity. Diabetic ketoacidosis is a very serious condition that can lead to coma and death. If you're having symptoms of this or any of the above diabetes complications, you need to seek medical attention without delay.

Conventional Treatments

If you are an adult at midlife or older and you've recently been diagnosed with diabetes, you more than likely have type 2. Your treatment may begin with dietary changes and an exercise program. If you weigh more than you should, your doctor may instruct you to slim down as well. He or she may suggest meeting with a nutritionist and/or a diabetes educator to help create a diabetes management plan just for you.

Sometimes these lifestyle adjustments are enough to rein in wayward blood glucose levels. With blood glucose under control, you're less likely to develop diabetes complications such as heart and circulatory problems and nerve, eye, and kidney damage.

If your blood sugar doesn't stabilize despite

your best efforts to modify your lifestyle, then the most likely next step is to add medication to your self-care plan.

Medications

Doctors use a number of medications to help manage diabetes. Which one your doctor prescribes for you depends on how the disease has manifested and how you've responded to the lifestyle modifications mentioned above.

Besides insulin, a number of oral diabetes medications are available. Often the two are used in combination.

Alpha-glucosidase inhibitors. Alpha-glucosidase inhibitors such as acarbose (Precose) and miglitol (Glyset) prevent enzymes in your gastrointestinal tract from breaking down carbohydrates. This slows the rate at which glucose enters your bloodstream. Potential side effects associated with this class of drugs are abdominal bloating, gas, and diarrhea, especially after a meal that is high in carbohydrates. In high doses, alpha-glucosidase inhibitors may cause liver damage.

Biguanides. Biguanides are considered especially useful for people with diabetes who are markedly obese. They work by inhibiting the production and release of glucose from the liver. Perhaps the best known of the biguanides is metformin (Glucophage, Glucophage XR). Among the potential side effects of these medications are loss of appetite, nausea, vomiting, a metallic taste in the mouth, abdominal bloating and pain, gas,

and diarrhea. Taking biguanides with food seems to reduce these side effects, which normally diminish over time.

A rare but much more serious potential side effect of the biguanides is the buildup of lactic acid in the body, a condition known as lactic acidosis. Symptoms of lactic acidosis include muscle aches, weakness, fatigue, and drowsiness. You are at increased risk for lactic acidosis if you have congestive heart failure or kidney or liver disease. If you are experiencing symptoms of lactic acidosis, you need to seek medical attention without delay. Untreated, the condition has a 50 percent fatality rate.

Insulin. Anyone with type 1 diabetes must use insulin. It also is prescribed for some people with type 2 diabetes, in order to replace the insulin that the body is unable to make.

The insulin used to treat diabetes is known as synthetic human insulin. Though it is manufactured, it is chemically identical to the natural hormone.

Since stomach enzymes break down insulin, the hormone must be injected with a syringe or an insulin pen injector. If you require a continuous supply of insulin, your doctor may suggest an insulin pump. About the size of a deck of cards, an insulin pump is worn outside the body. A tube from the pump carries insulin to a catheter under the skin of the abdomen. The pump may be adjusted to administer a larger or smaller amount of insulin.

Meglitinides. Meglitinides, such as

repaglinide (Prandin) and nateglinide (Starlix), are another class of medications commonly used to treat type 2 diabetes. Though chemically similar to sulfonylureas (described next), they are less likely to trigger low blood glucose. They also seem to be a better alternative for those with kidney problems. Potential side effects include headache, diarrhea, and a slightly elevated risk of cardiac events.

Sulfonylureas. Sulfonylureas prompt the pancreas to release more insulin. They work only if your body is able to make some insulin on its own. Examples of this class of medications are glipizide (Glucotrol, Glucotrol XL) and glyburide (DiaBeta, Glynase PresTab, Micronase).

The most common side effect of sulfonylureas is low blood glucose, which is most likely to occur during the first few months of treatment or if a patient is suffering from impaired liver or kidney function. Other potential side effects include weight gain and water retention.

Studies have shown that adults with type 2 diabetes who also take an ACE inhibitor appear to have greater protection from proteinuria, a kidney disease that's a potential diabetes complication.

These medications are not appropriate for people who are allergic to sulfa drugs. Since they may interact with other drugs, be sure to tell your doctor about all of the medicines—prescription and over-the-counter—that you're taking.

Thiazolidinediones. Also called TZDs or glitazones, thiazolidinediones make the body's tissues more sensitive to insulin, thereby improving their utilization of glucose. This class of medications includes rosiglitazone (Avandia) and pioglitazone (Actos).

Among the potential side effects of the TZDs are weight gain, swelling, fatigue, and anemia. They also may cause liver damage, which is why if your doctor prescribes a TZD, he or she should be checking your liver function every 2 months for the first 12 months of treatment. Further, if you experience any symptoms of liver damage (nausea, vomiting, abdominal pain, loss of appetite, dark urine, and yellowing of your skin and the whites of your eyes), you should see your doctor as soon as possible.

When compared to a placebo, rosiglitazone (Avandia) has been associated with a significant increase in the risk of heart attack as well as a borderline significant increase in the risk of death from cardiovascular causes. Additional studies are necessary to draw definitive conclusions about the drug's safety. You may want to discuss these risks with your doctor if he or she prescribes rosiglitazone for you.

Monitoring Blood Glucose Levels

Once you're diagnosed with diabetes, your doctor will give you very specific instructions for monitoring your blood glucose levels.

Generally, glucose tends to be more stable in people with type 2 diabetes, compared to those with type 1. So if you have type 2, you may need to check your blood glucose only once or twice a day—unless you're taking insulin, in which case your doctor may recommend more frequent monitoring.

A number of different kinds of monitoring devices are available. Ask your doctor for his or her opinion on which might be best for you.

Your doctor also may ask you to measure your glycosylated hemoglobin (HbA1c), considered to be a highly accurate indicator of overall diabetes control. Generally, the goal is to keep glycosylated hemoglobin below 7.0. Approved home testing kits are available for this purpose.

In a study involving patients with type 1 diabetes, researchers sought to compare the outcomes of intensive treatment versus conventional treatment. With intensive treatment, patients checked their blood glucose levels four times each day and adjusted their insulin based on their glucose readings. The goal was to keep blood glucose as close to normal as possible. Conventional treatment was less rigorous, with the objective of simply preventing glucose levels from rising too high or falling too low. The researchers found the prevalence of cardiovascular disease to be much lower in the group practicing intensive treatment. Based on this finding, it appears that keeping blood glucose as close to normal as possible can have long-term cardiovascular benefits.

Complementary Treatments

Like conventional medicine, complementary medicine advocates dietary modification and exercise as the primary strategies for both managing and preventing type 2 diabetes. Certain herbs, supplements, and relaxation techniques may be beneficial as well.

Ayurveda

The ancient Indian discipline known as Ayurveda takes a whole-body view of diabetes. A typical Ayurvedic "prescription" might include dietary changes, herbal remedies, relaxation techniques, and physical activities such as walking and yoga.

Gymnema (*Gymnema sylvestre*) is one of several herbal remedies used in Ayurveda to treat elevated blood glucose. Others include

If you are experiencing low blood glucose, you need to eat or drink something that contains a good deal of sugar, such as hard candy or fruit juice. If you are on insulin, you should carry a syringe containing glucagon, a hormone that stimulates the release of glucose into the bloodstream. Teach your family members and close friends how to give you the injection, in case you aren't able to do so.

guggul, which has been successful in improving insulin function; and banaba, an herb native to India, Southeast Asia, and the Philippines that has proven effective in lowering blood glucose in people with type 2 diabetes.

If you'd like to explore what Ayurveda has to offer, your best bet is to consult an Ayurvedic practitioner, who will create a treatment plan specific to your diabetes. The Ayurvedic Institute may provide names of practitioners in your area. Visit the institute's Web site at www.ayurveda.com.

Diet

Diet is so critical to proper diabetes management that, as mentioned earlier, it's best to work with a nutritionist to create an eating plan that is specific to your health status and your dietary needs and preferences. A nutritionist also will take into consideration lifestyle factors such as your work schedule and your physical activity level. With this information, he or she can formulate dietary recommendations to support optimal blood glucose control.

The basic dietary advice for diabetes is to eat a proper balance of complex carbohydrates and protein. Complex carbs—which include whole grains, fruits, and vegetables—help regulate both insulin and blood glucose. Further, these foods are good sources of fiber, which not only helps control blood glucose but also lowers blood cholesterol.

In a diabetes diet, very few calories come from simple carbohydrates—that is, sugar. While fruit is good for you, eating too much of the extra-sweet varieties, such as pears and bananas, may not be. The reason: They contain quite a bit of concentrated sugar. The same is true for dried fruit and fruit juices.

Cold-water fish such as salmon, mackerel, and herring can be beneficial for diabetes because of their abundant supplies of essential fatty acids. These good fats, which include the omega-3 fatty acids, help protect the heart and blood vessels. This is important, since diabetes raises the risk of heart disease. If you aren't fond of fish, you can get your essential fatty acids from walnuts, flaxseed oil, evening primrose oil, and black currant seed oil.

On the subject of fats, do your best to steer clear of trans fatty acids, which are common in packaged and processed foods. These bad fats contribute to diabetes as well as heart disease.

Garlic and onions help manage blood sugar by slowing the pace at which the body uses insulin. Garlic also is good for the heart, and it helps prevent yeast infections. Since yeast thrives in high-sugar environments, yeast infections are common in people with diabetes.

The trace mineral chromium helps insulin shuttle glucose into cells, where it can be used as fuel. In this way, chromium can help lower blood sugar. It also appears to reduce sugar cravings. Food sources of chromium include brewer's yeast, whole-wheat bread, and wheat bran.

The mineral zinc plays a role in insulin metabolism. To ensure that you're getting enough of this mineral in your diet, focus on food sources like pumpkin seeds, sunflower seeds, wheat germ, whole grains, brown rice, barley, and corn.

You may want to talk with your nutritionist about switching to a vegetarian diet. According to some recent research, this sort of diet can be very effective for managing diabetes and preventing its complications.

Exercise

As mentioned earlier, exercise is an important component of any diabetes management plan. It improves circulation, as well as the way in which the body uses insulin and burns fat. It also offsets stress and lowers blood pressure.

Exercising with diabetes does require a few precautions. Begin with a visit to your doctor, who can assess your fitness level and rule out any other underlying health issues, such as heart disease. If you have been relatively sedentary, don't try to do too much too soon. A daily 10-minute walk is a good starting point; over time, you can increase the duration and intensity of your workouts. You can vary your activities as well.

Just be careful not to overdo. Avoid prolonged or intense exercise, which actually may increase blood glucose. Also steer clear of activities that involve heavy lifting, which may raise blood glucose as well as blood pressure.

Before every exercise session, you'll need to check your blood glucose level. If it's below 100 mg/dL, eat a snack before you begin. If it is above 300 mg/dL, postpone your workout until later. Try to exercise with a buddy whenever possible, and always wear a medical ID bracelet.

Herbal Medicine

A number of herbs support insulin production, lower blood sugar, and help protect against diabetes complications. Always check with your doctor before adding any herb to your self-care regimen, to rule out potential interactions with any medication you may be taking.

Agave nectar. This natural sweetener is a derivative of the agave plant, a cactus native to Mexico. Because it is slowly absorbed into the bloodstream, it won't spike blood glucose levels. For this reason, agave nectar often is recommended as a sugar substitute for people with diabetes.

American ginseng. In recent studies, people with type 2 diabetes experienced smaller surges in blood glucose after taking 1 to 3 grams of American ginseng in capsule form 40 minutes before mealtime. It's believed that the ginsenosides in ginseng may stimulate the pancreas to make more insulin, which would help account for the effects on blood glucose. The typical dose of American ginseng is 200 milligrams daily of an extract standardized to 7 percent ginsenosides.

Bilberry. This herb helps protect against retinopathy and diabetes-related cataracts, perhaps by helping to normalize blood glucose levels. The recommended daily dose is one 100-milligram capsule, standardized to 25 percent anthocyanosides, three times a day.

Cinnamon. Research suggests that taking 1, 3, or 6 grams of cinnamon in capsule form per day can reduce blood glucose, triglycerides,

LDL cholesterol, and total cholesterol in people with type 2 diabetes.

Pine bark extract. Also known as pycnogenol, this herb—which comes from the French maritime pine—appears to help heal diabetic ulcers. In studies, the people who were taking pycnogenol showed greater improvement in their ulcers than those whose ulcers were only washed and disinfected. Take 80 milligrams daily, in divided doses of 40 milligrams.

Stevia. Stevia, or sweet leaf, comes from a plant that is native to Brazil and Paraguay. Because it is highly concentrated, it is much sweeter than sugar. Just a small amount can satisfy sugar cravings and therefore reduce sugar consumption.

You can find stevia in health food stores and some supermarkets. Try to limit total daily intake to 1 gram or less.

Naturopathy

Naturopathic doctors (NDs) advocate a holistic approach to managing diabetes. Their recommendations may include dietary modifications, nutritional supplements, and herbal remedies, along with exercise and other lifestyle strategies. To find a naturopath in your area, visit the Web site for the American Association of Naturopathic Physicians at www.naturopathic.org.

Nutritional Supplements

Many nutritional supplements have proven effective in helping to manage diabetes and protect against diabetes complications.

- B-complex vitamins: Take as directed on the label. Support sugar metabolism; necessary for ensuring normal nerve function and protecting against nerve damage (diabetic neuropathy).

- Vitamin C: 1,000 milligrams daily, in divided doses of 500 milligrams. Improves the body's ability to use glucose. It also fights infection and heals wounds.

- Vitamin D: 800 IU daily. In one recent study, the combination of vitamin D and calcium (below) lowered diabetes risk by 33 percent in the study participants, who were tracked over a 20-year period.

- Vitamin E: 400 IU daily. Improves glucose tolerance.

- Alpha-lipoic acid (ALA): 600 milligrams daily, in divided doses of 300 milligrams. Studies have linked ALA to a significant reduction in the severity of pain associated with diabetic neuropathy.

- Calcium: 1,200 milligrams daily. As mentioned above, taking calcium along with vitamin D appears to protect against type 2 diabetes.

- Chromium: 200 micrograms daily. Improves glucose tolerance, lowers insulin levels, reduces fasting glucose levels, lowers triglycerides and total cholesterol, and increases HDL cholesterol.

- DHEA: 25 milligrams daily. Increases insulin sensitivity and improves blood vessel function.

- Magnesium: 500 milligrams daily. Magnesium deficiency is common among people with diabetes. In the case of type 2 diabetes, running low on this mineral may interfere with blood sugar control.

- Zinc: 30 milligrams daily. Supports insulin metabolism.

Relaxation/Meditation

Excess stress and anxiety may cause blood glucose to rise dramatically or fall precipitously. Further, people who are stressed or anxious may struggle to stick with the dietary and lifestyle strategies that are necessary for optimal diabetes management.

Many physicians recommend relaxation techniques to patients with diabetes to help offset the effects of stress, balance their emotions, and lower their blood pressure. Disciplines such as deep breathing, meditation, visualization, and yoga are excellent for promoting relaxation; you can use them whenever you need them for stress reduction. Other effective techniques include biofeedback, qigong, and tai chi.

Here's a deep breathing exercise that you can try on your own. Begin by lying flat on your back, either on the bed or on the floor. Slowly inhale through your nose, pushing up your abdomen as though inflating a balloon. Then slowly exhale, allowing your abdomen to "deflate" as you do. Repeat the entire cycle 8 to 10 times. Practice this exercise as necessary.

Traditional Chinese Medicine

Traditional Chinese medicine (TCM) has a good track record for treating diabetes. Prac-titioners focus on the three Gs—great thirst, great hunger, and great urination, all of which are diabetes symptoms. They also consider emotional factors when creating a diabetes management plan.

Acupuncture is very effective for treating diabetes, though improvements come about very slowly. It works best when used in conjunction with conventional treatments.

Besides acupuncture, a TCM practitioner likely will recommend a nutritious diet and proper rest. Herbal remedies can help alleviate diabetes symptoms, as well as stress and anxiety.

To find a TCM practitioner in your area, visit the Web site of the National Certification Commission for Acupuncture and Oriental Medicine at www.nccaom.org or the American Association of Acupuncture and Oriental Medicine at www.aaaomonline.org.

Lifestyle Recommendations

Because of the risk of complications, people with diabetes need to closely monitor certain aspects of their health—in particular, their blood pressure and their eyes, feet, and gums. There are other lifestyle strategies to consider, too.

Get regular dental checkups. People with diabetes are more likely to develop gum infections. This is important, since research now suggests that gum disease has a direct link to cardiovascular disease, which often occurs in tandem with diabetes. Visit your dentist regularly for professional cleanings and exams. Practice good home care, too: Brush and floss at least twice a day. If your gums ever appear red and swollen, make an appointment to see your dentist as soon as possible.

Schedule annual eye exams. If you have diabetes, you should be getting annual screenings for retinal damage, cataracts, and glaucoma. People with diabetes are at increased risk for eye problems.

Tend to your feet. Diabetes can damage the nerves in your feet, thus reducing your ability to feel pain in the event of an injury. And since diabetes reduces bloodflow to the feet, wounds and sores may not heal properly.

To protect your feet, wash them and dry them thoroughly, then check for sores. Do this every day. Also wear good-fitting shoes at all times. You're less likely to injure your feet if you don't go barefoot.

Don't forget your vaccinations. Diabetes can weaken your immune system, leaving you more vulnerable to influenza and pneumonia. Be sure to get your vaccinations every year. Stay up-to-date on your tetanus booster shots, too.

If you smoke, quit. People with diabetes who smoke are three times more likely to die from cardiovascular disease or stroke. Smoking also increases your chances of developing kidney disease or nerve damage.

Check your blood pressure. Because people with diabetes are at increased risk for high blood pressure, you should see your doctor regularly for blood pressure screenings. You also might wish to invest in a blood pressure monitor (or sphygmomanometer) to track your readings at home.

Preventive Measures

Researchers have yet to find a way to prevent type 1 diabetes. On the other hand, since type 2 diabetes is largely a lifestyle disease, you can take steps to reduce your risk.

Overhaul your eating habits. According to an article that appeared in a 2002 issue of *Annals of Internal Medicine*, the typical Western diet—consisting of fatty meats, high-fat dairy products, sugar and refined grains, and fried foods—increases diabetes risk by 60 percent. Try to weed these foods from your diet, replacing them with lots of fruits, vegetables, whole grains, and nuts. This change alone can go a long way toward protecting against diabetes.

Get moving. People who exercise regularly are less likely to develop type 2 diabetes. Aim for at least 30 to 45 minutes of physical activity at least 5 or 6 days each week.

Slim down, if necessary. In light of the strong correlation between overweight and type 2 diabetes, it's in your best interest to get rid of any extra pounds that you may be carrying. This is especially true if those pounds have accumulated in your abdominal region, which is a risk factor for diabetes as well as heart disease.

Diverticulosis/ Diverticulitis

In diverticulosis, small bulging pouches called diverticula develop in the colon—usually along the left side, above the rectum, in what's known as the sigmoid colon. Diverticulosis is an extremely common medical condition. But since the diverticula usually don't cause any problems, most people are unaware that they have them.

For about 15 to 20 percent of people with diverticulosis, a diverticulum becomes infected or inflamed. This condition, called diverticulitis, may be caused by a small piece of stool lodging in the pouch and hindering bloodflow, or by a small tear in the pouch. Generally, the infection or inflammation remains localized around the diverticulum.

On occasion, small holes or perforations may develop in the infected diverticulum, and pus may leak through the holes into the abdomen. In rare instances, the diverticulum ruptures and intestinal waste enters the abdominal cavity. This may lead to inflammation of the lining of the abdominal cavity, a condition known as peritonitis. Peritonitis is a medical emergency that requires immediate care.

Causes and Risk Factors

Diverticula often occur after years of straining to pass stool. This can cause the colon wall to develop a weak spot, which eventually gives way to a bulge. Another potential contributor to diverticulosis is the typical American diet, which tends to have too little fiber. In the absence of fiber, stool becomes small, hard, and difficult to pass. This increases pressure inside the sigmoid colon.

The most significant risk factor for diverticulosis is age. In fact, by the time you reach 80, you're almost certain to have diverticula. As you get older, the outer, muscular colon wall begins to thicken, in turn narrowing the colon's inside passageway. The subsequent rise in pressure inside the colon increases the likelihood of pouch formation. It also slows the passage of food through the colon; the extra transit time places even more pressure on weak areas in the colon walls.

Signs and Symptoms

As mentioned earlier, in many cases diverticulosis produces no symptoms. Sometimes there's rectal bleeding, most likely because a weakened blood vessel in a diverticulum has burst. You may see dark blood in the stool or bright red blood in the toilet bowl. Generally, bleeding from a pouch lasts just a short time and stops without medical intervention.

You can buy home testing kits to detect rectal bleeding, but they aren't very reliable. If you suspect that you have diverticulitis, consult your doctor for a proper diagnosis.

Diverticulitis can produce severe symptoms such as pain, abdominal tenderness, constipation, diarrhea, nausea, and fever. Less common are rectal bleeding, frequent or painful urination, difficulty urinating, bloating, and vomiting. In the event of a flare-up of diverticulitis, you should seek medical attention right away, as it can lead to an intestinal obstruction. Once you've had one flare-up, there's a 30 percent chance of recurrence.

Conventional Treatments

For diverticulosis without symptoms, the standard treatment is a high-fiber diet. A flare-up of diverticulitis requires a few days of bed rest, along with a restricted diet (such as liquid or low fiber). This will reduce contractions in the colon and give it a chance to heal.

About half of all cases of diverticulitis require hospitalization. For example, if you are very nauseated or vomiting continuously, your doctor may advise you to not consume anything by mouth. Instead, you'll be given fluids intravenously. As your symptoms subside, you'll be able to reintroduce solid foods gradually.

To prevent a recurrence of diverticulitis, your doctor or nutritionist will provide instructions for increasing the amount of fiber in your diet.

Medications

If you know you have diverticulosis and you're prone to constipation, your doctor may recommend an over-the-counter stool softener. Diverticulitis may require a mild pain reliever, plus an antibiotic to kill any bacteria that are causing infection. Be sure to follow your doctor's prescription to the letter; if you're given an antibiotic, for example, take it as directed and complete the entire course. Patients with more complicated cases of

A Quick Guide to Symptoms

Diverticulosis
☐ Rectal bleeding

Diverticulitis
☐ Pain
☐ Abdominal tenderness
☐ Constipation or diarrhea
☐ Nausea
☐ Fever
☐ Rectal bleeding
☐ Frequent or painful urination
☐ Bloating
☐ Vomiting

diverticulitis may be given antibiotics intravenously.

Surgery for Diverticulitis

Ordinarily, dietary changes and medications work well to treat a first attack of diverticulitis. They aren't as effective for recurrences. In this case, your doctor may recommend surgery to remove the diseased section of the colon.

Approximately 20 percent of diverticulitis patients require surgery. The most common procedures are bowel resection with colostomy and primary bowel resection.

Bowel resection with colostomy. If you have extensive inflammation, you may need a bowel resection with colostomy. In this procedure, the surgeon removes the diseased section of the colon and makes a hole in the abdominal wall. The colon is connected to the hole, or stoma, and stool passes through the stoma into a bag attached to the abdomen.

Not all colostomies are permanent. Sometimes after a period of healing, the surgeon is able to reconnect the colon with the rectum, and the external bag no longer is necessary.

Primary bowel resection. In this procedure, which may be done traditionally or laparoscopically, the diseased portion of the colon is removed and the healthy sections are reconnected to each other. A traditional resection requires a long incision in the abdomen; for a laparoscopic resection, the surgeon makes several smaller incisions. Generally, patients recover much more quickly from the laparoscopic procedure than from the traditional surgery.

Surgery for Peritonitis

If the infection from diverticulitis leaks into the abdominal cavity—causing a condition known as peritonitis—it will require immediate surgery. An emergency situation like this almost always requires traditional surgery rather than a laparoscopic procedure. The goal of surgery is to identify and treat any infection or obstruction. Untreated, peritonitis can be fatal.

Complementary Treatments

Because diverticulosis is so closely linked to diet and lifestyle, changes in these areas may be enough to treat a mild case of the disease. Complementary therapies can help alleviate any symptoms that may arise, particularly pain from inflammation and gas.

Diet

A few key dietary strategies can help reduce pressure inside the colon. Begin by gradually increasing your consumption of fiber-rich foods such as fruits, vegetables, and whole-grain products. The word *gradual* is critical; by adding too much fiber too quickly, you raise your risk of uncomfortable gastrointestinal symptoms such as diarrhea, gas, bloating, and cramping.

Also be sure to get enough fluids. A good benchmark is eight 8-ounce glasses of water or other noncaffeinated, nonalcoholic beverages per day.

Herbal Medicine

Chamomile, ginger, peppermint, and slippery elm. Chamomile soothes and relaxes, which is beneficial for an agitated gastrointestinal tract. Ginger, a carminative (digestive aid), helps relieve gas; peppermint reduces intestinal spasms; and slippery elm protects the bowel lining. All of these herbs are readily available as prepared tea bags in health food stores and some supermarkets. Drink the tea of your choice as often as you wish, particularly after meals and before bedtime.

Garlic. Garlic fights infection through its antiseptic properties. The recommended dose for the fresh herb is two or three cloves per day, while the dose for supplements is 500 milligrams per day. If you have a choice, select fresh garlic over supplements; the supplements contain concentrated extracts, which may raise the risk of excessive bleeding. For this same reason, you should consult your doctor before using garlic supplements if you're on a blood-thinning medication (including aspirin), taking the herb ginkgo, or about to undergo surgery.

Nutritional Supplements

To increase your fiber intake, you might ask your doctor whether you could benefit from adding a natural fiber supplement containing psyllium seeds (such as Metamucil or Citrucel) to your self-care regimen. Follow the directions on the product label. The added bulk from the fiber stimulates intestinal contractions, softens stools, and supports proper digestive function.

If you do decide to try a fiber supplement, be sure to drink plenty of water. Otherwise, you may become constipated.

The following supplements also support optimal gastrointestinal function.

- *Lactobacillus acidophilus:* 200 milligrams daily. These beneficial bacteria help maintain intestinal health and combat yeast infections resulting from frequent antibiotic use. Look for a product that mentions "live" or "active" cultures on the label, with 1 billion to 2 billion organisms per capsule.

- L-glutamine: 400 milligrams three times daily, between meals. Necessary for proper intestinal function.

- Omega-3 fatty acids: 1,000 milligrams as fish oil daily. May help reduce inflammation associated with diverticulitis.

Lifestyle Recommendations

Regular exercise reduces pressure inside the colon and promotes normal bowel function. Try to set aside at least 30 minutes every day for physical activity. Any activity that gets you moving will be beneficial, so choose one

Fiber Content of Selected Foods

Use the following table to calculate the amount of fiber in your current diet and to increase your intake as needed.

Food	Serving Size	Fiber Content
Fruit		
Apple, fresh	1 medium	4 g
Peach, fresh	1 medium	2 g
Pear, fresh	1 medium	4 g
Tangerine, fresh	1 medium	2 g
Nonstarchy Vegetables		
Acorn squash, fresh	½ cup, cooked	7 g
Asparagus, fresh	½ cup, cooked	1.5 g
Broccoli, fresh	½ cup, cooked	2 g
Brussels sprouts, fresh	½ cup, cooked	2 g
Cabbage, fresh	½ cup, cooked	2 g
Carrot, fresh	1 medium, cooked	1.5 g
Cauliflower, fresh	½ cup, cooked	2 g
Romaine lettuce	1 cup	1 g
Spinach, fresh	½ cup, cooked	2 g
Tomato, fresh	1 medium, raw	1 g
Zucchini, fresh	1 cup, cooked	2.5 g
Starchy Vegetables		
Black-eyed peas, fresh	½ cup, cooked	4 g
Kidney beans, fresh	½ cup, cooked	6 g
Lima beans, fresh	½ cup, cooked	4.5 g
Potato, fresh	1 medium, cooked	3 g
Grains and Grain Products		
Bread, whole-wheat	1 slice	2 g
Cereal, bran flake	½ cup	5 g
Oatmeal, plain	½ cup, cooked	3 g
Rice, brown	1 cup, cooked	3.5 g
Rice, white	1 cup, cooked	1 g

Source: United States Department of Agriculture Web site, USDA National Nutrient Database for Standard Reference.

that you enjoy and that you can easily fit into your schedule.

If you have been relatively sedentary, walking might be a good "starter" activity for you. It requires no equipment other than a pair of good-fitting shoes, and it can be done just about anywhere. Begin with an easy 10-minute walk, and gradually increase the intensity and duration of your workouts.

If you have access to a heated pool, you might try walking in water. It offers a great cardiovascular workout while increasing your muscle strength and improving flexibility. The warm water is soothing and causes less muscular contraction.

Over time, you might incorporate other activities into your exercise program. Consider bicycling, dancing, or yoga.

Preventive Measures

Don't ignore your bowel. Delaying a bowel movement will leave stool harder and more difficult to pass. This adds to the pressure inside the colon.

Get more fiber. Just as increasing fiber intake can help treat diverticulosis, it also can help prevent it. The American Dietetic Association recommends consuming 20 to 35 grams of fiber each day. The average American doesn't get nearly that much.

To add fiber to your diet, build your meals around fiber-rich fruits, vegetables, and whole grains. Meanwhile, cut back on processed foods, which tend to have too little fiber.

You may experience some bloating as your body adjusts to your new, high-fiber eating habits. To reduce your risk of bloating, increase your fiber intake very gradually, over a period of 6 to 8 weeks.

Drink plenty of fluids. Fiber absorbs water to create soft, bulky stool. If you do not replenish your body's fluids, you may become constipated. Try to drink at least 2 quarts—that's eight 8-ounce glasses—of water or other noncaffeinated, nonalcoholic beverages each day.

Dry Skin

Dry skin, also known as xerosis or "winter itch," occurs when the top layer of skin lacks sufficient moisture. The skin may become flaky and itchy, and sections may appear reddish in color and feel rough to the touch. Dry skin is tight when you wash it. You're most likely to notice dry skin on your arms and legs, though it can affect any body part.

A Quick Guide to Symptoms

- ☐ Itching
- ☐ Flaking and peeling
- ☐ Irritation or infection

Causes and Risk Factors

The loss of moisture that's characteristic of dry skin may be due to a number of factors. First, as we get older, our skin is less able to retain water. As a result, too much water evaporates from the skin. A majority of older people experience dry skin.

Environmental factors may aggravate the situation. For example, indoor heat, dry or cold weather, and wind or sun exposure can dry out skin. So, too, will spending a lot of time in a chlorinated pool. Certain soaps, which remove oils from the skin, are very drying; bar soaps tend to be more drying than the liquid varieties. People who frequently wash their hands with bar soap or another drying soap will end up with very dry skin.

You're more likely to develop dry skin if you're skimping on your fluid intake, especially water. Dry skin also can be a side effect of certain medications (such as tretinoin, a topical preparation to prevent wrinkles) or a symptom of illnesses such as hypothyroidism and diabetes. If your dry skin is unusually severe or persistent, be sure to consult your doctor about it.

Signs and Symptoms

The primary symptom of dry skin is itching, which may range from mildly annoying to severely uncomfortable. Your skin also may flake and peel. If any of these symptoms causes you to scratch, you could end up with a skin irritation or infection. With an infection, your skin will be painful and warm to the touch.

Conventional Treatments

Treating dry skin requires a multifaceted approach. Begin by switching from ordinary bar soap, which can be drying, to a superfatted soap such as Dove or a moisturizing cleanser. Try to limit the length of your shower or bath, as excess showering and bathing deplete the oils in your skin. Warm water is less drying than hot.

After bathing, apply a moisturizing body lotion. Look for one that contains any or all of these ingredients: lactic acid, glycolic acid, urea, and/or alpha-hydroxy acids. Reapply the moisturizer as needed throughout the day.

Before going to bed, cover your hands and feet with generous amounts of moisturizing cream or petroleum jelly. Wear thin cotton gloves and socks overnight.

For skin that is especially red, itchy, and inflamed, you may benefit from a steroid ointment. Mild ointments are available over-the-counter; for a stronger formulation, you will need a prescription from your doctor.

Avoid skin and nail products that contain lanolin, a common allergen. Also steer clear of the following ingredients: camphor, benzoyl peroxide, acetone, alcohol, citrus juice, eucalyptus, menthol, and mint. All of these substances can dry or irritate your skin.

During the cold winter months, when you are heating your home, you might want to use a humidifier as well. At the very least, you should have one in your bedroom to run overnight. Just be sure to follow the maintenance instructions closely, as humidifiers tend to harbor bacteria and mold. As an alternative to a humidifier, you could place pans with water near your floor radiators.

Complementary Treatments

Practitioners of certain complementary therapies view dry skin as a sign of a buildup of waste products in the body and/or a lack of certain nutrients. Certain lifestyle habits may cause or contribute to dry skin, too. The goal of treatment is to increase moisture and strengthen the skin, which promotes healing.

Aromatherapy

Essential oils have properties that help regenerate and rejuvenate skin cells, replenish moisture, and clear away accumulated toxins. Some of the most beneficial for dry skin are frankincense, rosewood, sandalwood, vetiver, benzoin, and geranium. You can use any of these oils as a facial toner or a moisturizer, or in a warm bath. It's best to start with one essential oil and add others individually. Then you can tell if you're experiencing a skin reaction to a specific oil.

For a therapeutic bath, use no more than 10 drops of essential oil, either alone or in combination. You can make your own aromatherapeutic moisturizer by adding 10 drops of essential oil to an unscented moisturizing lotion. To make a facial toner, add up to 6 drops of essential oil to 8 ounces of water. Shake well, then apply to your face with a cotton ball.

Diet

In general, a nutritious, balanced diet with plenty of fruits, vegetables, and whole grains is essential for healthy skin. Avoid sugar, fried foods, and processed foods, which can contribute to skin problems.

Essential fatty acids, the best known of which are the omega-3 fatty acids, are as vital to the skin as they are to the rest of the body. The best sources of the omega-3's are cold-water fish such as bluefish, herring, salmon, and tuna. If you aren't fond of fish, you might try taking a tablespoon of flaxseed oil daily. Flaxseed is a rich source of alpha-linolenic acid (LNA), which the body converts to eicosapentaenoic acid (EPA) and docosahexaenoic acid (DHA). Both EPA and DHA are abundant in fish oil.

Dry skin can be a symptom of a nutrient deficiency—particularly vitamins A, B-complex, C, and E. Vitamin A comes from animal products such as eggs, dairy, and beef. Your body also can make its own vitamin A by converting beta-carotene, a compound found in most fruits and vegetables. In fact, beta-carotene is what gives these foods their color. It might be healthier to satisfy your body's vitamin A needs by eating lots of fruits and vegetables, especially dark leafy greens.

These greens also happen to be a good source of the B-complex vitamins, as are whole grains, oranges, avocados, beets, bananas, potatoes, dairy products, nuts, beans, fish, and chicken. Food sources of vitamin C—which helps to regulate the sebaceous glands that lubricate the skin—include strawberries, cranberries, melons, oranges, mangoes, papayas, peppers, spinach, kale, broccoli, tomatoes, and potatoes.

Vitamin E is found primarily in vegetable oils, nuts, seeds, and wheat germ, with smaller amounts available from leafy greens and whole grains.

Herbal Medicine

Aloe vera. Aloe vera can soothe, soften, and heal dry skin. If you have an aloe vera plant in your home, open a leaf and squeeze the gel directly onto the bothersome area. Commercial aloe vera gel is available in most drugstores as well.

Calendula. Calendula is available as a topical ointment. Look for products containing 2 to 5 percent calendula. Apply to the affected area four times per day.

Chamomile. Chamomile is used internally and externally to treat dry, flaky skin. You can find prepared tea bags in virtually any supermarket or health food store. To make a tea from the dried leaves, add 1 teaspoon to a cup of boiling water. Steep for 3 to 5 minutes, then strain and allow to cool before drinking. Also look for chamomile in a topical cream, which you can apply directly to the affected skin.

Nutritional Supplements

The following nutrients are necessary for healthy skin.

- Vitamin A: 10,000 IU daily. Vitamin A is an antioxidant that helps protect skin tissue. As mentioned earlier, a deficiency can lead to dry skin as well as skin aging.

- B-complex vitamins: Take as directed on the label. Prevents dry skin and skin aging.

- Vitamin C: 1,000 milligrams daily, as divided doses of 500 milligrams. Regulates the sebaceous glands and improves blood circulation to the skin.

- Vitamin E: 400 milligrams daily. An antioxidant, vitamin E helps protect against free radical damage to the skin. A deficiency may lead to dry skin.

- Omega-3 fatty acids: 4,000 milligrams of fish oil capsules daily or 1 tablespoon of flaxseed oil daily. Helps maintain healthy skin.

- Grape seed extract: 100 milligrams three times daily. Protects elastin and collagen, the proteins in skin tissue; prevents free radical damage. Look for an extract that's standardized to 40 to 80 percent proanthocyanidins or 95 percent OPC value.

- Selenium: 200 micrograms daily. Helps maintain healthy skin and protect against ultraviolet damage.

Lifestyle Recommendations

Wear gloves. Because it spends a good deal of time in water, the skin on your hands is especially vulnerable to dryness. Consider wearing plastic or rubber gloves when you are preparing meals, washing dishes, and performing household chores. Wear white cotton gloves under the rubber gloves for the best protection. Similarly, use appropriate gloves for gardening and outside chores. In cold weather, be sure to cover your hands with mittens or gloves.

Take a soothing bath. Add 3 cups of colloidal oatmeal (fine-ground powder) to lukewarm bathwater. Climb in and soak for 15 minutes, then gently pat dry with a towel. This will allow the absorbed water to remain in the skin. Using a moisturizer right after your bath will help seal the pores.

Try a botanical cleanser. Look for a water-based product that contains aloe vera, calendula, chamomile, or green tea, any of which can be soothing to the skin.

Preventive Measures

Avoid caffeine and alcohol. Because they act as diuretics, caffeine and alcohol can contribute to dehydration, causing fluids to be lost from your skin.

Drink plenty of water. At a minimum, you should be consuming 64 ounces—eight 8-ounce glasses—of water or noncaffeinated, nonalcoholic beverages each day.

Exercise. Exercise improves blood circulation, encourages bloodflow, and supports the removal of toxins from the body.

Get a good night's sleep. In order for skin cells to repair themselves, and for the rest of the body to restore itself, you need a sufficient amount of rest. At least 7 hours a night is ideal.

Increase the humidity in your home. If you cannot have a humidifier or you don't have radiators where you can place containers of water, you might increase the moisture content of the air in your home by leaving the bathroom door open when you bathe or shower. Even a small amount of steam is helpful. And turn down the thermostat; forced hot air can dilate the blood vessels and dry out the skin.

Houseplants may help increase the humidity in your home, as they release moisture that evaporates into the air.

Limit your time in the sun. The sun's ultraviolet rays are strongest from 10:00 a.m. until 4:00 p.m. It's best to avoid sun exposure during these hours. When you do go outside, apply a sunscreen with an SPF of at least 15 about 30 minutes beforehand. Reapply every few hours that you're outdoors. Choose a good-quality sunscreen that blocks both UVA and UVB rays.

Cut back on perfumes and aftershave lotions. These products may increase your skin's sensitivity to sunlight. They also may contain alcohol, which is very drying.

Stop smoking. The nicotine in cigarettes constricts blood vessels, depriving skin of necessary nutrients and oxygen. If you already have dry skin, smoking will only make it worse.

Emphysema

Emphysema is a form of chronic obstructive pulmonary disease (COPD) in which the air sacs, or alveoli, in the lungs lose their elasticity and their walls begin to break down. The air that is trapped inside overinflates the alveoli and causes them to rupture, thereby reducing the amount of surface area. The damage to the alveoli is permanent and irreversible; it prevents a person with emphysema from inhaling an adequate amount of oxygen and exhaling an adequate amount of carbon dioxide. As the disease progresses, the flow of air in and out of the lungs becomes more limited.

Emphysema is a fairly widespread health problem, affecting almost 2.8 million Americans—more men than women. People with emphysema are at greater risk for a number of other medical conditions, including asthma, acute and chronic bronchitis, pneumonia, and other respiratory problems.

Causes and Risk Factors

The vast majority of emphysema cases result from smoking—especially cigarettes, though smoking cigars and pipes also causes the disease. Smoking disrupts the chemical balance within the lungs, robbing the lungs of their ability to protect themselves against damage. People over age 40 who have smoked 20 cigarettes per day for 20 or more years are most likely to develop emphysema.

There is good evidence that long-term exposure to secondhand smoke may raise a person's risk for this condition. Exposure to air pollution, fumes, and dust (often on the job) also may play a significant role.

A far smaller number of emphysema cases are associated with an inherited disorder in which people are born with a deficiency of alpha-1-antitrypsin (AAT), a protein that protects against the damage caused by smoking or other pollutants. This may lead to an illness known as AAT-deficiency-related emphysema, which usually is diagnosed between ages 20 and 40. Most of those with AAT deficiency are of Northern European descent.

Signs and Symptoms

The first symptom of emphysema usually is an acute chest illness characterized by increased coughing, sputum, wheezing, and shortness of breath. As the disease progresses, shortness of breath may become more frequent; you may breathe harder than usual when you are exercising or running up stairs. Eventually, you will experience bouts of difficult breathing, with your exhalations taking twice as long as your inhalations.

Other common symptoms of emphysema include anxiety, weight loss, fatigue, and swelling of the legs, ankles, and feet. In addition, there may be an increase in the diameter of your chest, a condition known as barrel-shaped chest.

If you develop shortness of breath, you should see your doctor—especially if you are a smoker or you have a family history of the genetic form of emphysema. Shortness of breath is a symptom of a number of health problems and so requires proper medical evaluation.

Conventional Treatments

If you smoke, the first and most important step in treating emphysema is to quit. In addition, try to avoid exposure to secondhand smoke.

Medications

Antibiotics. Having emphysema places you at increased risk for respiratory infections, which will worsen your symptoms. Your doctor probably will recommend treating any infection with a course of broad-spectrum antibiotics, such as cephalosporin, ampicillin, tetracycline, or erythromycin.

Anti-inflammatory drugs (corticosteroids). To reduce inflammation in your lungs, your doctor may prescribe an anti-inflammatory medication such as prednisone. While these medicines are quite good at healing the delicate lining of the lungs, they can have a number of negative side effects, especially when used for an extended period. These include osteoporosis (in both men and women), weight gain, loss of lean body mass, and elevated blood pressure and blood sugar. Since inhaled steroids tend to have fewer side effects, they

A Quick Guide to Symptoms

☐ Onset of acute chest illness characterized by increased cough, sputum, wheezing, and shortness of breath
☐ Bouts of difficult breathing
☐ Anxiety
☐ Weight loss
☐ Fatigue
☐ Swelling of the legs, ankles, and feet
☐ Barrel-shaped chest

may be a better option than oral steroids.

Bronchodilators. Your treatment plan probably will include a bronchodilator, which relaxes the muscles around the airways. Examples of bronchodilators are albuterol, terbutaline, ipratropium bromide, and theophylline. Generally, these medications have few side effects.

Oxygen Therapy

If emphysema has severely impaired your lung function, and you are unable to obtain a sufficient amount of oxygen through normal respiration, your doctor may suggest oxygen therapy. It's helpful in treating shortness of breath and also may prevent heart failure.

Protein Therapy

If your emphysema is the result of an AAT deficiency, you might benefit from weekly intravenous infusions of the protein. This treatment may slow damage to your lungs.

Pulmonary Rehabilitation Program

A treatment plan for emphysema often includes participation in a pulmonary rehabilitation program. These programs combine education about emphysema with smoking cessation, nutrition counseling, physical activity, psychosocial support, and training in special breathing techniques. If you are interested in such a program, you should ask your doctor for a referral.

Surgery

For certain patients with emphysema, surgery may be necessary. Usually it involves one of two procedures: lung volume reduction surgery and transplant surgery.

Lung volume reduction surgery. This procedure may eliminate the need for supplemental oxygen. Once a CT scan has determined the location of the damaged lung tissue, the surgeon makes two or three small incisions in the chest, through which he threads a tiny camera to view the inside of the lungs. An instrument removes small wedges of damaged tissue—usually between 20 and 30 percent of each lung. Since there is less lung, there is less pressure on the diaphragm, and the remaining lung is able to return to a normal position. After this procedure, the contraction and relaxation of the diaphragm—and your breathing—should improve.

One study compared the outcomes of lung volume reduction surgery to those of medical management of emphysema. Though surgery did not affect overall mortality, the patients who'd undergone surgery showed improvement in their exercise capacity.

Transplant surgery. Because of the serious shortage of transplantable lungs as well as the invasiveness and high risk associated with the procedure, doctors generally recommend transplant surgery only as a last resort. It may be appropriate for younger patients who have no other serious health problems.

Complementary Treatments

For people with emphysema, practitioners of complementary therapies will focus their efforts on improving breathing and relieving any discomfort.

Aromatherapy

Eucalyptus has expectorant properties and can help loosen mucus. Place 2 drops of eucalyptus oil in a large pan of steaming water. Place your head over the bowl, cover with a towel, and slowly inhale through your nose. Lift your head away from the steam and exhale through your mouth. Reposition your face over the bowl, cover your head, and inhale again. Repeat up to five times per treatment.

Diet

Eat smaller but more frequent meals. With emphysema, obstructed air may become trapped in the enlarged lungs and push down on the abdominal area. Since less oxygen makes its way to the stomach, digesting large meals is harder.

Try to avoid foods that produce gas, such as legumes, cabbage, onions, broccoli, and radishes. These foods cause the abdomen to distend, which may hinder breathing. Likewise, steer clear of foods that produce excess mucus, such as dairy products and anything fried. People who have emphysema tend to collect mucus in their airways.

Remember, too, that drinking lots of fluids will help thin mucus secretions. Aim for at least eight 8-ounce glasses of water and other noncaffeinated, nonalcoholic beverages per day.

Herbal Medicine

Garlic. An antioxidant, garlic helps fortify the immune system and is effective for all chronic respiratory conditions, particularly for preventing pneumonia. The recommended dose of fresh garlic is two or three cloves per day, while the dose for supplements is 500 milligrams per day. If you have a choice, select fresh garlic over supplements, which contain concentrated extracts and so may increase the risk of excessive bleeding.

Mullein, coltsfoot, wild cherry bark, and peppermint. This blend of herbs may assist in loosening mucus and eliminating phlegm. To make a tea, fill a saucepan with water and add the herbs in equal amounts. Use 1 tablespoon of each herb per 1 cup of water. Bring the tea to a boil, then turn off the burner and allow to steep for at least an hour before straining. Drink 2 cups of the tea each day.

Nutritional Supplements

Antioxidant nutrients are helpful for strengthening lung tissue and detoxifying the body after exposure to harmful substances, including cigarette smoke and environmental pollutants.

- Multivitamin/mineral: Take as directed on the label. Look for a supplement product that contains the minerals magnesium, potassium, selenium, and zinc, which often are deficient in people with emphysema.

- Vitamin A: 10,000 IU daily. Aids in repairing lung tissue.

- Vitamin C: 2,000 milligrams daily, in divided doses of 1,000 milligrams. Heals inflamed lung tissue.

- Vitamin E: 400 IU daily. Delivers oxygen throughout the body.

Lifestyle Recommendations

Watch your weight. If you weigh more than you should, your body must work even harder to obtain extra oxygen.

Take a walk. While people with emphysema tire easily, any amount of walking is better than none at all. It will improve your endurance and build your muscle strength.

Practice breathing exercises. The following exercises can be beneficial in cases of emphysema, though you may wish to consult a respiratory therapist to learn proper technique.

Begin with diaphragmatic breathing. Lie on your back, with pillows under your head and knees for support. Position your fingertips on your abdomen, below your rib cage, so that you can feel your diaphragm lift with each inhalation. As your chest fills with air, push your abdomen against your hand. Slowly inhale through your mouth for a count of three, then exhale through pursed lips for a count of six.

Practice this technique until you are able to complete 10 to 15 cycles of inhaling and exhaling. Then try it while lying on your left and right sides in turn. Next perform the exercises while sitting in a chair, standing, and walking. Eventually, you should be able to do diaphragmatic breathing while you are climbing the stairs.

Along with diaphragmatic breathing, work on deep breathing. Sit or stand comfortably and inhale deeply. Hold your breath for a slow count of five while arching your chest. Then contract your abdominal muscles and force out the air. Repeat 10 times. Practice deep breathing once a day.

Alleviate stress. Studies have shown that stress increases the body's demand for oxygen. To help unwind and reduce your stress level, try relaxation techniques that incorporate deep breathing, such as meditation, tai chi, and yoga. Listening to music or a relaxation CD also can help relieve tension and anxiety.

Avoid wearing restrictive clothing and accessories. Because emphysema interferes with breathing, the chest and abdomen must be able to expand freely.

Protect your respiratory system from cold air. If you have emphysema, your respiratory tract is very sensitive to cold. Cover your face with a mask or scarf when heading outside in cold weather.

Reduce your exposure to air pollution. Inhaling airborne pollutants will only aggravate your condition. Pay attention to daily air quality reports, and stay inside as much as possible when the air quality is compromised.

Address respiratory infections. Because any type of respiratory infection will aggravate emphysema symptoms, you should contact your doctor at the first signs of a respiratory illness, such as a cold or the flu. Your doctor may be able to suggest medication that will reduce the severity of your symptoms.

Seek support from others. Emphysema is an emotionally difficult disease that can take a serious toll on you and your family. A few sessions with a counselor or therapist may help you better cope with your situation. So may joining a support group, in which you can commiserate with and learn from others who are facing similar challenges.

Set priorities. Don't expect your life to be the same as it was before emphysema. Learn to control what you can physically, emotionally, and psychologically. Continue to pursue the activities that are important to you, but with adjustments so that they require less effort.

Preventive Measures

Don't smoke, and if you do smoke, stop. Smoking is the primary cause of emphysema. Smokers are 10 times more likely than nonsmokers to develop the disease. The risk is even higher for smokers with an AAT deficiency.

Since it's possible to develop emphysema from exposure to secondhand smoke, try to steer clear of smoky environments, too.

Erectile Dysfunction

Erectile dysfunction, the current term of choice for what long was known as impotence, refers to the inability to obtain an adequate erection for sexual performance and satisfaction. Erectile dysfunction, or ED, is thought to be quite common, affecting between 20 million and 30 million American men (and their partners). An estimated 620,000 men between ages 40 and 70 have a bout of erectile dysfunction each year.

Causes and Risk Factors

Aging is the most significant risk factor for erectile dysfunction. Though study results tend to vary, a significant number of men over age 50 are believed to have the disease to some degree.

A number of physical conditions can make a man more likely to develop ED. For example, chronic disease of the kidneys, heart, liver, thyroid, lungs, or nerves can contribute to ED, as can multiple sclerosis, epilepsy, Parkinson's disease, stroke, and endocrine disorders such as diabetes. Atherosclerosis—that is, the accumulation of fatty deposits in the arteries—may impede bloodflow to the penis. Other possible medical causes include surgery to the pelvic area or spinal cord and surgery for rectal, bladder, or prostate cancer. A deficiency of the male hormone testosterone can be a risk factor, too.

Certain medications identify ED as a possible side effect. Among these are medicines for high blood pressure (especially diuretics and beta-blockers), cancer, and pain, as well as antidepressants, antihistamines, tranquilizers, sleeping pills, and antifungal drugs, particularly ketoconazole (Nizoral).

Chronic excessive alcohol consumption can contribute to ED, as can illegal drugs such as marijuana, heroin, and cocaine. Smoking can damage penile arteries. Sometimes men who ride their bicycles for prolonged periods experience temporary ED.

About 10 to 15 percent of all ED cases are believed to have a psychological cause, such as depression, anxiety, or stress. Often multiple psychological causes occur at once, or psychological causes occur along with physical ones. For example, a physical condition

ED and Heart Disease

According to one study that tracked 9,500 men—all over age 55—for 5 years, erectile dysfunction (ED) may be a harbinger of future cardiovascular disease. The men who had ED at the beginning of the study, as well as those who developed ED during the study, were at higher risk for cardiovascular disease than those who did not have ED. Any man with ED should talk with his doctor about the possibility of heart trouble.

may lead to ED, the onset of which can trigger anxiety that only aggravates ED.

Signs and Symptoms

With erectile dysfunction, you are unable to have an erection or to maintain an erection for a sufficient amount of time to have sex.

Every man should expect an occasional bout with erectile dysfunction, especially as he gets older. You should consult your doctor if ED persists for more than 2 or 3 months.

Conventional Treatments

Medications

Most men with ED will see improvement with one of the following medications.

Alprostadil. A synthetic version of the hormone prostaglandin E, alprostadil relaxes the smooth muscle in the penis, thereby enhancing bloodflow as necessary for an erection. The medication is available in several forms.

With injectable alprostadil (Edex, Caver-ject), you administer the medicine directly into the side of the penis using a fine needle. It produces an erection within 5 to 20 minutes, and the erection will last for about an hour. The pain from the injection is minimal, though you may experience other side effects such as prolonged erection, the formation of fibrous tissue in the penis, or bleeding at the site of the injection. Some doctors recommend using injectable alprostadil in combination with other prescription drugs such as phentolamine (Regitine) or papaverine. Do not inject yourself with alprostadil more than once a day or three times a week.

Alprostadil also is available as a tiny suppository that is inserted into the tip of the penis. The erectile tissue absorbs the drug, which increases bloodflow. The trade name for this delivery system is medicated urethral system for erection (MUSE). Possible side effects include minor bleeding in the urethra, pain, dizziness, and the formation of fibrous tissue in the penis. Do not use MUSE more than twice a day.

Then there is the topical cream form of alprostadil, sold under the brand names Topiglan and Alprox-TD. The cream is rubbed directly on the penis 15 minutes before intercourse.

Alprostadil is not appropriate for men who have severe circulatory or nerve damage or bleeding abnormalities, who take blood-thinning medication, or who have penile implants. Some female partners of men using alprostadil experience vaginal itching or burning. If this happens, try using a condom.

A Quick Guide to Symptoms

☐ **Unable to have an erection**
☐ **Unable to maintain an erection for a sufficient amount of time to have sex**

Sildenafil. Most people will recognize sildenafil by its brand name: Viagra. It works by increasing bloodflow to the genital area, producing an erection within 30 to 60 minutes after a pill is taken.

Not all men are good candidates for sildenafil. For example, anyone taking a nitrate or a nitrate-containing medication (including nitroglycerin) should not use sildenafil. Combining these medications—both of which dilate blood vessels—may cause low blood pressure, dizziness, and heart and circulatory problems.

Common side effects of sildenafil include headaches, indigestion, nasal congestion, dizziness, flushing, and blurred vision. About 2.5 percent of men who take sildenafil report seeing a blue haze or increased brightness, or briefly losing their vision, after taking sildenafil. Fortunately, these side effects appear to be temporary.

Sildenafil is best taken on an empty stomach, as combining it with food will diminish its effectiveness. Do not use it more than once a day, and do not combine it with other medications for erectile dysfunction. Likewise, sildenafil should not be taken at the same time as certain antibiotics, such as erythromycin, or certain acid blockers, such as cimetidine (Tagamet).

Vardenafil and tadalafil. While sildenafil probably has received the most media attention, there are other oral medications for erectile dysfunction. Two of them, vardenafil (Levitra) and tadalafil (Cialis), seem to work in much the same way as sildenafil.

But they do vary in dosage, duration of effectiveness, and possible side effects. As with sildenafil, neither of these drugs should be taken in combination with nitrate medications. Any man with a history of cardiac problems should use vardenafil or tadalafil with care.

Psychological Counseling

In the absence of any physical cause for ED, your doctor may recommend counseling. Ask for a referral to a professional with training and experience in addressing sexual issues. Generally, the goal of such treatment is to reduce any anxiety associated with sex.

Surgery

Penile implants. This procedure involves the surgical placement of implants on two sides of the penis. The implants may be some sort of inflatable devices, or somewhat rigid rods made from silicone or polyurethane. While the procedure generally is safe, there is a small risk of infection.

Vascular surgery. If erectile dysfunction is a result of damage to the arteries or other blood vessels, your doctor may recommend surgery. The two most common surgical procedures for ED are revascularization (bypass) and venous ligation.

During revascularization, the surgeon removes an artery from the leg and surgically connects it to the arteries in the back of the penis. This circumvents any arterial blockage and restores normal bloodflow. Sometimes a penile vein is used to create the bypass; this procedure is known as deep dorsal vein arterialization.

In cases where the penis isn't able to store enough blood to maintain an erection, doctors may opt for venous ligation. In this procedure, any veins that are causing too much blood to drain from the erection chambers are either tied off or removed. A related procedure, known as venous ablation, involves injecting ethanol into the deep dorsal vein, which is the primary vein for draining blood from the penis. This causes scarring, which closes smaller veins and stops blood from leaking.

Testosterone Replacement Therapy

If your doctor concludes that an inadequate amount of testosterone may be responsible for your ED, he or she may recommend treatment to increase blood levels of the hormone.

Vacuum Devices

Vacuum devices consist of an external vacuum and one or more tension rings (rubber bands). A hollow plastic tube is placed over the penis, and then a pump is used to create a vacuum inside the tube. This pulls blood into the penis. Once an erection occurs, usually in 3 to 5 minutes, a tension ring is placed around the base of the penis. This should sustain the erection long enough to have sexual intercourse.

Potential side effects of the vacuum devices include blocked ejaculation, minor bruising, and mild discomfort from both the pump and the tension ring. If you decide to use a vacuum device, ask your doctor to recommend one that has been medically approved. Those that aren't may not have the necessary safety elements, and so raise the risk of injury.

Venous Flow Controllers

If you are able to achieve an erection but it doesn't last, you may be a candidate for a venous flow controller. It's a simple constricting device with rings made from rubber or silicone, which are placed at the base of the penis to "trap" an erection. One example of a venous flow controller is Actis, a product made by the Vivus Corporation.

To avoid causing damage to the penis due to lack of oxygen, refrain from using one of these devices for more than 30 minutes at a time. They are not appropriate for men who have bleeding problems or who are taking blood-thinning medications.

Complementary Treatments
Acupuncture

Numerous studies have confirmed the benefits of electro-acupuncture for the treatment of erectile dysfunction. In electro-acupuncture, a mild electric current is run through the needles to help stimulate the appropriate acupuncture points.

To locate an acupuncturist in your area, visit the Web site of the National Certification Commission for Acupuncture and Oriental Medicine at www.nccaom.org.

Diet

Build your meals around fruits, vegetables, and whole grains. These foods support a healthy vascular system, which is essential for proper bloodflow to the penis. A diet of these nutritious foods also can help melt away extra pounds—an important benefit, since overweight is a risk factor for ED. Aim for at least four servings of fruits, five servings of vegetables, and six servings of whole grains per day.

As you shift your dietary focus to fresh, whole foods, you may be less inclined to eat anything fatty or sugary. That's a good thing, since these unhealthy foods not only contribute to weight gain, they also interfere with the absorption of essential nutrients. Also steer clear of anything containing caffeine. Though caffeine is a central nervous system stimulant, it actually relaxes muscles and may interfere with normal genital function.

The mineral zinc is necessary for your body to produce testosterone. Even a mild zinc deficiency can play a role in ED. Good food sources of zinc include pumpkin and sunflower seeds.

Herbal Medicine

The following herbs may be helpful for treating ED.

Asian ginseng. Asian ginseng helps maintain an erection and improves male potency. It is available in tea or capsule form. The recommended daily dose of Asian ginseng is 100 to 200 milligrams, standardized to 4 to 7 percent ginsenosides. The herb is not appropriate for anyone with high blood pressure, heart trouble, or hypoglycemia.

Damiana. This herb has a long history as an aphrodisiac, able to increase libido and calm jangled nerves. Damiana capsules generally contain 3 to 4 grams of the powdered leaves; take two capsules twice a day. When using damiana tincture, add 3 to 4 milliliters to an 8-ounce glass of water or juice and drink twice a day.

If you prefer, you can brew a tea from dried damiana leaves, which are available in some health food stores and organic grocery stores. Place 2 to 3 grams of dried leaves in a cup of boiling water and steep for 10 minutes, then strain and allow to cool. Drink 2 to 3 cups per day.

Garlic. The use of garlic as a medicinal herb dates back thousands of years. Studies have shown the herb to be effective for improving circulation. Fresh garlic works best; if you tolerate the herb well, try to eat one whole clove every day.

For garlic supplements, look for enteric-coated tablets or capsules with standardized allicin potential. Take 400 to 500 milligrams, once or twice per day, to provide up to 5,000 micrograms of allicin.

Garlic has anticoagulant properties, so if you are taking any blood-thinning medication, be sure to talk with your doctor before using the herb therapeutically. Also inform your doctor that you're taking garlic if you require any sort of surgery. You may need to discontinue treatment for at least 2 weeks prior to your procedure.

Ginkgo biloba. Ginkgo improves blood-flow to the penis as well as throughout the entire body. It is sold raw or in capsule form. The recommended dose is 120 milligrams, twice a day, of an extract standardized to 24 percent flavone glycosides and 6 percent terpene lactones. The terpene lactones are responsible for ginkgo's effect on circulation, while the flavone glycosides have antioxidant properties.

If you are taking any blood-thinning medication, be sure to consult your doctor before adding ginkgo to your self-care regimen.

Maca. Grown at elevations of 12,000 feet and higher in its native Peru, maca belongs to the same plant family as turnips and radishes. It is known for treating ED because of its ability to increase sexual desire and performance. It also is quite nutrient dense, which is beneficial for physical vitality, endurance, and stamina.

Maca is available in capsule form. The recommended dose is 550 milligrams, twice a day.

Sarsaparilla. In Central and South America, sarsaparilla has been used for centuries as an impotency treatment and as a general tonic. It is known for restoring the male reproductive organs.

You can buy packaged sarsaparilla tea in health food stores and organic grocery stores. Drink 1 cup of tea two or three times daily.

Siberian ginseng. Siberian ginseng increases energy and stamina. Look for the herb in capsule form, standardized to at least 0.8 percent eleutherosides. Take 100 to 300 milligrams daily.

Because of the herb's stimulant properties, avoid taking Siberian ginseng within 1 hour of going to bed. Anyone with hypertension should not use this herb.

Hypnotherapy

Hypnotherapy is beneficial for ED that is psychological rather than physical in origin. To learn more about hypnotherapy and to locate a practitioner in your area, visit the Web site of the American Society of Clinical Hypnosis at www.asch.net.

Kegel Exercises

Studies have shown that men who practice Kegels—which involve contracting and relaxing the muscles around the scrotum and penis—experience improvement in erectile function, if not a return to normal function. To try Kegels, you first need to identify your pelvic muscles, which can be done by slowing or stopping the urine flow while you are urinating. The muscles that allow you to do this are the same ones that you need to strengthen. Try to perform 5 to 15 Kegels, three to five times daily. Hold each Kegel for a count of 5 to start, and gradually work your way to a count of 10.

Nutritional Supplements

The following nutrients are necessary for normal sexual function in men.

- B-complex vitamins: Take as directed on the label. May help relieve anxiety.

- DHEA: 50 milligrams daily. Reduces the incidence of ED.

- L-arginine: 1,000 to 2,000 milligrams daily. Necessary for the body to produce nitric oxide, which is vital to a normal erection.

- Zinc: 30 milligrams daily. Supports normal sexual function in men.

Lifestyle Recommendations

Check your medications. As mentioned earlier, ED is a common side effect of medications. Read the labels or the product inserts of any medicines that you may be taking. If you see ED listed as a potential side effect, you might want to ask your doctor about reducing your dosage or switching to another medication.

Control your cholesterol. Studies have shown that high cholesterol may raise a man's risk of erectile dysfunction.

Adopt a healthy lifestyle. Beyond the dietary changes suggested above, other lifestyle strategies can help treat ED. Increase your physical activity. Get enough sleep. Cut back on caffeine and alcohol.

Reduce stress. Since stress may contribute to ED, find ways to relax and unwind. Even 10 minutes a day of uninterrupted "quiet time" can help. Just close your eyes, empty your mind, and breathe deeply.

Communicate. If you have been experiencing bouts of ED, you need to talk about it with your partner. Your chances of overcoming ED are much greater if the two of you work together.

Preventive Measures

The following lifestyle strategies can reduce your chances of experiencing ED.

Get regular exercise. Men in midlife who are in good physical shape are less likely to develop ED. Exercise not only increases testosterone but also improves oxygen and blood flow to the penis. Focus on activities that improve circulation, such as walking, running, and swimming.

Address emotional issues. Stress, anxiety, and depression contribute to ED. To help keep them in check—and thus avoid erectile issues—practice relaxation techniques such as deep breathing, guided imagery, and/or visualization.

Limit alcohol consumption. You're more likely to develop ED if you drink in excess. In fact, having more than one alcoholic beverage per day may depress your central nervous system and impair sexual function.

Quit smoking. Smokers are more likely than nonsmokers to develop ED.

Essential Tremor

As its name suggests, essential tremor involves abnormal shakiness. While it may manifest in any part of the body, it most often affects the head, voice box (larynx), hands, or arms. When essential tremor occurs in more than one member of a family, it is referred to as familial tremor.

Essential tremor is the most common movement disorder, affecting as many as 5 million Americans. Though it sometimes is confused with Parkinson's disease, it is an entirely different disorder and, in fact, is far more prevalent than Parkinson's.

Essential Tremor versus Parkinson's Disease

The symptoms of essential tremor differ from those of Parkinson's disease. With essential tremor, the symptoms tend to appear when you are using a particular part of your body, such as your hands. There is obvious shaking when you pick up a glass, for instance. In Parkinson's, the symptoms are most noticeable when you are resting. Also, essential tremor does not cause other medical conditions, while Parkinson's is known to contribute to problems such as rigid limbs, stooped posture, and slow movement.

Causes and Risk Factors

Essential tremor is the result of abnormal communication between different portions of the brain, including the cerebellum, thalamus, and brain stem. The two primary risk factors for the disorder are genetics and age.

Researchers believe that about half of all cases of essential tremor can be traced to genetic mutations. If one of your parents has the genetic mutation for essential tremor, you have a 50-50 chance of developing the disorder. Two genes—designated as ETM1 and ETM2—have been linked to essential tremor, though other genes may be involved as well. In imaging studies, people with essential tremor show increased activity in certain parts of the brain, such as those responsible for relaying pain and other sensory messages.

The risk of essential tremor rises as we get older. Though the mean age of onset is 45, the disorder is particularly common among those over age 60. It affects men and women about equally, though women appear more likely to develop essential tremor of the head.

Certain lifestyle factors may trigger essential tremor. Chief among these are tobacco use, excessive caffeine consumption, and alcohol withdrawal. The disorder can be a side effect of certain medications, such as some asthma, antidepressant, and antiseizure drugs, as well as lithium. It also is associated with medical conditions, including pheochromocytoma (a tumor of the adrenal glands), Wilson's disease (a rare condition in which copper accumulates in the brain and liver), and hyperthyroidism.

Signs and Symptoms

The most common symptom of essential tremor is trembling (or up-and-down movement) of the hands—or, in rare instances, of just one hand. You may have difficulty writing, holding a glass of water, or threading a needle. As mentioned earlier, essential tremor also may affect the head, voice box (larynx), arms, and on occasion other parts of the body. The tremors occur at a rate of 6 to 10 per second.

Fatigue, anxiety, and extreme temperatures tend to worsen symptoms. Conversely, symptoms tend to diminish with adequate rest.

Conventional Treatments

In many cases of essential tremor, there is no formal course of treatment. Doctors simply advise patients to avoid stressful situations and to limit consumption of caffeinated foods and beverages. If essential tremor is interfering with day-to-day living, however, treatment may be necessary.

Medication

Medications provide relief for about 40 to 60 percent of people with essential tremor.

Any of the following may be prescribed.

Antiseizure medications. These medicines—an example is Mysoline—may be helpful in cases of essential tremor that do not respond to beta-blockers (discussed next). Potential side effects include drowsiness, difficulty concentrating, nausea, poor gait, and flulike symptoms.

Beta-blockers. Beta-blockers are best known for treating high blood pressure, but they also have proven effective for about 50 percent of those with essential tremor. One commonly prescribed beta-blocker is propranolol (Inderal). Potential side effects of this class of drugs include dizziness, fatigue, nausea, erectile dysfunction, shortness of breath, nasal stuffiness, and—in some older adults—confusion and memory loss. Generally, anyone with asthma, type 1 diabetes, or certain heart problems should not use beta-blockers.

Botulinum toxin injections. Perhaps best known by their brand name, Botox, these injections not only erase wrinkles, they also alleviate certain types of essential tremor—especially tremor of the head or larynx. The injections work by blocking neuromuscular transmissions. Because they can cause weakness in the fingers, Botox injections generally are not used to treat tremor of the hands.

It is important to note that although these injections minimize tremors, they do not improve a patient's functioning.

Bronchodilators. In one study, researchers found that the bronchodilator theophylline reduced essential tremor as well as propranolol and significantly better than a placebo. No side effects were reported.

Tranquilizers. If anxiety seems to play a role in your tremors, your doctor may suggest taking a tranquilizer such as diazepam (Valium) or alprazolam (Xanax). Among the potential side effects of these drugs are memory loss and confusion.

Physical Therapy

Ask your doctor to refer you to a physical therapist, who can teach you exercises that will promote stability in your hands and wrists. After a few sessions, you will be able to practice the exercises at home, on your own.

Psychotherapy

Some people with essential tremor may struggle to cope with the disorder, experiencing emotional effects such as embarrassment and depression. In these cases, psychotherapy—which focuses on healing the mind and emotions—may prove helpful.

Your primary-care physician or your local hospital should be able to provide a referral to a trained psychotherapist. You also might try visiting the Web sites for the following professional organizations: the American Psychiatric Association (www.psych.org), the American Psychological Association (www.apa.org), and the National Association of Social Workers (www.naswdc.org).

Surgery

If your symptoms of essential tremor are severe or disabling, and they haven't responded to treatment with medication, you may require surgery. Here are two procedures that your doctor may recommend.

Deep brain stimulation (DBS). This procedure involves the surgical implantation of a device known as a thalamic stimulator in the thalamus of the brain. Then a pacemaker-like chest unit sends electrical pulses to the implant through a wire. These pulses stop the signals from the thalamus that cause the tremors. This procedure is not as risky as a thalamotomy (described next), and since it may be used on both sides of the thalamus, it may control tremors on both sides of the body.

Stereotactic thalamotomy. In this procedure, a small section on one side of the thalamus is destroyed. If the surgery is effective, as it is in about 70 to 80 percent of patients, it will relieve tremors on the opposite side of the body. Since operating on both sides of the thalamus poses a risk of speech loss and other complications, surgeons usually operate on only one side.

Complementary Treatments

Depending on the cause of the essential tremor, complementary treatments may be useful in reducing symptoms of this disorder.

Biofeedback

Biofeedback involves using an electric monitoring device, which provides data on certain of the body's vital signs, such as heart rate and blood pressure. In a biofeedback session, you will learn how to alter or slow these signs through the use of relaxation techniques. In cases where essential tremor is triggered or aggravated by nervousness, excitement, or tension, biofeedback may help control it.

Various health care professionals use biofeedback in their practices, including psychiatrists, psychologists, social workers, nurses, physical therapists, occupational therapists, speech therapists, respiratory therapists, exercise physiologists, and chiropractors. Try to find someone who has been certified through the Biofeedback Certification Institute of America. For help in locating a biofeedback instructor in your area, visit the BCIA Web site at www.bcia.org or contact your local hospital for a referral.

Lifestyle Recommendations

If you smoke, quit. Smoking may trigger episodes of essential tremor.

Avoid caffeine. Caffeine tends to make your body produce more adrenaline, which may intensify the tremors.

Don't use alcohol as medication. Many people with essential tremor report that their symptoms improve when they drink alcoholic beverages. But using alcohol as a treatment for essential tremor is dangerous and could lead to addiction.

Be safe. If your tremors are severe or not well controlled, take care when holding containers of hot liquid, for example.

Avoid heavy physical exertion. Intense physical activity can aggravate essential tremor. Try not to overdo it.

Reduce stress. Since emotional stress may worsen essential tremor, you need to find ways to offset stress and promote relaxation. Techniques such as deep breathing, guided imagery, and visualization can help alleviate tension and anxiety.

Join a support group. People who are unable to control their tremors often isolate themselves socially, leaving their jobs and spending most of their time at home. A support group not only provides much-needed social interaction and engagement, it also offers a setting in which you can share information and ideas and learn from the experiences of others.

Participate in a clinical trial. If you are having trouble controlling your symptoms, you might want to enroll in a clinical trial for testing of new medications, surgical procedures, and other treatments. Discuss your options with your doctor.

Fallen Bladder

Fallen bladder (cystocele) occurs when the structures that support a woman's bladder and urethra (the tube that carries urine from the bladder out of the body) weaken and drop into the space occupied by the vagina. This can lead to urine leakage and incomplete emptying of the bladder.

Doctors classify cases of fallen bladder as follows.

- Grade 1 cystocele—the bladder has dropped only slightly.

- Grade 2 cystocele—the bladder has reached the opening of the vagina.

- Grade 3 cystocele—the most severe form, in which the bladder bulges out through the opening of the vagina.

Though rarely discussed, fallen bladder is more common than most people realize. In fact, as many as 10 percent of women develop fallen bladder requiring surgical repair at some time during their lives.

Causes and Risk Factors

In women at midlife or older, a fallen bladder may be associated with a decline in the hormone estrogen, which helps strengthen the vagina and nearby muscles. The condition also may be the result of excessive straining—for example, while lifting a heavy object or having bowel movements.

Signs and Symptoms

Women who have a fallen bladder may experience a sensation of pressure in the vagina. Since the bladder does not empty fully during urination, it creates an ideal environment for the proliferation of infectious organisms, causing frequent and painful urination. In addition, urine leakage may occur upon lifting a heavy object, coughing, sneezing, or laughing—a condition known as stress incontinence.

Conventional Treatments

If you are only mildly bothered by the cystocele, your doctor will probably advise you to refrain from any behaviors, such as heavy lifting, that could worsen your condition. If

A Quick Guide to Symptoms

- ☐ A sensation of pressure in the vagina
- ☐ Frequent and painful urination
- ☐ Leakage of urine upon lifting a heavy object, coughing, sneezing, or laughing

this is not sufficient, there are other measures that may be recommended, including estrogen replacement therapy, the use of a pessary, and, in more severe cases, surgery.

Estrogen Replacement Therapy

If you are experiencing menopausal symptoms and are not already taking estrogen replacement therapy, a course of therapy may be recommended. Estrogen replacement therapy is known to strengthen the muscles around the bladder and vagina.

Pessary

In some instances, in conjunction with vaginal estrogen, your doctor may recommend a pessary, a plastic device that fits into the vagina. When properly inserted, a pessary returns your pelvic organs to the correct position. Pessaries are effective for about 80 percent of women. However, a pessary may lead to such complications as bleeding and open sores in the vaginal wall. If a pessary fits well, the chance of complications is reduced. Follow your doctor's instructions on how and when to clean and reinsert the pessary.

Surgery

If the fallen bladder is bothersome and does not respond to nonsurgical interventions, your doctor may recommend surgery, a procedure known as a cystocele repair. Before the surgery, you will be given a regional or general anesthetic. During the procedure, which is normally conducted through an incision in the vagina, a surgeon will lift and tighten the tissues around the bladder. This stops the bladder from pushing against the vagina. After the procedure, in order to give your bladder time to recover, you will need to wear a catheter for several days. For about 4 weeks after surgery, you may have smelly and/or bloody drainage from your vagina. For at least 2 weeks after surgery, avoid heavy activity. It may take as long as 4 to 6 weeks before you are able to return to normal activities.

Possible complications of this type of surgery include infection and bleeding. If your catheter becomes plugged and you stop passing urine, if you have heavy bleeding, or if you develop a fever, you should contact your surgeon or doctor immediately.

Complementary Treatments

By increasing estrogen levels through dietary and herbal products, practitioners of complementary medicine seek to reduce or eliminate the symptoms of fallen bladder. Strengthening the pelvic wall through exercise and chiropractic adjustments has also been shown to be beneficial.

Acupuncture

When the underlying cause of the fallen bladder is determined, acupuncture has been shown to be very effective. It is particularly useful in treating the symptoms of incontinence, painful urination, and retention of urine. It also helps relieve the pressure sensation in the vagina. To locate an acupuncturist in your area, visit the Web site of the National Certification Commission for Acupuncture and Oriental Medicine (NCCAOM) at www. nccaom.org.

Biofeedback

Biofeedback uses an electric monitoring device to monitor the muscle activity in the pubic area. Exercises are then taught that will help strengthen the muscles and reduce some of the symptoms associated with fallen bladder.

Chiropractic

By adjusting the bones and joints around the pelvis, chiropractic treatments have been successful in strengthening the bladder muscles. To locate a chiropractor in your area, visit the Web site of the American Chiropractic Association (www.amerchiro.org).

Diet

To compensate for the body's low estrogen production, it may be helpful to eat certain foods that are high in plant estrogens, such as soybeans, which come in many forms including miso, natto, soy flour, soy milk, soy oil, tamari, tempeh, and tofu. Other foods containing natural plant estrogens are alfalfa, apples, beans, beets, carrots, cherries, chickpeas, cucumbers, dates, eggplant, flaxseeds, garlic, lentils, olive oil, olives, parsley, peas, peppers, plums, potatoes, pumpkin, rhubarb, rice, sesame seeds, sunflower seeds, tomatoes, whole grains, and yams. These foods are also high in fiber, which can help reduce constipation. Chronic constipation can increase your risk of developing a fallen bladder.

Herbal Medicine

Black cohosh. Traditional Chinese medicine practitioners recommend this herb as one "that lifts the sunken." Widely used as a natural alternative to hormone replacement therapy, it may be taken in capsule form. The minimum recommended daily dose is 20 milligrams in the morning and 20 milligrams at night of standardized black cohosh (containing 1.0 to 2.5 milligrams of deoxyactein). However, your doctor may recommend a higher dose. Women dealing with breast cancer, fibroids, and/or ovarian cysts should not take black cohosh. Since black cohosh increases estrogen levels in the body, it may exacerbate these conditions.

Uva ursi. Uva ursi is beneficial for treating infections that may result from the inability to empty the bladder fully during urination. It contains arbutin, which acts as an antiseptic. Uva ursi may be taken in capsule or tea form. The recommended daily dose for capsules is 250 to 500 milligrams of standardized 20 percent arbutin, twice daily, once in the morning and once at bedtime. Or purchase the tea. Steep 1 teaspoon in 1 pint of boiling water for 30 minutes, and drink a half cup every 4 hours. For the most effective results during treatment, your urine must be alkaline, so avoid acidic fruit juices. Do not take uva ursi for more than 14 days; prolonged use may cause stomach distress.

Lifestyle Recommendations

Try double voiding. A good technique to empty the bladder completely is called double voiding. Urinate until you feel that you are done. Then, wait a moment; relax. Then, lean forward and void some more. Often, there is a little left that needs to be released. This technique helps to avoid leakage.

Practice Kegels. Kegel exercises, which help to strengthen the muscles of the pelvic floor that support the bladder and close the sphincters, were originally designed to assist women before and after childbirth. However, they have been found to be quite useful for at least the milder forms of cystocele.

Begin by identifying your pelvic muscles. This may be done by slowing or stopping the urine flow while you are urinating. These are the muscles you need to make stronger. Try to perform 5 to 15 contractions, three times each day. Hold each Kegel for a count of 5 to start, and gradually work your way to a count of 10.

Preventive Measures

Lifestyle changes may be helpful in preventing fallen bladder.

Avoid becoming constipated. If you repeatedly strain to have bowel movements, you increase the possibility of a fallen bladder. It may be helpful to try moving your bowels in a more natural squatting position with your knees raised. Place a small stool in front of the toilet, and rest your feet on it. If a stool is not available, you can use books or a box.

Do not lift heavy objects. Lifting heavy items increases the possibility that you will develop a fallen bladder.

Maintain a healthy weight. Obesity is a risk factor associated with a fallen bladder.

Fatigue

Fatigue is physical and/or mental tiredness or sensation of exhaustion. It is actually a symptom rather than a disorder. Fatigue is extremely common: Just about everyone feels fatigued at some point, although some people are fatigued all the time. According to one survey, up to 7.5 percent of adults report they are fatigued.

and some medications, such as beta-blockers, antihistamines, and anti-anxiety drugs. People who are coping with pain may be profoundly fatigued. Fatigue may be the result of treatment for a medical problem; for example, it is well known that some treatments for cancer cause fatigue. Fatigue may also be the first sign of an illness, as it may be with diabetes.

Causes and Risk Factors

Though it may be caused by a seemingly endless number of physical and psychological medical conditions, fatigue is more likely to occur when there is excessive physical or mental stress. Most often, it is a response to overexertion. Other common causes of fatigue include illness, lack of exercise, poor physical condition, insufficient sleep, excess weight, poor diet, stress, emotional or psychological problems,

Signs and Symptoms

The symptoms of fatigue include sensation of exhaustion, tiredness, indifference, and a lack of energy and/or motivation. Other symptoms include apathy and drowsiness.

Conventional Treatments

Treatments for fatigue will vary according to the cause of your fatigue. Thus, if your doctor determines that your fatigue is caused by an infection, then the infection will be treated with antibiotics. If you have fatigue from depression, then you will probably be offered medication and advised to seek psychotherapy.

If your fatigue does not appear to have a direct cause, you may be told to manage your stress more effectively and become more active. You may also be advised to eat a healthier diet and to obtain sufficient sleep. Also, your doctor will want to review your

A Quick Guide to Symptoms

- ☐ Sensation of exhaustion
- ☐ Tiredness
- ☐ Indifference
- ☐ Lack of energy and/or motivation
- ☐ Apathy
- ☐ Drowsiness

medications, because they may be contributing to your fatigue.

Complementary Treatments

Complementary medicine incorporates various approaches designed to address the physical, emotional, and spiritual components of the individual, including dietary modifications, exercise, bodywork therapy, and lifestyle changes.

Craniosacral Therapy

The gentle hands-on techniques of craniosacral therapy treat stress and restriction, thereby reducing fatigue. To search for a qualified therapist in your area, visit the Web site of the International Association of Healthcare Practitioners at www.iahp.com.

Diet

Eating a healthy diet full of whole grains, fruits, vegetables, nuts, and seeds is an excellent way to fight fatigue. Try to include a minimum of five servings of vegetables, four servings of fruit, and six servings of whole grains each day. These foods are high in the essential vitamins and minerals necessary to maintain optimal energy levels and a healthy immune system. Vitamin C, the B vitamins, magnesium, and essential fatty acids are particularly useful in fighting fatigue. All of these nutrients help to strengthen the immune system. Vitamin C also supports the adrenal glands, which regulate the production of stress hormones in the body. Good

If your fatigue is profound, if you are exhausted for no apparent reason, and if these symptoms are continuing for an extended period of time, you may have an illness known as chronic fatigue syndrome.

sources of vitamin C include almost all fruits and green vegetables, especially broccoli; cranberries; kale; mangoes; melons; oranges; papayas; peppers; potatoes, including sweet potatoes; spinach; and tomatoes.

In addition to strengthening the immune system and supporting the adrenal glands, the B vitamins are essential to a healthy nervous system. The B vitamins are found in dark green, leafy vegetables, whole grains, avocados, beans, beets, bananas, potatoes, dairy products, nuts, fish, and chicken. Many of these foods are considered complex carbohydrates (starchy foods and root vegetables) that are a good source of glucose, a fuel for the body.

Magnesium may be found in green leafy vegetables such as spinach, parsley, broccoli, chard, kale, and mustard and turnip greens. It is also in green peas, corn, lima beans, squash, yams, raw almonds, pumpkin seeds, sunflower seeds, sesame seeds, pistachios, walnuts, wheat germ, potatoes, tofu, and fruits such as bananas, papayas, prunes, raisins, and grapefruit and pineapple juice.

Essential fatty acids fortify the parts of the cells that help to fight fatigue and boost the immune system. The primary symptom of essential fatty acid deficiency is fatigue. In fact, it has been estimated that 80 percent of the population is deficient in essential fatty acids. Omega-3 (also known as linolenic acid) is an essential fatty acid that is made up of three types: EPA (eicosapentaenoic acid), DHA (docosahexaenoic acid), and ALA (alpha-linolenic acid). EPA and DHA are found in fish oil, particularly cold-water fish such as bluefish, herring, salmon, and tuna. Flaxseed oil is a rich source of ALA. Because your body converts ALA into EPA and DHA, taking flaxseed oil is another good way to reap the benefits of essential fatty acids.

Amino acids are the building blocks of protein. An unhealthy diet may cause low blood levels of amino acids, which in turn may cause fatigue. By eating a well-balanced, healthy diet, you will be sure to obtain sufficient amino acids. Including protein in your diet will ensure you consume all the amino acids you need. Good sources of protein are milk, eggs, lean red meat, soy, and poultry.

Finally, instead of three larger meals, try eating five or six smaller meals throughout the day. Large meals and overeating may disrupt sleep, and crash dieting may also cause fatigue. Instead, eat smaller portions of healthy foods and eliminate high-fat foods, caffeine, alcohol, and sugary products—these contribute to weight gain and upset sleep patterns.

Herbal Medicine

Panax ginseng fights fatigue by increasing stamina. Look for products standardized to contain at least 7 percent ginsenosides. Take 100 milligrams three times daily.

Nutritional Supplements

The following essential nutrients are necessary to relieve physical and mental exhaustion.

- Multivitamin/mineral: Take as directed on the label. Supplement should contain potassium and calcium as deficiency leads to increased fatigue. Should not contain iron.

- B-complex vitamins: Take as directed on the label. Important to regulation of energy and vitality. Often lost due to stress and unhealthy diet. Must be replenished as they are not stored in the body.

- Vitamin C: 1,000 milligrams daily, in divided doses of 500 milligrams. Supports adrenal glands and strengthens immune system.

- Magnesium: 500 milligrams daily. Deficiency of this mineral is linked to fatigue. Take before bed.

- Omega-3 fatty acids such as flaxseed oil or fish oil: 1 tablespoon of flaxseed oil daily or 4,000 milligrams daily of fish oil capsules. Fortifies the parts of the cells that help fight fatigue and boost the immune system.

- Zinc: 30 milligrams daily. Combats fatigue, improves muscle strength and endurance.

Polarity Therapy

Polarity therapy is a gentle and noninvasive approach that allows the body's natural healing energy to return to balance by moving blocked energy. Fatigue can be the result of suppressed emotions and internalized stress, which contribute to blocked energy. Energy blockages reside in muscles, bones, and internal organs. Polarity can provide deep relaxation, improve sleep, and thus improve your energy level.

Psychotherapy

Individual or group psychotherapy has been found effective in helping patients cope with fatigue due to anxiety or stress. The best way to find a psychotherapist is to ask your primary-care physician for a referral.

Relaxation/Meditation

Stress plays a large role in causing fatigue. It is essential for people suffering from fatigue to find ways to reduce the level of stress in their lives. A regular routine of guided imagery, meditation, or deep breathing exercises may promote relaxation, allowing the release of physical and emotional tension. If you don't have the time to take a short nap during the day, set aside time to allow your body and mind to relax. Even short breaks may be beneficial to relieving fatigue.

Therapeutic Massage

Therapeutic massage can help to alleviate fatigue as well as decrease anxiety. Massage reduces stress, promotes a restful night's sleep, and provides a general sense of well-being. To locate a massage therapist, visit the Web site of the American Massage Therapy Association at www.massagetherapy.org or the National Certification Board for Therapeutic Massage and Bodywork (NCBTMB) at www.ncbtmb.org.

Trager Approach

Since it releases patterns of tension and pain as well as muscular restriction, the Trager Approach has been found beneficial in relieving fatigue and promoting a sense of deep relaxation. Emotional tension is also released.

To locate a Trager therapist in your area, visit the Web site of the United States Trager Association (www.trager-us.org) or the Web site for the National Certification Board for Therapeutic Massage and Bodywork (www.ncbtmb.org).

Lifestyle Recommendations

Obtaining sufficient and refreshing sleep is the most important step in preventing fatigue. Going to bed at the same time each day helps to improve the quality of sleep.

Avoid sweets. When you are tired, don't try to obtain energy from eating candy and other sweets. Instead, eat complex carbohydrates such as nuts and fruits. Sweets reduce the levels of amino acids in your blood, which may increase fatigue. On the other hand, complex carbohydrates increase amino acid levels.

Get sufficient sunlight. Obtain adequate amounts of vitamin D through 15 minutes of daily exposure to sunlight. This may lift your spirits and give you an energy boost. Even when it is cold outside, take the time to bundle up and breathe in some fresh air.

Include exercise in your daily routine. You may think that exercise will increase fatigue. On the contrary, over time, if you exercise regularly, you will reduce your level of fatigue. Any form of gentle exercise that increases levels of endorphins (brain chemicals that serve as the body's natural opiate or painkiller) is beneficial in reducing anxiety and stress and promoting a general feeling of well-being and increased stamina.

If you have been relatively inactive, begin gradually with brief walks of 10 to 20 minutes per day. Work up to longer walks and other activities that enable you to get fresh air. Exercise may be particularly useful if you have a sedentary job or lead a sedentary lifestyle. Swimming, bicycling, tai chi, yoga, and qigong are other forms of movement that may be effective in reducing fatigue.

One caveat: Avoid exercising too late in the evening. It may impair your ability to obtain restful sleep.

Make time for adequate sleep. If you have trouble falling asleep, try creating a sleep routine. Before going to bed, drink a cup of chamomile tea and take a warm bath. To help your mind relax, listen to soothing music. Lie in bed and take deep, slow abdominal breaths: Let your belly become fully extended and slowly exhale through your mouth. Tell yourself that you are tired and ready to go to sleep.

Make your bedroom sleep-friendly. You will probably sleep better if your bedroom is cool, dark, and quiet. It should be peaceful and relaxing. Eliminate clutter and electronic equipment; don't bring work into the bedroom. It should be solely suited to sleep. Try to awaken around the same time each day. It is okay to nap, but keep your naps short and take them earlier in the day.

Simplify your lifestyle. Fatigue may be exacerbated by stress and inadequate amounts of sleep. To better manage your life, limit your responsibilities, if possible. Having too much to do may cause you to feel overwhelmed. It may be useful to make lists to help you stay focused and not feel that you need to remember everything. In addition, as you complete tasks, you can cross them off, which enables you to see progress.

Preventive Measures

Avoid caffeinated drinks. Caffeine may remain in your system for more than 10 hours, thereby causing a major disruption in your sleep pattern. Further, caffeine robs the body of magnesium, and magnesium deficiency is a major contributor to fatigue.

Change your routine. Spice up your life—change the furnishings in a room or make small variations to your daily routine. This may give you a psychological boost and relieve fatigue and the sense of being in a rut.

Eat breakfast. Don't skip breakfast—your body needs the fuel to get going for the day.

Get some ventilation. If you live or work in a warm, dry environment with poor ventilation, get some fresh air. Take necessary breaks to cool down. Drink plenty of fluids.

Pace yourself. When working or doing chores, make time for periodic breaks. Don't try to do everything at breakneck speed.

Stop smoking. By inhibiting the delivery of oxygen to tissues, smoking robs the body's energy, which only increases fatigue.

Take time for yourself. Each day, find a few minutes to do something for yourself. It may be as simple as 20 minutes of quiet reading, relaxing in a bath, or taking a walk to breathe in some fresh air. Whatever it is, it must be just for you.

Female Sexual Dysfunction

Simply described, female sexual dysfunction (FSD) is a disorder in which a woman has a problem with some aspect of sex. There are four types of FSD: desire, arousal, orgasmic, and pain. With desire disorders, there is a loss of interest in having sex. In arousal disorders, there is a lack of sexual response. Orgasmic disorders occur when a woman is unable to have an orgasm or has pain with an orgasm. With sexual pain disorders, a woman has pain during or after sex. Each of these types have three subtypes: lifelong versus acquired; generalized versus situational; and organic, psychogenic, mixed, or unknown etiologic origin. According to a report in the August 23, 2007, issue of the *New England Journal of Medicine*, about half of older adult women reported one bothersome sexual problem. However, only 22 percent of women reported having discussed sex with a physician since age 50 years.

Female sexual dysfunction is believed to be quite common. Though statistics vary, it has been estimated that almost 40 percent of all women report some form of FSD at some point in their lives.

Causes and Risk Factors

There are a number of physical and psychological causes for sexual dysfunction, and fre-quently, these interact with one another. The causes include medications, diseases such as diabetes or high blood pressure, alcohol use, depression, and vaginal infections. After menopause, with the loss of the female hormone estrogen and the thinning and shrinking of the vaginal tissues, women may have a diminished interest in sex. They may also have a slower response to sex and more vaginal dryness. Sex may be painful, and since the vaginal area is less acidic, there is an increased risk for infections. Female sexual dysfunction may also be caused by a present or past unhappy or abusive relationship or other emotional problems.

A survey of US adults on sexual behavior found that women who had less than a high school education were more likely than college graduates to have a lack of interest in sex. Compared to women who had never married or were widowed or divorced, married women had lower rates of FSD. White and Hispanic women had fewer issues with FSD than

Though there is a loss of the female hormone estrogen with menopause, testosterone continues to be manufactured. So many menopausal women do not experience a loss of interest in sex.

- ☐ **General disinterest in sex**
- ☐ **Difficulty with becoming aroused and having orgasms**
- ☐ **Vaginal dryness**
- ☐ **Pain with sex**

African American women. However, white women had slightly higher rates of sexual pain. Smoking increases the risk for all women.

Signs and Symptoms

There are several symptoms associated with female sexual dysfunction. These include a general disinterest in sex, difficulty with becoming aroused and having orgasms, vaginal dryness, and pain with sex.

Self-Testing

Easy to obtain online, the Female Sexual Function Index (FSFI) may help you to determine if you have female sexual dysfunction (you may find it at www.fsfiquestionnaire.com). However, if you have been experiencing the previously noted symptoms for more than a few months and believe that you may have the condition, you should discuss your situation and share the results of your completed FSFI with your doctor.

Conventional Treatments

Treatments vary according to the cause of the FSD.

Hormone Therapy

If your levels of estrogen are low, you may benefit from hormone replacement therapy. (See Menopause on page 368.) However, when a woman still has her uterus, estrogen therapy must be combined with progesterone, which is known to decrease sexual desire.

Since the hormone testosterone increases sexual desire, some people advocate that it be used for FSD, but the use of testosterone is controversial. And testosterone may have potential side effects, such as acne, weight gain, abnormal hair growth (hirsutism), lowering of high-density lipoprotein cholesterol, deepening of the voice, and enlarging of the clitoris.

Pain Relief

If female sexual dysfunction is associated with a good deal of vaginal pain, you may benefit from the use of lubricants, vaginal estrogens, moist heat to the genital area, and topical lidocaine. You may also consider experimenting with different sexual positions, until you find one that is more comfortable for you.

Psychotherapy

If the FSD is probably psychological, individual and couples therapy may be helpful.

Be sure that your therapist has training and experience in sexual dysfunction.

Complementary Treatments

Complementary medicine works toward reducing and eliminating the symptoms of sexual dysfunction while also determining the cause.

Acupuncture

Acupuncture releases endorphins, which have a positive effect on the nervous system and help with anxiety, depression, stress, and insomnia, all of which may result in sexual dysfunction. In addition, acupuncture rebalances the hormonal system.

Diet

Maintaining a low-fat, high-fiber diet that includes lots of fresh vegetables, fruits, and grains supplies the body with the necessary nutrients to maintain physical and emotional health. A healthy diet may also prevent conditions that cause sexual dysfunction, such as diabetes and high blood pressure, while helping to replace estrogen lost after menopause. To compensate for the body's low estrogen, it may be useful to eat certain foods that are high in phytoestrogens, particularly soy. Soy contains a class of phytoestrogens known as isoflavones (genistein, daidzein, and glycitein), which act as weak estrogen and decrease vaginal dryness. Soy milk, tofu, soybeans, tempeh, and miso are excellent ways to reap the benefits. Substituting soy protein for animal protein may also benefit the cardiovascular system.

Other foods containing phytoestrogens include alfalfa, almonds, anise seeds, apples, barley, beans, beets, berries, carrots, cashews, cherries, clover, cucumbers, dates, eggplants, fennel, flaxseeds, garlic, lentils, oats, olives, parsley, peanuts, peas, peppers, plums, pomegranates, rhubarb, sage, sesame seeds, sunflower seeds, tomatoes, yams, and whole grains.

Essential fatty acids (EFAs) are useful in maintaining hormonal balance and preventing vaginal dryness. EFAs may be found in salmon, bluefish, herring, mackerel, tuna, cod, almonds, peanuts, walnuts, and sunflower seeds. Flaxseed oil is also a good source of essential fatty acids.

Herbal Medicine

Black cohosh. Black cohosh, which is the natural alternative to hormone replacement therapy, may be taken in capsule form. The minimum recommended daily dose is 20 milligrams in the morning and 20 milligrams at night of standardized extract of 2.5 percent triterpene glycosides. Your doctor may advise a higher dose. Black cohosh can help reduce irritability, anxiety, and depression. Further, it lowers cholesterol levels and blood pressure. Expect to take black cohosh for about 4 weeks before you notice any improvement.

Chasteberry. Chasteberry contains estrogen- and progesterone-like compounds. Through its effect on the pituitary gland, chasteberry may balance hormones and alleviate depression. Look for products containing 0.5 percent agnuside, the active ingredient. Take 400 milligrams a day.

Dong quai and Asian ginseng. Dong quai and Asian ginseng are herbs with estrogenic properties that may increase libido. Dong quai promotes relaxation and strengthens blood vessels. The recommended daily dose is 200 milligrams three times a day of extract standardized to 0.8 to 1.1 percent ligustilide. However, if you are taking a prescription blood-thinning medication, be sure to consult your doctor before taking dong quai supplements. Asian ginseng is effective for decreasing mental and physical fatigue and increasing energy. The recommended daily dose is 100 to 200 milligrams, standardized to 4 to 7 percent ginsenosides. However, do not use ginseng if you have high blood pressure, heart disorders, or hypoglycemia.

Ginkgo biloba. Ginkgo improves bloodflow to the extremities and brain. It may alleviate fatigue and depression; it has been proven useful for sexual dysfunction caused by antidepressant medications. It is sold raw or in capsule form. However, if you are taking prescription blood-thinning medication, be sure to consult your doctor before taking ginkgo supplements. The recommended daily dose is 120 milligrams, twice a day, of extract standardized to 24 percent of flavone glycosides and 6 percent terpene lactones.

Maca. Maca is a perennial crop from Peru that has been used for centuries. It is grown at elevations of 12,000 feet and higher, is in the same family as turnips and radishes, and is a highly nutritious food. It has an overall nutritive effect that improves physical vitality, endurance, and stamina. Maca can be useful for the treatment of female sexual dysfunction because of its ability to fuel the endocrine system so that it can produce its own hormones. It is available in capsule form. The recommended daily dose is 550 milligrams twice a day.

Hypnosis

Hypnosis has been proven successful for treating sexual dysfunction and is most useful when the cause of the dysfunction is psychological rather than physical. For more information and to locate a practitioner in your area, visit the Web site of the American Society of Clinical Hypnosis (www.asch.net).

Nutritional Supplements

Nutritional supplements can help alleviate symptoms associated with sexual dysfunction.

- Multivitamin/mineral: Take as directed on the label. Necessary to maintain proper levels of nutrients. Should include magnesium and zinc.

- Vitamin A: 10,000 IU daily. Strengthens mucous membranes and reduces vaginal dryness. Take with vitamin E.

- B-complex vitamins: Take as directed on the label. Maintain energy and reduce anxiety, depression, insomnia, and loss of libido.

- Vitamin C: 1,000 milligrams daily in divided doses of 500 milligrams each.

- Vitamin E: 400 IU daily. Assists the body in maintaining synthetic or natural estrogen.

- Evening primrose oil: 3,000 milligrams daily in divided doses of 1,000 milligrams each to provide 240 milligrams of GLA (gamma-linolenic acid). Improves blood-flow and prevents vaginal dryness.

- Omega-3 fatty acids: 1 tablespoon flaxseed oil daily or 2,000 milligrams fish oil capsule twice a day. Reduces vaginal dryness.

Polarity Therapy

Polarity therapy has been shown to be valuable in the treatment of sexual dysfunction, particularly when the dysfunction is related to suppressed emotions. Suppressed emotions and internalized stress are some of the major causes of blocked energy. Energy blockages reside in muscles, bones, and internal organs. Polarity is a gentle and noninvasive approach that allows the body's natural healing energy to return to balance.

Relaxation/Meditation

Stress may have a direct effect on sexual function. Therefore, any form of meditation or relaxation in which the mind is focused on a particular object, sound, visualization, breath, or activity is useful for reversing the body's fight-or-flight response to stress. You may meditate while you are lying down or in a seated position. Be sure to sit properly—upright, with your back straight, on a chair or the floor. Yoga and tai chi are considered meditation in movement and help relax muscles, quiet the mind, and create inner peace.

Therapeutic Massage

Massage helps to reduce stress, promote relaxation, and increase circulation. To locate a massage therapist, visit the Web site of the American Massage Therapy Association at www.massagetherapy.org or the National Certification Board for Therapeutic Massage and Bodywork (NCBTMB) at www.ncbtmb.org.

Yoga

Studies have found that yoga is beneficial for insomnia, depression, and vaginal problems. The postures increase flexibility and improve coordination and balance while strengthening the muscles and increasing blood circulation. The deep breathing exercises that are part of a yoga session increase blood circulation and elevate the level of endorphins released in the brain.

Lifestyle Recommendations

As with many medical disorders, lifestyle changes coupled with treatment for a specific medical issue may be necessary.

Address any medical problems. If a medical problem is causing your FSD, obtain an appropriate treatment. For example, better management of diabetes should lead to improvement in your FSD symptoms.

Be realistic. To achieve sexual satisfaction, midlife women often need more time for foreplay.

Communicate. Share your feelings about sex with your partner. Which aspects of sex do you prefer? Which would you like to avoid? What makes it easier for you to become aroused?

Drink water. Drinking lots of water throughout the day may help decrease vaginal dryness.

Exercise. People who exercise regularly tend to be in better physical shape and have a more positive approach toward all aspects of life.

Help yourself sleep better. If you have been having trouble sleeping, don't exercise at night or drink caffeinated beverages after lunch. Learn some relaxation techniques, such as deep breathing and guided imagery.

Try over-the-counter lubricants. If you are experiencing vaginal dryness, purchase some over-the-counter water-based vaginal lubricants such as Astroglide or moisturizers such as Replens. And wheat germ oil, which contains vitamin E, may also be used as a lubricant. It may be combined with other soothing oils such as marigold, chamomile, or slippery elm.

Preventive Measures

Check for medication side effects. It may be useful to read the literature that accompanies your prescription drugs. One of the potential side effects may be the loss of libido. This is particularly notable for antidepressant medications. In fact, in one study, more than 70 percent of women on antidepressant medication experienced a loss of libido and other sexual dysfunction.

Decrease stress. In all probability, stress plays a key role in many instances of female sexual dysfunction. Find ways to incorporate stress reduction techniques into your daily life.

Don't smoke. Women who smoke are at an increased risk for female sexual dysfunction.

Limit your alcohol use and don't use illicit drugs. The excessive consumption of alcohol, as well as the use of illicit drugs, tends to impair sexual functioning.

Fibromyalgia

Fibromyalgia is a chronic condition characterized by widespread pain in the fibrous tissues of the muscles. There may also be an increased sensitivity to pain, sleep disturbances, and fatigue. Though you may be diagnosed with fibromyalgia without these problems, in general, at least 11 of 18 specific areas of your body feel pain when exposed to pressure. Moreover, the generalized pain continues for a minimum of 3 months. Though the symptoms tend to be persistent and may be disabling and last for extended periods of time, fibromyalgia is not a progressive disease and it is not life-threatening.

Fibromyalgia is believed to affect 6 million to 8 million people in the United States (about 2 percent of the American population). About 80 percent of those are women.

Over the years, fibromyalgia has been known by a number of different names, such as chronic muscle pain syndrome, psychogenic rheumatism, and tension myalgias. Today, it may also be called fibromyositis, fibrositis, and myofascial pain syndrome. Physicians tend to divide fibromyalgia into two main groups, primary and secondary fibromyalgia. With primary fibromyalgia, which is also called idiopathic fibromyalgia, the cause is not determined. On the other hand, with secondary fibromyalgia, the cause is identified.

Causes and Risk Factors

Researchers believe that there are a number of potential causes of fibromyalgia. Some say it is the result of chemical changes in the brain, specifically alterations in the regulation of certain brain chemicals known as neurotransmitters. Two commonly mentioned neurotransmitters are serotonin (low levels of which are linked to depression, gastrointestinal upset, and migraines) and substance P (which is associated with stress, pain, anxiety, and depression).

Other possible causes include injury to the upper spinal region, infection, and abnormalities in the autonomic (sympathetic) nervous system, the system that regulates body functions that are not consciously controlled. Since people with fibromyalgia tend to have low levels of the hormone called somatomedin C, which plays an important role in the processes by which the body rebuilds itself (as it does during sleep), it has also been speculated that fibromyalgia is linked to sleep disturbances.

Women, especially those between the ages of 20 and 60, have a higher risk of developing fibromyalgia compared to men. There is also an increased risk associated with disturbed sleep patterns or a family history of the disease.

Signs and Symptoms

While the symptoms of fibromyalgia tend to differ from person to person, there are a few that appear to occur more often. When pressure is applied to certain areas of the body, there may be widespread pain that persists for months at a time. The pain is often felt in the upper chest, upper back and neck, back of the head, elbows, hips, and knees. The pain is frequently accompanied by stiffness.

People with fibromyalgia are fatigued. They have sleep problems, such as restless legs syndrome or periodic leg movements of sleep (PLMS). With restless legs syndrome, there are spontaneous, continuous leg movements while at rest; there are also tingling sensations. With PLMS, there are involuntary jerking leg movements during sleep.

About 40 to 70 percent of people with fibromyalgia have irritable bowel syndrome (IBS), with symptoms such as constipation, diarrhea, abdominal pain, and bloating; about half have chronic headaches and facial pain; and about half have a heightened sensitivity to odors, noises, bright lights, changes in weather, and some foods. Other symptoms associated with fibromyalgia include dizziness, irritable bladder, difficulty concentrating, mood changes, chest pain, pelvic pain, dry eyes and mouth, sensation of swollen hands and feet, and numbness or tingling sensations in the hands and feet.

A Quick Guide to Symptoms

- ☐ Widespread pain that persists for months
- ☐ Stiffness
- ☐ Fatigue
- ☐ Sleep problems
- ☐ Irritable bowel syndrome (IBS) or irritable bladder
- ☐ Chronic headaches and facial pain
- ☐ Heightened sensitivity to odors, noises, bright lights, changes in weather, and some foods
- ☐ Dizziness
- ☐ Difficulty concentrating
- ☐ Mood changes
- ☐ Dry eyes and mouth
- ☐ Numbness or tingling sensations in the hands and feet

Conventional Treatments

Managing fibromyalgia usually begins with a mild exercise program. It is probably best if you work with a physical therapist who has experience in treating people with fibromyalgia. Be sure to start slowly—don't try to do too much too soon, which may overtax your body and leave you unable to exercise. Your routine should include aerobic and strength-training exercises.

Cognitive-Behavioral Therapy (CBT)

Cognitive-behavioral therapy (CBT) seeks to alter an individual's distorted impressions of the world and to stop self-defeating behaviors. For individuals who are dealing with the symptoms of fibromyalgia, it may help to prioritize responsibilities and focus on those that must be accomplished. Usually, cognitive-behavioral therapy includes 6 to 20 one-hour sessions with a therapist. Programs tend to include the following elements.

- **Keeping a diary.** By recording your daily events, you will be able to observe those factors that tend to exacerbate your symptoms. You may also be able to determine those factors that have beneficial effects on your symptoms.

- **Confronting your negative thoughts.** You will be shown how to deal with and reverse pessimistic feelings.

- **Setting limits.** You will learn how to assume manageable amounts of work and not overtax yourself with too much to do.

- **Pursuing pleasurable activities.** You will be taught how to select low-energy activities that you enjoy.

- **Prioritizing.** You will be trained to complete what is most necessary and drop or delegate what you do not need to do.

- **Accepting your relapses.** Relapses are part of your disease. When they occur, take extra care of yourself.

Medications

Antidepressants. Two main classes of antidepressants are used for fibromyalgia, tricyclics and selective serotonin reuptake inhibitors (SSRIs). The tricyclics tend to be better at reducing pain, while the SSRIs are more effective for depression. Often, the medica-

Differentiating between Fibromyalgia and Other Conditions

The symptoms of fibromyalgia may be similar to those of a number of other medical problems, including lupus, multiple sclerosis, osteoarthritis, hypothyroidism, peripheral neuropathy, sleep apnea, restless legs syndrome, rheumatoid arthritis, and some psychiatric disorders (such as major depression). If you have the symptoms of fibromyalgia, your doctor will likely want to perform tests that may help differentiate between fibromyalgia and these other disorders.

tions work best when they are combined. There is good evidence that amitriptyline, a tricyclic, may be quite useful, and fluoxetine, an SSRI, may be somewhat useful. Important characteristics of these drugs are as follows.

The most common tricyclic used for fibromyalgia is amitriptyline (Elavil, Endep). Since amitriptyline tends to lose its effectiveness over time, other tricyclics may be tried. These include imipramine (Tofranil), amoxapine (Asendin), doxepin (Sinequan), desipramine (Norpramin), and nortriptyline (Pamelor, Aventyl). Normally, low doses are prescribed, so any side effects are generally not severe. Still, reported side effects include blurred vision, dry mouth, weight gain, difficulty in urinating, drowsiness, dizziness, disturbances in heart rhythm, and sexual dysfunction. Overdoses may be life-threatening.

SSRIs increase the levels of serotonin in the brain, which improves sleep, fatigue, and sense of well-being. Examples are fluoxetine (Prozac), sertraline (Zoloft), fluvoxamine (Luvox), and paroxetine (Paxil). To avoid insomnia, SSRIs should be taken in the morning. Reported side effects include nausea, agitation, and sexual dysfunction.

Estrogen therapy. Menopausal women who take estrogen therapy tend to sleep better than those who do not. They have longer periods of REM sleep and fewer wakeful times. Estrogen should be taken at bedtime.

Muscle relaxants. Although it should not be used for more than 3 weeks, the muscle relaxant cyclobenzaprine (Flexeril) may bring relief from muscle spasms when taken at bedtime. Potential side effects include dry mouth, drowsiness, and dizziness. If you are taking a monoamine oxidase (MAO) inhibitor, a type of medication prescribed for depression, you should *not* take cyclobenzaprine.

Pain relievers. Mild fibromyalgia pain may be treated with acetaminophen (the active ingredient in Tylenol and other over-the-counter products). Since pain from fibromyalgia is not caused by inflammation, anti-inflammatory drugs, such as aspirin and ibuprofen (Advil and others), tend to be less useful.

Though some physicians prescribe opioids (narcotic pain relievers) for their patients with fibromyalgia, many believe that this practice is unwise. These drugs pose a serious risk of addiction. Instead, doctors may advise using the pain reliever tramadol (Ultram), which is less likely to be addictive. Potential side effects include gastrointestinal disturbances such as nausea and diarrhea, as well as mood changes.

Prepared from an extract of hot chili peppers, capsaicin ointment (Zostrix) may be helpful for the relief of muscle pain. It is thought to be useful for some people with fibromyalgia.

Sleep medications. There are two sleep medications that tend to be useful for those with fibromyalgia, zolpidem (Ambien) and zaleplon (Sonata). You may wish to discuss these with your doctor.

Psychotherapy

Individual or group psychotherapy has been found to be effective in helping patients cope with depression and the mood changes associated with fibromyalgia. Be sure to request a therapist who has experience treating patients with this disorder.

Stretching Techniques

There are two main types of stretching techniques for fibromyalgia. In both cases, they require the assistance of another person.

With the first technique, tender points are sprayed with either ethyl chloride (Chloroethane) or Fluori-Methane. These cool the blood vessels, thereby inactivating the tender points. The person who is assisting may then stretch the muscle.

In the second type of stretching, an anesthetic (such as lidocaine) is injected directly into the tender points. While the injections may cause sudden intense pain, once the medication takes effect, muscles are able to be stretched. Nevertheless, the tender points may be left with some residual soreness. These injections, which are administered by a medical professional, may be repeated two or three times over 6 to 8 weeks.

Complementary Treatments

Complementary medicine may play a leading role in alleviating and reducing many of the symptoms associated with fibromyalgia.

Acupuncture

Studies show that acupuncture is effective for the treatment of fibromyalgia in helping to decrease pain, anxiety, and fatigue. The National Institutes of Health recommends acupuncture as a treatment for fibromyalgia. People with fibromyalgia generally have lower than normal levels of endorphins (natural body chemicals that reduce pain). Acupuncture treatments help to release endorphins into the system. Individuals suffering from fibromyalgia may prefer the limited amount of touch involved in the approach, particularly during a period of severe hypersensitivity.

Aquatic Therapy

Therapeutic exercises conducted in warm water are beneficial for people with a number of the symptoms associated with fibromyalgia. In particular, Watsu, a form of shiatsu massage performed in chest-high warm water, is very useful for decreasing pain and promoting relaxation.

Biofeedback

Biofeedback uses an electric monitoring device to obtain data on vital body functions. During a session, you will be taught ways to use relaxation techniques to alter or slow the body's signals. Biofeedback is an appropriate treatment approach for the physical and emotional symptoms of fibromyalgia, such as anxiety, headaches, muscular pain, and stress-related disorders. Various health care professionals incorporate biofeedback into their practice, including psychiatrists, psychologists, social workers, nurses, physical therapists, occupational therapists, speech therapists, respiratory therapists, exercise physiologists, and chiropractors.

It is recommended that you seek a health care practitioner who has been certified through the Biofeedback Certification Institute of America (BCIA). To locate a practitioner in your area, look on the BCIA Web site at www.bcia.org, or check your local hospitals, medical clinics, or in the Yellow Pages under the practitioners mentioned above.

Craniosacral Therapy

Craniosacral therapy (CST) is the hands-on gentle manipulation of the craniosacral system—the brain, spinal cord, cerebrospinal fluid, dural membrane, cranial bones, and the sacrum. Craniosacral therapy can be useful for chronic fatigue, depression, anxiety, facial pain, and headaches, all of which are major symptoms of fibromyalgia. To search for a qualified therapist in your area, visit the Web site of the International Association of Healthcare Practitioners at www.iahp.com.

Diet

Eating a diet rich in whole foods, including lots of raw fruits and vegetables, is helpful for people with fibromyalgia. Try to include a minimum of five servings of vegetables, four servings of fruit, and six servings of whole grains each day. Highly processed foods and other foods containing additives and other chemicals will only aggravate this condition. Try to include a wide variety of organically grown foods in your diet.

Sugar, in particular, should be eliminated from the diet, as it interferes with the absorption of calcium and magnesium in the body, two minerals necessary for muscle health. People with fibromyalgia may already be deficient in these two minerals and do not need to lose any through drinking or eating products containing sugar.

Exercise

Exercise is a natural way of increasing the body's levels of endorphins and serotonin and improving sleep quality. Any form of gentle exercise is beneficial in reducing pain and stiffness in the muscles, as well as increasing flexibility and muscle strength. Walking, swimming, bicycling, tai chi, yoga, and qigong are forms of movement that are particularly effective for fibromyalgia. Try to exercise at least 40 minutes each day.

Herbal Medicine

Herbal medicine may be useful for boosting the immune system, removing toxins from the body, increasing energy, reducing anxiety and inflammation, and relieving insomnia, all of which may be associated with fibromyalgia.

If you suffer with irritable bowel syndrome, a cup of chamomile tea may help you relax and is soothing to the gastrointestinal tract. Drinking peppermint tea throughout the day may be useful for relieving abdominal spasms.

Grape seed extract. Grape seed extract contains flavonoids called procyanidolic oligomers or PCOs (also known as proanthocyanidins). Often referred to as PAC, grape seed extract is a valuable antioxidant that rids the body of damaging free radicals and helps protect muscle cells. Large numbers of those who suffer from fibromyalgia have lowered immune systems and constant muscular pain and tension. The typical recommended dose is 100 milligrams in capsule form, three times a day, of extract standardized to contain 92 to 95 percent PCOs.

Green tea. Green tea is a powerful antioxidant that may help boost the compromised immune systems of those with fibromyalgia. Try to drink several cups of green tea every day.

Panax ginseng. Siberian ginseng fights

fatigue by increasing stamina. Look for products standardized to contain at least 7 percent ginsenosides. Take 100 milligrams three times daily.

Passionflower and valerian root. Passionflower and valerian root calm the central nervous system, thereby relieving the anxiety and insomnia that may accompany fibromyalgia. They are available in prepared tea bags and tinctures and as dried herbs. For passionflower, look for products containing no less than 0.8 percent total flavonoids. As a tincture, take 1 to 4 milliliters in the evening to increase sleepiness. When using the dried herb, pour 1 cup of boiling water over 1 teaspoon of the dried herb, and steep for 10 to 15 minutes. Drink before bedtime. When taking valerian root, look for products containing 0.8 percent valeric/valerenic acid. Since valerian may have a bitter taste and strong odor, you may prefer to take it in capsule form. Take 400 to 450 milligrams 1 hour before bedtime. As with echinacea and goldenseal, passionflower and valerian are often rotated, using one for 2 weeks and then switching to the other. It may take several weeks of regular use for valerian to take effect. If you are taking other sleep-inducing products, before beginning a regimen of either passionflower or valerian, check with your doctor.

Nutritional Supplements

Many nutritional supplements help reduce symptoms associated with fibromyalgia as well as provide the necessary nutrients that are often deficient.

- Multivitamin/mineral: Take as directed on the label. Supplement should contain potassium and calcium as deficiency leads to increased fatigue. Should not contain iron.

- B-complex vitamins: Take as directed on the label. Important to regulation of energy and vitality. Often lost due to stress and unhealthy diet. Must be replenished as they are not stored in the body.

- Vitamin B_{12}: 1,000-microgram sublingual tablet daily. Necessary due to inability to absorb adequate amounts of B_{12}. Injections of B_{12} may be more beneficial for this condition.

- Vitamin C: 1,000 milligrams daily in divided doses of 500 milligrams each. Supports adrenal glands and strengthens immune system.

- Vitamin E: 400 IU daily. Stimulates immune system and helps reduce restless legs syndrome.

- Omega-3 fatty acids such as flaxseed oil or fish oil: 1 tablespoon of flaxseed oil daily *or* 4,000 milligrams daily of fish oil capsules. Aids in the reduction of inflammation.

- Evening primrose oil: 3,000 milligrams daily in divided doses of 1,000 milligrams each to provide 240 milligrams of GLA (gamma-linolenic acid). Aids in the reduction of inflammation.

- Magnesium: 500 milligrams daily. Deficiency of this mineral is linked to chronic fatigue. Take before bed.

- Zinc: 30 milligrams daily. Combats fatigue, improves muscle strength and endurance.

Polarity Therapy

A gentle and noninvasive approach that allows the body's natural healing energy to return to balance, polarity therapy is especially useful for patients suffering from severe muscular tenderness. By visiting the Web site of the American Polarity Therapy Association at www.polaritytherapy.org, you will be able to search for a practitioner in your area.

Relaxation/Meditation

If you have fibromyalgia, it is essential to find ways to reduce the level of stress in your life. A regular routine of guided imagery, meditation, or deep breathing exercises will promote relaxation, allowing the release of physical and emotional tension. To create a temporary escape, close your eyes and imagine being in a place or doing an activity that you enjoy. The goal is to tell your mind to enjoy itself instead of focusing on pain and worries. Find the forms of meditation that are easy for you to commit to and practice daily.

Therapeutic Massage

Several studies of the effects of therapeutic massage on patients with fibromyalgia have found that it helps alleviate symptoms. Therapeutic massage has been known to decrease pain, stiffness, anxiety, fatigue, depression, and difficulty sleeping.

Trager Approach

The Trager Approach releases patterns of tension and pain as well as muscular restriction, helping to reduce fatigue, release emotional tension, and promote a sense of deep relaxation. Movements are adjusted according to the specific needs of the individual. It is a passive treatment and enables muscle tightness to be released without pain. Over time, the body's nervous system is reeducated to respond in the proper manner to relieve pain and discomfort.

Yoga

The gentle stretches, postures, deep breathing, and meditation done during a yoga session offer an uplifting effect to the body without draining energy. It is an excellent form of exercise for fibromyalgia sufferers.

Lifestyle Recommendations

There are a number of measures you may take to make it easier to deal with fibromyalgia and its effects.

Change your lifestyle. Simplify your lifestyle. The symptoms of fibromyalgia are made worse by stress and inadequate sleep. Limit your responsibilities so that you can better manage your life. On the days that you feel better, don't overdo it. If you do, you will feel much worse the next day.

Consider an elimination diet. Attempt to determine which foods trigger your condition by trying an elimination diet. For the first 10 days, eliminate all citrus fruits and foods containing corn, dairy, egg, and gluten (wheat, oats, barley, and rye). After 7 to 10 days, if your symptoms remain unchanged, you probably do not have a sensitivity to these foods. If, however, your symptoms do improve and you find that you have more energy and a better mood, then you need to start returning these food groups back into your diet, one at a time, every 3 to 4 days. This will enable you to determine the culprit or culprits causing a reaction. During this time, keeping a food journal will help you track your symptoms.

Spend time outdoors. Fifteen minutes of daily exposure to sunlight will help you obtain adequate amounts of vitamin D. This may lift your spirits and give you an energy boost. Even when it is cold outside, bundle up and breathe in some fresh air.

Find time for yourself. Each day, find a few minutes to do something for yourself. It may be as simple as 20 minutes of quiet reading, relaxing in a bath, or taking a walk to breathe in some fresh air. Whatever it is, it must be just for you.

Get enough sleep. Try to establish a regular sleep routine. If you have trouble becoming sleepy, it may be useful to create a sleep environment. Drink a cup of chamomile tea and, right before going to bed, take a warm bath. To help your mind relax, listen to soothing music. Lie in bed and take deep, slow abdominal breaths, letting your belly become fully extended and slowly exhaling through your mouth. Tell yourself you are tired and ready to go to sleep.

If you need additional help, try taking 2 to 3 milligrams of melatonin 1 hour before bedtime.

Join a support group. When dealing with a chronic, debilitating disease like fibromyalgia, you may benefit from talking to others who are facing similar challenges. Support groups are excellent for this. You may also learn about new treatments and coping mechanisms.

Ensure proper hydration. Be sure to drink a lot of fluids, especially water. Proper hydration helps prevent constipation, which may cause fatigue. Water flushes the system and removes toxins from the body, a buildup of which may cause fatigue and muscular pain.

Stay active. Remaining as mentally and socially active as possible is an important part of recovery from fibromyalgia. People with fibromyalgia who leave their jobs and remove themselves from all social activity tend to have worse outcomes than those who remain more active.

Stop smoking. By inhibiting the delivery of oxygen to tissues, smoking robs the body of energy, which only increases fatigue. If you smoke, quit. And try your best to avoid secondhand smoke.

Flatulence

More commonly known as gas, flatulence is the passage of air or gas (flatus) from the intestines through the rectum. The gas is primarily composed of oxygen, nitrogen, hydrogen, carbon dioxide, and methane, which are all odorless substances. Flatulence becomes problematic when it occurs at socially unacceptable times or has a foul smell. The smell comes from other, sulfur-containing gases that are produced in the colon by decomposing food. Also, some people are more aware of gas than others, and they may be more bothered by it.

From the time you are a few days old until you die, your body produces gas. Each day, an average adult releases between a pint and a half-gallon of flatulence. In a study, 10 healthy adults were given a regular diet plus 7 ounces of baked beans. In a 24-hour period, they passed between 1 pint and 3 pints of gas.

Causes and Risk Factors

Intestinal gas comes from two main sources. Some gas enters the intestines through swallowing. Though this is more likely to occur when you eat or drink quickly, some people simply swallow air throughout the day, especially when they are under stress. Worry, anxiety, and tension may also cause you to swallow more air. In addition, during the digestive process, as food is broken down, gas is formed. Certain foods, such as beans, tend to produce more gas. Because fatty foods slow digestion, they may trigger flatulence as well. Artificial sweeteners, such as sorbitol and mannitol, are known gas producers, and naturally occurring sugar, such as trehalose (in mushrooms) and lactose (in dairy products), may produce gas. People who are constipated are more likely to have gas.

Gas forms more easily when you are lying down. When you are standing, gas is more likely to back up to the esophagus and leave through the mouth. Gas is fairly common after abdominal surgery and may be linked with the excessive use of laxatives or constipating drugs. Antibiotics, which disrupt the balance of intestinal bacteria, may cause gas.

Gas may occur with a number of medical problems such as stomach flu, food poisoning, diverticulitis, intestinal scar tissue (adhesions), internal hernias, irritable bowel syndrome, ulcerative colitis, or Crohn's disease. If people with celiac disease (an autoimmune disorder that requires the elimination of the grain protein gluten from the diet) continue to ingest gluten, they may have significant bouts of flatulence.

As people age, they tend to have more flatulence. Since the pelvic muscles may weaken with age, older adults may have a diminished ability to control flatulence. Prior abdominal surgery or pregnancies may further aggravate the situation.

Signs and Symptoms

With flatulence, there is abdominal bloating that may be accompanied by sharp pains and cramps in the abdomen. This pain is usually relieved when gas is passed. If nausea, vomiting, bleeding, weight loss, or fever accompanies the flatulence, or if the pain is prolonged or severe, you should see your doctor.

Conventional Treatments

Medications

Your doctor may recommend a medication that contains simethicone, such as Mylicon, which reduces stomach gas. Available over the counter, simethicone may help control intestinal gas, particularly for people who swallow air.

Complementary Treatments

Though you cannot prevent gas, you can reduce the amount of gas that you have and restore balance to the digestive system to relieve discomfort.

Aromatherapy

The essential oils of the following herbs have been shown to relieve flatulence: basil, ginger, peppermint, rosemary, and thyme. Place 2 or 3 drops of each in an unscented oil, such

A Quick Guide to Symptoms

☐ **Abdominal bloating**
☐ **Sharp pains and cramps in the abdomen**

as jojoba or almond oil. (If you do not want to purchase a special oil, common household oils such as canola or olive oil are fine.) To combine the oils, place them in a small bottle and gently roll the bottle between your hands.

Gently massage the oil mixture over the abdomen once a day. A warm bath is also helpful. Try any of the essential oils alone or make your own combination using 2 or 3 drops of each. In any of these treatments, whether combining oils or using a single oil, do not use more than a total of 10 drops. The number of drops varies depending on the essential oil; some are very strong and may require only 3 drops in a full bath.

Breathing Exercises

Deep breathing techniques may help relieve gas pain. Lie on your back in a comfortable position. Place a hand on your abdomen and inhale through your nose. If you are breathing correctly, you should feel your hand rise as your abdomen expands, like a balloon filling with air. Exhale slowly through your mouth and feel your abdomen fall as if air is being let out of the balloon. Make this a daily ritual; do it for 10 minutes every day. Deep breathing techniques may also reduce stress and quiet your mind.

Diet

Usually, the first course of action in preventing excess gas is modifying the diet. Reduce the amounts of gas-producing foods that you eat. Some well-known gas-producing foods include apples, apricots, bananas, beans, bran, brussels sprouts, cabbage, cucumbers, melons, oats, onions, peas, prunes, radishes, raisins, wheat, and whole-wheat bread. People who are lactose-intolerant will tend to have gas after eating dairy products. To decrease the amount of gas, it may be helpful to consume dairy products with solid foods or replace dairy with soy products.

If you would like to continue eating legumes or the vegetables previously mentioned, try soaking them in water before cooking. This reduces their gas-producing abilities. Cooking them in a pressure cooker may also be useful. You should also reduce your intake of carbonated beverages, including those containing alcohol, such as beer and sparkling wine.

Herbal Medicine

Carminative herbs. Carminative herbs prevent intestinal gas from forming and may also expel it. A few of these are anise, which may be brewed as a hot tea to relieve flatulence; peppermint, a popular tea that aids digestion; and fennel seeds, which may be sprinkled on food, taken in tea form, or simply chewed to bring relief. If you are using loose herbs to make a tea, place 1 heaping teaspoon of the herb or herbs in a tea strainer or tea ball, and place the strainer or ball in a cup of boiling water. Allow the tea to steep for 4 to 5 minutes.

Parsley. Parsley, which is often used as a garnish in restaurants, is a great digestive aid. Simply chew a sprig or two.

Turmeric. Turmeric is a culinary herb known to reduce flatulence. To make a tea, pour 1 cup of boiling water over 1 teaspoon of powdered turmeric and let steep for 5 minutes. Strain well and drink 2 or 3 cups daily.

Homeopathy

Carbo vegetabilis, *Nux vomica*, and *Lycopodium* are homeopathic remedies that are useful in relieving flatulence. Take one dose of 6C potency 15 minutes before eating and another dose 15 minutes after eating. Let the pellets dissolve under the tongue. While some homeopathic remedies may be available in liquid form, the pellets are very easy to use and may be carried in a purse or pocket for immediate use.

Hydrotherapy

Alternating the application of hot and cold compresses may soothe gas pain and stimulate normal intestinal movement. Soak a washcloth in hot water, ring out the excess water, and place it over your abdomen until it cools. Remove the washcloth and rub an ice cube briskly over the abdomen in a circular motion. (You do not need to follow the path of the colon.) Repeat this process as needed.

Nutritional Supplements

If you want to continue to eat gas-producing foods, you may wish to neutralize their effect with the enzyme alpha-galactosidase, widely sold as Beano. It is available in tablets and drops. Take Beano immediately before you consume the troublesome food. If you are lactose intolerant, take a lactase enzyme before eating a food that is high in lactose.

If the flatulence is the result of antibiotics, *Lactobacillus acidophilus* supplements may help restore the beneficial bacteria in your intestine that the antibiotics destroyed. Acidophilus is available in capsule and powder form and may be found in most health food stores. Simply follow the directions on the bottle. Yogurt and kefir are good sources of acidophilus as well.

Because of their absorptive ability, activated charcoal tablets are believed to reduce the amount of gas in the intestine. The usual recommendation is to take two to four tablets after meals or at the onset of symptoms. They may be taken with liquid or food, whole or chewed. However, because charcoal may also absorb vitamins, minerals, and other medications you are taking, it should be used sparingly.

To guard against possible drug interactions with current medications, to ensure proper dosing, and to avoid conflicts with medical conditions and/or lifestyle factors, consult with a knowledgeable doctor before beginning a regimen of dietary supplements.

Reflexology

Consider nightly foot massages. Either give yourself one or, even better, receive one from your spouse, partner, or friend. Almost the entire sole of the foot correlates to some part of the digestive system—the stomach, liver, gallbladder, pancreas, and intestines. Gently massaging the bottom of the foot may help the entire digestive process. It stimulates regular intestinal contractions, encourages the secretion of digestive enzymes through the pancreas, aids in the secretion of bile by the liver, and releases stored bile from the gallbladder. Be gentle. Pay attention to sensitive areas that feel like tiny crystals under the surface of the skin. Do not avoid these areas; rather, continue working them gently until the area feels smooth. Taking deep breaths may help you through the sore spots.

Yoga

Yoga has been shown to be effective in controlling or eliminating flatulence. Any posture that stretches or compresses the abdomen may stimulate digestion and reduce gas and bloating.

Lifestyle Recommendations

It may be helpful to keep a diary of all of the foods and beverages that you consume, and how your digestive tract responds. By recording the episodes of gas, you may be able to identify the foods that aggravate your digestive system, and then avoid them.

Preventive Measures

Drink peppermint tea. Drink a cup of peppermint tea with meals. Peppermint tea contains menthol, which seems to have an antispasmodic effect on the smooth muscles of the digestive tract. Unfortunately, while it may help with gas, it may foster heartburn and acid reflux. So, if you are dealing with heartburn and acid reflux, you should probably avoid this approach.

Reduce the amount of air you swallow. Take measures to reduce the amount of air you swallow. Chewing gum and eating hard candies are two habits that increase the amount of swallowed air. Further, many of these products may be flavored with sorbitol, which may produce gas. Eat more slowly, and chew thoroughly—when you eat quickly, you take in more air. Also, don't drink through straws, which draw more air into your body, or drink carbonated beverages.

Use digestive aids. Use products that aid digestion. If you are lactose intolerant, use a product such as Lactaid or Dairy Ease that helps with lactose digestion. If you have trouble with high-fiber foods, consider using Beano, which aids fiber digestion. All of these products should be taken immediately before the food is consumed.

Develop healthy eating habits. Chew food slowly and thoroughly, and sit up straight when eating. Do not overeat. Also, try to eat fewer different foods at one sitting. For instance, don't go to a buffet and have one of everything.

Floaters

Floaters are the gray or black spots and opaque dots that appear in your visual field. These spots and dots, which take a wide variety of shapes, may be particularly apparent when you are working at your computer, reading, or viewing a solid, light background. You are even able to see them when your eyes are closed, particularly if the lighting is very bright or you are sitting in the sun.

Generally, floaters are caused by the process of aging. As one ages, miniscule clusters of cells or gel may separate from the eye's vitreous humor (the fluid that fills the eyeball). Floaters are the shadow that these clumps cast on the retina, where the visual images are focused. Some floaters last for years; others may fade in a relatively short period of time.

Floaters are extremely common. Most people have them at one point or another. Though they may be annoying, in the vast majority of cases, floaters are harmless.

Causes and Risk Factors

Your chances of having floaters increase as you age. By the time you reach the age of 60, there is a one in four chance that you will have floaters. At least 65 percent of people in their eighties have them.

Floaters appear to be more common in people who are nearsighted, as well as those who have had cataract surgery. People with diabetes and those who have experienced a head injury are also at greater risk.

Signs and Symptoms

Anyone who has experienced floaters knows exactly what they are like. While you are reading or working at your computer, or sitting outside on a sunny day, spots appear. They seem like small specks or tiny clouds floating outside your eye. The name *floaters* is very appropriate—though they are actually inside your eye, floaters literally float through your field of vision.

Conventional Treatments

Normally, eye care professionals do not treat floaters. There are no medical or surgical treatments, and floaters typically pose no danger. Theoretically, an eye surgeon could perform a vitrectomy, an operation that removes the vitreous. But this operation is risky and poses the risk of complications such as retinal detachment and cataracts. Most surgeons will not perform a vitrectomy to remove everyday floaters. A vitrectomy would be considered only if the floaters seriously impair vision.

It has been suggested that one of the ways

Floaters and Retinal Detachment

Normally, if you see a few floaters, you should not be concerned, especially if you have been experiencing floaters for quite some time. However, if you suddenly note a significant increase in the number of floaters, if the floaters look like white flashing lights, if there is a loss of peripheral vision, or if the floaters appear in all four quadrants of your vision, you should seek immediate attention from an eye care professional. You may have a serious problem, such as a detaching retina.

Retinal detachment may occur when the vitreous fluid separates from the back wall of the eye. Though such a separation is benign, as the vitreous pulls, it may cause a tear in the retina. When there is such a tear, fluid may collect under the retina and result in a detachment. Although there is no pain, blood from the detachment may be leaking into the vitreous, triggering the relatively rapid development of a great many floaters. This is a medical emergency that is treated with surgery. If not treated promptly and properly, it may lead to permanent vision loss. As people age, their risk of retinal detachment increases. People with diabetes also have a higher than normal risk of retinal detachment.

If you are experiencing the symptoms of retinal detachment, you need to seek emergency assistance.

to "treat" floaters is to move your eyes up and down and side to side several times. This could shake up the vitreous and move the floaters out of the field of vision.

Complementary Treatments

Since the process of aging most often causes floaters, prevention requires maintaining a healthy lifestyle and dietary regimen.

Diet

A healthy diet that includes lots of whole grains, vegetables, and fruits and avoids foods high in hydrogenated fats, such as solid vegetable shortening, margarine, and deep-fried foods, is most beneficial in maintaining optimal eye health. Be sure to include foods that contain lots of the carotenoids lutein and zeaxanthin, such as spinach and kale. Try to have at least four or five servings each week; one serving each day is even better. Lutein and zeaxanthin are antioxidants in the carotenoid family and are the only known carotenoids that are present in the human eye, particularly the retina, the macula, and the lens.

Also, consume lots of foods with high amounts of vitamin C. The lens of the eye actually absorbs vitamin C. So, the more vitamin C you consume, the more the lens will contain. Dietary sources of vitamin C include oranges, melons, tomatoes, strawberries, red and green peppers, and sweet potatoes.

Herbal Medicine

Ginkgo biloba and bilberry extract are two herbal remedies that have been shown, through their antioxidant effects, to be useful in maintaining eye health. They both improve the delivery of oxygen to the eyes. The recommended dose of ginkgo is 120 milligrams of standardized extract (6 percent terpene lactones and 24 percent flavone glycosides), taken twice a day in capsule form. However, you should not use ginkgo if you are taking a blood-thinning medication. The recommended dose of bilberry extract is 100 milligrams of 25 percent anthocyanosides, three times a day.

Nutritional Supplements

A number of nutrients have been shown to have a direct effect on the health of the eyes. These nutrients protect the nerves, reducing oxidative damage from sunlight, reducing eye pressure, and preventing vision loss.

- Multivitamin/mineral: Take as directed on the label. Should include copper to balance zinc supplementation.

- Vitamin B_{12}: 100 micrograms daily. Protects nerves.

- Vitamin C: 1,000 milligrams daily in divided doses of 500 milligrams each. Prevents eye damage.

- Vitamin E: 400 IU daily. Protects against free radical damage to the eyes.

- Beta-carotene: 25,000 IU daily. Needed for proper eye function.

- Lutein: 10 milligrams daily. Helps support eye health.

- Selenium: 200 micrograms daily. Important antioxidant that works well with vitamin E.

- Zinc: 30 milligrams daily. Deficiency has been linked to vision disorders.

Reflexology

In reflexology, eye points are located at the base of the second and third toes. Stimulating the area on the toes will help improve circulation to the eyes as well as throughout the body. Tenderness in this area means that circulation to the eye area is blocked. You may even feel what seem to be tiny crystals when working in this area of the foot. If so, continue to apply gentle pressure, moving along the area until it feels smooth.

Traditional Chinese Medicine

Traditional Chinese medicine perceives floaters as a manifestation of congestion in the liver and kidneys. Acupuncture, relaxation techniques, and herbal remedies may all be beneficial. Acupuncture treatment focuses on eliminating the congestion, thereby clearing the eyes and strengthening the tissue of the retina and blood vessels of the eyes. Milk thistle is one of the herbs that is likely to be used—the active ingredient in milk thistle, silymarin, helps maintain healthy liver function. To locate a practitioner trained in traditional Chinese medicine, visit the Web site of the National Certification Commission for Acupuncture and Oriental Medicine (NCCAOM) at www.nccaom.org or the American Association of Acupuncture and Oriental Medicine at www.aaaomonline.org.

Yoga

Netra vyayam are yoga eye exercises that reduce stress and promote relaxation of the eye muscles. You shift your eyes in a series of motions, such as up, down, to the left, to the right, and in a circular motion. Breathing techniques are also used to relax the body and face. Between sets of exercises, the eyes are closed. Exercises are resumed when the eyes feel rested. The exercises end with palming, another yoga practice. Palming allows the eyes to feel soothed from the warmth of the hands. After briskly rubbing your hands together until you feel heat emanating from them, place the palms over your closed eyes in a cupping position. No pressure should be placed on the eyeballs. The warmth and darkness are a soothing end to the eye exercises.

Lifestyle Recommendations

Exercising increases the delivery of nutrients to the eyes and facilitates the removal of waste products. In addition, maintaining a regular exercise program helps reduce stress, which is a common risk factor in developing floaters. The most important type of exercise for promoting eye health is aerobic exercise. Consider walking on a regular basis.

Preventive Measures

When outdoors, wear a hat and sunglasses. Most eye professionals believe that ongoing exposure to sunlight increases the risk of floaters. It is a good idea to wear a protective hat and sunglasses that block out 100 percent of both ultraviolet-A (UVA) and ultraviolet-B (UVB) rays and filter out at least 85 percent of blue-violet sunrays. Be aware that some medications make the skin and eyes more sensitive to light. Ask your doctor if any of your medications have this potential. If you are taking such a medicine, you need to be extra vigilant with hats and sunglasses.

Gallstones

Gallstones are solid deposits that form in the gallbladder or adjacent bile ducts. The gallbladder stores bile, a substance produced in the liver that aids in the digestion of fat. When the body needs to digest fat, the gallbladder contracts and sends the bile into a tube known as the common bile duct. The common bile duct, in turn, carries the bile to the small intestine.

After forming inside the gallbladder, gallstones may leave the gallbladder via the bile ducts, which are collectively known as the biliary tree. The gallbladder and the ducts that transport bile and other digestive enzymes from the liver, gallbladder, and pancreas are collectively known as the biliary system.

If gallstones remain in any of the ducts that bring bile from the liver to the small intestine, they may interfere with the flow of bile. These ducts include the hepatic ducts, which carry bile from the liver into the cystic duct, which takes it to and from the gallbladder. The common bile duct transports bile from the cystic and hepatic ducts to the small intestine. If bile becomes trapped in these ducts, the gallbladder, the ducts, and (rarely) the liver may become inflamed. Since the pancreatic duct opens into the common bile duct, if a gallstone blocks the opening of that duct, there may be a significant amount of painful inflammation with a medical condition called gallstone pancreatitis. If these ducts remain blocked, there is the potential for a serious, life-threatening infection.

About 80 percent of gallstones are white or yellow in color and composed of cholesterol. A smaller percentage are dark brown or black pigment stones that consist of bilirubin (a breakdown product of hemoglobin and blood protein) and calcium salts. Gallstones may be as tiny as a grain of sand or as large as a golf ball. Some are smooth and round, but others are irregular in shape. There are also primary bile duct stones, produced in the bile duct, which tend to be soft and brown in color.

Though many people are unaware that they have them, gallstones are extremely common. It has been estimated that at any given time, they may be found in up to 20 million people in the United States. Approximately 1 million new cases are diagnosed each year.

Causes and Risk Factors

Gallstones are believed to be caused by a number of factors. It is known that gallstones may develop when bile contains too much cholesterol and too little bile salt. But other factors also appear to play a role. If the gallbladder does not release bile, bile may become overconcentrated within the gallbladder.

Also, proteins in the liver and bile may support or inhibit gallstone formation. In addition, people with cirrhosis of the liver have a higher than average risk of developing gallstones. If you have had one gallstone attack, there is a good chance you will have another, although it might not happen again for years.

Because people who are obese tend to have excess amounts of cholesterol in their bile, low bile salts, and lower levels of gallbladder emptying, obesity is thought to be a risk factor for gallstone formation. However, a very low-calorie diet, a rapid weight-loss diet, and prolonged fasting all seem to foster gallstone formation.

Estrogen replacement therapy may increase cholesterol levels in bile and lower gallbladder movement, so it may also be a culprit. Men receiving estrogen therapy as treatment for prostate cancer also have an increased risk for gallstones. Gallstones seem to be associated with diabetes as well. Moreover, when the gallbladder or bile ducts become inflamed or infected as a result of

Even though gallstones are usually composed mostly of cholesterol, there is no conclusive evidence linking blood cholesterol levels with gallstones.

the gallstones, they tend to hurt the nearby pancreas, which makes digestive enzymes and hormones such as blood sugar–regulating insulin.

Women between the ages of 20 and 60 are twice as likely as men of the same age group to have gallstones. Both men and women over the age of 60 have a greater risk than the population in general. Between the ages of 60 and 70, about 16 percent of men and women have gallstones. Certain Native Americans and Mexican Americans are at increased risk for gallstones, while African Americans are at lower than average risk. Because cholesterol-lowering medications increase the amount of cholesterol that is secreted in the bile, those who take these medications have a higher risk. Interestingly, the moderate consumption of coffee, defined as two to three cups per day, appears to reduce the risk in both men and women.

Signs and Symptoms

Most people with gallstones have no symptoms. In fact, only about 1 to 3 percent of those who have gallstones develop symptoms. Still, if a gallstone leaves the gallbladder and becomes stuck in a passageway, you may have severe pain in the upper right portion of your belly as well as in your upper back; this is called biliary colic. The pain generally starts suddenly and continues for as long as 5 hours. Since the gallbladder contracts to release bile in response to fat, pain is most likely to occur after a fatty or greasy meal. The contraction pushes the gallstone against the gallbladder outlet (cystic duct opening). This medical problem is known as a gallstone attack. The pain may occur at night and awaken you from sleep. You may have nausea and vomiting.

A complete or partial blockage from a gallstone may irritate and inflame your gallbladder, a condition known as acute cholecystitis. If this occurs, you may experience the same type of pain that you have during a gallstone attack, and it may continue for days. You may also have a fever. Your skin may turn yellowish in color (jaundice), your urine may be coffee-colored, and your stools may be clay-colored. Other possible symptoms include a rapid heartbeat, fast breathing, and mental confusion. In its most serious state, acute cholecystitis causes an infection that spreads throughout the body, a condition known as septicemia. In about 3 percent of the cases, there may be pus in the gallbladder, which is called empyema. Acute cholecystitis may also result in a perforation of the gallbladder, which is a potentially life-threatening medical problem; this occurs in about 2 percent of cases. The risk of perforation increases if gas has formed in the gallbladder (emphysematous cholecystitis). This occurs more often in people with diabetes. Acute cholecystitis is an emergency condition. When untreated, it may also cause gangrene.

If the stone is lodged in the common bile duct (choledocholithiasis), you may have symptoms similar to those of acute cholecystitis. Again, an infection or cholangitis may occur. This is a medical emergency.

There is also a condition called chronic cholecystitis, in which gallstones cause low-grade inflammation of the gallbladder. Although some people have no symptoms,

A Quick Guide to Symptoms

- ☐ Often no symptoms
- ☐ Severe pain in the upper right portion of the belly and the upper back
- ☐ Pain after a fatty or greasy meal
- ☐ Nausea and vomiting
- ☐ Inflamed gallbladder (acute cholecystitis)

this medical problem may cause symptoms such as gas, nausea, and abdominal discomfort after meals. One study found a correlation between chronic cholecystitis and chronic diarrhea, defined as having 4 to 10 bowel movements every day for at least 3 months.

If you are experiencing symptoms of a gallstone attack, you should seek emergency medical care without delay.

Conventional Treatments

In general, gallstones that have no symptoms require no treatment. These "silent stones" tend to be found during routine tests for other medical problems. Still, there are some people who are at very high risk for complications from gallstones and may wish to have gallstones treated before symptoms appear. This group includes those who have calcified gallbladders and are at greater risk of developing gallbladder cancer, Pima Native Americans, people who have stones larger than 3 centimeters, and those who have large polyps on the gallbladder. On the other hand, if you have symptoms from your gallstones, you need to be treated. In fact, you will be so uncomfortable that you will want to be treated.

If your doctor believes that you have an infection, especially one that is traveling throughout your body, your treatment will likely begin with the administration of intravenous antibiotics. And if you are in pain, you will be given pain medication.

Contact Dissolution Therapy

With contact dissolution therapy, the organic solvent methyl *tert*-butyl ether (MTBE) is injected directly into the gallbladder. Since this is a technically difficult and potentially hazardous procedure, it must be performed by an experienced physician. Still, MTBE does rapidly dissolve the stones. Possible side effects include severe, burning pain that usually lasts for a relatively short period of time.

Endoscopic Balloon Dilation

During endoscopic balloon dilation, which is appropriate for stones that are less than 8 to 10 millimeters in diameter, a tiny deflated balloon is passed into the bile duct to beyond the stone. The balloon is inflated and pulled back, thereby sending the stone and balloon into the small intestine. An endoscopic balloon dilation causes less trauma to the biliary

sphincter. However, sometimes it is not entirely effective and another procedure, such as a lithotripsy, must be used.

Extracorporeal Shock Wave Lithotripsy

In extracorporeal shock wave lithotripsy (ESWL), shock waves are used to break the stones into small crystals that are able to be passed through the bile duct into the intestines. The procedure is best for solitary stones that are less than 2 centimeters (about ¾ inch) in size. Usually, some form of local anesthesia is administered. Then, you are either placed on a soft cushion or partially submerged in water. An ultrasound device is used to generate shock waves that travel through your body and hit the stones. Though you won't feel the shock waves, they do create a great deal of noise. To protect your hearing, you will likely be given headphones or earplugs. Lithotripsy is often combined with bile acid treatment (bile salt tablets).

Potential complications include pain in the area of the gallbladder and the development of pancreatitis within a month of treatment. Further, not all of the stone fragments may clear the bile duct. About 35 percent of the people who undergo this treatment are left with fragments, and the chance of recurrence is high.

Medications

If your doctor believes that surgery is not a good option, bile salt tablets may be prescribed. These are most effective for small cholesterol stones. Ursodiol (Actigall) is one of the safest bile salt tablets, and it appears to have the fewest side effects. But it is expensive and the effects are not permanent. Within 10 years, about half the people who have taken this medication experience a recurrence of gallstones. To avoid a recurrence, ursodiol must be taken continuously.

Surgery

The preferred treatment for gallstones is removal of the gallbladder, a procedure known as a cholecystectomy. It is one of the most common surgical procedures performed in the United States. The gallbladder is not an essential organ; you can live well without it. After a gallbladder is removed, bile flows from the liver via the hepatic ducts into the common duct. From there, it goes into the small intestine.

Following surgery to remove your gallbladder, you may experience more frequent bowel movements and diarrhea. Typically, the symptoms lessen over time. If your diarrhea continues for more than a few weeks, try avoiding dairy products and fried and spicy foods, while gradually adding more fiber to your diet. Other potential complications include bleeding, infections, and injury to the common bile duct.

Laparoscopic cholecystectomy. About 75 percent of all cholecystectomies are performed with a laparoscope, a thin tube with a lighting system and miniature video camera. After making several small incisions in the belly, a surgeon uses a hollow instrument

Since removal of the gallbladder may alter the metabolism of cholesterol by the liver, following surgery you may have elevated levels of cholesterol. You should discuss this with your doctor and have your cholesterol levels periodically checked.

known as a cannula to insert the laparoscope into the abdomen. A magnified view of the inside of the abdomen is then shown on the monitor, and the gallbladder is removed. Because the amount of cutting is so small, recovery is usually fairly quick. You will probably spend no more than one night in the hospital. Within a few days, you should be noticeably better. Potential complications include injury to a bile duct that may result in liver damage, gallstones that are missed or spilled into the abdomen, and infection.

Open cholecystectomy. If the walls of the gallbladder are especially thick or if they have been scarred by previous surgery, the surgeon may recommend the removal of the gallbladder through a large abdominal incision, a procedure known as an open cholecystectomy. This is major surgery, and you will need to spend several days in the hospital. Allow yourself at least 3 weeks of at-home recovery.

In about 5 to 10 percent of the cases, the surgery begins as a laparoscopic cholecystectomy, but, during the procedure, the surgeon decides that an open cholecystectomy is needed. Among the reasons that this may occur are the presence of common bile stones that may not be removed with a laparoscope, injury to major blood vessels, internal structures that are not clearly visible, or unexpected problems that are not correctable with a laparoscope.

Minilaparotomy. The minilaparotomy, which is also known as a minimally invasive open cholecystectomy, is a type of open cholecystectomy in which the incision is much smaller. Patients tend to recover faster and are able to return to work sooner than after a standard open cholecystectomy. The procedure may not be used on people who are obese.

Percutaneous cholecystostomy. A procedure known as percutaneous cholecystostomy is used for people who are unstable and seriously ill with acute cholecystitis and who are medically unable to have emergency surgery. In this procedure, a needle removes fluid from the gallbladder, and a catheter is implanted for 6 to 8 weeks. At the end of that time, the gallbladder may be removed.

Complementary Treatments

Practitioners of complementary medicine attempt to eliminate gallstones, reduce the symptoms, and prevent recurrence through dietary and lifestyle changes, herbal remedies, and other therapies.

Acupuncture

Acupuncture may be extremely effective in stopping the pain associated with gallstones. It is particularly useful in treating the early stages when gallstones are small. To locate an acupuncturist in your area, visit the Web site of the National Certification Commission for Acupuncture and Oriental Medicine (NCCAOM) at www.nccaom.org.

Diet

Studies have shown that women who eat a vegetarian diet that is high in fiber and low in saturated fat have a 50 percent lower incidence of gallstones. Women are three times more likely than men to have gallstones. Therefore, eating a well-balanced diet consisting of lots of whole grains, fruits, vegetables, and soy protein is most beneficial. Further, studies show that people who have a higher intake of trans fatty acids increase their risk of developing gallstones. Try to avoid processed foods, which may be high in fat, and other fatty foods.

Studies have shown that vitamin C is also effective in reducing the risk of gallstones. Vitamin C helps convert cholesterol in the gallbladder into bile, which is then excreted into the intestines. Eating one large orange a day may reduce the risk of stones by 13 percent.

When bile is composed of the appropriate chemicals, stones may be less likely to occur. Turmeric encourages the liver to secrete this appropriate composition. Therefore, it may be helpful to add this herb to cooked foods. In addition, foods such as brewer's yeast, cabbage, cauliflower, chickpeas, egg yolks, lentils, rice, soybeans, and wheat germ contain lecithin, which may help prevent the formation of gallstones.

You may also wish to try an elimination diet or be tested for food allergies. An allergic reaction to certain foods may cause the bile ducts to swell. This, in turn, reduces the flow of bile and causes the pain associated with a gallbladder attack.

Herbal Medicine

Milk thistle. Milk thistle is considered a choleretic herb. Similar to turmeric, it encourages the liver to secrete the appropriate chemical composition of bile, thereby reducing stone formation. Milk thistle is available as an herbal extract, standardized to 70 to 80 percent silymarin. The recommended dose is 280 milligrams of silymarin per day. Since it stimulates gallbladder activity, there may be a mild laxative effect, which should stop in 2 or 3 days.

Peppermint. Peppermint is an herb that aids in the cleansing of the gallbladder and acts as an antispasmodic, soothing the muscles of the digestive tract. During an acute attack, it may be used safely for mild spasms. Take 200 milligrams, three times a day, in capsule form. Note that when there are no symptoms, people with gallstones should not take peppermint, as it may slow the passage of bile.

Naturopathy

Using a combination of dietary advice, herbal remedies, acupuncture, and lifestyle changes, a naturopathic physician may locate the underlying cause of gallstones while offering a variety of treatments to eliminate them.

Contact the American Association of Naturopathic Physicians at www.naturopathic.org to find a practitioner in your area.

Nutritional Supplements

Certain nutritional supplements guard against the development of gallstones as well as enhance the digestive process.

- Multivitamin/mineral: Take as directed on the label. Aids in the optimum function of organs and the digestive process.

- B-complex vitamins: Take as directed on the label. Aids in the digestive process by enhancing nutrient absorption essential to proper function of the digestive organs.

- Vitamin C: 500 milligrams daily. Reduces the risk of developing stones.

- Vitamin E: 400 IU daily. Promotes bile production.

- Lecithin: 500 milligrams before each meal. An essential fatty acid that helps prevent stones from forming.

Lifestyle Recommendations

Try to maintain a steady weight. Studies show that if you keep losing weight and then regaining it, you are placing yourself at higher risk for gallstones. If you need to lose weight, do it slowly—about a pound or two per week is reasonable.

Drink coffee with caffeine. In studies of men age 40 to 75 without a history of gallstone disease, researchers found that drinking 2 to 3 cups of caffeinated coffee per day decreased the risk of developing gallstones.

Preventive Measures

Drink plenty of fluids. Fluids help to dilute bile, inhibiting gallstone formation. Drinking at least eight 8-ounce glasses of water every day is recommended. Herbal teas and juices made from fresh fruit and vegetables are also beneficial.

Eat a healthier diet. Gallstones tend to occur more often in those who eat a high-fat, high-sugar, low-fiber diet.

Exercise. Even in people who are overweight, exercise appears to lower the risk of gallstones. At least three times a week, try to incorporate some form of aerobic exercise into your daily routine. A brisk walk, climbing stairs, swimming, jogging, and bicycling are good choices. If you have been sedentary for some time, you should consult your doctor before beginning any new exercise regimen.

Quit smoking. If you smoke, quit. Smoking has been shown to be a risk factor for developing gallstones.

Stimulate your gallbladder. Each morning, take 1 tablespoon of cold-pressed, extra-virgin olive oil. To eliminate the oily aftertaste, follow the olive oil with a small amount of fresh squeezed lemon. This acts as a jump start for your gallbladder, which will then begin the process of breaking down fats.

Take a daily baby aspirin. Some studies have shown that taking one baby aspirin a day may prevent the recurrence of gallstones. Check with your doctor before adding this to your daily routine.

Take turmeric. Turmeric, an herb that helps prevent gallstones, may be taken in capsule form. The recommended daily dose is 400 milligrams. However, if you are already suffering from gallstones, you should avoid turmeric.

Watch your weight. Especially for women, excess weight appears to play a key role in increasing the risk of gallstones. Being only 20 percent over your ideal weight may double your risk for developing gallstones. If you are already seriously overweight and your doctor recommends rapid weight loss, you may wish to take ursodiol or ursodeoxycholic acid (Actigall), medications that dissolve gallstones. This is a very useful method of prevention. Discuss this with your doctor.

Gastroesophageal Reflux Disease (GERD)

In people with gastroesophageal reflux disease (GERD; also known as acid reflux), the lower esophageal sphincter (LES), which controls the passage of food from the esophagus into the stomach, fails to function properly. As a result, stomach acids travel back into the esophagus, a process called reflux. Without the thin layer of mucus that protects the stomach from these acids, esophageal tissue may be injured and symptoms develop, most often heartburn (a burning feeling in the chest and throat). The regurgitation, or acid reflux, into the esophagus may cause coughing and leave an unpleasant taste in your mouth.

People who suffer from GERD may develop an inflammation of the esophagus known as esophagitis. As time passes, esophagitis may further erode the esophagus and cause bleeding and difficulty in swallowing. In about 10 percent of the people who have GERD, scar tissue forms in the lower esophagus. The scar tissue results in a narrowing of the food pathway and may cause swallowing problems. Because stomach acid has the potential to erode esophageal tissue, it may lead to the formation of painful ulcers, open sores that may bleed and make swallowing difficult.

Just about everyone has occasional bouts of heartburn and acid reflux. However, when these symptoms occur repeatedly over an extended period of time, they are classified as GERD. GERD is a relatively common disorder: It affects at least 5 percent of the world's population. Yet, it is frequently unrecognized and undiagnosed.

Barrett's esophagus, a potentially serious complication of GERD, occurs in about 5 percent of those who are affected. In this disorder, the normally pink-colored stratified squamous epithelium tissue of the lower esophagus changes to an intestinal-type epithelium, which is a salmon color. People with Barrett's esophagus are 30 to 125 times more likely to develop esophageal cancer.

GERD is associated with an increased risk for certain other medical problems. For example, people who have GERD frequently also have asthma and other respiratory disorders, such as chronic bronchitis, chronic sinusitis, and recurrent pneumonia. And because of the acid backing up into the mouth, people with GERD tend to have erosion of dental enamel.

Causes and Risk Factors

There are a number of factors that increase the risk for developing GERD. Though people of any age may develop GERD, about half of those diagnosed with GERD are between the ages of 45 and 64. To determine if there is a relationship between body mass index (BMI) and GERD, more than 10,000 women were studied. A strong positive association was found between the symptoms of GERD and BMI. In subjects who were normal weight and overweight, the risk of GERD symptoms increased with a rising BMI. Symptoms increased as the percentage of body fat increased. Some research has shown that obese people have higher levels of acid in the esophagus, which increases the chance for GERD.

Family history is also thought to play a role. Do you have close family members with this disease? If you do, you probably have a higher risk. People who have a hiatal hernia (a protrusion of part of the stomach into the lower chest so that the diaphragm no longer supports the LES) are more vulnerable. Smoking and drinking excess amounts of alcohol are known to raise the risk.

A Quick Guide to Symptoms

- ☐ **Heartburn**
- ☐ **Difficulty swallowing**
- ☐ **Chest pain**
- ☐ **Nausea**
- ☐ **Belching**
- ☐ **Acid regurgitation**
- ☐ **Throat problems (chronic sore throats or needing to clear the throat frequently)**

Signs and Symptoms

In addition to heartburn, GERD may cause a number of other symptoms, including difficulty swallowing, chest pain, nausea, belching, and acid regurgitation. You might also have throat problems, such as chronic sore throats, and you may need to clear your throat frequently.

Symptoms are more frequent at night. Further, they may appear when you are engaging in the following activities: lifting, lying down on your back, and bending over. Symptoms are also more likely to occur after a heavy meal.

Although Barrett's esophagus may cause precancerous changes in the esophagus, it may cause few symptoms. On the other hand, some people have severe heartburn without any damage to the esophagus.

Conventional Treatments

Conventional treatment for GERD may involve a number of approaches, among them lifestyle changes, a variety of medications, and surgery.

Lifestyle Changes

Treatment for GERD normally begins with several lifestyle changes. These include eating smaller meals, sitting or standing after you eat, limiting your consumption of fatty foods, avoiding foods and drinks that tend to be more problematic (chocolate, onions, citrus fruits, coffee, and carbonated beverages), wearing more comfortable clothing that is not tight around your stomach, losing weight, avoiding or limiting your consumption of alcohol, and raising the head of your bed. You may also be advised to stop smoking and make time for relaxation.

Medication may be another factor that contributes to GERD. Your doctor will want to review all your medications, as you may be taking a medication that tends to exacerbate GERD. These include nonsteroidal anti-inflammatory drugs (NSAIDs) such as aspirin, ibuprofen, naproxen, and ketoprofen; sedatives and tranquilizers; potassium tablets; vitamin C tablets; calcium-channel blockers (often prescribed for high blood pressure); anticholinergics (medications that relax smooth muscle, such as those used for chronic obstructive pulmonary disease); theophylline (an asthma drug); quinidine (used to treat heart arrhythmia); and alendronate (for osteoporosis). Don't discontinue any of these medications without consulting your doctor.

Medications

If you have not achieved sufficient relief from lifestyle changes and a medication review, your doctor may suggest medication. There are a number of different types that may be used.

Acid blockers. Acid blockers, which are also called H-2 blockers, reduce the secretion of stomach acid. They last longer than antacids and may prevent acid reflux and heartburn in about half the people who have GERD. Some acid blockers are available over-the-counter; others are sold by prescription only. The over-the-counter acid blockers have half the strength of those sold by prescription. Well-known examples are cimetidine

Self-Testing

There is no specific self-test for GERD. However, if you suspect that you may have GERD, the American College of Gastroenterology suggests that you ask yourself the following questions. If you answer "yes" to two or more of the questions, you may have GERD.

1. Do you frequently have one of the following:
   - ☐ An uncomfortable feeling behind the breastbone that seems to be moving upward from the stomach?
   - ☐ A burning sensation in the back of the throat?
   - ☐ A bitter acid taste in your mouth?
2. Do you often experience these problems after meals?
3. Do you have heartburn or acid indigestion two or more times per week?
4. Do you find that antacids provide only temporary relief from your symptoms?
5. Are you taking prescription medication to treat heartburn symptoms but still having symptoms?

(Tagamet HB) and famotidine (Pepcid AC). On occasion, these medications may have side effects such as dry mouth, dizziness, drowsiness, and bowel changes. Be sure to ask your doctor if they may interfere with other medications you are taking.

Antacids. Over-the-counter antacids, which neutralize gastric acid, are probably better for occasional heartburn than for GERD, but you may wish to see if they help you. Though they do not cure GERD, they may relieve your symptoms. Common examples are Tums and Rolaids. When antacids are consumed frequently, they may sometimes trigger constipation or diarrhea. Some antacids may interfere with other medications, particularly those for kidney and heart disease. Frequent use of antacids that contain calcium may place you at risk for kidney stones. Further, antacids that contain aluminum, calcium, or magnesium are known to interfere with the absorption of some medications, such as ciprofloxacin (Cipro), tetracycline, and propranolol (Inderal). To prevent these interactions, take these medications either 1 hour before or 3 hours after the antacid.

Proton-pump inhibitors (PPIs). Proton-pump inhibitors (PPIs), such as lansoprazole (Prevacid), omeprazole (Prilosec, Zegerid), and pantoprazole (Protonix), are the most effective medications for GERD. These medications block the production of acid, giving the tissue time to heal. But they may have potential side effects, such as diarrhea, headaches, flatulence, loose stools, and stomach or abdominal pain.

Surgery

The effectiveness of GERD medications has reduced the need for fundoplication surgery, but sometimes surgery may be the most reasonable course of action. Your doctor may recommend surgery if you have a large hiatal hernia, repeated narrowing of the esophagus, Barrett's esophagus, severe esophagitis (particularly with bleeding), or lung problems caused by the acid reflux. A study demonstrated that surgery does not eliminate the need for acid-reducing medications in all patients. In addition, the procedure does not lower the risk for esophageal cancer in patients with GERD and Barrett's esophagus. Surgery corrects about 85 percent of GERD-related respiratory symptoms.

Laparoscopic fundoplication. The open Nissen fundoplication (see below) has now largely been replaced with the laparoscopic fundoplication, in which only tiny incisions are made in the abdomen. The surgeon wraps the upper part of the stomach around the esophagus, creating the same collarlike structure that is found in the open Nissen fundoplication. Because of complications, in about 8 percent of the cases, the surgeon must discontinue the laparoscopic procedure and switch to the open Nissen fundoplication. Your chances of having a successful laparoscopic fundoplication procedure are greatly improved if you select a highly experienced surgeon.

Postoperative problems may include a delay in intestinal functioning, which may result in vomiting, gagging, and bloating. Typically, this lasts for no more than a few weeks. Though uncommon, there may be complications such as bowel obstruction; wound infection; respiratory problems, such as a collapsed lung; muscle spasms after food is swallowed; and an excessively wrapped fundus that causes difficulty swallowing or gas, bloating, or the inability to burp.

Open Nissen fundoplication. Until the early 1990s, open Nissen fundoplication was the surgery most often used for GERD. After making wide surgical incisions, the surgeon wraps the upper part of the stomach around the esophagus, thus forming a collarlike structure. By putting pressure on the LES, reflux is prevented. With this surgery, hospital stays average 6 to 10 days. Failure rates range from 9 to 30 percent. When the procedure fails, it needs to be repeated.

Repairing the lower esophageal sphincter (LES). Using endoscopy, physicians may repair the lower esophageal sphincter (LES). This may be accomplished in a number of ways. In the Bard Endoscopic Suturing System (Endocinch), a tiny "sewing machine" stitches weakened areas of the LES. In the Stretta System, radio-frequency energy heats and melts tissue in the malfunctioning valve and the area connecting the esophagus to the stomach. The scar tissue seems to tighten the valve. With both surgeries, it is possible to return home the same day. There may be some chest, stomach, or throat pain. You should not have either procedure if you have a hiatal hernia or Barrett's esophagus.

Complementary Treatments

Complementary approaches treat the symptoms of GERD, address the underlying cause, and promote dietary and lifestyle changes that are helpful in reducing or eliminating this problem.

Herbal Medicine

Chamomile and ginger. Chamomile, which has an antispasmodic effect, and ginger, a carminative (helps to relieve gas), may be taken as a tea three or four times a day between meals. Chamomile and ginger are readily available in prepared tea bags.

Coriander. Coriander, a stomachic (stimulates digestion) herb, has also been used for the relief of GERD. Steep 2 teaspoons of dried seeds in 1 cup of boiling water for 15 minutes. Drink 1 cup daily.

Devil's claw. Devil's claw is considered a bitter herb that helps neutralize stomach acid. It is available in a tincture, tea, or capsule. As a tea, 1 to 2 grams of the dried powdered root is steeped in a cup of boiling water for 5 to 10 minutes. Drink 3 cups per day. With a tincture, take 1 teaspoon three times a day. In capsule form, 400 milligrams is the recommended daily dose. (There is no standardization of devil's claw.)

Fennel seeds. Chewing fennel seeds can help reduce the burning sensation associated with GERD.

Licorice. Deglycyrrhizinated licorice (DGL) is an anti-inflammatory and helps coat the esophagus. Chew one or two 380-milligram wafers three times daily.

Turmeric. Turmeric reduces acid and breaks down fatty foods. It has long been used in India as a remedy for heartburn. To make a tea, pour 1 cup of boiling water over 1 teaspoon of powdered turmeric and let steep for 5 minutes. Strain well and drink 2 or 3 cups daily.

Hydrotherapy

Prior to eating, place an ice pack over your stomach for 5 minutes. This may reduce the probability of acid reflux.

Nutritional Supplements

Bromelain and quercetin help promote healing of GERD. You may wish to purchase a supplement that contains both bromelain and quercetin.

- Bromelain: 150-milligram capsule three times a day between meals. Anti-inflammatory digestive enzyme that enhances the action of quercetin. Take together.

- Quercetin: 500-milligram capsule three times a day between meals. Anti-inflammatory flavonoid that accelerates healing.

Lifestyle Recommendations

Change your nighttime routine. Since a large percentage of people who suffer from GERD have nighttime symptoms, consider some of these suggestions.

- Avoid bedtime snacks. In fact, don't eat for at least 2 hours before going to bed; 3 hours is even better.

- Take an after-dinner walk, or at least sit upright after eating.

- In bed, lie on your left side. When you sleep on your right side, the stomach is higher than the esophagus, which may put pressure on the LES.

- To raise the entire top half of your body, elevate the head of your bed with 4- to 6- inch blocks or a wedge support. This will help keep stomach acids in the stomach. Don't attempt to accomplish this goal with pillows—that raises only the head and increases your risk of reflux.

Preventive Measures

Make dietary changes. Avoid or reduce your consumption of chocolate, caffeine, spearmint, peppermint, alcohol, carbonated drinks, tomatoes, onions, garlic, and citrus fruits, all of which lower LES pressure. At the same time, increase your intake of whole grains, protein, and non-acidic fruits and vegetables. Remember to eat slowly and in a relaxed environment.

Quit smoking and reduce alcohol. If you smoke, quit. Also, reduce your consumption of alcoholic beverages. Both smoking and alcohol lower LES pressure, making acid reflux more likely to occur. Quitting smoking and reducing alcohol consumption are thought to be key elements in the prevention of GERD.

Reduce stress. Participating in regular exercise and relaxation techniques such as yoga, tai chi, qigong, and meditation may help reduce stress and improve digestion and other bodily functions.

Reduce your waistline. Large waistlines seem to increase the risk of acid reflux symptoms among white adults, according to a study of more than 80,000 members of the California Health Plan.

Glaucoma

Glaucoma is not a single illness but rather a group of diseases that damage the optic nerve of the eye. In almost all forms of glaucoma, an abnormally high pressure inside the eyeball causes damage to the optic nerve. A healthy optic nerve is crucial to good eyesight. Composed of about 1 million nerve fibers, the optic nerve connects the retina, a light-sensitive layer of tissue located at the back of the eye, with the brain. If the optic nerve is impaired, as it may be by glaucoma, you will eventually develop blind spots and suffer the loss of peripheral (side) vision. By the time you experience these symptoms, a significant amount of damage has occurred.

Glaucoma has the potential to lead to blindness. At present, there are no known means to correct the damage once it has occurred. Luckily, there are now easy methods to detect glaucoma early, and there are a number of treatments. In people who receive regular preventive eye care, glaucoma should be diagnosed fairly early, and they should be able to avoid the long-term consequences.

Because of internal pressure in the eye, known as intraocular pressure (IOP), the eye is able to function properly and keep its shape. Aqueous humor, a type of eye fluid, is key to this process. In a healthy eye, aqueous humor is produced and drained continuously through what is called the trabecular meshwork (or drainage angle). This process maintains normal pressure within the eye. If eye fluid is unable to drain properly, eye pressure builds and the optic nerve may be damaged, as it is in glaucoma.

In open-angle glaucoma (also known as primary open-angle glaucoma), the eye's means of drainage remains open, but the aqueous humor is draining too slowly. As a result, the fluid backs up and the IOP rises. Acute closed-angle glaucoma (also known as angle-closure glaucoma) is far less common than open-angle glaucoma, but is potentially more serious. In this type of the disease, part of the iris (the colored area of the eye around the pupil) pushes against the lens, closing off the drainage angle and leading to a rapid increase in IOP.

It is possible to have glaucoma without an increase in IOP, a condition known as normal-tension glaucoma. Or you may have a higher-than-normal IOP without injury to the optic nerve. So, in contrast to the prevailing perception that a high IOP is synonymous with glaucoma, a high IOP is actually only one possible component of a glaucoma diagnosis.

Affecting about 3 million Americans, glaucoma is a very common disorder. Almost all of those who have glaucoma have a chronic form of the most common type of glaucoma, open-angle glaucoma.

Causes and Risk Factors

It is believed that open-angle glaucoma is genetically linked. Thus, people with close relatives who have been diagnosed with glaucoma are at greater risk. Also, the incidence increases with age. Open-angle glaucoma is rarely seen among those under the age of 40. Once you turn 50, your risk for open-angle glaucoma doubles about every 10 years. Approximately 14 percent of people who are 80 years old have glaucoma.

African Americans are three to four times more likely than whites to have glaucoma, and they tend to develop glaucoma at younger ages. Asian Americans and Hispanic Americans are also at greater risk. Other factors that increase the risk include medical conditions such as diabetes, high blood pressure, heart disease, retinal detachment, hypothyroidism, eye tumors, and eye inflammation. People who have suffered trauma to the eye as well as those who are profoundly nearsighted are also more vulnerable. Eye abnormalities and prolonged use of corticosteroids also increase the chance that you will develop glaucoma.

A Quick Guide to Symptoms

Open-Angle Glaucoma
- [ ] **Loss of peripheral vision**
- [ ] **Problems with night vision**
- [ ] **Sensitivity to glare and lights**
- [ ] **Inability to distinguish differing shades of light and dark**
- [ ] **Frequent changes in eyeglass or contact lens prescriptions**

Closed-Angle Glaucoma
- [ ] **Severe eye pain**
- [ ] **Headache**
- [ ] **Eye redness**
- [ ] **"Halos" around lights**
- [ ] **Blurred vision**
- [ ] **Nausea and vomiting**

Signs and Symptoms

A large number of people with glaucoma do not realize they have a problem. The symptoms of open-angle glaucoma tend to be subtle and do not become more apparent until there is serious damage to the optic nerve. During this time, people lose more and more of their peripheral vision. Open-angle glaucoma tends to affect both eyes, though usually not at the same time. Other symptoms of open-angle glaucoma include problems with night vision, sensitivity to glare and lights, and an inability to distinguish differing shades of light and dark. It is not uncommon for people with open-angle glaucoma to require frequent changes in eyeglass or contact lens prescriptions.

Responding to a rapid rise in eye pressure, closed-angle glaucoma develops quickly. Symptoms include severe eye pain, headache, eye redness, "halos" around lights, blurred vision, and nausea and vomiting. Closed-angle glaucoma requires immediate attention. In only a few hours, there can be permanent vision loss, and blindness may occur in a day or two.

Conventional Treatments

There is no cure for glaucoma, and none of the treatments is able to reverse the damage caused by the disease. Yet, glaucoma may be controlled. If you have been diagnosed with glaucoma, you will need to become more aware of your vision, and you will become a more frequent visitor to your eye care specialist. Conventional treatments for glaucoma include medication and surgery. Recommendations vary according to the type of glaucoma as well as the individual's particular needs.

Medications for Open-Angle Glaucoma

To prevent further damage of the optic nerve, your eye care professional will probably prescribe medication in the form of eye drops; sometimes, he or she may advise more than one type of eye drop. These are designed either to reduce the amount of aqueous fluid produced by the eye or allow better drainage of the fluid in the eye. It is very important to administer these drops exactly as your doctor advises.

Beta-blockers. Beta-blockers reduce the production of aqueous humor. The most common beta-blocker is timolol (Betimol, Timoptic). Timolol is long acting and has excellent efficacy for the treatment of glaucoma. It also has few ocular side effects. Though generally used without any problems, beta-blockers must be taken with caution by anyone with a breathing or heart problem.

If you are experiencing any of the symptoms of open-angle glaucoma and believe that you may have the disease, visit an eye care professional for testing. If you think you may be having symptoms of closed-angle glaucoma, seek medical help immediately.

Carbonic anhydrase inhibitors. Carbonic anhydrase inhibitors reduce the production of aqueous humor and are available in oral and eye drop forms. Dorzolamide (Trusopt) is an example of a carbonic anhydrase inhibitor. When taken orally, some common potential side effects are frequent urination and tingling in the fingers and toes. Depression, stomach problems, fatigue, weight loss, and sexual dysfunction have also been noted from the oral form. Since carbonic anhydrase inhibitors are a form of sulfa medication, people who are allergic to sulfa drugs should not take them.

Prostaglandin analogues. These hormone-like medications increase the outflow of aqueous humor. Latanoprost (Xalatan) is an example of a prostaglandin analogue. They have the potential to cause allergic reactions, inflammation within the eye, blurred vision, fatigue, and headache. In some people, they cause blue, green, or hazel eyes to permanently change to brown, and they cause eyelashes to grow longer.

Miotics. By reducing the size of the pupil and pulling the iris away from the drainage network, miotics allow better drainage of fluid. But they also cause a dimming of vision and problems seeing at night or in a darkened room. Other potential side effects include allergic reactions, teary eyes, and eye pain. Pilocarpine (in Piloptic and other medications) is an example of a miotic.

Alpha-2 adrenergic agonists. These agents reduce the production of aqueous humor and increase its outflow. Apraclonidine (Iopidine) is an example of an alpha-2 adrenergic agonist. While their most common potential side effects are dry mouth and altered sense of taste, they may also cause an allergic reaction, with red and itching eyes and lids.

Tips for Using Eye Drops

The eye is able to hold only about 20 percent of the amount of fluid in a standard eye drop. Therefore, put only one eye drop in your eye at a time. If you have been instructed to use more than one eye drop, wait about 5 minutes between the drops. This will allow more of the drops to be absorbed and will reduce waste.

To minimize the amount of eye drops absorbed into your bloodstream, after putting the drops in your eyes, close your eyes for a minute or two. While your eyes are closed, lightly touch the corner of your eyes closest to your nose. This will help close the tear ducts, which keeps the drops from getting into your nose and being absorbed through the blood vessels in the nasal mucosa. End the process by wiping excess eye drops from your eyelid.

Medications for Acute Closed-Angle Glaucoma

As has been noted, acute closed-angle glaucoma is an emergency situation. Doctors generally administer medications to reduce eye pressure. After that, surgery is normally required.

Medications for Normal-Tension Glaucoma

Since the IOP does not rise to an abnormal level with this form of glaucoma, this is a more challenging situation for eye care professionals and their patients. However, it has been determined that the usual IOP-reducing medications do slow the development and progression of the disease.

Surgery for Open-Angle Glaucoma

If the medications are poorly tolerated or ineffective, your eye care professional may recommend surgery. Types of surgery for open-angle glaucoma include laser trabeculoplasty and conventional incisional surgery. It should be noted, however, that while surgery may be helpful, it does not actually cure glaucoma. More than half of the patients who undergo surgery require medication within 2 years. None of these surgeries are without risk, and there may be complications. Selecting a highly trained and experienced eye surgeon may reduce the risk of these.

Conventional incisional surgery. This procedure is also referred to as trabeculectomy or filtering surgery. After you receive medication to help you relax, eye drops, and an anesthetic injection to numb your eyes, your physician uses an operating microscope to open a small hole in the sclera or white part of the eye. Fluid is able to drain from the small bubble, or bleb, that forms over this opening. Filtering blebs are at risk for leaking and infection, and retinal swelling may blur or reduce vision.

If there is scar tissue from the glaucoma, a physician may prefer an alternative surgical technique in which a plastic valve is implanted. This provides a means by which eye fluid may drain. After this procedure, expect several follow-up visits. About one-third of the people who have this type of surgery develop cataracts within 5 years, but it is not certain whether or not the cataracts are related to the surgery.

Laser trabeculoplasty. In a trabeculoplasty, a physician uses a laser to burn tiny spots in the trabecular meshwork, a drainage area located in the front of the eye. These spots tend to improve the eye's ability to drain. With improved drainage, the damage to the optic nerve may be halted.

Before the office procedure, which requires less than 30 minutes, the doctor numbs the eye with drops. During the surgery, you sit at a slit lamp and are fitted with a special eye lens. The doctor aims the laser beam through the lens. You may see flashes of green or red light. One or two hours after the surgery, the doctor checks your eye pressure. For a few days after the procedure, you may have blurred vision and a sensitivity to light, but there should be no pain. Anticipate follow-up appointments to check eye pressure. Unfortunately, the benefits of a trabeculoplasty may be limited: There's evidence that in more than half of all cases, the eye pressure rises to an unsafe level within 2 years of surgery.

Surgery for Acute Closed-Angle Glaucoma

This condition is a medical emergency. If you have symptoms of acute closed-angle glaucoma, seek help from an eye care professional immediately. In an attempt to lower the eye pressure as quickly as possible, the physician will probably administer several medications. Then, the eye surgeon will make a tiny opening in the eye's iris, thereby enabling the aqueous fluid to flow more freely. This may be done either with a laser (iridotomy) or conventional surgery (iridectomy). Since it is likely that if you have acute glaucoma in one eye the other eye will also develop this disorder, physicians generally recommend surgery in the second eye as well. Recovery may take up to 8 weeks, and during this time your vision may be blurred.

Complementary Treatments

By incorporating dietary measures, lifestyle changes, and herbal medicine, practitioners of complementary medicine seek to boost the body's natural healing powers. A number of nutrients also hold promise for people with glaucoma.

Diet

Studies have shown that people with glaucoma may be deficient in certain vital nutrients, such as vitamins A, B_{12} (cobalamin), C, and E, plus the minerals magnesium and selenium. These substances are essential for protecting the optic nerve, reducing eye pressure, and preventing vision loss.

Vitamin A may be found in yellow, orange, and dark green vegetables and fruits, such as carrots, broccoli, spinach, winter squash, sweet potatoes, and cantaloupe. Further, it is found in liver, eggs, cheese, and butter. Vitamin B_{12} is best obtained from animal-based food such as meat, fish, livers, eggs, milk, and oysters. Vitamin C is found in all fruits and vegetables, such as those that contain vitamin A. Good sources of vitamin E include green leafy vegetables, liver, whole-grain cereals and breads, and dried beans.

Magnesium is found in virtually all raw, green leafy vegetables, as well as in almonds, cashews, soybeans, most seeds, and whole grains. You may obtain selenium from seafood, chicken, meat, whole-grain cereals, egg yolks, and garlic.

Increasing your intake of foods rich in these nutrients may aid in reducing the effects of glaucoma. Dark green, leafy vegetables such as spinach, kale, and broccoli contain phytochemicals known as carotenoids, including beta-carotene, lutein, and zeaxanthin, which play an important role in eye health. The body converts beta-carotene into vitamin A, the "eye vitamin." Studies have shown that lutein and zeaxanthin in particular slow vision loss associated with glaucoma and even help improve eyesight. A healthy diet that includes lots of whole grains, vegetables, and fruits may help to avoid many of the risk factors associated with glaucoma, such as diabetes, high blood pressure, and heart disease.

Studies have shown that coffee may reduce bloodflow to the retina. If you presently have retinal damage, you may want to reduce your consumption of coffee or eliminate it altogether. Moreover, drinking a quart or more of any liquid within a half-hour period should be avoided. People with glaucoma should drink lots of fluids, but not a lot at any given time; just drink smaller amounts throughout the day.

Herbal Medicine

Ginkgo and bilberry are two herbal remedies that have shown promise for the treatment of glaucoma.

Bilberry. Bilberry acts as an antioxidant. By stabilizing collagen, decreasing capillary fragility, and improving the delivery of oxygen to the eyes, bilberry has a protective effect. Bilberry extract is available as a dietary supplement. The recommended dose is 100 milligrams of bilberry extract (standardized to 25 percent anthocyanosides), three times a day.

Ginkgo biloba. Ginkgo contains a variety of bioflavonoids and also acts as an antioxidant. It increases the oxygen supply to the eyes, assists in improving circulation to the optic nerve, and reduces oxidative damage. One study found that people with decreased ocular bloodflow experienced a mild improvement after taking 160 milligrams of ginkgo extract (standardized to 24 percent flavone glycosides and 6 percent terpene lactones) for 4 weeks, then 120 milligrams a day for an indefinite period of time. However, a dose as low as 40 milligrams per day is often recommended. The flavone glycosides give ginkgo its antioxidant benefits; the terpene lactones increase circulation and have a protective effect on nerve cells. You should not use ginkgo if you are taking a blood-thinning medication. Consult with your doctor.

Hydrotherapy

Alternating hot and cold compresses over the eyes for a short period of time may help to increase circulation in the eyes. Hot compresses relax the nervous and circulatory systems; cold compresses stimulate the circulation in the eyes. Begin with 2 minutes using a hot compress, then follow that with 1 minute using a cold compress. This procedure may be repeated two or three times, but always end the treatment with a cold compress.

Nutritional Supplements

The following nutrients decrease IOP and protect the optic nerve by neutralizing free radicals and aid in maintaining healthy eyes.

- Vitamin A: 10,000 IU daily. Reduces visual impairments such as night blindness, an early symptom of open-angle glaucoma.

- Vitamin B_{12}: 100 micrograms daily. Protects the optic nerve and prevents visual loss. One Japanese study reported that people with glaucoma who took 1,500 micrograms of B_{12} daily over a 5-year period regained some sight and showed no visual deterioration.

- Vitamin C: 1,000 milligrams daily in divided doses of 500 milligrams each. Antioxidant that helps prevent cell damage. Do not take with selenium.

- Vitamin E: 400 IU daily. Neutralizes free radicals and protects optic nerve.

- Beta-carotene: 25,000 IU daily. Aids in maintaining healthy eyes.

- Fish oil (essential fatty acid): 3,000 milligrams daily in divided doses of 1,000 milligrams. Reduces inflammation.

- Magnesium: 500 milligrams daily. Increases blood supply to the optic nerve.

- Selenium: 200 micrograms daily. Decreases IOP and protects the optic nerve. Take with vitamin E for better absorption.

Traditional Chinese Medicine

Practitioners of traditional Chinese medicine have used acupuncture, tai chi, and herbal medicine (particularly the herb *Salvia miltiorrhiza*) to lower IOP. In Chinese medicine, the eyes are a reflection of the strength of the liver. The acupuncture treatment is focused on nourishing and strengthening that organ. Acupuncture is very effective in treating the early stages of glaucoma. It is also useful in treating other symptoms associated with glaucoma, such as headaches and vomiting. To locate a practitioner trained in traditional Chinese medicine, visit the Web site of the National Certification Commission for Acupuncture and Oriental Medicine (NCCAOM) at www.nccaom.org or the American Association of Acupuncture and Oriental Medicine at www.aaaomonline.org.

Lifestyle Recommendations

Aerobic exercise appears to be a factor in the control of IOP. Studies have shown that people with glaucoma who take a brisk, 40-minute walk 5 days a week are able to reduce their eye pressure by 2.5 milliliters, which is equivalent to the reduction expected from beta-blockers. When exercise is discontinued, the pressure increases. This form of exercise also aids in lowering cholesterol, reducing high blood pressure, and improving circulation to the retina.

Preventive Measures

Limit your intake of coffee. One study found that coffee produced a reduction of up to 13 percent in the retinal bloodflow. This is particularly damaging to those who are already in the process of losing vision.

Protect your eyes. Wear a protective hat and sunglasses that block out 100 percent of the sun's ultraviolet-A (UVA) and ultraviolet-B (UVB) rays and filter out at least 85 percent of blue-violet rays.

Quit smoking. If you smoke, quit. And avoid exposure to secondhand smoke. Smokers have an increased risk for developing glaucoma. If you have glaucoma and you smoke, your disease will probably progress more rapidly. Studies have shown that retinal bloodflow is reduced by 16 percent by the nicotine in cigarettes.

Reduce stress. It is believed that stress may trigger acute closed-angle glaucoma. Relaxation and meditation involve deep-breathing exercises, muscle relaxation, and focused attention, all of which work together toward shutting down the anxiety-producing "fight-or-flight" response of the body and reducing IOP. Some of these techniques include tai chi, yoga, biofeedback, and various forms of meditation.

Watch what you eat. Eliminate trans fatty acids and avoid refined foods such as white sugar and white bread and saturated fats. This type of diet can lead to diabetes, a condition that can then lead to glaucoma.

Watch your blood pressure. Elevated blood pressure is a risk factor for developing open-angle glaucoma.

Gout

Recognized as an illness for more than 2,000 years, gout (also known as acute gouty arthritis) is an arthritic condition that causes inflammation of the joints. When the body has more uric acid than it can manage, it may convert some of it into needlelike crystals (tophi). These may then be stored in the joints. But elevated uric acid alone does not cause gout. Many people with elevated levels never have this disorder.

Uric acid is a by-product of the breakdown of purine, a substance that is part of human tissue and is found in a number of foods, among them organ meats, sardines, anchovies, and meat gravies. Normally, uric acid is dissolved in the blood and eliminated from the body via urine or broken down in the gut and eliminated via the stool. If the body starts to produce excess amounts of uric acid, if the kidneys fail to eliminate sufficient amounts, or if you start to eat large amounts of food with high amounts of purine, levels of uric acid in the blood may rise. This is a condition known as hyperuricemia. Then, if uric acid forms crystals that collect in joint spaces, you may develop gout. Once in the joints, the crystals may cause inflammation, including swelling, redness, and intense pain. Under the skin, the collection of crystals may look like lumps.

Because uric acid crystals may collect in the kidneys, if you have gout, there is a 10 to 40 percent chance that you will also develop kidney stones. About 25 percent of people who have chronic hyperuricemia develop progressive kidney disease. People with gout frequently have cardiovascular problems such as high blood pressure, coronary artery disease, and congestive heart failure, and they have higher rates of cataracts and dry eye syndrome.

Gout is a relatively common disorder: More than 2 million Americans have it. It affects more men than women (especially men 40 and older), but after menopause, women's risk increases.

Causes and Risk Factors

A number of factors are believed to play a role in the development of gout. Family history (genetics) helps determine your risk. Do you have family members with this disorder? If you do, you may be at increased risk. In some cases, there is an enzyme defect that interferes with the way the body breaks down purines. Because people who are overweight have more tissue to turn over and break down, excess weight is associated with an increased risk. Also, alcohol interferes with the removal of uric acid from the body, so drinking too much alcohol raises your risk. Lead in the environment may trigger gout, and there is some evidence that people with thyroid problems are at greater than normal risk.

Some medical conditions raise the risk of gout, including hypertension (high blood pressure), hyperlipidemia (high levels of fat in the blood), and arteriosclerosis (narrowing of the arteries). Uric acid levels in the body may rise because of surgery, immobility due to bed rest, and severe or sudden illness. As chemotherapy treatments break down abnormal cells, they may cause purine to be released into the blood and increase the risk of gout.

Certain medications interfere with the body's ability to remove uric acid, so they increase the amount of uric acid in the body. These include diuretics (taken for hypertension, edema, and heart disease) and anti-inflammatory medicines made from salicylic acid, such as aspirin. Other suspect medicines include niacin, levodopa (used for Parkinson's disease), and cyclosporine (which suppresses the body's immune system and is given to recipients of an organ transplant). That explains why people who have undergone organ transplantation are at greater than normal risk for gout.

Signs and Symptoms

The majority of people first realize that they may have gout when they have excruciating pain in the great toe or knee. Gout is less likely to occur initially in the ankle, wrist, finger, elbow, or instep. There are four basic stages of the disease.

1. In the first stage, known as asymptomatic hyperuricemia, you have an elevated uric acid level, but experience no symptoms. During this time, you will not know that you have gout. For a fortunate few, the disease never advances beyond this stage.

2. With the second stage, known as acute gout or acute gouty arthritis, you have uric acid deposits in the joints. You will experience a sudden (between 8 and 12 hours) onset of intense pain and swelling in (usually) one joint, which tends to be warm and tender. The skin over the area may be taut, red, and shiny, and, after a few days, it may peel. There also may be chills and a mild fever. You may not want to eat, and you may feel generally ill. Acute attacks tend to occur at night and may be triggered by stress, alcohol, drugs, or another illness. The pain may be so severe that you are unable to endure the weight of your blanket on your toe. Most early attacks subside within 3 to 10 days, even without treatment. It may be months or years before another attack.

3. Most people with untreated gout will have a second attack within 2 years. With time, attacks last longer and occur more often. The period between acute attacks is known as intercritical gout.

4. The final stage of gout, known as chronic tophaceous gout, develops over an extended period of time. However,

gout that is properly treated may not advance to this stage. In chronic tophaceous gout, the intercritical periods become shorter and the attacks longer. There is permanent joint damage, chronic low-grade pain, and mild to acute inflammation. Several joints may be affected. Knobby crystal deposits may appear on the curved ridge on the edge of the ear, the forearms, elbows, knees, hands, feet, and (rarely) around the heart and spine. If you have chronic tophaceous gout, the cartilage and bone at the affected joints may be destroyed. Tophi may grow as large as handballs. Though it is rare, if the crystals lodge in the spine, there may be serious damage.

Conventional Treatments

Designed to relieve pain, reduce inflammation, and prevent damage to the affected joints, there are several treatments for an acute attack of gout. Conventional treatment for gout includes resting and protecting the affected joint with a splint. Applying ice packs four times a day for 30-minute intervals may bring quite a bit of relief. Whenever possible, treatment should begin at the very first sign of an attack. It is always advisable to keep a supply of your medication on hand, as you never know when you might have an attack.

Since asymptomatic hyperuricemia doesn't always lead to gout, it is not normally treated. However, treatment may be recommended if very high uric acid levels pose a threat to the kidneys.

A Quick Guide to Symptoms

☐ Excruciating pain in the great toe or knee
☐ Taut, red, and shiny skin over the affected area
☐ Chills and a mild fever

Medications

During the intercritical period between acute attacks and to prevent further attacks, your doctor may recommend low doses of either anti-inflammatories or colchicine. Antihyperuricemic drugs help reduce the amount of uric acid.

Antihyperuricemic drugs. Because your doctor may want to reduce the amount of uric acid, a drug classified as an antihyperuricemic may be prescribed. These drugs dissolve monosodium urate (MSU) crystals and tophi. They are more likely to be recommended if you have had two or more acute gout attacks, if your x-rays show damage from gout, if your gout attacks are severe, if more than one joint is affected, if you are considered at risk for tophaceous gout, or if your hyperuricemia is caused by an identified inborn metabolic deficiency. Still, if you do not have normal kidney function, you should not take these drugs.

Before prescribing an antihyperuricemic drug, your doctor will want to determine if your high levels of uric acid are caused by an overproduction of uric acid or by your body's failure to eliminate a sufficient amount of uric acid. To do this, your doctor may ask you to collect your urine for 24 hours. If you produce too much uric acid, you may be prescribed allopurinol (Zyloprim); if you excrete too little uric acid, you may be prescribed a uricosuric (probenecid or sulfinpyrazone).

Before you begin antihyperuricemic therapy, your doctor will want to have your most recent attack of gout under complete control. The joints should no longer be inflamed. Some doctors advise waiting a month.

Anti-inflammatory drugs. Younger people with no serious health problems are typically started on high doses of nonsteroidal anti-inflammatory drugs (NSAIDs), such as indomethacin (Indocin) and naproxen (Anaprox, Naprosyn). NSAIDs reduce inflammation caused by the uric acid crystals, but they do nothing to alter the amount of uric acid in the body. COX-2 inhibitors may also be effective medications to reduce the inflammation during an acute attack. If you are unable to tolerate the gastrointestinal side effects of NSAIDs, then oral corticosteroids may be recommended or a steroid preparation may be injected into the affected joint. The most frequently prescribed oral corticosteroid is prednisone.

When taken over an extended period of time, these medications are likely to cause gastrointestinal side effects. Other possible side effects include increased blood pressure, dizziness, ringing in the ears, headache, skin rash, and depression. If you experience any of these problems, you should report them to your doctor.

Be aware, too, that NSAIDs—particularly aspirin and other salicylate drugs—diminish the effectiveness of uric acid medications.

Colchicine. In some cases, if you do not respond to NSAIDs or corticosteroids, your doctor may consider colchicine. This is a urate blocker that is most useful when taken within the first 12 hours of an attack. It is not recommended for adults who have kidney or liver problems. Possible side effects include nausea, vomiting, diarrhea, and blood and/or kidney problems.

Surgery

On occasion, surgery is used to remove large tophi. With gout, it is rarely necessary to replace a joint.

Complementary Treatments

Complementary medicine treatments focus on removing excess uric acid from the body. Nutrition and herbal medicine are the main approaches to reduce and eliminate the symptoms of gout.

Diet

Purine is a compound in the body that breaks down to form uric acid. Eating foods high in purine may raise the levels of uric acid in the body, causing gout in people who are susceptible to this condition. The following foods are high in purine and should be eliminated from the diet: organ meats, anchovies, sardines, mackerel, herring, fish roes, and meat extracts. Because they have moderate amounts of purine, limit your consumption of other meats and fish as well as lentils, whole-grain cereals, beans, peas, asparagus, cauliflower, mushrooms, and spinach.

To lower your uric acid levels and prevent an attack, eat a half pound of fresh or frozen cherries every day for 2 weeks. The antioxidants that they contain have been shown to be effective in lowering uric acid levels. Other beneficial antioxidants are hawthorn berries, blueberries, strawberries, and other dark red-blue berries. Noncitrus juices and vegetable juices such as celery, parsley, and carrot juice are also recommended. Vegetables such as cabbage, kale, and other green leafy vegetables may be valuable.

Herbal Medicine

Bilberry and grape seed extract. Bilberry and grape seed extract, also referred to as proanthocyanidin (PAC) bioflavonoids, are both antioxidants that are useful in the relief of gout. Bilberry eliminates uric acid, and grape seed extract reduces inflammation. The recommended daily dose of bilberry is one 100-milligram capsule, standardized to 25 percent anthocyanosides, three times a day. Take one daily 100-milligram capsule of grape seed extract, standardized to contain 95 percent procyanidolic oligomers (PCOs).

Devil's claw. Devil's claw, which is an anti-inflammatory agent, relieves joint pain and reduces uric acid levels. It is available in a tincture, tea, or capsule. As a tea, 1 to 2 grams of the dried powdered root is steeped in a cup of boiling water for 5 to 10 minutes. Drink 3 cups per day. With a tincture, take 1 teaspoon three times a day. In capsule form, 400 milligrams is the recommended daily dose. (There is no standardization of devil's claw.)

Flaxseed and charcoal poultice. Another useful herbal remedy is a poultice made of flaxseed and charcoal. To prepare, combine equal amounts of flaxseed powder and activated charcoal powder. Both of these are available in health food stores. Gradually add hot water until a paste is formed. Place the paste on the afflicted joint and cover it with plastic wrap. This will draw out toxins. Replace the poultice every 2 to 4 hours.

Juniper berries and nettle. Juniper berries and nettle are two diuretic herbs, effective in reducing uric acid. Juniper berries are available in tincture form; take 0.5 to 1.0 milliliter, three times a day. It should be noted that due to their stimulating effect on the kidneys, juniper berries should be avoided by people with kidney disease. Stinging nettle supports kidney function. The recommended daily dose for nettle is 250 milligrams.

Nutritional Supplements

Nutritional supplementation aids in maintaining proper levels of nutrients, prevents the production of uric acid, and has anti-inflammatory effects.

- Multivitamin/mineral: Take as directed on the label. Ensures proper levels of essential nutrients.

- B-complex vitamins: Take as directed on the label. Assist in proper digestion.

- Bromelain: 200 to 400 milligrams three times a day between meals. Anti-inflammatory. Often found in capsules with quercetin as they should be taken together for better absorption.

- Folic acid: 5 milligrams daily. Helps inhibit the production of uric acid.

- Omega-3 fatty acids: 1 tablespoon of flax-seed oil daily. Decreases inflammation and tissue damage of gout.

- Quercetin: 250 to 500 milligrams three times a day between meals. Bioflavonoid that inhibits the enzyme that produces uric acid and prevents release of inflammatory compounds.

Lifestyle Recommendations

Elevate the painful joint. During an attack, keep the painful joint elevated.

Lose weight. If your doctor has indicated that excess weight is contributing to your gout, you need to lose some of the pounds. Ask your doctor for some suggestions or a referral to a weight-loss program.

Preventive Measures

Sip coffee. Canadian researchers found that coffee consumption, both caffeinated and decaffeinated, lowered uric acid levels, which reduces the risk of gout.

Don't smoke. Smoking increases blood pressure and cholesterol, two risk factors of gout.

Drink nonalcoholic and noncaffeinated fluids. Drink plenty of nonalcoholic and non-caffeinated fluids throughout the day. Fresh juices made from raw fruits and vegetables are best, particularly during an attack. Juices made with blueberries, carrots, celery, cherries, parsley, strawberries, and any other dark red-blue berries are most beneficial, as all of these help to neutralize uric acid. This dilutes and promotes the excretion of uric acid in urine. You also need to keep your fluid intake up in order to avoid dehydration, which can trigger a gout attack.

Exercise. Exercising and stretching regularly increase circulation, which helps to remove uric acid and other excess toxins from the body. Any type of exercise that does not irritate the affected joint is beneficial. Swimming, walking, and bicycling are all recommended. Tai chi, yoga, and qigong are other forms of exercise that increase circulation and remove excess uric acid.

Reduce alcohol consumption. Reduce your consumption of alcohol. Studies have shown that a daily glass of red wine may provide some health benefits without increasing the risk of gout or an attack as compared to consuming beer or hard liquor.

Gum Disease

Gum disease is an infection of the gums or the tissues that surround and support the teeth. It is caused by plaque, a sticky film of bacteria, which may harden into a substance called tartar (calculus). Toxins emitted by the bacteria damage the gums.

In the early stage of gum disease, which is called gingivitis, the gums tend to be red and swollen, and they may bleed easily. Still, this type of gum disease is reversible. In the more advanced forms of gum disease (periodontitis), the inner layer of the gum and bone recede and form pockets, called periodontal pockets. Spaces between the teeth and gums have the tendency to collect debris and become infected. Gums and the bones supporting the teeth become profoundly damaged. Teeth may fall out or require extraction by a dentist.

In addition to harming your teeth and their supporting bones, periodontal (gum) disease places you at increased risk for other medical problems. For example, if you have periodontal disease, you have a greater risk for respiratory infection. Moreover, people with periodontal disease are almost twice as likely to have coronary artery disease, and there is also an association between gum disease and stroke.

Gum disease is extremely common. It has been estimated that more than 75 percent of Americans over the age of 35 have some level of this disorder.

Causes and Risk Factors

While gum disease may be caused by inadequate oral hygiene, there are also a number of other factors that may play a role. One of the key causes is the use of tobacco. People who smoke are far more likely than nonsmokers to have gum disease. Moreover, smoking reduces the likelihood that any treatment will be effective. Other possible contributing factors are hormonal fluctuations, stress, poor nutrition, poor-fitting fillings and crowns, anatomical tooth abnormalities, illness, and clenching and grinding of the teeth.

People who are living with HIV/AIDS or autoimmune conditions such as rheumatoid arthritis and Crohn's disease are known to have higher rates of gum disease, as do those who have inadequate amounts of vitamin C in their diet. Diabetics are more likely to suffer from periodontal disease. Likewise, people with diabetes who have periodontal disease experience increases in their blood sugar, which means they have a greater risk for complications.

Since saliva is protective of the teeth and gums, medications that reduce the levels of saliva in the mouth may foster gum disease. The antiseizure medication diphenylhydantoin (Dilantin) and the drug nifedipine (Nimotop, a calcium-channel blocker used to treat cardiovascular disease) may cause gum tissue to grow abnormally.

Your risk for gum disease increases as you age. More than half of those over age 55 have periodontitis. Furthermore, it is believed that up to 30 percent of the American population may have a genetic tendency for gum disease. Those who are predisposed may be up to six times more likely to develop some level of gum disease than those who do not have this predisposition.

Signs and Symptoms

Even if you don't notice symptoms, you still may have gum disease. That is one of the reasons that regular visits with a dentist are so important. However, many people with gum disease do have symptoms. These may include receding gums; gums that bleed during and/ or after brushing the teeth; frequent bad breath or bad taste in the mouth; red, swollen, or tender gums; loose or shifting teeth; abscesses; deep pockets or pus between teeth and gums; and changes in your bite or the fit of your partial dentures.

Conventional Treatments

The goal of treatment is to stop the progression of gum disease and control infection. Your dentist will suggest how often you should brush and floss your teeth. Since brushing removes only the plaque from the outside of the teeth, flossing is very important. It gets under the gumline and between the teeth. In some instances, to obtain a better cleaning, your dentist may advise using a special toothbrush that has motorized heads.

During a checkup, your dentist or dental hygienist will remove plaque and tartar that are above and below the gumline. If there is evidence of gingivitis, more frequent cleanings will most likely be advised. Your dentist may also suggest that you use a toothpaste or mouthwash that is FDA-approved for gingivitis. Colgate Total, which contains the mild antimicrobial triclosan, has received FDA approval for that use. You will need a prescription from your dentist for a mouthwash that contains chlorhexidine, which has received similar approval.

If your dentist determines that there has been bone loss and your gums have receded, you will probably be referred to a periodontist, a dentist who specializes in gum disease and dental implants. It is at the periodontist's office

A Quick Guide to Symptoms

- ☐ Receding gums
- ☐ Gums that bleed during and/or after brushing the teeth
- ☐ Frequent bad breath or bad taste in the mouth
- ☐ Red, swollen, or tender gums
- ☐ Loose or shifting teeth
- ☐ Abscesses
- ☐ Deep pockets or pus between teeth and gums
- ☐ Changes in your bite or the fit of your partial dentures

that you will have a more intensive, deep cleaning, which is called a scaling and root planing (or SRP). To reduce the discomfort, before the procedure, you will be given a local anesthetic. During a scaling, the periodontist performs a deeper scraping of the plaque and tartar above and below the gumline. Root planing smoothes the roots of the teeth and aids in the removal of bacteria. With a smooth, clean surface, gums are better able to reattach to the teeth.

In conjunction with an SRP, you will probably be given a prescription for doxycycline hyclate (Periostat), an oral medication. It curtails the action of collagenase, an enzyme that is instrumental in the destruction of teeth and gums.

Choosing Floss

Avoid using very thin floss, which may cut the gum. Fortunately, it has become increasingly more difficult to locate. If you have little room between your teeth, try a floss made of Gore-Tex. It will slide more easily and not tear as quickly. If you have bridgework, you may want to consider a floss threader, a device that resembles a needle with a large loop. After floss is threaded into the loop, it may be placed between the bridge and the gum. It may then clean under the false tooth and along the sides of the adjacent teeth. A Proxabrush, a tiny narrow brush, is also useful for cleaning areas under bridges.

Surgery

If you have significant gum disease, surgery may be advised. Surgery allows for a more extensive deep cleaning of the root surface as well as the removal of diseased tissue. Bones, gum, and tissues supporting the teeth may be repositioned and shaped.

Bone grafting. If there has been severe bone loss, it may be useful to attempt to encourage the regrowth and restoration of bone tissue. During a bone-grafting procedure, either your bone or bone from a donor (decalcified freeze-dried bone allografts or DFDBAs) is used to replace lost bone and stimulate new bone growth.

Gingivectomy and gingivoplasty. In a gingivectomy, a periodontist removes gum tissue. This procedure is followed by a gingivoplasty, in which gum tissue is reshaped. Since the size of the periodontal pockets is significantly reduced, bacteria have a less desirable environment in which to grow, and the gums may be restored to good health.

Guided-tissue regeneration. In the beginning of this procedure, which is used to stimulate bone and gum tissue growth, the root surfaces and diseased bone are carefully cleaned. Special absorbable or nonabsorbable

If you have a history of mitral valve prolapse or rheumatic heart disease, tell your dentist. You may be prescribed an antibiotic before you undergo any dental work. This is done to prevent bacterial endocarditis, a life-threatening illness in which there is a bacterial infection in the heart valves.

fabrics are used to cover any holes in the bone. Gum is sewn over the fabric. In about 4 to 6 weeks, the nonabsorbable fabric must be removed.

Implants. Some patients who have lost teeth as a result of periodontal disease want dental implants. Endosteal implants are the most common type; they are positioned in the jawbone. Subperiosteal implants are placed on the jaw and are used when there is minimal bone height, due to age or disease.

Open flap curettage. During this procedure, small incisions are made in the gums, and the gums are lifted away from the teeth and bone. The diseased root surfaces are curetted (cleaned and scraped), and the pocket depth is minimized. Bone may be recontoured. Gum tissue is then positioned into the proper place.

Medications

After periodontal procedures, your dentist or periodontist may recommend continued treatment with antibiotics or other medications. Some antibiotics or other medications are applied directly to the gums; other antibiotics are taken orally.

Agents applied directly to the gums. Actisite is a thin strip that resembles dental floss, but contains tetracycline hydrochloride, an antibiotic to kill bacteria. Threads are generally inserted between a tooth and the gum and secured with dental adhesive, a type of glue. Steady concentrations of tetracycline are released into the gum. After 10 days, the threads are removed.

While the Actisite is in place, avoid foods that may loosen or dislodge the strips. These include peanuts, raw vegetables, crusty breads, and sticky items. When brushing or flossing your teeth, avoid the areas with Actisite. Also, be aware that tetracycline medication increases your sensitivity to the sun. So, as long as you are using it, be sure to wear sunscreen and, during the sunniest times of the day, try to stay out of the sun.

Other products include Atridox, which conforms to the surface of the gums and solidifies and releases antibiotics, and PerioChip, a chip that is placed inside the gum pocket after it is scaled. It releases the powerful bacteria-killing antiseptic chlorhexidine. Elyzol is either a gel or strip that is placed on the gum. It contains metronidazole, which is useful against bacteria and parasites. Since they only work locally and do not affect other areas of the body, topical products are generally the preferred method.

Oral antibiotics. A 10-day course of treatment with doxycycline (Periostat) has been found useful for acute inflammation and infection. Sometimes, a low-dose form of doxycycline is prescribed for a number of weeks. Though the dose is too low to fight bacteria, it blocks the actions of collagenase, the enzyme that harms the connective tissues that hold the teeth. Taking a nonsteroidal anti-inflammatory drug (NSAID) such as aspirin or ibuprofen (Advil) with doxycycline appears to improve the effectiveness of doxycycline.

There is also evidence that chronic periodontal disease responds to a combination of metronidazole and amoxicillin. These are administered for 1 week per month for 4 months. Potential side effects include yeast overgrowth, stomach upset, allergic reactions, and sensitivity to sunlight.

Complementary Treatments

By addressing the underlying causes, complementary medicine has been successful in providing approaches that stop the progression of gum disease and control gum infection.

Ayurveda

Because of its strong antibacterial and anti-inflammatory properties, Ayurvedic practitioners often recommend the use of neem powder to fight gum disease. In addition, neem prevents plaque and is an excellent agent in fighting periodontal disease. Neem is available as a toothpaste, as a mouthwash, and as a gum.

Biofeedback

Biofeedback uses an electric monitoring device to obtain data on vital body functions. During a session, you will be taught ways to use relaxation techniques to alter or slow the body's signals. Biofeedback has been shown to be valuable for people who have gum disease caused by clenching or grinding their teeth. Various health care professionals incorporate biofeedback into their practice, including psychiatrists, psychologists, social workers, nurses, physical therapists, occupational therapists, speech therapists, respiratory therapists, exercise physiologists, and chiropractors.

It is recommended that you seek a health care practitioner who has been certified through the Biofeedback Certification Institute of America (BCIA). To locate a practitioner in your area, look on the BCIA Web site at www.bcia.org, check your local hospitals and medical clinics, or check the Yellow Pages under the practitioners mentioned above.

Diet

Gums and teeth always benefit from a healthier diet. The absence of antioxidants in your diet can lead to an increase in free radicals, which increase bacteria and inflammation of the gums. Be sure to include lots of fruits and vegetables that contain vitamin C, such as broccoli, brussels sprouts, cantaloupe, grapefruit, oranges, and strawberries. Deficiency in vitamin C is directly linked to gum disease. Additionally, many smokers have lower levels of vitamin C, which may increase the risk of developing gum disease even further. Limit your intake of processed foods and foods that are high in sugar and saturated fat. An unbalanced, poor diet may weaken the immune system, which may cause receding gums and bone loss.

Oral treatments, or medications you ingest by mouth, have the potential to cause side effects such as gum redness, swelling, pain, aching, throbbing, soreness, and bleeding. If you are experiencing more than mild discomfort, you should contact your dentist or periodontist.

Herbal Medicine

Herbs may be found in all dental care products, such as toothpaste, mouthwash, dental floss, dental picks, and lip balm. Because of their antiseptic and antibiotic properties, there are many herbs that are helpful in treating gum disease. Others are used for their invigorating and fresh taste. They safely and effectively provide the same benefits as ingredients found in conventional dental products. Instead of artificial flavors and sweeteners, such as saccharine or glycerine, natural toothpaste may freshen breath with natural ingredients such as fennel or peppermint. Peppermint also has antiseptic and antibiotic properties that treat gum infections. Clove is useful in relieving toothaches and is invigorating to the mouth and gums, as is ginger. Chamomile has anti-inflammatory properties that soothe the mucous membranes in the mouth. Eucalyptus is a germicide, antiseptic, and astringent; myrrh repairs painful bleeding gums; and calendula eases toothache pain.

Aloe vera. To help reduce pain and inflammation, rub a small amount of aloe vera gel directly on the gums. Aloe vera is available as a prepared ointment, a liquid drink, or a gel. To accelerate the healing of irritated gums, the natural gel or prepared ointment should be rubbed directly on the gums.

Echinacea and goldenseal. When used in mouthwashes, echinacea and goldenseal are as effective against germs as are conventional mouthwashes that contain alcohol.

Horsetail and bloodroot. Horsetail and bloodroot have been found to be extremely helpful in preventing and treating gum disease. The gel from the silica of the horsetail plant is particularly effective for periodontal disease caused by years of smoking. It also protects against bacteria, fungi, and viruses. Bloodroot has been shown to inhibit oral bacteria, diminish plaque, and stimulate the flow of saliva. The enzyme in the saliva breaks down plaque and flushes out food particles, so bloodroot is useful in the treatment of gingivitis.

Sage. Because of its antiseptic and astringent properties, sage is another herb that is beneficial in mouthwash.

Tea tree oil. Tea tree oil is a powerful antiseptic, germicide, and fungicide commonly found in dental products. It is particularly useful for combating bacteria that cause gum disease.

Nutritional Supplements

Deficiency in essential vitamins and minerals can increase the risk for periodontal disease.

- Multivitamin/mineral: Take as directed on the label. Should contain 200 IU of vitamin D for its anti-inflammatory effects, which can help reduce susceptibility to gum disease.

- Vitamin C: 1,000 milligrams daily in divided doses of 500 milligrams each. Deficiency leads to gum disease.

- Calcium: 1,000 milligrams daily in divided doses of 500 milligrams each. Needed for strong teeth.

Lifestyle Recommendations

Check your town's fluoride levels in drinking water. A study reported in the April–June 2007 issue of the *Indian Journal of Dental Research* stated that when excess fluoride was added to the drinking water, incidence of gum disease increased. Interestingly, for the study, fluoride levels were brought up to the level commonly used in many US cities, 4 ppm (parts per million).

Choose natural dental care products. Natural ingredients are able to perform the same functions as the chemicals and additives found in conventional dental products. Calcium carbonate (natural chalk) polishes teeth without harsh abrasives. In addition to cleaning and whitening, by hardening the tooth enamel, baking soda remineralizes and strengthens the teeth as effectively as fluoride. Sea salt also remineralizes the teeth and makes them stronger. Peroxide is particularly useful for fighting gingivitis.

Drink sufficient water. Drink at least eight 8-ounce glasses of water every day. That will enable your mouth to produce sufficient amounts of saliva, which reduces mouth inflammation. This becomes increasingly more important as one ages. In addition, an adequate amount of daily water may reduce bad breath, tooth decay, and infection.

Replace your toothbrush about once a month. Brushes that are worn are less effective in removing plaque. Look for an American Dental Association (ADA) seal on your toothbrush and always choose a toothbrush with a soft head.

Use correct brushing technique. Begin by brushing your teeth with a dry brush for about $1\frac{1}{2}$ minutes. Brush where the gum meets the tooth. The bristles should rest at a 45-degree angle to the teeth. Brush the inside of the bottom teeth first, and then the inside of the top teeth and the outside of the teeth. Don't forget also to brush the biting surfaces of the teeth. After applying a paste to the toothbrush, repeat the entire process. Conclude the process by brushing the tongue for about 30 seconds. Thoroughly rinse your toothbrush and follow the brushing with flossing.

In choosing a toothbrush, it is important that you find the right one for you. There are scores of different options. Experiment with the various shapes, and replace the brush when the bristles become frayed. You do not need to brush hard.

Use correct flossing technique. In spite of the proven benefits, about two-thirds of people do not floss. Yet, flossing is one of the most important things you can do for your teeth. Begin with about 18 inches of dental floss. Wind it around the middle fingers of both hands. Holding the floss between your thumbs and forefingers, glide it gently back and forth between your teeth. At the gum line, curve it around each tooth and slide it against the gum. Then, rub it up and down the teeth.

Preventive Measures

Brush often. Brush your teeth at least twice a day. Use a soft-bristled toothbrush that is in good condition and toothpaste and mouth-washes containing natural ingredients that strengthen teeth and prevent decay. At least once each day, clean between your teeth with floss or an interdental cleaner.

Cut down on sugar. Sugar helps the bacteria that create plaque to multiply.

Get outside. Vitamin D, which is absorbed through direct sunlight, is needed for healthy gums. Try to get 15 minutes of sun per day to give your body an adequate amount of vitamin D.

Get regular dental checkups. Keep regular visits with your dentist. This will improve the chances that problems will be caught early, when they are easiest to treat. Also, professional cleanings are vital in the prevention of periodontal disease.

Massage the gums. To help strengthen your gums and improve their overall health, use a sulcus brush, which is a toothbrush with a stimulator. These are sold wherever toothbrushes are sold. The brush should be used without toothpaste to massage the gums. By stimulating lymphatic flow, this will improve circulation and help remove waste products. It is recommended that you do this 2 to 3 minutes every day.

Another option is to massage your gums with the tip of a finger onto which you have applied a small amount of eucalyptus or witch hazel. Massage in a circular motion for 5 minutes each day.

Reduce stress. Take measures to reduce stress and to deal with the stress that you cannot avoid. Excess stress and worry may lead to higher levels of the stress hormone cortisol in the saliva. Cortisol lowers immunity, which in turn may lead to gum disease.

Stop smoking. If you smoke, stop. Smoking contributes to gum disease. Studies have shown that smoking is the number one cause of periodontal disease. More than half of periodontal cases are linked to smoking.

Use a tongue scraper. Remove as much bacteria from your tongue as you can. The tongue is a breeding ground for bacteria. In fact, 90 percent of bad breath is from bacteria on the tongue. To combat the buildup of bacteria, you may wish to use a tongue scraper. It removes bacteria from the tongue crevices. To avoid gagging, start at the tip of the tongue and gradually work your way to the back, scraping toward the tip.

Take your time to brush. The American Dental Association recommends brushing your teeth for 2 minutes to ensure adequate removal of plaque. Plaque is a thick, sticky substance similar to peanut butter. If you try to wipe peanut butter from your counter surface, you will find that it does not remove with one easy swipe of a paper towel or sponge. Many toothbrushes, both manual and electric, have built-in timers that beep to let you know when you have reached 2 minutes.

Hair Loss

If you're under the impression that your hair grew better when you were young, you're probably right. When you're young, each individual strand of hair grows for between 2 and 6 years. When the strand finally falls out, it is quickly replaced by a brand-new hair that grows in the very same follicle. But as people age, their hair grows at a slower pace, and some of the individual hairs are not replaced by new strands.

Most people are familiar with male-pattern baldness, which begins with the thinning of the hair and the recession of the hairline from the forehead, crown, and temples. At first, the receding hair tends to follow an M-shaped pattern. In time, more hair falls out, and the remaining hair forms a horseshoe pattern that covers the head. For women who experience hair loss, the picture is somewhat different. In a condition known as female-pattern baldness, women's hair simply thins, or there may be an enlargement of the part in the center of the scalp. In women, hair loss may begin as early as adolescence. Before women reach their 50th birthday, about half have some degree of hair loss. Most of these women have normal menses and hormone levels.

Hair loss is extremely common. Under normal conditions, a person loses at least 100 of the 100,000 hairs on their scalp every day. By midlife, both men and women are at greater risk for hair loss. Women's hair is more likely to thin. Men tend to go bald. By the time a man is age 60, there is about a 66 percent chance that he will be balding or bald.

Causes and Risk Factors

Both male- and female-pattern baldness are known as androgenetic alopecia, and both are caused by hormonal changes and heredity. However, excess hair loss may be caused by other factors. These include illness, stress, surgery, inadequate diet, anemia, nutritional deficiencies, thyroid disease, diabetes, lupus, chemicals in hair dyes and permanents, excess consumption of vitamin A, and scalp infections. Sometimes, hair loss due to such causes may be delayed. For example, hair loss may occur 3 or 4 months after an illness or surgery. Medications are a well-known cause of hair loss. Among the medications that may trigger hair loss are anticoagulants (blood thinners), antidepressants, and chemotherapy agents.

Signs and Symptoms

If you are losing significant portions of your hair, there's a good chance that you will know it. You will notice more hair on your clothes, on the bathroom floor, on your comb or brush, and in the shower drain. Your hair may feel thinner or even fall out in chunks in your hands. Men who are losing their hair may note their receding hairlines.

Conventional Treatments

If your hair loss is caused by an underlying medical problem or the use of certain medications, the medical problem will need to be addressed or the medication changed, if appropriate. Typically, these actions should stop hair loss. If your hair loss is due to chemotherapy treatments for cancer, your hair should start growing again after treatment is completed. However, it may take up to a year for adequate hair regrowth to occur, and the hair might initially be different in color and texture from the hair that was lost.

If hair loss is caused by male- or female-pattern baldness, you do not necessarily need to take any action. These are physically benign conditions. Still, if you are uncom-fortable with your appearance, you may wish to seek treatment.

Medications

The FDA has approved one drug for baldness in both men and women and a second drug for baldness in just men. Minoxidil (Rogaine), which is approved for both men and women, is an over-the-counter topical solution that increases bloodflow to the scalp. Increased bloodflow is believed to foster hair growth. Expect to use minoxidil for at least 3 to 6 months before you see any results. Minoxidil does not help everyone. Approximately 20 to 25 percent of those who use minoxidil will experience hair growth, but that hair tends to be short. A majority will note that hair loss slows down. If you decide to try minoxidil, the recommended use is twice a day. Watch out for headaches, a known side effect. If you do experience headaches, report this to your doctor. When minoxidil treatment is discontinued, hair loss recurs.

Finasteride (Propecia), a daily oral medication, has been approved only for male-pattern baldness. It blocks the formation of dihydrotestosterone (DHT), the male hormone that reduces the duration of the growing phase of hair. Excess amounts of DHT trigger both the thinning of hair and hair loss. About half of the men who take this drug experience increased hair growth within a year, so it typically offers better results than minoxidil. When men stop taking finasteride, the benefits last no longer than 1 year. Fewer than 2 percent of men who

A Quick Guide to Symptoms

- ☐ **More hair on your clothes, on the bathroom floor, on your comb or brush, and in the shower drain**
- ☐ **Hair may feel thinner or even fall out in chunks**
- ☐ **Receding hairline**

take this drug experience some form of sexual dysfunction as a side effect, and a small number of men experience some breast tenderness. Because finasteride may be absorbed through the skin, a woman who is pregnant or of reproductive age should *never* touch one of these pills. Even minimal exposure may cause abnormal growth in the genitalia of developing male fetuses.

Surgery

Several types of surgery can address hair loss, primarily hair loss resulting from male-pattern baldness. Take special care when selecting a physician to perform any of these procedures. Not every physician who practices surgery for hair loss has adequate training. You may wish to check with the American Board of Hair Restoration Surgery at www.abhrs.org.

Hair transplantation. In a hair transplant, a physician removes tiny plugs of hair from areas of the scalp that have hair and grafts them in areas of the scalp that have lost hair. The procedure will likely take place either at your doctor's office or at an outpatient surgical center. Before the procedure, you will be given a sedative, and your scalp will be anesthetized. Following the procedure, you may have a headache and bruising around your eyes, but this should resolve within a few days. Pain is managed with over-the-counter or prescription medication. Sometimes, the donor areas have minor scarring, and there's a small risk of infection in the grafted areas.

Days after the procedure, the grafted hair begins to fall out. During the first month, you can expect only minimal hair growth to replace this. It takes about 3 months for hair from the transplanted follicles to begin showing real growth.

Generally, these transplants are done in stages and completed during a few office visits. The procedures are both time-consuming and expensive.

Laser hair transplantation. Instead of using a scalpel to make the holes in which the hair is grafted, some physicians use a laser. Beams from the laser vaporize scalp tissue. The physician doesn't use the laser to harvest the donor hairs. These are harvested with a scalpel. Those who favor the use of lasers maintain that they reduce bleeding, shorten the time it takes to complete the surgery, and lessen the chances that the scalp will have a "lumpy" look. Those who are opposed to the use of lasers contend that they produce more scarring and destroy more tissue. You should be aware that when lasers are used, individuals tend to have less hair growth.

Scalp reduction surgery. In this surgery, bald areas of the scalp are removed and replaced with grafts of skin covered with hair. Generally, this technique requires a number of separate procedures that are performed in a physician's office under local anesthesia. This surgery is controversial; some call it outdated and barbaric. And it has a number of possible complications, such as infection, bleeding, and scarring at the site of the reduction.

Complementary Treatments

Enhancing bloodflow to the scalp may reduce hair loss. This is done through dietary changes, nutritional supplements, and various complementary medicine approaches.

Acupuncture

Health care practitioners use acupuncture to treat hair loss because of its ability to increase the circulation of blood in the scalp. To locate an acupuncturist in your area, visit the Web site of the National Certification Commission for Acupuncture and Oriental Medicine (NCCAOM) at www.nccaom.org.

Aromatherapy

Essential oil of rosemary fosters hair growth, clary sage may minimize hair loss, and cedarwood is said to do both. You can create your own shampoo blend with these oils by adding them to a natural, unscented shampoo. Add 10 drops of each to 8 ounces of the unscented shampoo and use daily.

For a hot oil treatment, add 6 drops of each oil to 1 ounce of jojoba oil. Place the oil in a clean container and gently blend. Place the container in a pan of hot (not boiling) water until it is warm, then gently massage into your hair. Wrap your hair in a towel and wait 20 minutes before rinsing.

Ayurveda

Ayurvedic medicine addresses hair loss through a combination of diet, herbs, meditation, and massage. The focus is on balancing the *pitta* dosha (an Ayurvedic constitutional type). Individuals with excess *pitta* have too much heat in their bodies, including in the sebaceous glands at the root of the hair. This excess heat may cause the hair to thin and fall out.

An Ayurvedic practitioner may recommend a number of solutions. A half cup of aloe vera juice, which is cooling to the system, may be taken daily; it reduces heat and strengthens hair. Used as a massage oil, coconut oil may be applied every night to the scalp, palms of the hands, and soles of the feet; this calms the *pitta* dosha.

As additional heat will only aggravate your condition, you should avoid spicy foods. On the other hand, feel free to enjoy dairy products, especially yogurt. Eating yogurt with 2 tablespoons of white sesame seeds or almonds every day promotes hair growth.

Diet

Many nutrients are essential for maintaining healthy hair, improving hair growth, and preventing hair loss. The B vitamins, for example, play an important role in hair growth and hair loss. Vitamins B_3 (niacin) and B_5 (pantothenic acid) are essential for hair growth. Deficiencies in biotin, folic acid, inositol (a cofactor of B vitamins that helps them convert food into cellular energy), and the minerals magnesium, zinc, and sulfur may contribute to hair loss. You do not need to have deficiencies in all of these vitamins to experience hair loss. An insufficient amount of any one of them could trigger a problem. It should be noted that if hair loss is due to a deficiency in the B vitamins, it may be reversed when these essential nutrients are added to the diet. However, it may take 2 to 4 months to see the results.

The B vitamins may be found in avocados, bananas, beans, beets, chicken, dairy products, dark green leafy vegetables, fish, nuts, oranges, potatoes, sunflower seeds, and whole grains. Magnesium is found in nuts (almonds, peanuts, peanut butter, and walnuts) and beans (kidney, white, pinto, and lima). Cooked broccoli and spinach are also good sources, as are soy milk and tofu. Zinc is contained in the same nuts mentioned for magnesium, but high amounts are also found in raw, canned, or smoked oysters.

Since healthy hair is related to the status of your immune system, it may be possible to stimulate hair growth by enhancing immune function. In addition to zinc, the antioxidant vitamins C and E are necessary to strengthen the immune system. Vitamins C and E also improve circulation to the scalp, which fosters hair growth. Vitamin C may be found in almost all fruits and vegetables. Vitamin E is in nuts (almonds, hazelnuts, and peanuts), sunflower seeds, and oils such as wheat germ, sunflower, safflower, peanut, corn, and almond.

Iron-deficiency anemia may cause hair loss. If you eat a healthy diet that includes dark green, leafy vegetables, whole grains and cereals, raisins, dates, and lean red meat, you should be getting the iron you need.

It should be noted that a lack of protein in the diet might also cause hair, which is composed of protein, to enter a resting phase, during which new growth stops. If you eat cheese, eggs, fish, meat, milk, poultry, and yogurt, you probably have sufficient protein in your diet. Soy protein, found in tofu and soy milk, strengthens the hair and stimulates growth.

You should be aware of any possible underlying health concerns that may cause or contribute to hair loss and that can be addressed through nutrition. For example, people with kidney disease must be careful to monitor their protein intake. Do not make radical changes in your diet without first consulting with your doctor.

Herbal Medicine

Ginkgo biloba. Ginkgo is an antioxidant that supports circulation. It is available in capsule form. However, if you are taking prescription blood-thinning medication, be sure to consult your doctor before taking ginkgo supplements. The recommended daily dose is 120 milligrams, twice a day, of extract standardized to 24 percent of flavone glycosides and 6 percent terpene lactones. The flavone glycosides give ginkgo its antioxidant benefits, while terpene lactones increase circulation and have a protective effect on nerve cells.

Kombucha. Kombucha stops hair loss and

is a popular herb that is added to green tea. It is found in commercially prepared tea bags in health food stores and natural grocery stores. Drink 2 to 3 cups daily. Refer to Traditional Chinese Medicine (below) for additional herbal suggestions.

Homeopathy

To determine the best remedy for your particular symptoms, it is best to consult a homeopathic practitioner. However, the following are examples of remedies that work for hair loss. Phosphorus (6C potency) is recommended for hair that falls out in clumps. *Phosphorum acidum* 1X is for hair loss that is due to depression. Selenium 6C is for hair loss that is accompanied by a tender scalp that is painful to touch. And *Fluoricum acidum* 6C is for brittle hair that falls out in smaller amounts. To find a practitioner trained in homeopathy, visit the Web site of the National Center for Homeopathy at www.homeopathic.org.

Nutritional Supplements

Nutritional supplementation can help prevent deficiencies that can lead to hair loss; it can also help maintain healthy hair.

- B-complex vitamins: Take as directed on the label. Essential for health and growth of hair. Deficiency in certain B vitamins may result in hair loss. As the B vitamins work best when taken together, take a B-complex.

- Vitamin C: 500 milligrams daily. Improves circulation, nourishing the scalp.

- Vitamin E: 400 IU daily. Improves circulation to the scalp.

- Copper: 2 milligrams daily. Take with zinc for absorption and to aid in hair growth.

- Zinc: 30 milligrams daily. Promotes hair growth and slows the loss of hair. Take with copper.

Relaxation/Meditation

Try to incorporate some form of relaxation or meditation into your daily schedule. These techniques not only help to relieve stress and tension, but by relaxing the body they improve circulation. Some relaxation techniques, such as yoga, tai chi, and qigong, may even strengthen and tone the vital organs of the body and detoxify the blood. You may try sitting or lying still for 15 minutes each day and concentrating on inhaling and exhaling slowly and deeply. This focus on the breath quiets the mind and relieves tension.

Therapeutic Massage

A gentle head massage may stimulate circulation to the scalp, which is essential for hair growth. Start at the front of the head in the middle of the scalp, and using the pads of the fingers, apply pressure in a circular motion, slowly working toward the back of the head. Then, bring the hands to the front of the head, a little lower than the middle of the scalp. Keep going until you have covered the entire head. Repeat the process using your knuckles, only using the amount of pressure that is comfortable. Next, hold a chunk of hair very close to the scalp and give it a gentle tug. Work your way around your entire head, tugging as you go.

In a standing position, bend your knees slightly and slowly lean forward at the waist until your head is just below your waist. Massage your entire head with your fingers and knuckles. Pay special attention to the back of your head and neck. Slowly raise your body. (If you have any health concerns with your back, heart, or blood pressure, do not do this part of the routine.) Next, massage the neck muscles. Releasing tension in the neck helps the blood circulation to the scalp. Using the pads of your fingers only, apply easy strokes and circular motions to the sides and back of your neck. Using your right hand, massage and squeeze the left shoulder area. Repeat on the opposite side.

End the session by sitting straight in a chair. Grab under the seat of the chair, and pull upward on the chair as hard as you can. This tightens the neck and shoulder muscles. While pulling, turn your head slowly to the left, back to the center, and then slowly to the right. Return to the center and lift your chin up toward the ceiling, being careful not to overextend to an uncomfortable position, and then move it down to your chest. Return to the center, and roll your head gently in a circle. This stretches the muscles and increases circulation to the neck and upper body, allowing freer circulation to the head. Repeat this three times. In the beginning, do this routine for 5 minutes; then try to work up to 10 minutes each day.

Traditional Chinese Medicine

Practitioners of traditional Chinese medicine attempt to determine the underlying weakness in the body that is causing hair loss. Once they learn what is causing it, they try to correct the problem by strengthening the weakness. Practitioners believe that the hair is directly related to the blood. Since the kidneys play a role in cleansing the blood, treatments focus on strengthening the kidneys to improve the quality of the blood, thereby preventing hair loss. This may be accomplished through the use of herbs, acupuncture, diet, and scalp massage.

Oriental tonics promote new hair growth by toning the kidneys and liver with herbs such as Chinese yam, lycium fruit, and Chinese foxglove root. Psoralea seeds have been shown to stimulate hair growth; the recommended dose is to eat at least 3 grams of seeds each day. Biota is an herb that may help prevent further hair loss as well as thicken existing hair. Drynaria may stimulate hair growth. A traditional Chinese medicine practitioner will be able to guide you to the proper dosage and combination of herbs. To locate a practitioner trained in traditional Chinese medicine, visit the Web site of the National Certification Commission for Acupuncture and Oriental Medicine (NCCAOM) at www.nccaom.org or the American Association of Acupuncture and Oriental Medicine at www.aaaomonline.org.

Preventive Measures

While hair loss due to genetic reasons cannot be prevented, the following may be helpful in minimizing further hair loss.

Reduce exposure to chlorine and salt water. These may damage your hair, leaving it dry and brittle. This increases the risk of hair loss. If you cannot keep your head out of the water or wear a bathing cap, be sure to rinse your hair immediately after swimming.

Reduce stress. There is a definite relationship between stress and hair loss. During stressful periods, the body may stop making hair. If you are able to decrease the stress in your life, you may reduce the amount of hair you are losing.

Take better care of your hair. Reduce the physical stress on your hair. If you tend to wear your hair in cornrows or tied back tightly in a bun, you may be exposing it to too much tension. Consider wearing your hair in a style in which there is less tension. Also, frequent exposure to heat from the use of blow-dryers and curling or straightening irons places stress on the hair, causing it to dry, become brittle, and fall out. Chemicals used in most hair colors and permanents may irritate the scalp, causing an allergic reaction; in addition, they may stunt hair growth.

Use natural shampoos and conditioners. Pick your shampoo wisely. Avoid shampoos and conditioners with artificial chemicals and try to find shampoos with natural ingredients and low acid pH.

Hearing Loss

Hearing loss is the diminished ability to hear sounds in one or both ears. It's hardly surprising that so many of us experience hearing loss as we age. After all, hearing is a complicated and delicate affair. The ear is divided into three components: the outer ear (auricle and external ear canal), the middle ear (eardrum, middle ear bones, and middle ear space), and the inner ear (the cochlea, semicircular canals, and internal auditory canal). Sound waves are trapped by the auricle and channeled through the external ear canal to the eardrum. The sound waves cause the eardrum to vibrate, leading to motion in the middle ear bones. This motion triggers fluid waves within the cochlea, which are then transformed into nerve impulses in the auditory nerve. The auditory nerve transmits these impulses to the brain, where the messages are organized into sounds.

Hearing loss is generally classified as either sensorineural or conductive in origin. Sensorineural hearing loss is due to problems in the inner ear or auditory nerve. This form of hearing loss, which may be the result of head injury, tumors, illness, the use of certain prescription drugs, poor circulation, stroke, high blood pressure, or birth defects, may not be reversible. Conductive hearing loss is due to problems in the outer or middle ear that block or limit sounds from the tympanic membrane (eardrum) from reaching the inner ear. Blockage may be caused by the presence of fluid in the middle ear, abnormal bone growth, earwax in the ear canal, or a middle-ear infection. Conductive hearing loss is often correctable.

The most common type of hearing loss in aging adults is presbycusis, which is sensorineural in origin and is caused by changes in the inner ear (the cochlea and semicircular canals). As we age, hair cells in the cochlea die and are not replaced. As a result, there is a reduced transmission of electrical messages from the outer ear to the brain. Hair cells that receive high-frequency sounds are the first to deteriorate.

Tinnitus is another common form of hearing loss, which is usually sensorineural in origin. With tinnitus, you hear ringing, roaring, or other sounds inside your ears. The condition may be caused by a number of factors, such as the overuse of aspirin, the use of antibiotics, earwax, an ear infection, or a nerve disorder. However, doctors are frequently unable to locate a cause. The progression of tinnitus is variable: It may stop entirely, periodically reappear, or remain more or less constant.

Hearing loss is quite common. A total of about 28 million Americans of all ages have some degree of hearing loss. By the age of 55, about 20 percent of all Americans are affected. A decade later, at the age of 65, that figure climbs to 33 percent.

Causes and Risk Factors

The process of aging increases your risk for hearing loss. Genetics is also believed to play a role, and environmental factors are extremely important. Those who have been exposed to loud sounds for extended periods of time are at greatly increased risk.

An increasingly common cause of hearing loss is the exposure to loud noise, a sensorineural condition that is called noise-induced hearing loss. While this may be due to sudden exposure to loud noise such as an explosion, noise-induced hearing loss is most often seen in people who are exposed to persistent loud sounds, such as those who work (or previously worked) in noisy environments. Musicians, construction and airport workers, and tree cutters are among those particularly prone to noise-induced hearing loss.

More than 1 million Americans, primarily women over the age of 40, have Ménière's disease, an inner-ear sensorineural disorder. Though it is known for causing episodes of dizziness, nausea, vomiting, tinnitus, and vertigo, this condition may also result in spells of hearing loss that may come and go. It is believed that Ménière's disease is triggered by the buildup of excess fluid in the inner ear, eventually resulting in the bursting of inner ear membranes. Over time, hearing loss may become profound.

Medications That May Cause Hearing Loss

The following are some of the prescription medications that may cause hearing loss.

☐ **Beta-blockers such as metoprolol (Lopressor) and propanolol (Inderal), which are frequently used for high blood pressure**

☐ **Aminoglycoside antibiotics, such as gentamicin (Geramycin, G-Mycin, Jenamicin 2), neomycin, and tobramycin (Nebcin)**

☐ **Diuretics such as furosemide (Lasix, Myrosemide) and ethacrynic acid (Edecrin), prescribed for high blood pressure and congestive heart failure**

☐ **Chloroquine, a malaria drug (the hearing loss is usually reversible)**

☐ **Aspirin (the hearing loss is usually reversible)**

☐ **Quinidine (Cardioquin, Quinaglute, Quinidex, Quin-Release), used to treat irregular heartbeat**

☐ **Cisplatin (Platinol), a cancer chemotherapy agent**

Signs and Symptoms

If you have hearing loss, you are having difficulty hearing what other people say. You may have a problem hearing the other person on the telephone. It may seem as if others are mumbling or the radio or television volume is too low. You may have trouble hearing when there is noise in the background. If more than two people are talking at the same time, you may be unable to follow a conversation. You may have tingling or ringing in your ears.

Do you often misunderstand what people are saying? Do others tell you that the TV or radio volume is too loud? Are you finding that you are frequently asking others to repeat what they just said? These are all signs of hearing loss.

Conventional Treatments

If your doctor determines that your hearing loss is caused by an ear infection, then the appropriate antibiotic may be prescribed. Similarly, if the loss is from impacted earwax, your doctor will remove it. This process begins with putting a few drops of baby oil, mineral oil, or glycerin into the affected ear to loosen the wax. Then, using a bulb syringe, your doctor squirts warm water into your ear. On occasion, the procedure needs to be repeated several times before the wax falls out. At times, a doctor may use a suction device or a small instrument known as a curette to scoop out the wax.

Other treatments for hearing loss, depending on their cause and nature, may include the use of hearing aids and surgery.

Hearing Aids

The vast majority of adults with age-related hearing loss benefit from wearing a hearing aid. It is important to remember that hearing aids make sounds louder, but they do not make them any clearer. However, you don't want the hearing aid to make sound too loud, which could further damage your ears. So, take care to find a reputable dealer; ask your doctor to recommend one. Allow yourself at least 4 to 6 weeks to adjust to a hearing aid.

The following is a brief outline of the main types of available hearing aids.

• Completely in-the-canal (CIC): The size of a jellybean, this is the smallest and least visible style. It fits into the ear canal. This type of hearing aid is useful for mild to moderate hearing loss. Since the volume is preset, you may need to return to the dealer several times for adjustments. Also, this type is not for people with a lot of earwax.

• In-the-canal (ITC): This type of hearing aid fits into the opening of the ear canal. It is useful for people with moderately severe hearing loss. Though the volume control device is small and may be difficult to use for someone who has arthritis in the fingers, the user may adjust the volume. As with CIC devices, these hearing aids are not for people with a lot of earwax or fluid that drains from the ear.

• In-the-ear (ITE): While far more noticeable than the previous two types of hearing aids, these have controls that are easier to adjust. They are also the smallest type that may be used by people who have a buildup of earwax or fluid in the ears. They are useful for people with moderately severe hearing loss.

- Behind-the-ear (BTE): These are the largest and most powerful type of hearing aid. They may be useful for people with severe hearing loss. It is easy to change the batteries and adjust the volume controls.

- Implantable bone-conducting hearing aids: For people who are unable to use any of the previously noted hearing aids, this type is another option. With this type, a metal screw is implanted into the skull behind the ear. The hearing aid may then be attached to the protruding metal. Unlike the other types of hearing aids that amplify sound, these devices conduct sound into the inner ear by vibrating against the mastoid bone. Implantation requires two surgical procedures.

In addition to selecting a style of hearing aid, be prepared to choose a type of circuitry. Circuitry determines the quality of sound that you will obtain from your hearing aid. The oldest type, analog circuitry, amplifies all the sounds. It is better for people who are home more and who tend to have one-on-one conversations. Programmable circuitry is more flexible and is a better choice for someone who lives in a variety of sound environments. The newest circuitry is digital circuitry, which provides the best sound but is also the most expensive.

Surgery

If your hearing loss has been caused by abnormal bone growth or trauma to the ear, it may be corrected by surgery. You will need to consult with an otolaryngologist, a physician specializing in disorders of the ear, nose, and throat, who will be able to determine if you would benefit from a surgical intervention.

Adults with severe sensorineural hearing loss who have obtained little or no benefit

Self-Testing

If you suspect that you have a diminished ability to hear, ask yourself the following questions. Positive answers may mean that you have lost some of your hearing.

☐ Do you find yourself straining to understand conversations, especially if several people are talking?
☐ Do you find yourself having trouble hearing people on the telephone?
☐ Do you seem to hear better in one ear than the other?
☐ Are you misunderstanding what other people are telling you?
☐ Have other people told you that the radio or TV is too loud?
☐ Do you sometimes fail to hear your telephone ringing?
☐ Do you frequently ask people to repeat what they have said?
☐ Do you work or have you worked in a noisy environment?
☐ Do you have a great deal of difficulty hearing the voices of women and children?
☐ Have you found yourself avoiding social situations because of communication problems?

from hearing aids may wish to consider a cochlear implant. A cochlear implant consists of a microphone, speech processor, transmitter and receiver/stimulator, and electrodes. During the procedure, an otolaryngologist makes an incision behind the ear and mastoid on one side of the head. Some bone is removed and electrode wires are inserted through the middle ear into the cochlear or inner ear. About 6 weeks after the surgery, you will be fitted with the remaining parts. The small microphone picks up sounds from the environment and the speech processor, then selects and arranges the sounds. A transmitter and receiver/stimulator converts signals from the speech processor into electric impulses, and the electrodes collect impulses from the stimulator and send them to the brain.

Since the procedure requires surgery under general anesthesia, you should be in overall good health. Once you have a cochlear implant, you will need to work with an audiologist to learn how to interpret the sounds. Rehabilitation for an adult may take 6 months to a year.

Complementary Treatments

Individuals suffering from hearing loss should seek the care of a specialist. Complementary medicine treatments may be used as an adjunct to this care and are generally concerned with the moving of blockages, such as fluid, mucus, or earwax, and with stimulation of the auditory nerve. Lifestyle changes with diet, nutrition, and herbs may be beneficial.

Acupuncture

Acupuncture improves the flow of stagnant *qi* (life energy), which is associated with hearing loss. Specialized treatments may decrease the symptoms of tinnitus and remove blockages to the middle ear. To locate an acupuncturist in your area, visit the Web site of the National Certification Commission for Acupuncture and Oriental Medicine (NCCAOM) at www.nccaom.org.

Alexander Technique

Keeping the head in the correct position in relation to the spine may improve circulation to the inner ear and has been shown to ease the symptoms of tinnitus, such as dizziness and nausea. A practitioner trained in the Alexander Technique may teach you the proper method. To locate an Alexander Technique teacher, visit the Web site of the American Society for the Alexander Technique at www.alexandertech.org.

Aromatherapy

The essential oil of basil reduces mucus buildup, helping to combat inner-ear infections. Basil oil may be used as a hot compress and applied to the ear. Pour 1 quart of hot water into a bowl and add 3 drops of basil oil. Soak a small washcloth in the water, ring out the excess water, and hold against the ear for 10 minutes. Apply as needed throughout the day.

Chiropractic

Chiropractic adjustment and manipulation of the neck and spine may increase circulation to the inner ear and relieve blockages affecting the nerves that supply the inner ear. To locate a chiropractor, visit the Web site of the American Chiropractic Association (ACA) at www.amerchiro.org.

Craniosacral Therapy

Imbalances and discrepancies in the rhythm of the cerebrospinal fluid lead to impaired body functions, which may result in chronic ear infection and hearing loss. The practitioner works to reestablish a balanced rhythm and normal function of the cerebrospinal fluid. To search for a qualified therapist in your area, visit the Web site of the International Association of Healthcare Practitioners at www.iahp.com.

Diet

Preliminary studies have shown that deficiency in folate (folic acid or B_9) and B_{12} contributes to age-related hearing loss. Good sources of folate are cooked asparagus, black beans, black-eyed peas, chickpeas, kidney beans, lentils, baby lima beans, navy beans, and cooked spinach. B_{12} is found mostly in meat, fish, and eggs, and some breakfast cereals are fortified with B_{12}. Since the B vitamins work best when taken together, taking a B-complex supplement is recommended.

Eating plenty of raw fruits and vegetables may help clear mucus that is clogging the ears. Garlic, which dilates tiny capillaries, including those that supply the inner ear, should be eaten freely.

Since it causes retention of water in the middle ear, which may cause hearing loss, you should avoid or greatly reduce your consumption of sodium (salt). Saturated fats, processed meats, and other meats place stress on the body and constrict the arteries. Sugar narrows the blood vessels of the inner ear. As a result, these foods should be avoided. Also, dairy products have been linked to recurrent middle-ear infections, which may cause hearing problems.

If you have Ménière's disease or tinnitus, avoid caffeine, chocolate, alcohol, salt, and sugar. This may help reduce the frequency of attacks.

Herbal Medicine

A number of herbs have been shown to be useful for hearing loss.

Black cohosh. Black cohosh has been shown to be effective in decreasing the symptoms of tinnitus. It is available in capsule form. The recommended daily dose is 20 milligrams, twice a day, of standardized extract containing 1 milligram of deoxyactein per tablet.

Echinacea and goldenseal. Echinacea and goldenseal are antioxidant herbs that fight infection, which may reduce the dizziness often associated with hearing loss. These may be taken in capsule form, but a tincture of echinacea with goldenseal is also available. The recommended daily dose is 500 milligrams of standardized extract per day. If taken in liquid extract form, 1 teaspoon, three times each day, is the recommended dose. When taking an echinacea and goldenseal tincture combination, follow the directions recommended on the label. To avoid building up immunity to the herbs, they should be used for relatively short periods of time, such as 2 weeks. Take them when you have symptoms or when you believe that your immune system has been compromised.

Ginger. Ginger improves circulation and bloodflow to the ear and aids in reducing nausea from tinnitus and Ménière's disease. It is advised that you consume a $\frac{1}{4}$-inch slice of fresh ginger each day. It may be grated over a salad or added to a stir-fry or any other meal where the flavor would work well. Ginger is also available in tincture form as well as tea bags. For the tincture, follow the directions on the label.

Ginkgo biloba. Ginkgo is an antioxidant that supports circulation, increases bloodflow to the inner ear, and relieves dizziness. It is available in capsule form. However, if you are taking prescription blood-thinning medication, be sure to consult your doctor before taking the ginkgo supplements. The recommended daily dose is 120 milligrams, twice a day, of extract standardized to 24 percent of flavone glycosides and 6 percent terpene lactones. The flavone glycosides give ginkgo its antioxidant benefits, while terpene lactones increase circulation and have a protective effect on nerve cells.

Nutritional Supplements

Deficiency of certain vitamins can lead to hearing loss. Supplementation also supports ear function and reduces symptoms associated with hearing loss.

- Vitamin A: 10,000 IU daily. Stimulates auditory nerve and aids in proper functioning of the cochlea.

- B-complex vitamins: Take as directed on the label. Deficiency linked to ear problems. Reduces tinnitus and stabilizes fluid in inner ear.

- Vitamin B_{12}: Injections or a 1,000-microgram sublingual tablet daily. Deficiency found in many individuals with hearing loss. Injections of B_{12} have been more effective with this condition.

- Vitamin D: 400 IU daily. Supports the cochlea, prevents damage to bones of the middle ear, and may restore some hearing loss.

- Zinc: 30 milligrams daily. May restore some hearing and control symptoms of tinnitus.

Lifestyle Recommendations

It is important to minimize loud background noise as it can cause hearing loss. For example, when mowing the lawn, use adequate hearing protection.

Be aware of HRT. Several studies have linked hormone replacement therapy to an increase in hearing loss by 20 to 30 percent in comparison to women not using HRT.

Be observant. Acute hearing loss caused by loud noise, such as from a concert or parade, should go away within 2 days. If your hearing loss persists, consult your doctor.

Exercise. Regular aerobic exercise may improve circulation, boost the immune system, and disperse blockages.

Fluid drainage. If fluid starts to drain from an ear, let it flow; this is a good sign and a natural process, which indicates that the excess buildup of fluid may be releasing.

Reduce noise exposure. Reduce background noise. At home, turn off the TV and/or radio when you are not watching or listening. When dining outside the home, try to sit in the least busy/noisy area of the restaurant.

Communicate more effectively. When you are speaking with others, face them directly and ask them to speak directly to you. That should improve your ability to hear what is being said. Further, so that facial expressions and gestures may be observed, it is useful to have good lighting.

Tell people not to shout at you. Rather, tell them to lower the pitch of their voices—high-pitched sounds are more difficult to hear.

Because it makes you raise the tone or pitch of your voice, talking loudly is often counter-productive. Also, ask people to speak at a normal speed. It is not necessary to speak slowly.

Watch what you eat. Pass up foods and drinks that contain caffeine, chocolate, alcohol, salt, and sugar to reduce the frequency of attacks of Ménière's disease and tinnitus.

Preventive Measures

Protect your hearing. Much of hearing loss is permanent and can't be restored. Whenever possible, take measures to protect your hearing, especially from environmental factors such as loud noises. After all, hearing damage can occur at noise levels of just 85 decibels. For comparison, a normal conversation is around 60 decibels, while a chain saw operates at approximately 100 decibels.

If you are working in a noisy environment, wear sound-reducing earmuffs or earplugs, which can help prevent hearing damage.

Quit smoking. Studies have shown that there is a direct correlation between smoking and an increased risk of hearing loss.

Heart Palpitations

Heart palpitations are the uncomfortable sensation that your heart is beating irregularly, forcefully, or rapidly. Normally, you are unaware of your heart beating. If you have palpitations, however, you feel your heart beating and skipping beats. Palpitations may be associated with a heart that beats faster than 100 beats per minute or a heart with a normal rate that has an occasional early beat. They may be felt in the throat, chest, or neck.

Heart palpitations are very common. One study found that 16 percent of outpatient internist or cardiologist patients reported experiencing palpitations.

Causes and Risk Factors

Heart palpitations may be caused by a number of different medical conditions, including anemia, anxiety, fever, hyperthyroidism, problems with the heart's nervous system, and mitral valve prolapse (mild deformity in a valve of the heart). Other things that might trigger heart palpitations include caffeine in foods such as soda, tea, and coffee, as well as the nicotine in cigarettes. Exercising too strenuously may result in palpitations. Some diet pills and decongestants may have stimulants that trigger them. Higher than needed doses of thyroid hormone medications as well as certain antidepressants may cause palpita-

tions, as may the illegal drug cocaine. In addition, palpitations may be seen in individuals with depression and panic disorder. Palpitations are more common in people over age 40.

If, during a single episode, you experience heart palpitations for an extended period of time or if your palpitations are accompanied by chest pain, sweating, fainting, shortness of breath, or dizziness, you may be having a heart attack or another serious heart event. Call 911 or seek emergency assistance immediately.

Signs and Symptoms

If you are experiencing palpitations, your heart feels as if it is pounding or racing. It might also seem as if your heart is fluttering, thumping, or jumping around in your chest. You may feel as if you have butterflies in your

A Quick Guide to Symptoms

- ☐ **Heart feels as if it is pounding**
- ☐ **Heart feels as if it is racing, fluttering, thumping, or jumping around the chest**
- ☐ **Feel butterflies in chest**

Though there are no self-tests for heart palpitations, you will probably know if you are having them. Keep a record of all your episodes. Note how long they last, and list what you were doing when they occurred. Were you experiencing any unusual stress? Were you exercising? What other symptoms did you have? Also, note any medications that you were taking and what you had been eating and drinking.

chest. The symptoms may last for a few seconds or continue for as long as a few minutes.

Conventional Treatments
Addressing the Underlying Cause

Heart palpitations are generally treated by addressing the underlying cause. If your palpitations are from a stimulant in a medication, your doctor may recommend an alternative medication. If you have been taking too high a dose, your doctor may recommend a lower dose. If the cause is anxiety, you may be advised to take anti-anxiety medications and undergo psychotherapy. Relaxation techniques such as meditation are also useful. If you have anemia, your doctor will want to determine the source. If you have an overactive thyroid, you will require treatment for that condition.

If there is a problem with the heart's nerve conduction system, then further evaluation and testing are needed. These should be conducted by an electrophysiologist, who finds or "maps" the nerve that is causing the problem. When that location is determined, then radiofrequency ablation (radio waves) will be used to destroy the specific site of the conduction problem.

Medications

If you have been diagnosed with an abnormal heart rhythm, you may be referred to a physician who specializes in heart rhythm problems. Most likely, this physician will review your past tests, conduct additional tests, and suggest treatments. If tests determine that you have a problem with your heart, you may be treated with an anti-arrhythmic medication such as a beta-blocker or a calcium-channel blocker.

Anticlotting medication. If you have a type of abnormal heart rhythm known as atrial fibrillation, your doctor may recommend that you take low-dose aspirin or another anticlotting medication. Aspirin inhibits the activity of blood platelets, thereby helping to prevent blood from clotting. Still, you should realize that the prolonged use of aspirin may increase your risk for gastrointestinal ulcers and bleeding. Other medications that suppress the activity of blood platelets include clopidogrel (Plavix) and ticlopidine (Ticlid).

Beta-blockers. Beta-blockers reduce the heart rate and lower arterial pressure. Examples of beta-blockers are propranolol (Inderal), atenolol (Tenormin), and carvedilol

(Coreg). Potential side effects of beta-blockers include moderate lowering of levels of high-density lipoproteins (HDL or "good" cholesterol), fatigue, and lethargy. There have been reports of unusually vivid dreams, nightmares, memory loss, sensations of cold in the extremities, and depression. Some people experience a diminished capacity for exercise, decreased heart function, sexual dysfunction, or gastrointestinal upset.

Calcium-channel blockers. Calcium-channel blockers reduce the heart rate and dilate the blood vessels. Examples of calcium-channel blockers are verapamil (Calan, Isoptin), nifedipine (Adalat, Procardia), nicardipine (Cardene), diltiazem (Cardizem, Tiazac), and amlodipine (Norvasc). Withdrawal from calcium-channel blockers should be gradual, and you should not mix them with grapefruit juice, which may increase their effects.

Complementary Treatments

When addressing the underlying cause of heart palpitations, complementary medicine offers a number of treatment options that may reduce or eliminate the symptoms.

Diet

Many processed and refined foods contain a high level of preservatives, artificial colors and flavors, saturated fats, caffeine, and other chemicals that may lead to heart palpitations. It is best to eat a healthy diet that is as close to nature as possible. Your diet should include lots of fruits, vegetables, whole-grain foods, and foods that are high in fiber. Try to include a minimum of five servings of vegetables, four servings of fruit, and six servings of whole grains each day.

Be sure to wash fruits and vegetables carefully to remove pesticides and other chemicals that may have been used. Better yet, buy organic products that have been grown without the use of pesticides and chemicals. If you consume animal-based foods such as poultry, pork, or red meat, select organically raised, free-range varieties.

Potassium is a nutrient that is essential for healthy heart rhythm. It is found in many fruits, vegetables, and whole grains. If you consume a diet that contains plenty of these foods, you will eat sufficient amounts of potassium. Since it may affect the potassium level in your body, be sure to limit your salt intake.

Herbal Medicine

Because it strengthens the action of the heart and helps to alleviate sleeplessness due to anxiety, hawthorn is particularly good for heart palpitations. It is available in tea and capsule form. To make tea, steep 2 teaspoons of the herb in a cup of boiling water for 10 minutes and drink slowly. Drink 2 cups of tea each day. Hawthorn is also available in capsule or tincture form, standardized to 2.2 percent total bioflavonoid content. The recommended dose of hawthorn capsules varies widely, ranging from 100 to 300 milligrams, two or three times per day. Be aware that higher doses may significantly lower blood pressure, which may cause you to faint. In tincture, the recommended dose of hawthorn is 4 to 5 milliliters, three times per day. It may take up to 2 months before you see the effects of this herb.

Nutritional Supplements

The following nutrients have been shown to be effective in reducing or eliminating heart palpitations.

- Multivitamin/mineral: Take as directed on the label. Ensures proper levels of essential nutrients.
- Calcium: 1,000 milligrams daily in divided doses of 500 milligrams. Helps with the absorption of magnesium.
- Magnesium: 500 milligrams daily. Essential for normal heart function and regulates heart rhythm.
- Potassium: Before taking potassium supplements, consult with your doctor. Effective for reducing or eliminating heart palpitations.

Relaxation/Meditation

If you find that your heart palpitations are triggered by anxiety, stress, or other emotional issues (such as anger), it is important to find some coping mechanism. Any practice that addresses the mind/body connection may be useful. These techniques assist in reinforcing a calm and relaxed mind, which in turn relaxes the body and helps restore the heart to a normal rhythm.

Deep breathing exercises allow the mind to focus only on the breath—where it begins, how long to inhale, how long to exhale, and where to feel the exhalation. This slows the mind and the bodily responses that are affected by an anxious mind. Autogenic training is also particularly useful for reducing and eliminating heart palpitations. The repetition of a series of specific phrases takes you through a systematic process of relaxing the entire body. Other techniques to aid in reducing stress and other emotional issues include biofeedback, psychotherapy, yoga, and meditation.

Therapeutic Massage

Swedish massage may be an excellent source of relaxation for both treating and preventing heart palpitations brought on by emotional issues. The rhythmic movements, along with gentle pressure, may loosen tense muscles, allowing a freer flow of blood throughout the body. During a Swedish massage, you will be encouraged to focus on your breathing, thereby reducing anxiety and returning the heart to a normal rhythm.

Lifestyle Recommendations

Keep a journal. Since it may be difficult to determine the underlying cause of heart palpitations, maintaining a daily journal may be useful. Record your intake of foods, beverages, and nutritional supplements; the duration and frequency of physical activity; and how you feel emotionally, mentally, and physically. Be sure to list specific times you exert yourself and any special circumstances. Also, record when you have heart palpitations. You may find that they are the result of a food intolerance, vigorous exercise, or emotional stress. If you are able to note a pattern, you may be able to make lifestyle changes that reduce or eliminate the palpitations. However, if the palpitations continue, you should consult with your doctor.

Quit smoking. The nicotine in cigarettes, which is a stimulant, may cause heart palpitations. Smoking also increases blood pressure and reduces the amount of oxygen to the heart.

Reduce or eliminate caffeine. Caffeine may be found in coffee, tea, chocolate, soft drinks, over-the-counter stimulants, pain medica-tions, cold medications, and appetite sup-pressants. If you are consuming these products, they may be contributing to your heart palpitations. You may benefit from reducing your intake or eliminating them completely.

Reduce stress. Reduce the stress in your life and take measures to control the stresses you cannot eliminate. Consider meditating or some other way to calm yourself. Any form of meditation in which the mind is focused on a particular object, sound, visu-alization, breath, or activity is helpful in reversing the body's fight-or-flight response to stress. Yoga and tai chi are considered meditation in movement and help to relax muscles, quiet the mind, and create inner peace. You can also meditate while you are lying down or in a seated position. When you meditate while seated, be sure to sit properly—upright on a chair or the floor, with your back straight.

Hemorrhoids

Also known as piles, hemorrhoids are clusters of dilated veins in the anus. Located in the lowest section of the rectum and anus, hemorrhoids develop when repeated straining or pressure causes the veins in the rectum to enlarge.

There are two types of hemorrhoids, internal (inside the rectum) and external (around the anus). While internal hemorrhoids are usually not painful, passing stool may irritate them and cause them to bleed. Blood may appear on stool or toilet tissue, or in the toilet bowl. Sometimes, straining may push an internal hemorrhoid out through the anal opening. This is known as a prolapsed hemorrhoid. With a prolapsed hemorrhoid, you may have constant, dull, aching pain, as well as itching and bleeding. External hemorrhoids tend to be quite painful. The blood inside may collect and form a clot (thrombus), which may trigger severe pain and inflammation. When irritated, external hemorrhoids tend to itch and/or bleed.

Hemorrhoids are extremely common. By the age of 50, about half of all men and women have some evidence of this disorder.

Causes and Risk Factors

Hemorrhoids are caused by a number of factors. These include the straining or pressure associated with constipation, diarrhea, and the expulsion of diarrhea stools, waiting too long to have a bowel movement, pregnancy, sitting too long on the toilet, frequent coughing or sneezing, heavy lifting, injury to the anus, some liver diseases, and sitting or standing for extended periods of time.

You may also inherit the tendency to develop hemorrhoids. Stress increases the risk of a hemorrhoid flare-up, as does the excess intake of alcohol. With age, the risk for hemorrhoids increases. And people who are obese have a greater risk.

A Quick Guide to Symptoms

☐ Itching and burning
☐ Bleeding consisting of bright red blood
☐ Tenderness and swelling around the anus
☐ Painful bowel movements
☐ Lumps around the anus

Signs and Symptoms

While hemorrhoids may be symptom-free, they are often associated with a number of symptoms. These include itching, burning, bleeding of bright red blood, tenderness and swelling around the anus, painful bowel movements, and lumps around the anus that may be as large as a walnut.

Conventional Treatments

Dietary Modifications

Eating lots of high-fiber foods coupled with drinking a good deal of water helps to prevent constipation. Good sources of fiber are raw and cooked vegetables, such as cabbage and carrots, and whole-grain cereals with bran.

Medications

If you have mild to moderate pain, your doctor may prescribe a cream or ointment that contains witch hazel, zinc oxide, hydrocortisone, or petroleum jelly, and/or medicated suppositories that are placed inside the rectum.

Nonsurgical Procedures

Hemorrhoid banding or rubber band ligation. In these procedures, used to treat protruding internal hemorrhoids, the doctor places a tight band around the enlarged vein. The vein is then cut open, and the blood clot is removed. Within a few days, the vein heals and the scab falls off.

Other nonsurgical treatments. Your doctor may use freezing, electrical or laser heat, or infrared light to destroy a hemorrhoid. Or it may be shrunk by injecting a chemical around the vein (sclerotherapy).

Sitz Baths and Cold Packs

Try sitting in lukewarm water for about 15 minutes, two or three times a day. You may also want to place a cloth-covered ice pack on the anus for 10 minutes, four times a day.

Surgery

If you are in severe pain from hemorrhoids and none of the previously noted nonsurgical methods has provided sufficient relief, your doctor may recommend the surgical removal of the hemorrhoids (hemorrhoidectomy). Before the procedure begins, you will be given general or spinal anesthesia or the anus area will be injected with an anesthetic. In some instances, the procedure may require a 1- or 2-day hospitalization.

Complementary Treatments

Some of the most effective remedies and treatments for hemorrhoids are the ones that you may practice yourself. Dietary changes, exercise, and over-the-counter herbal supplements may not only relieve symptoms associated with hemorrhoids; they may also eliminate the condition.

Diet

Be sure to eat a diet that includes complex carbohydrates, fiber, and flavonoids. These foods may help strengthen the veins, promote regular bowel movements, and decrease the severity of irritating symptoms. Foods containing complex carbohydrates include beans, peas, vegetables, and whole grains. Flavonoids are the substances that give fruits and vegetables their color. Eat lots of fresh fruits and vegetables every day to obtain these substances to help decrease the swelling, inflammation, and bleeding associated with hemorrhoids.

It is important to increase high-fiber foods gradually. If you rapidly increase your intake of these foods, you may have uncomfortable symptoms such as diarrhea, gas, bloating, and cramping. High-fiber foods help to create stool that is soft, bulky, and easier to pass. Bran is a good source of fiber, but it has a tendency to bind with minerals such as calcium and zinc, which may result in deficiencies of these minerals. Limit or avoid foods that have little or no fiber, such as cheese, meat, and processed foods.

You should also increase your intake of fluids. Each day, try to consume about eight 8-ounce glasses of fluids—plain water is best—that do not contain caffeine or alcohol, substances that may promote dehydration.

Herbal Medicine

To help alleviate symptoms and speed healing, a number of herbs have been proven appropriate for internal use and for topical use as an ointment.

Butcher's broom. Butcher's broom tones the veins and reduces inflammation, helping to shrink hemorrhoids. In capsule form, the recommended daily dose is a standardized extract that provides 50 to 100 milligrams of ruscogenins (the active ingredient) per day. It may also be taken as a liquid extract, 1 teaspoon twice a day.

Horse chestnut. Horse chestnut has been found useful in reducing pain and alleviating the swelling associated with hemorrhoids. The recommended daily dose is 50 milligrams, three times a day, of 16 to 21 percent of standardized extract of aescin. It is also available in a tincture and as a topical cream. Be sure to avoid the leaves and nuts, which are toxic. If you suffer from liver or kidney problems, you should not use this herb.

St. John's wort. This herb is used as a topical ointment applied directly on hemorrhoids to reduce pain and inflammation.

Witch hazel. To ease discomfort and shrink hemorrhoids, witch hazel may be used in a sitz bath. Add 1 cup of distilled witch hazel to 6 inches of lukewarm bath water. Sit in the water for 15 minutes. Distilled witch hazel may be purchased over-the-counter at any pharmacy. For emergency use, a bottle of witch hazel may be kept in the refrigerator. Soak a cotton ball with cold witch hazel and dab directly on the external hemorrhoid. As witch hazel causes blood vessels to contract, this may be especially effective on bleeding hemorrhoids.

Homeopathy

Various over-the-counter homeopathic remedies may be useful depending upon the type of hemorrhoids you have and their symptoms. There are remedies to reduce inflammation, bleeding, and itching. They are readily available at natural and organic health food and grocery stores. Homeopathic practitioners will also take into account your constitution (emotional, physical, and psychological makeup) in addition to your symptoms when suggesting a remedy and dose.

Nutritional Supplements

Certain supplements can promote the healing process by strengthening the immune system and tissues.

- Vitamin C: 1,000 milligrams daily in divided doses of 500 milligrams. Helps shrink hemorrhoids and tone the veins.
- Vitamin E: 400 IU daily. Promotes healing.
- Zinc: 30 milligrams daily. Helps the recovery process.

Lifestyle Recommendations

Add additional fiber. To help regulate bowels and keep stools soft, it may be necessary to add additional fiber to your diet. Dissolve 1 tablespoon of psyllium seed powder in 8 ounces of water or juice; drink twice a day. A tablespoon of ground flaxseed may also be used.

Avoid dry, colored, or scented toilet paper. Dry toilet paper may cause further irritation. So, after a bowel movement, wipe with moist towelettes or wet toilet paper. A towelette that contains horse chestnut and/or witch hazel may relieve some symptoms and speed healing. Colored or scented toilet paper may increase irritation as well.

Avoid scratching. Scratching at inflamed hemorrhoids may actually irritate the walls of the veins and increase inflammation, thereby aggravating the condition.

Exercise. Participating in some form of regular exercise will help to keep the blood flowing in your veins, regulate bowel movements, and help to avoid constipation. Regular exercise reduces the pressure inside your colon, moves food along faster, and promotes the normal functioning of the bowels. One of the best exercises for constipation is a daily 20- to 30-minute walk. Regular exercise also helps maintain a healthy weight. Due to the excess pressure placed on the lower extremities, overweight individuals are more prone to hemorrhoids.

Preventive Measures

Exercise. Exercise may help to prevent constipation. Individuals who are constipated have higher risk for hemorrhoids.

Avoid long periods of sitting or standing. To help keep your blood flowing, periodically move around.

Dietary modifications. The same dietary modifications that are used to treat hemorrhoids may be used to prevent them—increase the fluid and fiber content of your diet.

Don't strain. Straining to pass a stool places increased pressure on the veins in the lower rectum. Straining due to lifting heavy objects has the same effect.

Limit the use of laxatives. Diarrhea may irritate the anus area.

Respond to your bowel. When you feel the urge to pass a bowel movement, don't delay. If you wait too long, the urge may pass and the stool will become drier and harder to pass.

Try an inflatable doughnut cushion. The cushion may be useful for hemorrhoid sufferers who are required to sit for long periods of time.

High Blood Pressure

Blood pressure is the amount of pressure that blood exerts against the arteries as it travels through the circulatory system. Three key organs are involved in the regulation of blood pressure: the heart, arteries, and kidneys. Your heart pumps the blood that flows throughout your body. If your heart must work harder to move the blood, it exerts more force on the arteries. As blood rushes through arteries, they expand and contract. If your arteries have narrowed or lost their elasticity, then your heart must use more force to propel your blood where it needs to go. Your kidneys regulate the amount of water-retaining sodium in your body. When excess salt leads to extra fluid in your body, your blood pressure may increase. Other factors such as stress can also affect your blood pressure.

In the United States today, high blood pressure is an extraordinarily common medical problem. It affects approximately 30 percent of adults. Every year, approximately 2 million additional cases are diagnosed.

If high blood pressure, which is also known as hypertension, is not treated, it has the potential to do serious harm to the body.

Measuring Blood Pressure

The measurement of blood pressure involves two numbers. The first number is known as systolic pressure. This represents the amount of pressure in your arteries when the heart contracts and ejects blood into the aorta (the main blood vessel leading from the heart). The second number is the diastolic pressure, which indicates how much pressure remains in the arteries between heartbeats, when the heart is relaxed and filling with blood. The two numbers are written as if they are a fraction, with the systolic pressure on the top and the diastolic pressure on the bottom. The systolic number is higher than the diastolic one.

Ideal blood pressure for adults is 120/80 mm Hg or less ("mm Hg" refers to the number of millimeters that a column of mercury will reach in response to a given level of pressure). Though not necessarily ideal, a reading of up to 129/84 or less is considered normal. Systolic pressures between 130 and 139 mm Hg and diastolic pressures between 85 and 89 mm Hg are viewed as high-normal or borderline. When your blood pressure is higher than that, you may be diagnosed with high blood pressure.

Blood pressure readings tend to fluctuate throughout the day. They increase when your heart is working harder, such as during periods of physical exercise or during times that are particularly stressful. Your doctor will probably request a number of separate blood pressure readings before deciding whether you have high blood pressure. Try to take these around the same time each day.

High blood pressure has been linked to heart failure, kidney failure, damage to arteries, arteriosclerosis, aneurysm, coronary artery disease, left ventricular hypertrophy, eye problems, stroke, heart attack, and premature death. It is believed that high blood pressure contributes to three-fourths of all strokes and heart attacks, and it causes about 30 percent of all cases of kidney failure. Every year, high blood pressure plays a direct or indirect role in more than 10 percent of the deaths in the United States. Nevertheless, many of those who have high blood pressure are unaware that they have this potentially life-threatening condition. Only about half of those who know that they have high blood pressure are receiving treatment, and only about 25 percent of people with high blood pressure have it under control.

In the vast majority of cases, high blood pressure develops slowly. Though it is rare, high blood pressure may also happen quickly, a condition known as malignant or accelerated hypertension. It occurs more often in people with uncontrolled high blood pressure or heart failure and requires emergency treatment.

There are two main forms of high blood pressure, essential and secondary. About 95 percent of adults with high blood pressure have the essential form, in which no single cause of the hypertension is identified. On the other hand, with secondary high blood pressure, there is a known underlying cause, such as a hormone abnormality or kidney disease. So, when the medical problems lead-ing to secondary high blood pressure are managed, the blood pressure will often drop.

Causes and Risk Factors

As might be expected, some people are more vulnerable to high blood pressure than others. In the United States, African Americans who live in the Southeast have the highest incidence of all groups in the country. But all African Americans seem to have a higher risk for this disorder. They are almost twice as likely as whites to have high blood pressure. Although in traditional societies throughout the world, where people are leaner and more active, blood pressure tends to remain the

Medications as a Cause of Hypertension

If you are being evaluated for high blood pressure, be sure to tell your doctor about all the medications and supplements that you are taking. Some medications have the ability to cause high blood pressure; others will further raise existing elevated pressure. The following are groups of medications that may be of particular concern.

☐ **Monoamine oxidase inhibitor (MAOI) antidepressants**
☐ **Steroids**
☐ **Appetite suppressants**
☐ **Cold remedies and nasal decongestants**
☐ **Cyclosporine**
☐ **Oral contraceptives**

same throughout life, in the United States, where older people have more body fat and are less active, the risk for developing hypertension increases with age. High blood pressure is relatively uncommon in people under 35. At the same time, more than half of people who are 65 or older have high blood pressure. Americans who are now 55 years of age or older have a 90 percent chance of developing high blood pressure during their lifetimes.

It is well known that high blood pressure runs in families. If either of your parents has or had high blood pressure, consider yourself to be at higher risk. Young and middle-age men have a higher risk than women. But after midlife and menopause, women and men have about the same risk.

The following factors also place people at higher risk.

- Obesity
- Excess alcohol consumption
- Smoking

- Sodium sensitivity (Each individual's blood pressure responds differently to the intake of sodium.)
- Lack of exercise
- High cholesterol
- Diabetes
- Emotional disorders, such as anxiety or depression
- Heart failure

It is important to note that the degree of risk that these factors add may be reduced through changes in behavior, diet, and medication.

One study looked at whether there is an association between sleep-disoriented breathing (apnea) and hypertension. Researchers followed more than 700 people with sleep-disoriented breathing for more than 4 years. Individuals with even a few periods of apnea had a 42 percent higher chance of having hypertension, compared with those without apnea. Those with 15 or more apnea events for every hour of sleep had three times the risk for hypertension compared with those without apnea.

A Quick Guide to Symptoms

- ☐ **Often no symptoms are apparent**
- ☐ **Nosebleeds**
- ☐ **Dizziness**
- ☐ **Ringing in the ears**
- ☐ **Blurred vision**
- ☐ **Headaches**

Signs and Symptoms

Because high blood pressure rarely has any symptoms, it has frequently been called "the silent killer." Still, there are a few subtle symptoms such as nosebleeds, dizziness, ringing in the ears, blurred vision, and headaches. Then again, these symptoms are so common among the population at large that it may be hard to connect them to high blood pressure. Less than 1 percent of people with high blood pressure—usually those who are faced with the life-threatening malignant or accelerated hypertension—do have noticeable symptoms. These include nausea, loss of vision, headache, confusion, and drowsiness.

Conventional Treatments

There are essentially two main ways to reduce blood pressure: lifestyle modifications and medications.

Lifestyle Modifications

Unless the situation requires immediate intervention, most doctors advise beginning with lifestyle modifications. These include eating a more healthful diet, losing weight, exercising regularly, reducing your intake of sodium, quitting smoking, limiting alcohol consumption, and developing better methods to deal with stress. Many people who make these lifestyle changes have been able to avoid taking medication or are able to take reduced doses of medication.

Medications

If lifestyle modifications do not sufficiently reduce blood pressure, the next step is likely to be some type of medication. There are many types of high blood pressure medication, which are also known as antihypertensives. You and your doctor may need to try a few before finding one that is suitable for

Self-Testing

Blood pressure is measured in an easy, painless manner with an instrument known as a sphygmomanometer. The sphygmomanometer has an inflatable cuff that wraps around your arm, an air pump, and a column of mercury (or a digital device that performs the same function). Some allow you to monitor your own blood pressure, and your doctor may ask you to purchase one so that you can take periodic readings at home. If you do buy one, be sure to select a sphygmomanometer that is easy to use. Consider an automatic version in which the results are digitally displayed.

To improve the accuracy of your tests, do not eat a big meal, drink caffeine or alcohol, or smoke for at least 30 minutes beforehand. These actions may raise your blood pressure and give a false reading.

you, and some people take a combination of drugs. The following are the most common categories.

ACE (angiotensin-converting enzyme) inhibitors. Angiotensin-converting enzyme (ACE) inhibitors prevent the body from producing a substance that causes the arteries to constrict. As a result, arteries remain wider, and blood may flow more freely. Though ACE inhibitors seem to have relatively few side effects, about 20 percent of the people who take them develop a dry cough. This is more likely to occur with women than men. Sometimes, the cough will become so annoying that a change in medication may be needed. Other potential side effects include reduced appetite, rash, and a changed sense of taste. ACE inhibitors are usually not advised for people with serious kidney problems.

Alpha-blockers. In addition to lessening the constriction of arteries, alpha-blockers mildly reduce the levels of total blood cholesterol as well as triglyceride levels. Since they also improve urine flow, men who have prostate problems may benefit from them. Alpha-blockers are available in both short- and long-acting forms. They may have side effects. When an alpha-blocker is first prescribed, it may cause you to feel dizzy or even faint. Therefore, your doctor will probably start you on a very low dose, which should be taken at bedtime. As you adjust to the medication, the dose may be increased. Other potential side effects include weakness, a pounding heartbeat, nausea, and headache.

Angiotensin II receptor blockers. Angiotensin II receptor blockers are among the newest drugs being used to treat high blood pressure. They prevent arteries from constricting and the kidneys from retaining water and salt. About as effective as ACE inhibitors, they do not trigger an annoying cough. Though side effects are relatively rare, some people report pain in the back and legs, diarrhea, indigestion, insomnia, dizziness, and nasal congestion.

Beta-blockers. Although originally developed to treat coronary artery disease, beta-blockers are now commonly used to treat high blood pressure. Beta-blockers block the effects of the hormone norepinephrine and cause a dilation of blood vessels as well as a decrease in heart rate. Additionally, they slow the kidneys' release of renin, an enzyme that is integral to the production of angiotensin II, a hormone that narrows blood vessels, thus increasing blood pressure.

The two most common side effects of beta-blockers are fatigue and a diminished capacity for exercise. Other potential side effects include the loss of sex drive, erectile dysfunction, depression, sleep problems, small increases in the triglyceride level in the blood, a minor lowering of HDL levels, and cold hands. Because of the possibility of negative side effects, people with asthma, heart failure, peripheral vascular disease, insulin-dependent diabetes, chronic obstructive pulmonary disease, and Raynaud's disease may be advised not to take some or all beta-blockers.

Calcium-channel blockers. These medications relax arterial walls, and some also lower the heart rate. There are two main types of calcium-channel blockers, short-acting and long-acting. Short-acting calcium-channel blockers reduce blood pressure quickly, but they must be taken several times a day. Long-acting forms require a longer time to lower blood pressure, but the pressure remains lower for an extended period of time. Potential side effects from calcium-channel blockers include rapid heartbeat, constipation, rash, and swelling of the gums and the feet and/or lower legs.

If you are taking the calcium-channel

blockers felodipine (Plendil), nifedipine (Nimotop), nisoldipine (Sular), diltiazem (Cardizem and others), or verapamil (Norvasc), consume grapefruit or grapefruit juice with enormous care. In fact, you may wish to avoid grapefruit products entirely. Grapefruit contains a substance that prevents an enzyme from breaking down calcium-channel blockers. As a result, they may accumulate in the blood. Blood levels may become too high and trigger side effects, such as angina, headaches, palpitations, and ankle swelling.

Centrally acting drugs. These medications stop the brain from sending messages to the nervous system to increase the heart rate and narrow blood vessels. As a result, the heart rate slows and blood flows more freely. Examples are methyldopa and clonidine (Catapres). Unfortunately, centrally acting drugs may have negative side effects such as extreme fatigue or drowsiness. In addition, they have been correlated with weight gain, impaired thinking, erectile dysfunction, dry mouth, headaches, and psychological problems such as depression. Also, when centrally acting drugs are discontinued, they may cause blood pressure to rise to dangerous levels. If you have been taking one and must stop, work with your doctor to find a method that is safe for you.

Diuretics. Diuretics are some of the most frequently prescribed medications for high blood pressure. Effective and inexpensive, they are often the first hypertension medication prescribed by doctors. Diuretics prompt the body to excrete water and salt. Thus, less fluid presses against artery and vein walls. But these drugs also remove potassium, so if you are on a diuretic, you may need to eat some potassium-rich foods such as nectarines, tangerines, watermelon, oranges or orange juice, bananas, mangoes, strawberries, apricots, and cherries.

Complementary Treatments

There are many complementary approaches for reducing blood pressure. Most may be used in conjunction with or even, in the case of diet, as part of conventional treatment.

Acupuncture

Acupuncture is very effective in treating hypertension. For best results, it is often combined with conventional medicine. Along with treatments, physical exercise will probably be encouraged. To locate an acupuncturist in your area, visit the Web site of the National Certification Commission for Acupuncture and Oriental Medicine (NCCAOM) at www.nccaom.org.

Aquatic Therapy

Aerobic exercise and relaxation techniques have been shown to lower blood pressure. Aquatic therapy is a gentle way to begin an aerobic exercise program and reduce stress. Water is an ideal environment to promote relaxation. The rhythmic movements and simple stretches help the mind and body to unwind and reduce stress.

Diet

Doctors who work with people who have hypertension often recommend the Dietary Approaches to Stop Hypertension (DASH) diet. In research studies, it has been proven to reduce blood pressure. The DASH diet is high in whole grains, fruits, and vegetables. In fact, it recommends seven or eight servings of grains each day and eight to 10 servings of fruits and vegetables; four or five servings of legumes, nuts, and seeds are also advised. Dairy products are limited to two or three servings a day, and these should be low-fat or fat-free. And there are no more than two servings each day of lean red meat, fish, or poultry without the skin.

The DASH diet advises no more than 2,400 milligrams of sodium per day, which is less than the 3,000 to 4,000 milligrams that many Americans consume. On a daily basis, your body actually needs only 500 milligrams of sodium. An important part of controlling sodium is limiting your salt intake (ordinary table salt is a form of sodium; it is 40 percent sodium and 60 percent chloride). The recommended maximum of 2,400 milligrams a day is about the amount contained in a single teaspoon of table salt. Some doctors suggest an even lower figure—about 1,500 milligrams of sodium per day. As you attempt to estimate your salt intake, remember that prepared foods, including restaurant foods, tend to contain higher amounts of salt than the food you make at home. Soy sauce generally has high amounts of salt, and there may even be salt in your antacid.

Since some recent studies have shown that sugar increases blood pressure in both animals and humans, it is also recommended that those with high blood pressure limit their intake of sugar. Be sure to check prepared foods for sugar content as well.

Herbal Medicine

Garlic. The use of garlic as a medicinal herb dates back thousands of years. Research has determined that ingesting 600 to 900 milli-

---

Reducing the Sodium in Your Diet

There are many simple, commonsense ways to reduce the amount of sodium in your diet.

☐ **Reduce your consumption of processed food and try to use as many fresh foods as possible. If you must use frozen or canned food, try to use those without added salt.**

☐ **Eat fresh meat, poultry, and fish rather than the canned or processed varieties, such as prepared cold cuts and hot dogs.**

☐ **Check ingredient labels whenever you purchase canned soups, packaged mixes, broths, and salad dressings. All of these tend to be high in salt.**

☐ **Prepare foods such as pasta and rice without adding salt to the water.**

☐ **Remove the saltshaker from the table.**

☐ **Don't add salt to cooked food.**

☐ **Limit your consumption of condiments such as ketchup and mustard.**

☐ **Watch your intake of olives and pickles. They may be high in salt.**

grams of garlic extract daily for a 4-week period significantly lowers blood pressure. While fresh garlic is the most effective, garlic supplements may also be useful. When taken fresh, garlic may be used liberally. If you can tolerate it, chew one clove daily. With garlic supplements, look for enteric-coated tablets or capsules with standardized allicin potential. To get up to 5,000 micrograms of allicin, take 400 to 500 milligrams of garlic, once or twice per day. Since garlic has anticoagulant properties, if you are taking prescription anticoagulant medication, check with your doctor before increasing your intake of garlic or beginning a garlic supplementation regimen. If you are planning to have surgery, you should inform your physician about your intake of garlic. It may be best to discontinue garlic for at least 2 weeks prior to surgery.

Ginkgo biloba. Ginkgo is an antioxidant that supports circulation. It is available in capsule form. The recommended daily dose is 120 milligrams twice a day of extract standardized to 24 percent of flavone glycosides and 6 percent terpene lactones. The flavone glycosides give ginkgo its antioxidant benefits, and terpene lactones increase circulation and have a protective effect on nerve cells. However, if you are taking prescription blood-thinning medication, be sure to consult your doctor before taking ginkgo supplements.

Grape seed extract. Grape seed extract contains flavonoids called procyanidolic oligomers or PCOs (also known as proanthocyanidins). Often referred to as PAC, grape seed extract is a valuable antioxidant that rids the body of damaging free radicals and has been shown to reduce blood pressure. The typical recommended dose is a 100-milligram capsule three times a day of extract standardized to contain 92 to 95 percent PCOs.

Green tea. Green tea contains high levels of substances called polyphenols, which have powerful antioxidant properties. It also helps to decrease cholesterol, lower blood pressure, and prevent the clogging of arteries. Green tea may be taken as a tea or in capsules. Prepared tea bags are readily available in grocery and health food stores. You may also brew a tea from leaves. Steep 1 teaspoon of the leaves in 1 cup of boiling water for 2 to 3 minutes. Green tea can become bitter if steeped too long. Drinking 3 cups of tea per day may provide 240 to 320 milligrams of polyphenols. In capsule form, standardized extract of EGCG (a polyphenol) may provide 97 percent polyphenol content. This is the equivalent of drinking 4 cups of tea per day without the caffeine.

Hawthorn. Hawthorn works to decrease cholesterol and lower blood pressure. In addition, hawthorn helps to strengthen the heart muscles, improve circulation, and rid the body of unnecessary fluid and salt. Hawthorn is available in capsule or tincture form, standardized to 2.2 percent total bioflavonoid content. The recommended daily dose of hawthorn capsules varies widely, ranging from 100 to 300 milligrams two to three times per day. Be aware that higher doses may significantly lower blood pressure, which may, in turn, cause you to faint. In tincture, the recommended dose is 4 to 5 milliliters three times per day. It may take up to 2 months before you see the effects of this herb.

Hibiscus. Recent studies are showing that hibiscus tea may be as effective as captopril, a popular drug used to treat mild to moderate hypertension. It was also reported that results can be obtained quickly. Study participants had more than a 10 percent drop in both systolic (top number) and diastolic (bottom number) pressure in just 2 weeks. You should have your blood pressure monitored carefully to ensure that it does not drop too low, particularly if you are presently taking blood pressure–lowering medications.

Nutritional Supplements

Some nutritional supplements have a favorable effect on hypertension. If you are on prescription medication, check with your doctor before beginning a nutritional supplement regimen.

- Calcium: 1,500 milligrams daily in divided doses of 500 milligrams. Effective against high blood pressure.

- Coenzyme Q_{10}: 100 milligrams daily in divided doses of 50 milligrams. Lowers blood pressure.

- Magnesium: 750 milligrams daily in divided doses of 250 milligrams. Deficiency linked to high blood pressure.

- Omega-3 fatty acids: 1 tablespoon of flax-seed oil daily. Lowers blood pressure, triglyceride levels, and cholesterol.

Relaxation/Meditation

Many doctors recommend various relaxation/meditation techniques to help patients with high blood pressure reduce their stress. Results from a study sponsored by the National Institutes of Health (NIH) and published in 2007 showed that transcendental meditation lowered high blood pressure. Other clinical trials have found a combination of biofeedback, yoga, and meditation to be successful in reducing blood pressure. Also effective for the treatment of hypertension include the gentle movement therapies of qigong and tai chi.

When meditating, finding the right mix of elements is a subjective process. Your goal is to create a setting that allows you to sit or lie down comfortably. Some people like to listen to soft music, while others prefer a sound such as ocean waves or a low hum. Still others prefer complete quiet. You may want to light a candle to gaze at, which may help pull you away from your busy thoughts.

Next, focus on your breathing. Inhale through your nose as if smelling a rose; then exhale with enough force to blow out a candle. Continue as long as you wish. Such deep, cleansing breaths create an overall sense of relaxation and openness.

Lifestyle Recommendations

Begin exercising. One of the key elements in controlling high blood pressure is moderate exercise. Exercise strengthens your heart, which enables it to pump greater amounts of blood with less effort. If the heart does not need to work as hard, then there is less force placed on the arteries. Try to make time for at least 30 minutes of aerobic activity, such as walking or running, as often as possible. Exercising every day is ideal. However, before beginning any exercise routine, it is best to check with your doctor.

Drink concord grape juice. The polyphenols found in grape juice help lower blood pressure. Studies suggest this may be due to their relaxation effect on artery walls. If sugar is a problem, concord grape juice is available unsweetened.

Limit your caffeine consumption. The relationship between high blood pressure and caffeine consumption is still the topic of some debate. However, it is known that caffeine temporarily raises blood pressure, which can stay elevated for up to 2 hours.

Reduce alcohol consumption. If you consume alcohol, do so in moderation. Excessive alcohol intake raises blood pressure, but drinking smaller amounts does not appear to raise blood pressure. Moderate drinking is considered safe. For men, that is no more than two drinks per day; for women or small-framed men, that is no more than one drink per day. However, if you have been drinking larger amounts of alcohol, do not suddenly stop. It is safer to reduce slowly, as stopping suddenly could send your blood pressure soaring.

Other alcohol-related issues include the fact that, when mixed with alcohol, certain blood pressure medications may have undesirable side effects. For example, beta-blockers slow heart rate and relax blood vessels. So, if you drink alcohol around the same time you take a beta-blocker, you might feel light-headed. You may have a similar response if you mix alcohol and ACE inhibitors or calcium antagonists. Drinking some extra water may help to alleviate the symptoms. Since alcohol and central-acting agents are sedatives, mixing the two could make you feel depressed.

Stop smoking. If you smoke, stop. It has been estimated that about a third of the people with high blood pressure smoke. People who have high blood pressure and smoke are three to five times more likely to die from a heart attack or heart failure than people who do not smoke. And they die of a stroke more than twice as often as those with high blood pressure who do not smoke.

Preventive Measures

In the industrial world, the lifetime risk for hypertension exceeds 90 percent. Excessive weight, elevated blood fats, diabetes, insulin resistance, and aging are other risk factors associated with hypertension. Preventive measures are key to a more healthful life.

Avoid loneliness. Research has shown that being lonely can elevate your blood pressure by as much as 30 points. Make sure you take the time to stay connected socially, especially if you live alone.

Consider a vegetarian diet. Studies have

shown that a vegetarian diet can significantly lower the risk of hypertension. Soy, a staple in vegetarian diets, has been shown to reduce blood pressure, LDL cholesterol, and triglycerides. A study published in the May 2007 issue of the *Archives of Internal Medicine* stated that participants who ate $\frac{1}{2}$ cup of soybeans each day for 8 weeks lowered their blood pressure and cholesterol levels.

Get moving. In addition to being useful for people who already have high blood pressure, exercise may prevent your blood pressure from becoming too high. Recent studies show exercise improves the nerve reflexes that control blood pressure and heart rate. Researchers noted that weakened nerve reflexes are a risk factor for sudden death after a heart attack. If you do not have hypertension and remain sufficiently active, you may never develop this disorder; studies show that men who are physically active can reduce their risk of developing hypertension up to 70 percent.

Lose excess weight. Excess weight is associated with high blood pressure. In fact, it is related to a number of chronic medical problems, including diabetes and stroke. If you are overweight, ask your doctor to determine if there is a medical reason, such as a thyroid imbalance. If no medical reason is found, you may wish to begin a weight-loss program.

Reduce stress. By itself, stress does not necessarily cause high blood pressure. Many people lead stressed lives, but their blood pressure remains normal. And there are people who are generally relaxed who have high blood pressure. Nevertheless, stress may, at least temporarily, raise your blood pressure. When you are stressed, your body releases hormones that narrow your blood vessels and increase your heart rate. If this happens frequently, it has the potential to damage your brain, kidneys, heart, eyes, and arteries. Try to reduce some of the stresses in your life. Develop some stress-coping mechanisms that work for you. You may wish to learn relaxation techniques such as deep breathing and meditation.

Use your senses to create a relaxing environment. By combining your senses of smell, sight, and hearing, you can create a therapeutic environment that is conducive to relaxation. Essential oils that may actually lower blood pressure are clary sage, lavender, lemon, marjoram, and ylang-ylang.

Try filling your bathtub with warm water and adding a few drops of the above oils. Then dim the lights, and light a blue or green candle, as both of these colors have a relaxing, calming effect on the body. Finally, play some relaxing music, lie back, and enjoy. When you are finished, wrap yourself in a blue or green towel, and climb into bed for a good night's sleep.

High Cholesterol

Cholesterol is a naturally occurring substance in the blood. Your body needs it to support nerve cells, produce hormones, and manufacture vitamin D on the skin's surface. The majority of the cholesterol in your blood is made by your liver from the carbohydrates, proteins, and fats that you consume. Large amounts of cholesterol are found in animal foods such as dairy products and red meats.

High cholesterol, or hypercholesterolemia, is a condition in which the level of cholesterol in your blood is too high. When this occurs, deposits of fat, called plaque, form inside the walls of the blood vessels. Over time, the blood vessels thicken and narrow, creating a medical problem known as atherosclerosis. This results in reduced bloodflow and increases your risk for heart disease and stroke. Heart disease is the most common killer of both men and women in the United States. Every year, about 1 million Americans have a heart attack and about 500,000 die from heart disease. High levels of cholesterol have also been linked with Alzheimer's disease.

High cholesterol is extremely common. About half of all Americans have it.

Causes and Risk Factors

A number of factors affect your cholesterol levels. Some you are unable to alter, such as your age and sex. As you age, your cholesterol levels tend to rise. Before menopause, women generally have lower total cholesterol levels than men, but after menopause that difference dwindles. In addition, genes play a role in

Two Types of Cholesterol

There are two primary components of cholesterol, low-density lipoprotein (LDL) and high-density lipoprotein (HDL). Both LDL and HDL carry cholesterol through your blood. LDLs leave fatty deposits on the vessel walls, thereby contributing to heart disease. On the other hand, HDLs clean artery walls and eliminate excess cholesterol from the blood, reducing the risk of heart disease. That is why LDL is often referred to as "bad" cholesterol and HDL is said to be "good" cholesterol. You should aim for higher levels of HDLs and lower levels of LDLs. Ideally, total cholesterol should be less than 200 milligrams/dL (milligrams of cholesterol per deciliter of blood), HDL should be 60 milligrams/dL or higher, and LDL should be less than 100 milligrams/dL. Some authorities use the ratio of total cholesterol to HDL cholesterol to more accurately predict individuals at greater risk for coronary heart disease. Though authorities vary on the ideal ratio, depending upon other risk factors such as tobacco use, age, and high blood pressure, men should strive for a ratio of less than 6.4; women should try to keep theirs below 5.6.

cholesterol—high cholesterol runs in families.

But there are cholesterol-altering factors that you *can* control. If you eat a diet that is high in cholesterol and saturated fat, you increase your risk. People who are overweight or who have hypothyroidism, type 2 diabetes, or metabolic syndrome—a constellation of factors that includes high blood sugar, blood pressure, and triglycerides as well as excess abdominal fat—are also at greater risk.

Signs and Symptoms

Most often, high cholesterol is a silent disease. You will experience no symptoms until there is a dramatic event, such as leg pain while walking that is caused by the narrowed or blocked arteries in your legs or the chest pain of a heart attack.

Conventional Treatments

The goal of lowering your cholesterol is to reduce the risk for heart disease and stroke. Most likely, you will begin with therapeutic lifestyle changes (TLCs)—various forms of dietary modifications, physical activity, and weight management. If those fail to achieve the desired result, you will probably be advised to take medications.

Dietary Programs

A number of dietary programs might prove helpful for dealing with high cholesterol.

The DASH (Dietary Approaches to Stop Hypertension) diet. Doctors who treat high cholesterol often recommend the Dietary Approaches to Stop Hypertension (DASH) diet. In addition to reducing blood pressure, it has been shown to lower cholesterol. The DASH diet is high in grains, fruits, and vegetables. In fact, it recommends seven or eight servings of grains each day and eight to 10 servings of fruits and vegetables; four or five servings of legumes, nuts, and seeds are also advised. Dairy products are limited to two or three servings of low-fat or fat-free items a day. And there should be no more than two servings a day of lean meat, fish, or poultry (without the skin). Oily fish, such as salmon, is considered especially beneficial.

Mediterranean diet. The Mediterranean diet focuses on heart-healthy fiber and nutrients such as omega-3 fatty acids and antioxidants. Though it has a relatively high fat content of between 35 and 45 percent, the vast majority of the fat is monounsaturated and polyunsaturated. The diet includes olive oil, which improves insulin and blood glucose levels and reduces blood pressure, and canola oil, which is filled with omega-3 fatty acids. Avoid high-fat dairy and meat products, and rely on fish as the primary source of protein. The diet relies heavily on fresh fruits and vegetables and relatively high amounts of nuts, legumes, beans, and

A Quick Guide to Symptoms

☐ **Often, you will experience no symptoms**
☐ **First sign may be a dramatic event, such as chest or leg pain while walking or the chest pain of a heart attack**

whole grains. Enjoy a daily glass or two of wine, and season food with garlic, onions, and herbs.

The Ornish program. If you're following the Ornish program (named after its creator, Dean Ornish, MD), you'll need to severely limit your intake of saturated fats. Only 10 percent of the diet may be obtained from even the healthier types of fat. At the same time, carbohydrates compose 75 percent of the diet. So, most of your meals will consist of lots of whole grains, legumes, and fresh fruits and vegetables. If you follow this diet, you will need to couple it with regular stress reduction techniques and at least 90 minutes of exercise three times each week. You will not be allowed to smoke. And you can't consume more than 2 ounces of alcohol each day.

The TLC diet. This diet focuses on eating low-saturated fat, low-cholesterol foods. If you elect to follow this diet, less than 7 percent of your calories can come from saturated fats. And you should eat no more than 200 milli-grams of dietary cholesterol per day. This diet includes higher amounts of soluble fiber and foods that contain plant stanols or plant sterols (naturally occurring substances that are believed to reduce the absorption of cho-lesterol from the gut), such as cholesterol-lowering margarine and salad dressings.

Foods that are low in saturated fat include skinless poultry, whole grains, lean meats, fish, fat-free or 1 percent fat dairy products, fruits, and vegetables. Use liquid margarine or margarine that is in a tub. Since some margarines contain unhealthy trans fats, be sure to read the label. Restrict your intake of full-fat dairy products, organ meats, and egg

Self-Testing

There are a number of cholesterol self-tests sold in pharmacies, discount stores, and online sites. Some test only for total cholesterol, while others determine total cholesterol, HDL cholesterol, and LDL cholesterol. In order to use the kits, you must obtain a few drops of blood from your finger. All the supplies that you need are included, but be sure to read the instructions carefully. However, you should be aware that many doctors question the accuracy of these tests. If the test results indicate that your cholesterol is not within the normal range, schedule an appointment with your doctor.

yolks. Good sources of soluble fiber include oranges, pears, brussels sprouts, carrots, dried peas, beans, and oats.

Physical Activity

You need at least 30 minutes of physical activity almost every day. It has been deter-mined that burning at least 250 calories a day raises HDL levels, thereby protecting against coronary artery disease. This may be accomplished by 45 minutes of walking or 25 minutes of running. Plus, resistance (weight) training reduces LDL levels.

Weight Management

If you are overweight, losing weight may help lower your LDL levels. This is particularly important if your triglycerides are high and your HDL level is low, and if you are a man with a waist measurement over 40 inches or a woman with a waist measurement over 35 inches. When it comes to health, carrying most of your excess weight in your hips and thighs or lower body (pear shape) is considered better than carrying most of your excess weight in your waist (apple shape).

In general, 1 pound of fat equals about 3,500 calories, so you can lose approximately 1 pound a week if you reduce your intake of calories by about 500 calories each day.

Medications

If you are unable to achieve sufficient improvement in your cholesterol levels from diet and exercise, your doctor will likely recommend medications. It is important to realize that medications should be used in conjunction with lifestyle changes, not instead of them.

Bile-acid binding resins. Bile-acid binding resins attach to bile in the digestive tract and the bile is then excreted in the feces. With less bile in the body, the liver uses greater amounts of cholesterol to produce more bile. So, more cholesterol is removed from the bloodstream and LDL levels drop. Examples are cholestyramine (Questran, Questran Light), colestipol (Colestid), and colesevelam (Cholestagel, Welchol). With these medications, there are frequent reports of side effects such as heartburn, gas, constipation, and other gastrointestinal problems. Colesevelam, the newest bile-acid binding resin, seems to have the fewest number of side effects. Nevertheless, after 1 year, about 40 percent of people on these medications stop taking them.

Bile-acid binding resins may contribute to calcium loss as well as deficiencies of vitamins A, D, E, and K. There have been rare reports of liver toxicity. Do not take bile-acid binding resins at the same time that you take digoxin (Lanoxin), warfarin, beta-blocker drugs, or any of a number of medicines used to treat hypoglycemia. Take these medications at least 1 hour before or 4 to 6 hours after taking your bile-acid binding resin.

Nicotinic acid. If your HDL is very low, your doctor may recommend nicotinic acid, the active component found in niacin (vitamin B_3). Examples are Niacor, Nicolar, and Slo-Niacin; there is also an extended-release form called Niaspan. When used in high doses, nicotinic acid raises HDL more than any other anticholesterol medication and also lowers both LDL and triglycerides. However, many find the side effects too uncomfortable. These include flushing of the face and neck, itching, headache, blurred vision, gastrointestinal problems, dry skin, darkening of the skin, and dizziness. Because of the side effects, after 1 year, about 40 percent of those who start nicotinic acid stop taking it.

About 3 to 5 percent of those taking nicotinic acid develop liver abnormalities. Fortunately, these disappear when the medication is stopped. If you have a chronic liver problem, you should not take any form of this medication. Since nicotinic acid elevates uric acid, if you have gout, you should not take it.

Statins. The statins—such as lovastatin (Mevacor), pravastatin (Pravachol), simvastatin (Zocor), fluvastatin (Lescol), and atorvastatin (Lipitor)—work directly in the liver to block a substance needed for the production of cholesterol. These are the most effective drugs for treating high cholesterol. While especially useful for lowering LDL, the statins also raise HDL and reduce triglycerides. There is evidence that they reduce inflammation in the arteries and help curtail blood clotting. Statins are generally considered the first choice for most people with high cholesterol and are particularly helpful for those who have type 2 diabetes.

A study published in the *New England Journal of Medicine* reported that intensive therapy with statin drugs not only lowered levels of LDL cholesterol, but also lowered a substance known as C-reactive protein. This is helpful because in people with coronary artery disease, the progression of the disease is apparently slowed by reducing both LDL cholesterol and C-reactive protein.

Statin drugs tend to be well tolerated. Nevertheless, reported side effects include gastrointestinal discomfort, skin rashes, headaches, muscle aches, sexual dysfunction, drowsiness, dizziness, nausea, constipation, and peripheral neuropathy (numbness or tingling in the hands or feet). Since statins may affect the liver, liver function tests should be given periodically. Statins should be taken with caution by anyone with liver problems, and they may interact with other cholesterol-lowering medications. If you are taking a statin medication, do not consume grapefruit juice or sour oranges, found in marmalades, as these may increase the potency of your medication.

Complementary Treatments

Complementary medicine treats high cholesterol in much the same way as conventional medicine, including dietary and lifestyle changes.

Tips for Taking Nicotinic Acid

There are ways to reduce the side effects of nicotinic acid. The following are a few suggestions.

☐ **Avoid hot drinks.**
☐ **Start with lower doses and slowly work up to the dose recommended by your doctor.**
☐ **Try taking a low-dose aspirin about 30 minutes before taking nicotinic acid. This seems to prevent flushing.**
☐ **Try the extended-release form.**

Diet

Beans and legumes contain pectin, a water-soluble fiber that helps move cholesterol out of the body. Eat one serving of beans (1½ cups) each day. Especially good choices are soybeans, lima beans, kidney beans, navy beans, pinto beans, black-eyed peas, and lentils.

Fruits also contain pectin and should be eaten regularly. Carrots, cabbage, broccoli, and onions have pectin in the form of calcium pectate, which helps remove cholesterol. Starting your day with half a grapefruit and eating two raw carrots at lunch is an ideal way to begin lowering your cholesterol.

Recent research has shown that certain nuts and seeds contain high levels of phytosterols, a group of chemicals found in plants that are known to reduce blood cholesterol levels. Nuts with the highest levels of phytosterols are pistachios, sunflower seeds, pumpkin seeds, pine nuts, almonds, macadamia nuts, and black walnuts.

A compound found in skim milk may actually inhibit cholesterol production in the liver.

It's a good idea to curtail large amounts of red meat. However, moderate amounts of lean red meat, with all visible fat removed, may be included in the diet.

Herbal Medicine

Garlic. Garlic has the ability to reduce cholesterol. Fresh garlic is the most effective, but garlic supplements may also be useful. However, some deodorized garlic supplements do not lower cholesterol. Look for enteric-coated tablets or capsules with standardized allicin potential. Take 400 to 500 milligrams, once or twice per day, to provide up to 5,000 micrograms of allicin. Since garlic has anticoagulant properties, if you are taking prescription anticoagulant medication, check with your doctor before increasing your intake of garlic or beginning a garlic supplementation regimen. If you are planning to have surgery, you should inform your physician about your intake of garlic. It may be best to discontinue garlic for at least 2 weeks prior to surgery.

Green tea. Green tea contains high levels of substances called polyphenols, which have powerful antioxidant properties. Green tea also helps to decrease cholesterol, lower blood pressure, and prevent the clogging of arteries. The tea may be taken as a beverage or in capsules. Prepared tea bags are readily available in grocery and health food stores. You may also brew a tea from leaves. Steep 1 teaspoon of the leaves in 1 cup of boiling water for 2 to 3 minutes. Green tea can become bitter if steeped too long. Drinking 3 cups of tea per day may provide 240 to 320 milligrams of polyphenols. In capsule form, standardized extract of EGCG (a polyphenol) may provide 97 percent polyphenol content. This is the equivalent of drinking 4 cups of tea per day without the caffeine.

Hawthorn. Hawthorn works to decrease cholesterol and lower blood pressure. In addition, hawthorn helps to strengthen the heart muscles, improve circulation, and rid the body of unnecessary fluid and salt. Hawthorn is available in capsule or tincture form, standardized to 2.2 percent total bioflavonoid content. The recommended daily dose of hawthorn capsules varies widely, ranging from 100 to 300 milligrams, two or three times per day. Be aware that higher doses may significantly lower blood pressure, which may, in turn, cause you to faint. In tincture, the recommended dose is 4 to 5 milliliters, three times per day. It may take up to 2 months before you see the effects of this herb.

Nutritional Supplements

The following supplements help lower total cholesterol and raise HDL cholesterol.

- Vitamin C: 1,000 milligrams daily in divided doses of 500 milligrams. Prevents plaque buildup in arteries. Improves HDL cholesterol, decreases LDL and triglycerides.

- Vitamin E: 400 IU daily. Works with vitamin C in preventing plaque buildup and raising HDL.

- Calcium: 1,500 milligrams daily in divided doses of 500 milligrams. Lowers total cholesterol.

- Magnesium: 750 milligrams daily in

divided doses of 250 milligrams. Works with absorption of calcium.

- Niacin: 100 milligrams daily. Lowers total cholesterol.

Lifestyle Recommendations

Add psyllium powder to your diet. Studies have shown that adding psyllium powder to your diet helps lower cholesterol. Psyllium powder is derived from the husks of the seeds.

Drink concord grape juice. The polyphenols found in grape juice help lower LDL cholesterol. If sugar is a problem for you, concord grape juice is available unsweetened.

Red wine, another grape product, has similar benefits. A number of studies have found that drinking one or two glasses of red wine each day improves cholesterol.

Stop smoking and stay away from smokers. Cigarette smoking lowers HDL levels. When you stop smoking, your HDL levels will naturally rise. However, secondhand smoke also lowers HDL levels, so you don't want to spend too much time around smokers. In addition, smoking as few as 20 cigarettes a week may increase your total cholesterol level.

Preventive Measures

Begin exercising. Becoming physically active is as close as you can get to having a magic solution for preventing high cholesterol. A regular exercise program not only raises HDL levels, it also helps decrease total blood cholesterol, blood pressure, body fat, and risk of heart disease and diabetes, and helps you maintain a healthy weight. Begin a regular exercise program before you are diagnosed with high cholesterol; include both weight-bearing and resistance exercises. Try to do some form of aerobic exercise for at least 30 minutes five times a week.

Change your diet. Reduce your consumption of saturated fats and eat lots of fresh fruits and vegetables, whole grains, and fish and poultry. Add more soluble fiber to your diet. Foods high in soluble fiber include oat bran, oatmeal, beans, peas, rice bran, barley, citrus fruits, strawberries, barley, prunes, and apples. Eat more fish, especially fish that are high in omega-3 fatty acids, such as salmon, mackerel, and herring. Eat more soy products, which contain isoflavones, substances that regulate cholesterol. Soy has been shown to reduce LDL cholesterol and triglycerides. A study published in the May 2007 issue of the *Archives of Internal Medicine* stated that participants who ate ½ cup of soybeans each day for 8 weeks lowered their LDL cholesterol level by as much as 11 percent. If you make these modifications, you may avoid the disorder completely.

Drink tea. The catechins (flavonoid phytochemical compounds) found in green, oolong, and black tea may help keep cholesterol in the normal range. Because of how it's processed, green tea has the most catechins; oolong has the second highest. Black tea has the least because its fermentation process makes the catechins less potent. While regular tea drinking may be beneficial, it must be combined with other dietary recommendations.

Reduce stress. Studies have shown that transcendental meditation can help to significantly reduce total cholesterol levels.

Hip Fracture

A hip fracture is a break at the top of the femur (thighbone) near the area where the femur fits into the hip socket. The most common direct cause of such a break is a fall. But the actual cause is probably a weakening of the structure of your bones, a condition called osteoporosis.

There are two main types of hip fractures: femoral neck fractions and intertrochanteric fractures. Femoral neck fractures occur 1 to 2 inches from the joint, while intertrochanteric fractures are located 3 to 4 inches from the joint.

Every year approximately 320,000 Americans are hospitalized for hip fracture. This is a common medical problem that will probably increase in frequency as the baby boomers continue to age.

A Quick Guide to Symptoms

- ☐ **Severe pain in the hip or groin area**
- ☐ **Inability to stand on the leg**
- ☐ **The painful leg is shorter than the other leg or it turns inward or outward**
- ☐ **Stiffness, bruising, and/or swelling in the hip**

Causes and Risk Factors

Since women lose bone density at a much faster rate than men, on average, women are two or three times more likely than men to have a hip fracture. In fact, the average woman has a one in seven risk of having a hip fracture during her lifetime. In contrast, that risk is one in 17 among men. Small-boned, slender women have the greatest risk. There is also a genetic component to hip fracture, particularly in Asians and whites. And people with some form of mental impairment, such as Alzheimer's disease and dementia, or who have chronic physical ailments like arthritis are more vulnerable. Your risk for hip fracture increases as you age.

Signs and Symptoms

A number of symptoms are associated with hip fracture. The most dramatic symptom is severe pain in the hip or groin area. You are unable to stand on the leg. In addition, the painful leg may be shorter than the other leg or turn inward or outward. And there may be stiffness, bruising, and/or swelling in the hip. If you are experiencing any of these and believe that you may have sustained a hip fracture, you need to seek emergency medical assistance.

Conventional Treatments

In the vast majority of cases, surgery is the best method for repairing a hip fracture.

Depending upon the nature of the hip fracture, there are different types of procedures.

Surgery for Femoral Neck Fractures

There are three types of surgery for femoral neck fractures: hemiarthroplasty, internal fixation, and total hip replacement.

Hemiarthroplasty. If the bones are damaged or the ends are not properly aligned, then the head and neck of the femur may be replaced with a metal prosthesis.

Internal fixation. If the hip fracture bones are still properly aligned, your surgeon may use metal screws to hold the bones together.

Total hip replacement. If the joint was already damaged before the fall (by arthritis or another medical problem), there is a good chance you will have a total hip replacement. During the surgery, which usually takes 2 to 3 hours, the surgeon replaces the damaged hip joint with artificial parts.

Hip replacement surgery, unfortunately, can lead to a number of complications. The most frequent complication is dislocation of the new joint. To reduce the risk that this will occur, you should not bend at the hip more than 90 degrees. Also, you should not allow your leg to cross the midline of your body. Other complications are infections at the incision and near the prosthesis. While these are generally treatable with antibiotics, a severe infection near the prosthesis may require further surgery. Following surgery you will have limited mobility for at least a temporary period of time. For that reason,

blood clots are a potentially serious complication. To reduce your risk for blood clots, you will be given blood-thinning medications, and you will probably have some form of compression device on your lower legs.

Long-term complications of hip replacement surgery include the loosening of the prosthesis within the bone. This is caused by an inflammatory reaction from the tiny particles that wear off the surfaces of the artificial joint. To reduce the risk of this complication, you may be advised to take an anti-inflammatory medication. Another potential complication is a break of the prosthesis. With both types of complications, additional surgery may be required.

If you have hip replacement surgery during your midlife years, there is a reasonable chance that your artificial hip parts may wear out and you may require revision surgery after 15 to 20 years. You should know that revision surgery tends not to be as successful as first-time hip replacement surgery.

If you have had hip replacement surgery, it is usually recommended that you have an antibiotic before any routine dental work. This reduces the risk of developing an infection near the prosthesis.

Surgery for Intertrochanteric Fractures

Surgery for intertrochanteric fractures normally includes the surgical insertion of a compression hip screw (a metal screw) across the fracture. The screw is attached to other screws that stabilize the bone. As the injury heals, the bone pieces compress, and the edges grow together.

Complementary Treatments

A combination of a healthy diet, nutritional supplements, exercise, and movement therapies is effective in preventing and treating hip fractures.

Acupuncture

Acupuncture has been shown to be effective for the rehabilitation of hip fractures. It may accelerate the healing process and decrease the amount of pain. To locate an acupuncturist in your area, visit the Web site of the National Certification Commission for Acupuncture and Oriental Medicine (NCCAOM) at www.nccaom.org.

Aquatic Therapy

Without placing stress on muscles, bones, and joints, exercise in a heated pool, with the buoyancy and resistance of water, is an ideal environment to develop strength, flexibility, and endurance. In addition, by calming the nerves, increasing circulation, and decreasing muscle stiffness, aquatic therapy exercises are useful during the hip fracture rehabilitation process.

Diet

Eating a low-fat, well-balanced diet that contains lots of whole grains, fresh fruits, and calcium-rich foods helps keep your body strong and healthy. Since vitamin D and the mineral magnesium play a role in the body's absorption and metabolism of calcium, your diet should include foods rich in these nutrients. Milk that is fortified with vitamin D is a very good source of calcium. However, since whole milk is high in fat, you should select a low-fat or skim alternative. If you prefer not to consume cow's milk, rice and soy milk are both fortified with vitamin D. Other foods that are high in calcium include shrimp, blackstrap molasses, calcium-fortified tofu, almonds, sardines, beans, oranges, raisins, and green leafy vegetables such as kale and broccoli.

Relatively few foods contain significant amounts of vitamin D. The best sources are fish such as salmon, tuna, Atlantic mackerel, oysters, shrimp, herring, and halibut. The livers and oil from these fish have high amounts of vitamin D. Other sources include milk, chicken liver, eggs, Cheddar cheese, and Swiss cheese.

It's easy to consume an adequate amount of magnesium because it's found in many different healthful foods. Good sources include whole grains, legumes, nuts, potatoes, seeds, dark green vegetables, bananas, and tomatoes.

Soy products, which contain plant estrogens known as isoflavones, are believed to support bone density. Calcium-fortified tofu is considered a good source. Three ounces of tofu have 60 percent of the daily calcium requirement.

Since it helps you hold on to the calcium in your bones, vitamin K may be another important bone-supporting part of the diet. Studies have shown that women who consume higher amounts of vitamin K have fewer hip fractures. Eating fruits and vegetables will give you the extra vitamin K that you may require. Especially good sources are strawberries, broccoli, spinach, parsley, cauliflower, brussels sprouts, blackstrap molasses, and collard greens. In addition, by eating lots of fruits and vegetables, you supply your body with boron, a trace element that has been found to assist in calcium absorption. Boron is found primarily in apples, dates, grapes, peaches, and pears.

Movement Reeducation Therapies

Since they help people to relearn proper body movements, the Alexander Technique, the Feldenkrais Method, tai chi, qigong, and the Trager Approach have been successful in the rehabilitation of hip fracture. These therapies also result in decreased pain, greater mobility, improved posture, and freer movement.

Nutritional Supplements

The combination of these nutrients helps maintain bone density and reduce the risk of fractures.

- Vitamin D: 400 IU daily. Promotes healthy bones. Deficiency causes bone weakening. Regulates absorption of calcium.
- Boron: 750 micrograms daily. Aids in metabolism of calcium and magnesium.

Especially effective with vitamin D deficiency or calcium absorption problems.

- Calcium: 1,500 milligrams in divided doses of 500 milligrams (the body is unable to absorb more than 500 milligrams of calcium at a time). Essential for healthy bones.
- Magnesium: 750 milligrams daily in divided doses of 250 milligrams. Works well with calcium.

Calcium supplements are available in a variety of forms, including calcium carbonate, calcium citrate, and calcium gluconate. Each contains a different concentration of calcium: Calcium carbonate is 40 percent calcium, calcium citrate is 24 percent calcium, and calcium gluconate is only 9 percent calcium. They also differ in their absorbability. Calcium citrate is better absorbed than most other types of calcium, and it increases the absorption of iron. Calcium citrate also contains acids, so it does not need stomach acid to be absorbed; as a result, it may be taken any time of the day. On the other hand, calcium carbonate requires stomach acid to be absorbed, so it must be consumed with food. It is recommended that calcium gluconate be taken between meals or at night. Finally, if you are on thyroid medication, be sure to allow a few hours between the thyroid medication and calcium supplementation. Otherwise, calcium will reduce the efficacy of the thyroid medication. If you would like to test the absorbability of your calcium supplement, place it in a glass of white vinegar. Does it break up within 30 minutes? If not, you may wish to try another form of calcium supplement.

Therapeutic Massage

By increasing the range of motion and circulation to the hip area and by promoting flexibility and relaxation, therapeutic massage is effective in the rehabilitation of hip fracture.

Lifestyle Recommendations

Allow recovery time. Recovery from a hip fracture may be a lengthy process. While you should follow the exercises recommended by your therapists, don't become discouraged when your rehabilitation seems to take a longer time than you anticipated.

Be careful with your hip. After you have been surgically treated for hip fracture, you will want to be especially careful with your hip. You should probably avoid any high-impact activities such as jogging, tennis, or basketball. Exercises that are safer for your hip include walking, swimming, and stationary bicycling.

Get your protein from vegetables and legumes. Studies show that postmenopausal women who consume higher amounts of vegetable protein than animal protein have a decreased risk of hip fracture.

Get out of bed. Following any form of surgery for hip fracture, you will be tempted to remain in bed. It is important to realize that you will recover faster and reduce your chances for complications if you remain more active.

Preventive Measures

Alcohol or medications can make you unsteady and at higher risk for falls and hip fracture.

Be aware of medication side effects. Some medications may make you feel dizzy or weak, increasing the risk for a fall. Ask your doctor to describe the side effects of your medications.

Be realistic with footwear. If you believe that you are at risk for a hip fracture, wear sensible shoes that are not too slippery, sticky, or spiky.

Begin exercising. Bone health usually requires exercising several times a week. Include aerobic, weight-bearing exercises such as walking, as well as strength or resistance training. An optimal exercise program includes 50 minutes of walking, three times a week, or 30 minutes, five times a week. If you have been relatively inactive, before beginning an exercise program, you should check with your doctor.

If you have osteoporosis, there are certain exercises you should *not* do. Do not do exercises that may hurt your spine (such as jumping, jogging, or running) or exercises in which you must bend forward from the waist with a rounded back (such as abdominal crunches, sit-ups, toe touches, or bringing the knees to the chest). When exercising, your back should be supported and stable. Strong abdominal muscles are necessary for maintaining back stability—they will take pressure off the hips and help you keep your balance and prevent falls. Since sit-ups are contraindicated, isometric exercises (using elastic stretch bands) work best. If you have osteoporosis, do not participate in any exercise in which you could easily fall, such as step aerobics. And don't do any exercise in which you need to move your leg sideways against resistance. Some resistance-exercise machines require such actions. Under pressure, a weakened hip could break.

Movement therapies that improve balance, coordination, muscle strength, and joint range of motion are useful for those who have osteoporosis or who are interested in prevention. Examples of movement therapies are yoga, tai chi, and qigong. Because the slow, graceful movements of these therapies focus on balance, coordination, and flexibility, they may aid in preventing falls.

Improve safety within your home. You may wish to remove area rugs and install grab bars in the bathroom. Be sure you have treads on steps and handrails along the stairways. Also, try to reduce clutter and keep your home well lit. Better lighting will enable you to see more, and you will be less likely to fall.

Limit alcohol intake. Alcohol not only interferes with the absorption of calcium in your body, but it also robs your body of this necessary nutrient.

Reduce coffee consumption. The caffeine in coffee has a diuretic effect, and more calcium is excreted in the urine. If you are a woman who has been drinking large amounts of coffee, consider reducing consumption or switching to another beverage.

Remain active. If you participate in regular exercise, you lower your risk for bone loss. Exercise also improves your balance and overall strength.

Spend time in the sun. Your body uses sunlight to produce vitamin D, a vitamin that is critical to bone production. Spending only a few minutes in the sun—about 15 minutes, whenever it is convenient, several times a week—may help prevent bone loss. While you are out in the sun, you should use sunscreen on your face but not on your arms and legs. Exposure should be direct, not filtered through a window. After this brief period in the sun, if you remain outside, you should cover your arms and legs with sunscreen.

Stop smoking. There is a direct relationship between smoking and decreased bone density. As a result, there is also a direct association between smoking and risk of fracture. All women who smoke have higher rates of spine and hip fractures than women who do not smoke. This is particularly true for postmenopausal women. Also, if women who take hormone replacement therapy smoke, they lose the bone-protective effect of the therapy. Male smokers also have lower levels of bone density. On the positive side, when people stop smoking, even later in life, they reduce the loss of bone.

Hyperthyroidism

Hyperthyroidism is a condition in which there is too much thyroid hormone in the body. The thyroid is a gland that is shaped in the form of a butterfly. Located in the front of the neck, slightly below the Adam's apple, it has two lobes that are joined together in the middle by an isthmus of thyroid tissue.

Using iodine, the thyroid makes two hormones—thyroxine (T4) and triiodothyronine (T3)—that are released into the bloodstream and carried throughout the body. These two hormones control the metabolism of all the body's cells. When there is too much thyroid hormone in the body, cells function too quickly. When there is too little, cells function too slowly, a condition known as hypothyroidism. Both of these conditions are abnormal.

While thyroid hormones are produced and stored in the thyroid, the pituitary gland, which is located in the base of the brain, determines the rate at which thyroid hormones are released. When the pituitary gland senses that the body needs more thyroid hormone, it will release more thyroid-stimulating hormone (TSH); when it senses that the body already has an adequate amount, it will release less TSH.

By conservative estimates, approximately 13 million Americans have some form of thyroid disease. In reality, the figure may be closer to 20 million. It is believed that more than half of these people remain undiagnosed. In the United States, about 275,000 new cases of hyperthyroidism are diagnosed each year.

Causes and Risk Factors

Most often, hyperthyroidism happens because of general overactivity of the thyroid gland, an autoimmune disorder more commonly known as Graves' disease, or diffuse toxic goiter. However, it is possible for the body to have too much thyroid hormone for other reasons. In a condition known as toxic nodular or multinodular goiter, one or more nodules in the thyroid gland may become overactive. Thyroiditis (inflammation of the thyroid) may also trigger hyperthyroidism. Researchers don't know what causes one or more of the thyroid nodules to become overactive, or why thyroiditis occurs.

It's even possible to develop hyperthyroidism from taking too high a dose of thyroid medication. If an individual triggers hyperthyroidism through the voluntary and excessive consumption of thyroid medication, there is probably a mental health problem. This condition is known as exogenous hyperthyroidism. Sometimes people take excessive thyroid medication to lose weight. To determine whether this is the case, a doctor will feel the thyroid gland. Unlike the other forms of hyperthyroidism, which tend to cause the thyroid gland to swell, the thyroid gland of those who purposefully overdose remains normal size.

The vast majority of people with thyroid disease are women. In fact, women are at least eight times more likely to have thyroid disorders than men. Times of hormonal fluctuations place women at greater risk. So, it should not be surprising that in the years prior to menopause and during the menopausal years, women are more vulnerable to thyroid disease.

Hyperthyroidism runs in families. For example, if one of a pair of identical twins has Graves' disease, the other has a 50 percent chance of having it as well. It is also strongly suspected that environmental factors, such as severe emotional stress, play a role in Graves' disease.

Signs and Symptoms

While there are different types of hyperthyroidism, they all produce similar symptoms. Of course, you will probably not experience all the symptoms, but you may have several. People with hyperthyroidism tend to feel warm and perspire, often when others do not feel warm. Their hands may be moist, and their fingers may have a tremor. They may have a sense of weakness and lose weight, though not intentionally.

When hyperthyroidism is caused by Graves' disease, the thyroid gland tends to be symmetrically enlarged and firm. If a single nodule is causing the overactivity, the nodule will be large, while the remainder of the gland shrinks. If there are multiple nodules involved, the thyroid will feel like there are several lumps.

The symptoms of hyperthyroidism include an increased pulse rate, which is why people with hyperthyroidism may have heart palpitations. Food may move more quickly through your body, and you may have more frequent bowel movements or diarrhea. Since your urinary system will also be working at a faster rate, you may need to urinate more often.

A Quick Guide to Symptoms

☐ Feel warm and perspire, when others are not warm
☐ Moist hands
☐ Tremors in fingers
☐ Sense of weakness
☐ Unintentional weight loss
☐ Enlargement of the thyroid (Graves' disease)
☐ Increased pulse rate
☐ Heart palpitations
☐ More frequent bowel movements or diarrhea
☐ Frequent urination
☐ Abnormal protrusion of the eyes
☐ Dry and irritated eyes
☐ Reduced range of movement of the eyes

There is a self-test that determines the amount of thyroid-stimulating hormone (TSH) in the blood. However, it is not believed to be accurate. If you are experiencing the symptoms of hyperthyroidism, you need to be evaluated by your doctor.

Approximately half of those with Graves' disease develop eye problems. The tissue behind the eyeballs may become inflamed and cause an abnormal protrusion of the eyes. The eyes may become dry and irritated and look as if they are popping out of their sockets. If the eye muscles are affected, the eyes may have reduced range of movement.

Conventional Treatments

There are several types of conventional treatments for hyperthyroidism. You and your doctor will work together to determine what will be effective for you. You may begin with one treatment and later switch to another.

Medications

Beta-blockers. To control symptoms, such as a racing heartbeat, your doctor may place you on a beta-blocker. Examples are propranolol (Inderal), atenolol (Tenormin), or metoprolol (Lopressor). Though beta-blockers do not affect the thyroid itself, they do make people feel better fairly quickly. For thyroiditis, a beta-blocker may be the only therapy. With other types of hyperthyroidism, these drugs may be used in conjunction with another therapy.

Propylthiouracil and methimazole. PTU (propylthiouracil) and methimazole (Tapazole) are two drugs that are frequently used to decrease thyroid hormone production. With respect to patient compliance, methimazole, with only one daily dose, has an advantage over propylthiouracil, a medication that needs to be taken three times a day. Also, methimazole has less severe side effects.

However, these drugs may also lower levels of white blood cells, which are essential for fighting infection. So, while you are on either of these medications, your doctor will probably want to test your blood for the level of white blood cells. Other potential side effects are swollen, stiff, and painful joints, skin rash, fever, and sore throat.

Radioactive iodine. If your medical condition does not resolve or if your symptoms worsen, your doctor may suggest destroying some of the hormone-producing cells in the thyroid gland. One of the ways this may be done is with radioactive iodine. In this treatment, your doctor administers a capsule or drink containing radioactive iodine. The radioactive iodine then concentrates in the thyroid and gradually destroys the overactive cells. Over the course of several weeks, as the cells die, thyroid hormone production falls. Though physicians make every effort to determine the exact dosage, sometimes an insufficient amount of radioactive iodine is used and the procedure needs to be repeated. Far more often, the dosage is too high, and too many cells are killed. Then, the person is left with hypothyroidism, a condition that requires daily thyroid medication. (For more information, see Hypothyroidism on page 307.)

Surgery

As a last resort, your doctor may wish to refer you for thyroid surgery. This is more likely to be advised if you have a large goiter, have a reaction to medication, or prefer not to use radioactive iodine. If only one nodule is involved, the surgeon will remove that nodule and leave the remainder of the thyroid intact. The thyroid usually returns to normal function. Then again, if several nodules are affected or the entire thyroid is overactive, the surgeon removes most, if not all, of the thyroid. In this case, you will require thyroid supplementation for the rest of your life.

Though generally safe, thyroid surgery has the potential for complications. You will want to locate a highly trained and experienced surgeon who specializes in thyroid surgery. If possible, find one who works at a major medical teaching center.

Complementary Treatments

Complementary medicine treatments attempt to relieve symptoms associated with hyperthyroidism and to assist in the proper functioning of the thyroid gland. They are not meant to replace conventional thyroid treatments.

Diet

It is important to eat foods that naturally help to suppress thyroid hormone production, such as broccoli, brussels sprouts, cabbage, cauliflower, kale, peaches, pears, soybeans, spinach, and turnips. It is equally valuable to avoid products that stimulate thyroid hormone production, such as dairy products and foods and drinks that contain caffeine and alcohol.

Homeopathy

The two remedies generally used for the symptomatic treatment of hyperthyroidism are *Iodum* and *Natrum muriaticum* (chloride of sodium). A homeopath can prescribe the proper potency based on individual symptoms. It should be noted that homeopathy is also effective for the treatment of the early stages of Graves' disease. To find a practitioner trained in homeopathy, visit the Web site of the National Center for Homeopathy at www.homeopathic.org.

Nutritional Supplements

A higher metabolic rate can lead to insufficient absorption of essential nutrients.

Relieving Eye Symptoms of Graves' Disease

☐ **Cover your eyes.** While sleeping, if your eyes do not close completely, cover them or close them with paper adhesive tape. This will help prevent damage from too much exposure to air.

☐ **Keep your eyes lubricated.** Use over-the-counter artificial tears.

☐ **Take care with contacts.** Limit or discontinue your use of contact lenses.

☐ **Wear sunglasses.** Whenever you are outside, wear sunglasses for protection.

● Multivitamin/mineral: Take as directed on the label. A high metabolic rate results in absorption of few nutrients.

● B-complex vitamins: Take as directed on the label. Recommended for proper thyroid function.

Lifestyle Recommendations

Exercise. While dealing with the symptoms of hyperthyroidism, you may not feel sufficiently well to exercise. Also, you may not want to raise your heart rate even further. However, after you begin to improve, and with your doctor's approval, you may wish to reintroduce exercise into your life. Start slowly—a short, 15-minute daily walk would be good. As the weeks pass, increase your amount of exercise and include both aerobic and weight-bearing exercises several times a week. Any shortness of breath should be reported to your doctor.

Preventive Measures

Quit smoking. Smoking triples your risk for thyroid disease. If you have thyroid disease and you smoke, you will tend to have more pronounced symptoms.

Reduce stress. Consider regular relaxation, exercise, yoga, or meditation to reduce the stress in your life.

Hypothyroidism

The thyroid is a gland that is shaped in the form of a butterfly. Located in the front of the neck, slightly below the Adam's apple, it has two lobes that are joined together in the middle by an isthmus of thyroid tissue. Using iodine, the thyroid makes two hormones, thyroxine (T4) and triiodothyronine (T3). These are released into the bloodstream and carried throughout the body. They control the metabolism of all the body's cells. When there is too little thyroid hormone in the body, cells function too slowly. This condition is known as hypothyroidism.

Thyroid hormones are produced and stored in the thyroid. However, the pituitary gland, which is located in the base of the brain, determines the rate at which thyroid hormones are released. When the pituitary gland senses that the body needs more thyroid hormone, it releases more thyroid-stimulating hormone (TSH). When it senses that the body already has an adequate amount, it releases less TSH.

In people with hypothyroidism, the thyroid gland releases an insufficient amount of thyroid hormone. Without an adequate amount of thyroid hormone, the body's metabolism slows. This may lead to a host of different symptoms such as fatigue, depression, and mental fogginess. When untreated, hypothyroidism may have a number of ill effects on the body. For example, hypothyroidism directly and indirectly has a negative impact on the heart. It is also correlated with high LDL ("bad") cholesterol levels, high blood pressure, and heart failure in people who already have heart disease. Hypothyroidism may worsen headaches in people who are prone to them. And in people with depression, untreated hypothyroidism may be quite profound and debilitating.

Thyroid disorders are actually far more common than most people realize. Many people do not realize they have a thyroid problem and suffer needlessly for years. By conservative estimate, approximately 13 million Americans have some form of thyroid disease. In reality, the figure may be closer to 20 million. Some estimate that as many as one in 10 adults has a thyroid disorder, and it is believed that more than half of these people remain undiagnosed.

Causes and Risk Factors

In adults, hypothyroidism is most often caused by Hashimoto's thyroiditis, an autoimmune disorder that results in inflammation of the thyroid gland. The peak incidence for this disorder is between 30 and 50 years, and eight to nine females are affected for each male. The inflamed, often enlarged, thyroid gland is left unable to produce proper amounts of thyroid hormone.

Some treatments for hyperthyroidism—slowing down the overactive thyroid—may result in hypothyroidism. Obviously, the surgical removal of the thyroid leaves an individual with hypothyroidism. And, within 5 years of treatment, between 25 and 50 percent of people who receive radiation to the head and neck areas develop hypothyroidism.

In a small percentage of cases, hypothyroidism occurs not because of a problem with the thyroid but rather because of a dysfunction of the pituitary gland, which is located in the brain. This condition, known as secondary hypothyroidism, can result from a tumor, surgery, or a history of radiation exposure. Similarly, a problem with the hypothalamus, which regulates the pituitary gland, can lead to what's known as tertiary hypothyroidism.

The vast majority of people with thyroid disease are women. In fact, women are at least eight times more likely to have thyroid disorders than men. On average, over a lifetime, one in every eight women will develop a thyroid disorder. Times of hormonal fluctuations place women at greater risk, so it should not be surprising that women are more vulnerable to thyroid disease during the years prior to menopause as well as during the menopause years.

Signs and Symptoms

Symptoms associated with hypothyroidism include aching muscles and joints; brain fog or poor memory and concentration; anemia; constipation; depression; weight gain; feeling cold and intolerance of cold; dry, scaly, itchy skin and scalp; excess sleeping; loss of hair; husky voice; leg cramps; loss of energy; menstrual irregularities; diminished sex drive (libido); puffiness of face, lower legs, and feet; and brittle fingernails that may have lines and grooves.

While these symptoms do not necessarily mean that any particular individual has

A Quick Guide to Symptoms

☐ Aching muscles and joints
☐ Brain fog or poor memory and concentration
☐ Anemia
☐ Constipation
☐ Depression
☐ Weight gain
☐ Milky discharge from breasts
☐ Feeling cold and intolerance of cold
☐ Dry, scaly, itchy skin and scalp
☐ Excess sleeping
☐ Loss of hair
☐ Husky voice
☐ Leg cramps
☐ Changes in skin pigmentation
☐ Loss of energy
☐ Menstrual irregularities or increased menstrual flow
☐ Diminished sex drive (libido)
☐ Puffiness of face, lower legs, and feet
☐ Tingling in wrists
☐ Brittle fingernails that may have lines and grooves
☐ Slow reflexes

hypothyroidism, they should be reason for concern. If you haven't been feeling well for a few weeks, you should visit your doctor. Still, it is possible to have hypothyroidism without any apparent symptoms. And there is a type of hypothyroidism, known as borderline hypothyroidism, in which there are no symptoms, though blood tests indicate some degree of abnormality.

Conventional Treatments
Medications

Hypothyroidism is treated with levothyroxine, a synthetic derivative of thyroxine (T4). Several brands are available, including Levothroid, Levoxyl, Synthroid, Unithroid, and Euthyrox. There are also a number of generic brands. Once you begin taking levothyroxine, it slowly normalizes your levels of TSH and T4. Adults commonly take 3 to 6 weeks to notice changes, but there are reports of faster responses. Weight loss, reduced puffiness, and improved pulse rate generally happen first. It takes longer for the anemia to resolve and the skin, hair, and voice tone to improve.

Your doctor will probably start you on a relatively low dose of levothyroxine. Most people begin on a daily dose of 50 micrograms and generally increase to a daily dose of 100 to 150 micrograms. If you remain fatigued, mentally foggy, and cold, your dose may be too low. If you begin to experience a rapid heartbeat, agitation, and palpitations, your dose may be too high. In either case, you

Self-Testing

It is possible to purchase a self-test that determines the amount of thyroid-stimulating hormone in the blood. However, the test is not believed to be accurate. If you are experiencing the symptoms of hypothyroidism, you need to be evaluated by your doctor.

If you are a woman concerned that your menopausal symptoms may be masking a hypothyroid condition, you may wish to try this easy test.

Stand before a mirror, and hold your head back slightly.

Drink a little water and swallow it.

Look at your neck. Are there any bulges? Does it look like something is protruding? If so, then you should visit your doctor.

should contact your doctor, who can adjust the dose.

Normally, thyroid medication should be taken upon awakening in the morning. Ideally, after taking the medication, you should not eat or drink (except water) for at least 30 minutes. An hour's wait is even better. It is especially important to wait a few hours before consuming any calcium supplements. Calcium can interfere with absorption of your thyroid medication.

Many other drugs interact with levothyroxine. Some decrease its effectiveness, others enhance it. Drugs that bind bile acids to lower cholesterol levels inhibit thyroid hormone. Anyone who takes both of these kinds of drugs should take them at least 4 hours apart. Similarly, iron is known

Generic vs. Brand-Name Thyroid Medication

There is some debate over generic versus brand-name thyroid medication. In the past, there were some problems with the quality control of the manufacturing of levothyroxine. New FDA requirements are now in place. As a result, many people say that the generics are as good as the brand-name drugs. Others, however, continue to prefer the brand names.

to interfere with the absorption of levothyroxine. Meanwhile, thyroid hormone decreases the effectiveness of the heart medication digoxin. People on digoxin who also take levothyroxine may require larger doses of digoxin. To prevent drug interaction problems, you should always tell your doctor about all the medications you are taking.

Eventually, taking thyroid supplementation will become part of your daily routine. In all probability, you will be on thyroid supplementation for the rest of your life. But since your thyroid requirements may change, about 6 months after beginning your medication, you should probably be reevaluated. After that, an annual evaluation is a good idea. Levothyroxine is identical to the thyroxine that your body manufactures. As long as

the dosage is appropriate, there are no known side effects.

Complementary Treatments

Treatments that naturally boost the body's ability to restore thyroid function are used to complement conventional treatment. Dietary changes may be very effective in lessening the symptoms of hypothyroidism.

Diet

The thyroid uses iodine to produce hormones. Foods rich in iodine, such as kelp, eggs, milk, cheese, ocean fish, molasses, parsley, apricots, dates, and prunes, should be part of your diet.

Since the following foods interfere with the body's ability to absorb iodine, they should be limited: broccoli, brussels sprouts, cabbage, cauliflower, kale, lima beans, mustard greens, peaches, peanuts, pears, radishes, rutabagas, soy beans and other soy products, spinach, sweet potatoes, and turnips. If you are experiencing severe hypothyroid symptoms, you may wish to avoid them entirely.

Herbal Medicine

Bladder wrack is known to assist in glandular diseases, especially goiter. Steep 2 tablespoons of bladder wrack in 1 cup of boiling water for 20 minutes. This tea may be taken four times a day, once before each meal and again before bed. Because bladder wrack contains iodine, consult with your doctor before beginning to use it.

Hydrotherapy

Alternating hot and cold compresses may be useful in stimulating thyroid function. Immerse a washcloth in hot water, squeezing out any excess water. Apply over the front of the neck and hold in place for 3 minutes. Then take a second washcloth that has been placed in cold water and hold over the same spot for 1 minute. Repeat this process two more times. This procedure may be done once in the morning and once in the evening.

Nutritional Supplements

These nutritional supplements help regulate thyroid hormone production but should not be regarded as a replacement for treatment. These supplements are effective if you are deficient in these particular vitamins.

- Vitamin A: 10,000 IU daily.
- B-complex vitamins: Take as directed on the label.
- Vitamin C: 1,000 milligrams daily in divided doses of 500 milligrams.
- Vitamin E: 400 IU daily.
- Selenium: 200 micrograms daily.
- Zinc: 30 milligrams daily.

Lifestyle Recommendations

Before your hypothyroidism was diagnosed and treatment begun, you may have been too tired to exercise. However, shortly after you begin thyroid medication treatment and with your doctor's approval, you may want to reintroduce exercise into your life. Start slowly—a short walk is usually good. As the weeks pass, increase your amount of exercise to include both aerobic and weight-bearing exercises several times a week.

Preventive Measures

If you smoke, quit. Smoking triples your risk for thyroid disease. If you have thyroid disease and you smoke, you tend to have more pronounced symptoms.

Incontinence

Involuntary leakage of urine before reaching the toilet is a common problem. It can happen if your bladder muscles contract abruptly or if the muscles controlling the urethra unexpectedly relax. Incontinence can be either a temporary medical problem or a chronic debilitating and embarrassing disorder that continues for years. It may range from the occasional leakage of a small amount of urine to the inability to hold any urine at all.

Though people often have more than one type of incontinence, doctors divide incontinence into four groups, according to the type of malfunction: stress incontinence, urge incontinence, overflow incontinence, and mixed incontinence.

Stress incontinence. Stress incontinence occurs when movements such as coughing, laughing, or sneezing put pressure on the bladder and cause leakage. In women, the muscles supporting the bladder may be weakened, so the bladder pushes downward. Muscles that shut the urethra are unable to squeeze as tightly as they once did or they are weakened, and urine leaks. Because estrogen deficiencies cause the urethra to thin, after menopause the incidence of stress incontinence tends to rise. Men may also have stress incontinence. Normally, in men stress incontinence results from sphincter muscle impairment caused by treatments

for prostate cancer or benign prostatic hyperplasia (BPH). In fact, most men undergoing these treatments should anticipate at least a temporary period of stress incontinence.

Urge incontinence. If you suddenly feel the need to urinate and then immediately urinate, you probably have urge incontinence, also known as hyperactive or irritable bladder. This condition causes you to lose the ability to control the flow of urine, even temporarily. Most often, inappropriate bladder muscle contractions cause urge incontinence. If your condition is a result of overactive nerves that control the bladder, your doctor might refer to this condition as "reflex incontinence." The malfunctioning nerves may result from a number of medical problems, such as damage to the spinal cord and brain, Alzheimer's disease, BPH, multiple sclerosis, Parkinson's disease, stroke, hysterectomy, infections, emotional disorders, and injury. With urge incontinence, the bladder might empty when you hear water running or even while you are sleeping, a condition known as nocturnal enuresis.

Overflow incontinence. People who have bladders that are so full that they frequently leak urine may have overflow incontinence. This type of incontinence tends to be caused by weak bladder muscles or a blocked urethra. The bladder is unable to empty fully. Diabetes is often a cause of weak bladder muscles, and a urinary stone or tumor may block the urethra. This type of incontinence is fairly common in men who have an enlarged prostate gland that constricts the urethra.

Mixed incontinence. Those who have mixed incontinence have involuntary leakage associated with exertion, sneezing, or coughing. This is the most common type of urinary incontinence in women.

A far more common problem than many people realize, it has been estimated that more than 13 million Americans are incontinent. As many as 10 to 30 percent of women and 1.5 percent to 5 percent of men up to age 64 have urinary incontinence.

Causes and Risk Factors

Risk factors for urinary incontinence include a history of childhood bedwetting, morbid obesity, engaging in high-impact physical activities, smoking, chronic cough, diabetes, depression, constipation, pregnancy, and heredity.

Signs and Symptoms

If you are unable to reach the toilet in time to urinate, you may be experiencing incontinence. Other symptoms include leaking urine in your underwear, wetting the bed at night, straining while attempting to urinate, and a slow urine stream.

A Quick Guide to Symptoms

- ☐ Unable to reach the toilet in time to urinate
- ☐ Leaking urine in your underwear
- ☐ Wetting the bed at night
- ☐ Straining while attempting to urinate
- ☐ A slow urine stream

Conventional Treatments
Behavioral Techniques

Although behavioral techniques do not work for functional incontinence, they may well be successful for other types of incontinence. All of the behavioral techniques focus on strengthening or retraining the bladder. They are even useful for men recovering from prostate surgery.

Crossing the legs. If you feel that you are about to sneeze, cough, or laugh, try crossing your legs. It may prevent urine leakage.

Pelvic floor muscle (Kegel) exercises. These exercises, which help to strengthen the muscles of the pelvic floor that support the bladder and close the sphincter, were originally designed to assist women before and after childbirth. However, they have been found to be quite useful for stress and urge incontinence in both men and women.

Begin by identifying your pelvic muscles. This may be done by slowing or stopping the urine flow while you are urinating. These are

Self-Testing

Though there are no self-tests for incontinence, if you are dealing with this disorder, you probably know it. Before visiting your doctor, record the following information. It will help your doctor assess your condition.

☐ **When did your problem begin?**
☐ **When does the problem occur—for example, during laughing, coughing, or physical activities?**
☐ **How frequently do you urinate?**
☐ **What is your daily fluid intake?**
☐ **How much caffeine and alcohol are you consuming?**
☐ **Is there blood in your urine?**
☐ **Does your urine have an unusual smell?**
☐ **How often are you urinating during the night?**
☐ **After you urinate, does your bladder feel empty?**
☐ **Do you have any pain or burning sensation during urination?**
☐ **How forceful is your urine stream?**

Also, it is a good idea to keep a voiding diary. For a few days, record everything you eat and drink, and list every time you void. Since it is useful if you have a sense of how much you are voiding, measure your urine with a measuring cup. In addition, log every incident of incontinence and estimate how much urine you lost.

the muscles you need to make stronger. Try to perform 5 to 15 contractions, three to five times daily. Hold each Kegel for a count of 5 to start, and gradually work your way to a count of 10. But don't do too many: Women who overexercise these muscles may make

them too tight. Once you learn to do Kegel exercises, try to avoid them when you are urinating, because this practice has the tendency to weaken muscles.

You will need to commit to Kegel exercises for your lifetime. If you discontinue them, any benefits you have achieved will disappear. Also, it may take several months of Kegel exercises before you see any improvements.

Collagen Injections

Your doctor may inject bulking materials, such as animal or human collagen, into the juncture of the bladder and urethra. This is done either through the urethra via the penis or through the bladder via the abdomen. The bulking materials tighten the seal of the sphincter. For a few days after the procedure, you will need to withdraw your urine with a urinary catheter. Since bulking materials such as collagen are reabsorbed over time, the procedure will probably need to be repeated every 6 to 18 months. Potential complications include infection and urinary retention. People with certain cardiac conditions may be advised not to have this procedure.

Electrical Stimulation of the Pelvic Floor

In this procedure, a probe is inserted into the anus or vagina. This causes a contraction of the pelvic floor muscles. It requires frequent visits to your doctor, and you will not see any results for 2 to 3 months. For urge incontinence, success rates range from 50 to 90 percent. Unfortunately, this therapy is usually not covered by insurance, and it may have unpleasant side effects such as abdominal cramps, diarrhea, bleeding, and infection.

Extracorporeal Magnetic Innervation Therapy

Extracorporeal magnetic innervation therapy, which is used for stress incontinence, triggers the pelvic muscles to perform Kegel exercises. During a treatment, you will sit on a special chair and remain fully dressed. Highly directed magnetic fields penetrate your pelvic area and stimulate the nerves. You will need twice-weekly sessions for about 6 to 8 weeks.

Medications

If your incontinence is caused by an infection, then you will likely be prescribed an antibiotic. Be sure to take all the medicine, as indicated by your doctor. Don't discontinue it after your symptoms improve. There are a number of medications that increase sphincter or pelvic muscle strength or relax the bladder. Since they help the bladder hold urine, these medications are most useful for urge incontinence.

Alpha-blockers. Alpha-blockers, which relax smooth muscle and improve the flow of urine, are useful for men who are incontinent as a result of BPH. Examples of these are terazosin (Hytrin), doxazosin (Cardura), tamsulosin (Flomax), and alfuzosin (Xatral).

Anticholinergics. Anticholinergics inhibit the voluntary contractions of the bladder. They also increase the capacity of the bladder and slow down the initial urge to void. Included in this group are propantheline (Pro-Banthine), oxybutynin (Ditropan), and tolterodine (Detrol). They potentially have some uncomfortable side effects, such as dry eyes, dry mouth, headaches, rapid heart rate, confusion, and constipation. In rare instances, they may precipitate glaucoma.

Antidepressants. Since there is some indication that urge incontinence may be associated with changes in the levels of serotonin and noradrenaline, neurotransmitters that play a role in depression, tricyclic antidepressants may be used to treat this disorder. They may also be useful for stress incontinence. Tricyclic antidepressants strengthen the internal sphincter and relax the bladder. Examples are imipramine (Janimine, Tofranil), doxepin (Sinequan), desipramine (Norpramin), and nortriptyline (Pamelor). The potential side effects are similar to those for the anticholinergic drugs. They may also cause drowsiness, low blood pressure, and overflow incontinence.

Antispasmodics. Antispasmodic medications may relax the bladder muscle. To avoid high amounts of urine retention, before they are prescribed, your doctor will want to evaluate you for possible ureter obstruction. A commonly prescribed antispasmodic medication is dicyclomine (Bentyl). These medications may potentially have a number of undesirable side effects, such as drowsiness, dry mouth, weakness, dizziness, hallucinations, impotence, and restlessness.

Estrogen. Topical estrogen has been used to restore the urethral lining, which tends to thin as women age, and to desensitize the bladder. Thus, it is useful for both stress and urge incontinence. Improvements may be seen in as few as 6 weeks. One product, the vaginal estrogen ring, is inserted into the vagina every 3 months.

Surgery for Stress Incontinence

Of the many surgical procedures that may be employed for incontinence, the vast majority reposition the bladder neck and urethra to correct stress incontinence. Generally, surgery is not effective for urge incontinence in middle-age individuals.

Retropubic surgery. Used for mild to moderate stress incontinence, retropubic suspension (also known as bladder neck suspension or bladder suspension) sews the bladder neck and urethra to nearby structures, such as the surrounding pelvic bone. This type of surgery requires a local or general anesthetic. Though people leave the hospital after 2 or 3 days, they must use a urinary catheter for about 10 days. Possible complications include adhesions or scar tissue that obstructs the urethra, prolapsed vagina, damage to surrounding tissue, difficulty urinating, and poor wound healing.

Sling procedure. In a sling procedure, after a small incision is made in the vagina, a strip of tissue is used to support the urethra and bladder neck and close the urethra during actions such as coughing that cause stress incontinence. The sling procedure is also used for men with incontinence triggered by prostate removal surgery (prostatectomy). Potential complications include infection, bleeding, and the formation of fistulas.

One study compared the effectiveness of two kinds of sling procedures: the Burch colposuspension procedure for stress incontinence and the pubovaginal sling procedure. Six hundred fifty-five women with stress incontinence were randomly assigned to either the Burch procedure or the sling procedure. The researchers determined that 24 months after the procedures, the success rates were higher for women who underwent the sling procedure. However, women who had the sling procedure had a higher incidence of urinary tract infections, greater difficulty with urination, and more postoperative urge incontinence.

Sphincter function surgery. If the urinary sphincter is not functioning properly, your doctor may advise the implantation of an artificial internal sphincter. This sphincter consists of three parts: an inflatable cuff that fits around the urethra, a balloon that regulates the pressure of the cuff, and a pump that controls the inflation and deflation of the cuff.

During surgery, the cuff is positioned around the urethra, and the balloon is placed beneath the abdominal muscles. The pump is then put just under the skin of the abdominal wall or thigh, or in the scrotum (for men) and the labia (for women). To use the sphincter, you will need to compress the pump. That diverts fluid from the urethral cuff to the balloon. This action allows the sphincter to relax and enables you to urinate. Within a few minutes, the cuff re-inflates.

There are a few problems with this system, however. The artificial sphincter may malfunction. If that happens, you will likely need another surgery. Also, there is a risk for infection, which may further erode the urethra or bladder neck.

Urge Incontinence Treatments

Percutaneous Stoller afferent nerve stimulation (PerQ SANS) system. In this procedure, a surgeon inserts a thin needle above the anklebone to the tibial nerve, which connects to the sacral nerve complex. (Located in the tailbone, the sacral nerves play a role in regulating bladder control.) For 3 months, 30 minutes of low-frequency radiation is applied weekly. At the end of that time, treatments may be every other week.

Sacral neuromodulation. Several therapies stimulate the sacral nerves to encourage better control over the bladder. One of these is the sacral nerve stimulation system (InterStim). A battery-operated generator is implanted under the skin in the abdomen, with a wire connected to the sacral nerves in the lower back. The generator sends electrical impulses to the nerves, which controls the hyperactivity of the bladder. Possible complications include pain at the implant site, infection, and lower back pain. But there is no nerve damage and, if necessary, the system can be removed.

Vaginal Cones

Vaginal cones are sets of weights designed to improve the effectiveness of Kegel exercises. Usually, the set consists of five cones that range in weight from 20 grams (less than 1 ounce) to 65 grams (more than 2 ounces). Beginning with the lightest weight, a woman places a weight in her vagina while she is standing, and she tries to prevent it from falling out. This strengthens the muscles that control incontinence. With sufficient practice, most women are able to work their way up to the heavier weights.

Complementary Treatments

Practitioners of complementary medicine attempt to stop incontinence by eliminating the cause, adjusting dietary habits, and strengthening the pelvic muscles and urinary system.

Acupuncture

Acupuncturists direct treatments toward restoring circulation and regulating the bladder. When the underlying cause of incontinence is determined, acupuncture may be extremely effective. To locate an acupuncturist in your area, visit the Web site of the National Certification Commission for Acupuncture and Oriental Medicine (NCCAOM) at www.nccaom.org.

Biofeedback

Biofeedback may help you learn to control muscle contraction and relaxation to avoid leakage during a bout of coughing or any unexpected activity that would trigger involuntary bladder release. It is also effective in teaching people to control the urge to urinate.

When combined with biofeedback, the effectiveness of Kegel exercises may be enhanced. With biofeedback for incontinence, in the privacy of your home, you insert a vaginal or rectal probe that transmits information to the monitoring equipment. You isolate the pelvic floor and bladder muscles, and perform Kegel exercises. The monitor indicates how strongly you are contracting the pelvic floor muscles and how successfully the bladder muscles are released. It may require several months of use before you see any results.

Herbal Medicine

Uva ursi strengthens the sphincter muscles and prevents the loss of bladder control. It is also a good herb for any bladder or kidney problem. Drink 1 cup of tea every morning. The tea is readily available in health food stores.

Homeopathy

Two remedies regularly used with good results for involuntary urination are *Pulsatilla* 6C and *Causticum* 6C. *Causticum* also helps relieve irritation of the urinary tract lining. To find a practitioner trained in homeopathy, visit the Web site of the National Center for Homeopathy at www.homeopathic.org.

Lifestyle Recommendations

Be vigilant about hygiene. To prevent skin problems, when you have a urinary accident, clean the area. After you bathe, use a moisturizer along with an occlusive cream, which will help protect the sensitive skin in the genital area from irritation. Most occlusive creams contain petrolatum, zinc oxide, or lanolin. Do not apply the cream inside the urethra.

For yeast infections, you should use an antifungal cream that contains miconazole nitrate. To reduce the odor associated with incontinence, there are deodorizing tablets that you may take orally; ask your doctor about them.

Preventive Measures

Avoid becoming constipated. Constipation may be a contributing factor to incontinence. The accumulation of stool pressed against the bladder and urethra, as well as the straining movements induced by constipation, may put undue force on the bladder, triggering leakage. Eating a high-fiber diet with plenty of fresh fruits and vegetables may be beneficial.

Drink more fluids. While you may believe that reducing your fluid intake will lower your risk for incontinence, the opposite is, in fact, true. If you reduce your fluid intake, the lining of the urethra and bladder may become irritated, which may increase leakage. However, stop drinking fluids at least a few hours before you go to bed.

Drink cranberry juice. Cranberry prevents bacteria from building up on the lining of the bladder, which reduces the risk for urinary tract infection. Drink four 4-ounce glasses of pure cranberry concentrate throughout the day. However, avoid cranberry juice cocktail, which is diluted and filled with sugar.

Eliminate problem foods. The following foods are believed to increase the risk of incontinence in some people.

- Caffeinated beverages and medications that contain caffeine
- All types of coffee and tea
- Carbonated beverages
- Citrus fruits and juices
- Chocolate
- Foods that contain sugar and honey
- Artificial sweeteners
- Milk and milk products
- Spicy foods
- Alcoholic beverages
- Corn syrup

Establish voiding habits. Do not hold your urine. Go when you have the urge. Even if you do not have the urge, get in the habit of trying to void. Begin by trying every half hour. Gradually lengthen the time between attempts to every hour, then every 2 hours, and then every 3 hours. Continue this pattern until you are able to void every 3 to 6 hours, which is the normal time period.

When you urinate, empty your bladder completely. A good technique to accomplish this is called double voiding. Begin voiding and go until you feel that you are done. Wait a moment and relax. Then, lean forward and void some more. Often, there is a little left that needs to be released. This technique helps to avoid leakage.

Lose weight. If you are overweight, try to lose the excess pounds. Your added weight may aggravate and weaken bladder muscles.

Quit smoking. If you smoke, quit. The persistent cough that many smokers have may cause urinary leakage. In addition, it has been shown that nicotine causes irritation to the bladder.

Indigestion

Indigestion is that uncomfortable or burning feeling in your upper abdomen. Also known as dyspepsia, this condition often appears with other medical problems such as belching, abdominal bloating, nausea, and, on occasion, vomiting. Bending over or lying down tends to make the pain worse.

Indigestion is quite common. Though some believe that the figure is higher, it has been suggested that about one in four people experience indigestion each year.

Causes and Risk Factors

Indigestion is frequently the result of certain behaviors, such as eating too much, eating too quickly, and eating high-fat foods. Other causes of indigestion include eating while dealing with a stressful situation, living a stressful life, excess consumption of alcohol, fatigue, and taking medications that tend to upset the stomach (such as anti-inflammatory drugs).

Indigestion may also be caused by a medical problem, such as a gastric or duodenal ulcer or gastroesophageal reflux disease (GERD). A gastric ulcer is an open sore on the inside lining of the stomach, and a duodenal ulcer is a similar sore on the lining of the beginning portion of the small intestine. There is a good chance that the ulcer was caused by the bacterium *Helicobacter pylori*. In GERD, the acid from the stomach backs up into the esophagus, the tube that connects the mouth to the stomach. When people with celiac disease, an autoimmune disorder, ingest foods that contain gluten (wheat, oats, barley, or rye), they may have significant indigestion. On rare occasions, indigestion is triggered by stomach cancer.

Sometimes, there is no apparent cause for indigestion. In such cases, the condition is known as functional or nonulcer indigestion. People with this form of indigestion may have a problem with the motility or muscular squeezing action of the stomach, which leads to a delayed emptying of the stomach.

Indigestion tends to occur more often as you age. If you are overweight or if you smoke, you are also at increased risk.

A Quick Guide to Symptoms

☐ **Gnawing and burning sensation in the upper middle part of abdomen**
☐ **Burping**
☐ **Nausea**
☐ **Stomach feels bloated and excessively full**

Signs and Symptoms

With indigestion, there is a gnawing and burning sensation in the upper middle part of your abdomen. You may burp and feel nauseated. Your stomach may feel bloated or excessively full.

Conventional Treatments

Lifestyle Changes

Treatment for indigestion normally begins with several lifestyle changes. These include eating smaller meals, sitting or standing after you eat, limiting fatty foods, avoiding foods and drinks that tend to be more problematic (such as citrus fruits and chocolate), losing weight, and avoiding or limiting alcohol. You may also be advised to stop smoking and make time for relaxation.

Since some medications may contribute to indigestion, your doctor will probably want to review all your medications. Some medications that are known for causing indigestion include nonsteroidal anti-inflammatory drugs (NSAIDs), such as aspirin, ibuprofen, and naproxen.

Medications

If you have not achieved sufficient relief from lifestyle changes and changes in medication, your doctor may suggest a medication.

Acid blockers. Acid blockers (also called H-2 blockers) reduce the secretion of stomach acid. Some acid blockers are available over-the-counter, while others are sold only by prescription. Well-known examples of these drugs are cimetidine (Tagamet HB) and

> **Since indigestion may be a sign** of a more serious illness, if you have symptoms such as weight loss, appetite loss, black tarry stools, blood in vomit, recurrent vomiting, and severe pain in the upper abdomen, see your doctor.

famotidine (Pepcid AC). On occasion, these medications may have side effects such as dry mouth, dizziness, drowsiness, and bowel changes. Be sure to ask your doctor if they might interfere with other medications you are taking.

Antacids. Over-the-counter antacids, which neutralize gastric acid, may relieve

Indigestion and Heart Attacks

It is well known that as people age, they may confuse a bout of indigestion with a heart attack. Many people have rushed to hospital emergency departments believing that they are having a heart attack, only to be diagnosed with indigestion. But it is also true that some people who are having a heart attack misinterpret their symptoms as indigestion and delay going to the hospital. If you experience intense pain in the center of the chest, and if it spreads to one or both arms and the lower jaw, you may be having a heart attack. You need to seek emergency medical care.

your symptoms. Common examples are Tums and Rolaids. However, when antacids are consumed frequently, they may trigger constipation or diarrhea. Also, some antacids may interfere with the effectiveness of other medications, particularly those prescribed for kidney and heart disease. Antacids that contain magnesium may cause a buildup of magnesium in the body, which may contribute to kidney disease, especially in people who have diabetes. And consuming too much calcium, which can also be found in antacids, may place you at risk for kidney stones. Antacids are also known to interfere with the absorption of some medications such as ciprofloxacin (Cipro), tetracycline, and propranolol (Inderal). To prevent these interactions, take these medications either 1 hour before or 3 hours after the antacid.

Antibiotics. If you have a history of peptic ulcer disease, active gastric ulcer, or an active duodenal ulcer with evidence of *H. pylori*, your doctor will probably want to eradicate the infection. Curing *H. pylori* is usually associated with a higher rate of ulcer healing and a reduction in complications and recurrences. There are at least four different treatment regimens for *H. pylori* infection that range in duration from 10 to 14 days. Typically, a proton-pump inhibitor (**see below**) or acid blocker is used in combination with two antibiotics and the possible addition of an antacid. Some of the recommended antibiotics include amoxicillin, metronidazole, clarithromycin, and tetracycline.

Prokinetics. If your doctor believes that your indigestion is caused by the motility or muscular squeezing action of your stomach, he or she may prescribe a medication to control this action. These are known as prokinetic drugs. They may help GERD by counteracting some of the physical abnormalities that may be present. Drugs such as metoclopramide (Reglan) may increase the pressure of the lower esophageal sphincter, improve emptying of the stomach, and encourage the normal digestive muscular contractions.

Proton-pump inhibitors. Proton-pump inhibitors are a newer class of drugs that block the final stage of acid production. Omeprazole (Prilosec) and lansoprazole (Prevacid) are examples. Potential side effects include headache, diarrhea, and abdominal pain.

Itopride. In one study done in Germany, researchers gave people with a type of indigestion known as functional dyspepsia three different strengths of itopride as well as a placebo. They randomly assigned individuals with dyspepsia to one of three drug treatments or placebo for a period of 8 weeks. Although the symptoms of dyspepsia improved in all groups, including the placebo treatment group, itopride produced superior symptom relief in those taking the medication. Itopride is currently unavailable in the United States.

Surgery

Unless your indigestion is caused by certain specific types of GERD or stomach cancer, your doctor is unlikely to consider surgery as a treatment option for this medical problem.

Complementary Treatments

Complementary medicine aims to find the underlying cause of indigestion and ultimately make appropriate nutritional and lifestyle changes in order to reduce it.

Aromatherapy

The essential oils of coriander, ginger, peppermint, and thyme aid the digestive process, helping to relieve indigestion. These oils help ease discomfort and aid digestion when added to a carrier oil, such as canola oil, and rubbed over the abdomen. Canola oil is a good choice because it is relatively inexpensive and easy to find. Other recommended oils are grape seed, sunflower, and sesame. Though jojoba oil also makes an excellent carrier oil, it may be more expensive, and you may already have one of the other oils in your home for cooking.

Start with a single oil before creating a combination in order to check for any adverse skin reactions. Add 10 drops of the essential oil to 1 ounce of carrier oil. If you do create a combination oil, stay within the recommendation of 10 total drops of essential oil per ounce of carrier oil.

Avoid thyme oil if you have high blood pressure or hyperthyroidism. Peppermint oil may counteract homeopathic remedies. If you are using peppermint oil, wait a few hours before taking any homeopathic remedy.

Diet

Individual constitutions are so specific and symptoms of indigestion so subjective that it is hard to pinpoint and recommend general dietary advice. Some people have trouble digesting wheat or lactose (found in dairy products). To determine if you have a food intolerance, you might wish to list everything you eat in a food journal. Keeping track of what you eat, when you eat, how you feel when you eat (such as stressed, relaxed, or rushed), and how you feel after you eat may help find trigger foods that are causing indigestion. You can then begin the process of eliminating specific foods that you feel are causing your problem. Do you feel better when you don't eat them? You may be able to reintroduce these foods after certain changes are made, such as eating in a relaxed environment, eating slowly, or chewing your food completely. You may also find relief from indigestion when digestive enzyme supplements are added to your daily supplement regimen.

Herbal Medicine

Herbs may be helpful either in relieving specific symptoms of indigestion or as a general tonic. You can use herbs for indigestion either individually or in combination. Herbs known as carminatives help to expel gas and prevent it from forming in the intestines. Antispasmodic herbs aid in preventing involuntary muscle cramps. And herbs known as stomachics stimulate digestion and tone the stomach.

Chamomile and peppermint. Chamomile is an antispasmodic and stomachic. It also fosters relaxation and reduces stress, which is a trigger for indigestion. Peppermint is a stomachic and carminative and is extremely useful for indigestion that is caused by overeating. It reduces acidity in the stomach and accelerates the stomach's emptying process by more than 40 percent. These two herbs are popular teas and may be taken to relieve indigestion. Both chamomile and peppermint are available as a dried herb or in prepared tea bags. When using the dried herb, pour 1 cup of hot water over 1 tablespoon of the herb, and steep for 10 minutes. When using the tea bags, follow the directions on the package. Peppermint tea may be taken throughout the day, but save chamomile for the evening, because it is especially good for relaxing before bedtime.

Fennel. Fennel seeds have a calming effect on the digestive system, and chewing them after a meal may eliminate indigestion. For quick relief, carry some fennel seeds in a tin to chew at any time on the road or at work.

Goldenseal. By increasing the flow of gastric juices, goldenseal promotes good digestion. To create a powerful treatment to relieve bloating or gas, add a few drops of goldenseal tincture to a cup of chamomile or peppermint tea. Goldenseal's antiseptic properties have been shown to be very effective against intestinal bacteria. However, if you suffer from high blood pressure, goldenseal should be used sparingly.

Slippery elm. The inner bark of the slippery elm tree (*Ulmus rubra*) contains mucilage that helps protect the throat and digestive tract. It also soothes irritated mucous membranes and neutralizes the excess stomach acid that may lead to indigestion. Prepare a tea from 1 tablespoon of the dried herb or 1 tablespoon of liquid extract poured over a cup of hot water. Drink 1 to 3 cups daily.

Homeopathy

Homeopathy may provide excellent results for treating the various symptoms associated with indigestion. The remedies are specific to the type and severity of symptoms. Natural health food stores carry remedies for milder conditions, while a homeopathic practitioner may prescribe stronger remedies.

Hydrotherapy

A moist heating pad or hot water bottle placed over the abdomen after meals may relieve symptoms of indigestion.

Nutritional Supplements

Digestive enzymes, available in a wide variety of over-the-counter preparations, may be helpful in battling indigestion. Lactase, for example, is a digestive enzyme necessary to break down the milk-sugar lactose found in dairy products. Some people who produce inadequate amounts of this enzyme take a lactase enzyme such as Lactaid prior to eating dairy products. There are other specific enzymes that are made in the body to digest protein, fats, and carbohydrates. Bromelain and papain, two enzymes that digest protein, are found in pineapple and papaya. Some products have a combination of enzymes to break down fats, protein, and carbohydrates. Take these products as directed on the label.

Relaxation/Meditation

To relieve stress, which directly affects the digestive process, practice relaxation, meditation, or deep breathing techniques. To work efficiently, the digestive system needs a large supply of blood. When the body is in a state of stress, it redirects the blood and uses it in other areas, such as the muscles, heart, and lungs, for the "fight-or-flight" response. This disturbs the digestive process, causing problems such as indigestion. A regular routine of meditation, deep breathing, tai chi, or yoga may reduce stress. Biofeedback may help you target why and how stress is affecting you and ways to reduce it.

Preventive Measures

Keep a food diary. Take note of those foods that trigger indigestion, then try eliminating them from your diet to see if your symptoms subside.

Avoid medications that irritate the stomach. Some common medications, such as aspirin, ibuprofen, and naproxen, are known to upset the stomach. If you need to take these types of medications, ask your doctor to suggest alternatives that are not as harsh on the stomach. If there are no alternatives, be sure to take these medications with food.

Avoid swallowing air. To avoid excessive bloating or belching, do not chew with your mouth open, talk while eating, or chew gum.

These all cause you to swallow air, which will increase your symptoms.

Don't eat before bedtime. Since lying down increases the chances of acid reflux, try to avoid snacking before bedtime. It may be useful to raise the head of your bed by 3 inches—this small change in elevation may prevent acid reflux.

Don't eat too much at one meal. Smaller meals are less likely to cause indigestion.

Don't exercise or lie down after eating. If you exercise after eating, you will divert blood away from your stomach, thereby hindering digestion. Schedule your exercise either before eating or at least 30 minutes after eating. It is fine to relax after eating, but don't lie down for 2 to 3 hours.

Don't rush your meals. Eating quickly increases your risk for indigestion. Take time to eat and chew your food properly.

Don't smoke. People who smoke increase their risk for indigestion since smoking can irritate the stomach lining.

Don't wear tight clothing. Clothing that is too tight may aggravate stomach discomfort after a meal and increase the symptoms of indigestion.

If you are overweight, lose the extra pounds. Your indigestion may improve if you lose excess weight.

Watch what you eat. Reduce your intake of acidic foods, spicy foods, fatty foods, carbonated beverages, and caffeine. These have all been correlated with indigestion. Caffeine, in particular, increases gastric secretions and irritates intestinal muscles.

Influenza

Also known as the flu, influenza is a contagious illness caused by the influenza virus. Most often passed from person to person in respiratory droplets of coughs and sneezes, the flu may also be spread when a person touches respiratory droplets on another person or object and then touches his or her mouth or nose. While some people infected with the flu virus do not experience symptoms, most symptoms tend to begin 1 to 4 days after infection. So, you may begin spreading the flu a day before you actually feel symptoms and continue spreading the flu for another 3 to 5 days. Most people recover within a week or two, although older people may take longer.

Every year, millions of people in the United States become sick with influenza. It has been estimated that between 5 and 20 percent of the population become ill with this disease. About 200,000 people who catch influenza require hospitalization, and 36,000 die from it.

There are two types of influenza virus, A and B. Type A causes the most severe influenza epidemics. Type B also causes epidemics, but they are milder than type A. Cases of influenza generally appear in the late fall, winter, and early spring.

Causes and Risk Factors

Influenza comes on suddenly and attacks the respiratory tract—nose, throat, and lungs. Though anyone may become ill with the flu, very young people, people with chronic medical problems, and those over the age of 65 are most at risk for complications, such as pneumonia, bronchitis, postinfectious cough, and sinus and ear infections. Complications often occur after you are feeling better.

Signs and Symptoms

The symptoms of influenza include fever at 101°F or above, headache, tiredness, dry cough, sore throat, nasal congestion, chills, and body aches. Symptoms of flu-related complications are high fever, shaking chills, chest pains with each breath, and coughing that produces thick, yellow-greenish-colored mucus.

A Quick Guide to Symptoms

- ☐ **Fever at 101°F or above**
- ☐ **Headache**
- ☐ **Tiredness**
- ☐ **Dry cough**
- ☐ **Sore throat**
- ☐ **Nasal congestion**
- ☐ **Chills**
- ☐ **Body aches**

Conventional Treatments

For fever and muscle aches, your doctor will probably recommend aspirin, acetaminophen, or ibuprofen. Be sure to rest and drink plenty of liquids. To treat your congestion, cough, and nasal discharge, try an over-the-counter decongestant and antihistamine.

Antibiotics

If you have an influenza-related complication such as pneumonia or a sinus or ear infection, your doctor may prescribe antibiotics. Antibiotics are used to treat infections caused by bacteria. Since the flu is a viral infection, antibiotics are not routinely used to treat it.

Antiviral Medications

Your doctor may suggest taking antiviral drugs, taken within the first 2 days of becoming ill. The adamantanes include amantadine (Symmetrel) and rimantadine (Flumadine). The newer medications are the neuraminidase inhibitors zanamivir (Relenza) and oseltamivir (Tamiflu). Amantadine and rimantadine are older medications that treat only type A influenza and are associated with several toxic side effects. Oseltamivir and zanamivir are useful for both types A and B influenza. These medications may reduce the symptoms, shorten the duration of the illness, and make you less contagious to others. Only oseltamivir has been found to reduce some of the complications that require antibiotics. Neuraminidase inhibitors are also useful for helping to prevent infection with the flu virus. Trials of long-term prophylactic use of zanamivir and oseltamivir in healthy adults, adolescents, and the elderly have shown reductions in the incidence of influenza. So, you may ask your doctor for a prescription if the flu is prevalent in your community or workplace or if a family member has the flu. Potential side effects include stomach upset, insomnia, and nervousness.

Precautions with Antiviral Medications

If you have a chronic lung disease such as asthma, you need to share that information with your doctor. And you need to use zanamivir (Relenza) with care. It may cause bronchospasm. After using zanamivir, you may have trouble breathing. Be sure to have a fast-acting reliever bronchodilator on hand.

Complementary Treatments

Complementary medicine is extremely beneficial in helping to relieve the symptoms associated with the flu. By supporting and strengthening the immune system, the body is better able to fight the flu virus.

Aromatherapy

The essential oils of eucalyptus and menthol have been shown to be effective in reducing nasal congestion associated with the flu. To clear your nasal passages, try placing a few drops on a handkerchief and breathing in before bed. You may want to place a few drops on a lamp in your bedroom and let the heat of the lightbulb disperse the essential oils into the air.

Diet

Eat light, easily digestible foods such as vegetable soups, broth, salads, and rice. Consume liberal amounts of garlic and onion, which have antiviral and immune-boosting properties.

Drink plenty of liquids. Make sure you get a good eight to ten 8-ounce glasses of fluids daily. Laboratory studies have shown that the tannins contained in grape juice may kill viruses. In addition, grape juice is rich in vitamin C, which may help boost the immune system. Other good choices include any juice high in vitamin C, such as orange juice, cranberry juice, and grapefruit juice, as long as the acidity does not bother the gastrointestinal tract. However, you should avoid juices containing high amounts of added sugar. Stay away from caffeine and alcohol as these can contribute to dehydration. Alcohol also robs the body of vitamin C.

Herbal Medicine

Astragalus. Astragalus root has been shown to increase the production of white blood cells, which help fight invading viruses. Because it helps strengthen the body against disease, astragalus should be taken at the first onset of symptoms. Take one 500-milligram capsule, four times a day, until symptoms abate, and then reduce dosage to one capsule, twice a day, for 1 week. Products should contain standardized extract of the root with 0.5 percent glucosides and 70 percent polysaccharides.

Echinacea. Echinacea also stimulates the immune system and increases white blood cell production and should be taken at the onset of symptoms. A study using 900 milligrams of *Echinacea purpurea* daily showed that, in 3 days, there was a significant decrease in body aches, headache, cough, and lethargy. For best results, echinacea should be used for 1 to 2 weeks at a time. When echinacea is used for an extended period of time, the body tends to build up a tolerance, making it less effective. The recommended daily dose to decrease flu symptoms is 500 milligrams of standardized extract per day containing at least 3.5 percent echinacosides, the active ingredient. If taken in liquid extract form, 1 teaspoon, three times a day, is the recommended dose. Echinacea tincture is often combined with goldenseal, a very effective herb for preventing the flu as well as a treatment at the onset of flu symptoms. Goldenseal contains berberine, which helps to activate white blood cells to destroy the flu virus.

Elderberry. Elderberry flowers contain properties that help stop the flu virus from infesting cells of the respiratory tract. The most effective treatment using elderberry is a patented drug called Sambucol. Clinical trials have shown that 90 percent of people with flu who took Sambucol recovered after 3 days. In 24 hours, 20 percent showed considerable relief from muscular aches and fever, and after 48 hours, 73 percent reported feeling better. The recommended dose is 4 tablespoons, three times a day, for 3 days.

Garlic. Garlic stimulates the immune system and is also effective in preventing respiratory complications such as bronchitis. Garlic cloves may be eaten raw, cooked in food, or taken as a capsule or tincture. Garlic is available in enteric-coated tablets or capsules to prevent stomach upset. The recommended daily dose is 500 milligrams, twice a day. Or take 2 to 4 milliliters of garlic tincture three times daily. If you have a choice, select fresh garlic over supplements. The supplements contain concentrated extracts, which may increase the risk of excessive bleeding.

Other herbs. Combine the herbs coltsfoot, mullein, peppermint, and wild cherry bark in equal amounts and brew a tea to assist in releasing mucus and eliminating phlegm. Fill a saucepan with water and add equal amounts of the herbs. For each cup of water, use a tablespoon of each herb. Bring the mixture to a boil, turn off the stove, and let the mixture steep for at least 1 hour. Drink the tea throughout the day. Due to their antiviral properties, other teas helpful in relieving the flu are forsythia, honeysuckle, and lemon balm.

Homeopathy

Oscillococcinum (Oscillo) is a homeopathic remedy, manufactured by Boiron, that speeds up the recovery process from the flu virus. The active ingredient in Oscillo is Anas barbariae hepatis et cordis extractum 200CK. Inactive ingredients are sucrose and lactose. Following the directions on the package, take Oscillo at the first sign of flu symptoms. Homeopathic remedies often make symptoms more severe for the first day or two, but recovery from the virus is much quicker.

Nutritional Supplements

Since zinc boosts the immune system, it has widely been used at the first sign of flu symptoms. When taken immediately, zinc can help the body recover from influenza quicker. The recommended dose for influenza is a zinc gluconate lozenge every 2 hours as needed.

High doses of vitamin C taken at the onset of symptoms or right after exposure to someone with the flu can help shorten the duration of your illness. Take 1,000 milligrams (divided doses of 500 mg each) of vitamin C daily.

Lifestyle Recommendations

Eat chocolate. Theobromine, a chemical found in chocolate, has been found to be more effective at calming persistent coughs than codeine.

Get vaccinated. The best way to prevent becoming ill with influenza is to obtain a flu shot between early October and mid-November each year. Ideally, you want to be vaccinated 6 to 8 weeks before the flu season begins. Since the actual virus changes from year to year, you need a new shot every year. Some people (fewer than one-third) who get a flu shot will have some soreness around the site of the injection. In rare instances, there may be aches, pains, and fever.

In 2003, the FDA approved FluMist, an influenza vaccine that is administered nasally. It is approved only for healthy people between the ages of 5 and 49. Do not take FluMist if you meet any of the following specifications.

- You have a metabolic disorder such as diabetes or kidney dysfunction.

- You have a lung condition, such as asthma, or a heart condition.

- You have an immunodeficiency disease or are on immunosuppressive treatment.

- You have had Guillain-Barré syndrome.
- You are pregnant.
- You have a history of being allergic or very sensitive to eggs or any part of FluMist.

Because the viral material in flu vaccines is grown in eggs, if you are allergic to eggs, you should not have a shot. You should also avoid a shot if you have a history of Guillain-Barré syndrome.

Minimize exposure. During flu season, avoid crowds and crowded spaces, because the flu virus spreads easily. In fact, individuals can spread the virus even before they are symptomatic. To help prevent the spread of the virus, always sneeze into a tissue. If you live with someone suffering from the flu, do not share items that can easily spread the virus, such as towels, clothing, blankets, cups, dishes, and utensils.

Pay attention to your diet. During the flu season, it is especially important to pay attention to what you eat. Avoid fried foods and refined sugars, as these foods may place an added burden on your immune system.

Reduce stress. Avoid overexertion and don't get run down. Both physical and emotional stress may impair your immune system, making you more susceptible to the flu.

Relieve coughing. A tablespoon of warm honey with a sprinkling of cinnamon is effective in clearing the sinuses and relieving chronic coughs. Take 1 tablespoon a day to relieve flu symptoms. Gingerroot has been used for centuries as a natural cough suppressant. To help control a cough, chew a small, dime-size piece of raw gingerroot. It lubricates the throat by stimulating the salivary glands.

Preventive Measures

Quit smoking. According to the Centers for Disease Control and Prevention, research shows an increase in influenza in smokers as compared to nonsmokers. There is a higher mortality rate for smokers from the flu as compared to nonsmokers. Smoking suppresses the immune function, causing more upper and lower respiratory tract infections.

Take supplements. In addition to a daily multivitamin/mineral supplement, it is important to begin boosting your immune system in the fall months to ward off any impending influenza outbreak. Take additional vitamin C (1,000 milligrams daily), as well as echinacea, goldenseal, and astragalus as recommended in the herbal medicine section. Take them for 1 to 2 weeks, and then discontinue for 1 to 2 weeks. Repeat this on-again, off-again schedule until the flu season is over. This program will help stimulate your immune system, but it will avoid building up a tolerance to these supplements.

Wash your hands. Wash your hands thoroughly with soap and water for a minimum of 20 seconds several times throughout the day. To help reduce your chance of infection, avoid touching your eyes, nose, and mouth, as these are open passageways for germs to enter the body.

Insomnia

If you have insomnia, you are obtaining inadequate or poor-quality sleep. And it may occur in a few different ways. You may have difficulty falling asleep, or you may have a problem staying asleep, or you may awaken too early in the morning and be unable to go back to sleep. As a result of your disrupted sleep, you are tired during the day.

Almost everyone has occasional problems with sleep. Some types of insomnia, such as insomnia from jet lag or the noise of a thunderstorm, are relatively brief. Insomnia that lasts from a few days to a few weeks is termed transient. When the bouts with insomnia happen from time to time, they are called intermittent. Insomnia that continues for a month or longer is considered chronic. People with chronic insomnia spend a good deal of time worrying about whether or not they will be able to get the sleep they need, and that only adds to the insomnia problem.

Insomnia is very common. Every year, about one in three adults is affected, and approximately 10 to 20 percent of these cases are severe. Insomnia also takes a physical toll on the body. It is believed to increase the risk of heart failure, stroke, high blood pressure, coronary artery disease, obesity, and diabetes.

Causes and Risk Factors

Older adults are at greater risk for insomnia. They are more sensitive to noise, and they awaken more easily. As people age, they are more likely to have trouble falling into the deeper stages of sleep, and there is a good chance they will have a medical problem or be on a medication that may disturb sleep. It is often said that the need for sleep decreases with age. That is not true. Rather, as we grow older, we tend to lose the ability to sleep as well as we did when we were younger.

Insomnia may also be caused by a number of other factors. Women, especially women past menopause, are more at risk than males. It is well known that hot flashes disrupt sleep. Transient and intermittent insomnia tend to be the result of stress, extreme temperatures, environmental noise, time changes, and the side effects of medication, particularly drugs containing caffeine.

Chronic insomnia is more multifaceted and may have a number of contributing factors. A frequent cause of chronic insomnia is depression. Other causes are heart failure, asthma, anxiety, hyperthyroidism, kidney disease, arthritis, restless legs syndrome, sleep apnea, Parkinson's disease, and narcolepsy.

Some people clearly have a genetic tendency. About 35 percent of people dealing with chronic insomnia have a positive family history. Most often, the mother is the affected family member.

Still, behavioral factors play a role in chronic insomnia, including chronic stress and misuse of caffeine or alcohol. Cigarette smoking before bedtime or napping in the afternoon or evening may also be sources of chronic insomnia. Additionally, humans are designed to work during the day and sleep at night. People who do nighttime shift work or work in a position that requires frequent shift changes may be plagued by insomnia.

Signs and Symptoms

Insomnia is characterized by three main symptoms. You may have an inability to fall asleep, you may awaken frequently during the night and have trouble returning to sleep, or you may awaken too early in the morning and find yourself unable to fall back to sleep. The next day you are tired. In fact, you are so tired that you may be irritable and have difficulty concentrating on your work.

Conventional Treatments

Transient insomnia and intermittent insomnia are normally not treated. However, if they impact daily activity, your doctor may prescribe short-acting sleeping pills.

There are several methods for treating chronic insomnia. Your doctor will probably begin by looking for any medical or psychological causes. Sometimes, when these are addressed, the insomnia stops. For example, if your insomnia is caused by depression, then treating the depression may end the insomnia. Or if your insomnia is a result of menopause-related symptoms, as it is in many women in their late forties and fifties, hormone replacement therapy may be advised. Similarly, if your insomnia is a result of anxiety, treating the anxiety may improve your sleep. Also, your doctor will attempt to determine if any of your behaviors, such as smoking at bedtime or drinking alcohol, may be contributing to the situation.

Behavioral Techniques

Stimulus control. Treating chronic insomnia may require a reinterpretation of how you view your bed. Don't use your bed for anything other than sleeping or sex. Go to bed only when you are very tired, and try to think comforting thoughts. If you find that you are unable to sleep in 15 to 20 minutes, get out of bed and do not return until you are very sleepy. It is best to establish set times for going to bed and awakening. Also, do not nap during the day. Avoid nighttime activities that could produce anxiety, such as bringing work home or watching television programs that you might find disturbing. Another suggestion is listening to audiotapes of soothing

A Quick Guide to Symptoms

☐ **An inability to fall asleep**
☐ **Awaken frequently during the night and have trouble returning to sleep**
☐ **Awaken too early in the morning and find yourself unable to fall back to sleep**

sounds or music that facilitate deep breathing, which promotes relaxation.

Progressive muscle relaxation. Spend about 10 minutes a day practicing the following form of relaxation.

- Concentrate on a specific muscle group in your body, such as the muscles in your left foot.

- As you inhale, tense the muscle group for about 8 seconds.

- Quickly release the muscle group and let it stay limp for about 15 seconds.

- Repeat the sequence.

- Then, go on to other muscle groups in your body. Typically, you should go from the bottom portion of your body to the top.

Sleep restriction therapy. While dealing with insomnia, some people spend many hours in bed trying to sleep. They may be helped by a program that limits how much time they are allowed to be in bed. As their sleeping pattern improves, they will be permitted additional time.

Sleep restriction therapy begins by keeping a sleep diary for 2 weeks. Divide the amount of time that you sleep by the time in bed—the answer is your sleep efficiency number. So, if you spend 8 hours in bed, but you sleep only 5 hours, then your sleep efficiency number is 62.5 percent. Your goal should be to take actions that will increase your number to 85 to 90 percent.

Begin by going to bed 15 minutes later than usual. Until an 85 percent sleep effi-

Self-Testing

You may wish to keep a sleep diary. Every morning, record how you slept during the previous night. How long were you in bed? How much time did you actually sleep? How often did you awaken? What time did you get up in the morning? In addition, comment on the quality of your sleep. Keeping such a diary provides a better sense of how you are sleeping. You should share this information with your doctor.

ciency is reached, decrease the amount of time in bed by 15 minutes every week. However, do not reduce the time in bed to fewer than 5 hours. When a 90 percent efficiency is reached, start increasing the time in bed by 15 minutes every week.

Medications

In order to break your pattern of chronic insomnia, your doctor may prescribe a short course of low-dose benzodiazepine sleeping pills. While you are taking these pills, your doctor may wish to monitor you carefully, and possibly lower the dose slowly. When certain sleeping medications are suddenly stopped, they may trigger a few nights of insomnia and produce side effects such as nausea, nightmares, dizziness, and headaches. These medications should never be mixed with alcohol.

While the older forms of sleeping pills, such as barbiturates, were known to be quite dangerous and had the potential to cause death when taken in high doses, the more recent medications are significantly safer. They have fewer side effects and are less likely to be addictive. Zaleplon (Sonata) is useful for individuals who have difficulty falling asleep. An intermediate-acting medication, eszopiclone (Lunesta), helps those who have trouble staying asleep. Studies have generally supported the efficacy of these medications, including improvement in the time needed to fall asleep, decrease in awakenings, and improvement in sleep quality and total sleep time. But there may be side effects, such as dizziness, drowsiness, and problems with coordination. Anyone on sleep medications should be carefully monitored by a doctor. Sleeping pills should always be viewed as short-term solutions. They should never be used for a prolonged period of time.

Sleep Apnea and Narcolepsy

In sleep apnea, breathing periodically stops throughout the night. Episodes may last for as long as a minute and occur hundreds of times during the night. By morning, people with sleep apnea are tired and confused. Usually, sleep apnea is caused by partial blockage of the upper airway. Obesity aggravates the condition, and men are far more at risk for sleep apnea than women. People with this condition may be advised to lose weight. They may also be told to wear an apparatus known as a CPAP (continuous positive airway pressure) every night, which provides an air splint to the upper airway, thereby keeping the airway open. Though it is not comfortable, for many with sleep apnea it is a solution. Sleep apnea is a risk factor for cardiovascular disease.

Narcolepsy is a central nervous system disorder in which a person has difficulty sleeping at night, but is excessively sleepy during the day. Some daytime sleeping episodes occur very quickly and cannot be prevented, so a person with narcolepsy may dose off in the middle of a sentence. Daytime sleep is often accompanied by dreams. People with narcolepsy may also be plagued by a condition known as cataplexy in which they collapse on the ground, conscious but temporarily paralyzed. Narcolepsy, which commonly first appears in early adulthood, is treated with a number of medications.

Complementary Treatments

Complementary therapies assist in finding the underlying cause of insomnia and provide lifestyle changes and behavioral approaches that can promote better sleeping habits.

Acupuncture

Studies show that acupuncture and acupressure are very successful for the treatment of insomnia. They both increase production of serotonin, a relaxing hormone; promote relaxation; enhance sleep quality; and decrease awakening during the night. To locate an acupuncturist in your area, visit the Web site of the National Certification Commission for Acupuncture and Oriental Medicine (NCCAOM) at www.nccaom.org.

To find a practitioner trained in acupressure, visit the following Web site: www.aobta. org (American Organization for Bodywork

Therapies of Asia) and www.ncbtmb.org (National Certification Board for Therapeutic Massage and Bodywork).

Aromatherapy

Several essential oils are helpful in stimulating the brain's neurotransmitters for relaxation, including chamomile, lavender, marjoram, and rose. They may be used individually or in combination. Add these oils to a warm bath, using 3 to 10 drops of each, or diffuse the oils into the air. They may also be diluted in a carrier oil, such as almond oil, and applied to the neck, shoulders, and wrists before bedtime. To do this, place 10 drops in 1 ounce of oil. (If you do not want to purchase a special carrier oil such as almond or jojoba, common household oils such as canola or olive are fine.) Combine the oils, place them in a small bottle, and gently roll the bottle between your hands to warm and mix the oils before applying.

Ayurveda

Ayurvedic medicine treats insomnia by restoring balance to the *vata* dosha (according to Ayurvedic constitutional type). Maintaining a regular nightly routine is also important. A successful treatment routine includes massaging the scalp and soles of the feet with sesame oil. It is also useful to rub the areas around the forehead and eyes with a paste made of nutmeg and *ghee* (a cooked, clarified butter with all the moisture removed). Other ways to relax the *vata* dosha include a warm bath followed by a warm glass of milk containing the Ayurvedic herb Amrit Kalash, relaxing music, and comforting reading.

Diet

Eating a well-balanced diet that limits the amount of sugar, caffeine, and processed foods helps to reduce insomnia. Calcium, magnesium, and vitamins B_6 and B_{12} are all useful nutrients for their ability to calm the nervous system. Foods high in calcium and magnesium are milk and milk products (select low-fat or skim); tofu; shrimp; almonds; green leafy vegetables, such as spinach, kale, or broccoli; black beans; and potatoes. Meat, fish, and eggs are foods that naturally contain B_{12}. Vitamin B_{12} is also often added to breakfast cereal. Poultry and fish are the best natural sources for B_6.

About an hour before bedtime, consume some foods containing the amino acid tryptophan. In the brain, tryptophan converts into serotonin, which helps foster sleep. Since milk contains tryptophan, consider drinking a small glass. Other tryptophan-containing foods are cheese, bananas, and turkey.

Herbal Medicine

A number of herbs may help relieve anxiety, calm an overactive mind, and induce sleep and improve the quality of sleep.

Chamomile, hops, and vervain. These are relaxing teas to drink before bedtime. They are readily available in prepared tea bags. People who suffer from depression should not take hops. When taken for a prolonged period of time, hops may disrupt the menstrual cycle.

Passionflower and valerian root. Passionflower and valerian root calm the central nervous system, relieving anxiety and insomnia. They are available in prepared tea bags, tincture, and as dried herbs. For passionflower, look for products containing no less than 0.8 percent total flavonoids. As a tincture, take 1 to 4 milliliters in the evening to increase sleepiness. When using the dried herb, pour 1 cup of boiling water over 1 teaspoon of the dried herb, and steep for 10 to 15 minutes; drink before bedtime. When taking valerian root, look for products containing 0.8 percent valeric/valerenic acid. Since valerian may have a bitter taste and strong odor, you may prefer to take it in capsule form. Take 400 to 450 milligrams an hour before bedtime. Passionflower and valerian are often rotated, using one for 2 weeks and then switching to the other. If you are taking other sleep-inducing products, before beginning a regimen of either passionflower or valerian, check with your doctor.

If there is any chance that you are pregnant, do not take passionflower.

Homeopathy

Various over-the-counter remedies for insomnia are readily available at natural and organic health food and grocery stores. *Coffea* is an effective homeopathic remedy for an overactive mind that will not shut down at night. *Nux vomica* is used for anxiety and is best taken at night. Take *Muriaticum acidum* for irritability and restlessness.

Melatonin

The supplement melatonin, a natural hormone produced at night by the pineal gland in the brain, is commonly used for insomnia. There have been different reports on its effectiveness, however. There is some indication that, under certain circumstances, people fall asleep faster on melatonin, but it does not appear to affect total sleep or feelings of fatigue during the day. Melatonin has some reported adverse side effects, such as nightmares, drowsiness, severe headaches, depression, low sperm count, and blood vessel constriction. If you decide to use melatonin, the typical recommended dose is 1 to 3 milligrams, 1 to 2 hours before bedtime. Start with a lower dose and increase as needed. Melatonin takes up to 2 weeks to affect a sleep pattern.

Nutritional Supplements

Nutritional supplements can help reduce stress, relax muscles, and have a calming effect.

- B-complex vitamins: Take as directed on the label. Effective for nervous system function and reducing stress.

- Calcium: 1,500 milligrams daily in divided doses of 500 milligrams. Natural sedating effects. Take with magnesium after meals and take the last dose 45 minutes before bedtime.

- Magnesium: 750 milligrams daily in divided doses of 250 milligrams. Helps relax muscles.

Therapeutic Massage

By relieving muscular tension, calming the nervous system, and improving circulation, therapeutic massage relaxes the body and the mind. So that you will experience these effects closer to bedtime, it is best to schedule massage appointments in the late afternoon or early evening.

Lifestyle Recommendations

Try a soak before turning in. Taking a shower or bath before bedtime is generally helpful in inducing restful sleep.

Begin exercising. Exercise is known to help with insomnia. Experts especially recommend brisk walks, runs, or bike rides late in the afternoon. They believe that afternoon exercise helps deepen sleep. Exercise raises body temperature. About 6 hours later, when the temperature falls, sleep will come more easily. So, people who exercise require less time to fall asleep. But avoid exercising at or right before your bedtime. Exercising 2 to 3 hours before bedtime may increase the chances of insomnia.

Consider yoga. The gentle stretches, deep breathing exercises, and guided imagery that make up a yoga routine are extremely beneficial in improving both the amount and the quality of sleep.

Practice deep breathing. Deep breathing can provide sound relaxation and improve your ability to fall asleep. While lying flat on your back, place both hands on your abdomen. Slowly inhale through your nose, pushing your abdomen up as if blowing up a balloon. Then, exhale slowly through your mouth, and feel your abdomen deflate. Practice this breathing process as often as possible.

Preventive Measures

Avoid fruit juice and high-sugar snacks before bedtime. High or low fluctuations in blood sugar levels can disrupt your sleep.

Control bedroom light and noise. Bright lights and loud noises disrupt sleep. If bright lights are streaming into your bedroom, you may wish to purchase light-blocking shades or lined drapes. You may even wish to try an eye mask. Excess outside noise that intrudes on the bedroom may be reduced with heavy curtains or drapes or by installing double-pane windows. Wearing earplugs and running a fan to create soothing white noise are other options.

Eat moderately at dinner. Eating a heavy meal for dinner tends to disturb sleep. On the other hand, a small bedtime snack is generally fine.

Establish a relaxing routine. Set up a prebedtime relaxing routine. Consider relaxation exercises or soaking in warm or hot water about $1\frac{1}{2}$ to 2 hours before bedtime. Don't take a hot bath too close to bedtime as it increases alertness. Consider reading or meditation before going to bed.

Keep a comfortable bedroom temperature.

Although there is some disagreement among researchers, it is usually believed that the bedroom should be slightly cool. So, turn the thermostat down in the winter and consider an air conditioner, fan, or dehumidifier for the summer.

Make lists. Before going to bed, write down all the things that you accomplished throughout the day. Next, make a "to do" list of those items that you did not get a chance to complete and include any other items that popped up in your day. This helps to empty your mind by seeing your accomplishments and by knowing that you are ready for the following day. You can rest easy and not stay awake thinking about all the things you have to do or didn't do.

Limit alcohol consumption. While alcohol consumption directly before bed will calm you and help you fall asleep, drinking alcohol at bedtime increases the amount of times you awaken at night.

Limit caffeine consumption. Caffeine is contained in a number of foods, including chocolate, cola drinks, teas, and regular coffee. While some people dealing with insomnia may be able to consume foods that contain caffeine early in the day, others may need to eliminate all caffeine from their diets. Certainly, if you have insomnia, you may wish to avoid any caffeine-containing foods for at least 6 hours before bedtime. It may be better not to consume any caffeine-containing foods after lunch.

Limit evening fluid intake. If you drink a good deal of fluid during the evening hours, you may awaken to use the bathroom. After using the bathroom, you may then have difficulty falling back to sleep.

Stop smoking. Cigarettes contain nicotine, which is a stimulant. Smoking before bedtime increases the risk of insomnia. As you sleep, you experience nicotine withdrawal and the need for nicotine may awaken you. People who smoke are also known to have more nightmares.

When you first stop smoking, you increase your risk of insomnia. But that risk will soon fade, and you will reap the benefits of not smoking.

Hormone Replacement Therapy and Sleep

If your hormone replacement medication involves taking estrogen and progesterone separately, then take the progesterone in the evening. Progesterone has a sedative effect, and it may help you sleep better.

Irritable Bowel Syndrome

People with irritable bowel syndrome (IBS) are faced with a host of uncomfortable symptoms. These include diarrhea (IBS with diarrhea) or constipation (IBS with constipation), gas, abdominal pain or cramping, a bloated feeling, and mucus in the stool.

Irritable bowel syndrome is a "functional" disorder of the large intestine (colon). While the large intestine appears physically normal (without infectious, inflammatory, or structural abnormality), it fails to function in a normal manner. IBS is also known as spastic colon, colitis, mucous colitis, nervous stomach, nervous bowel, irritable colon, spastic colitis, and spastic bowel.

In order to receive a diagnosis of irritable bowel syndrome, you must have experienced abdominal pain or discomfort for at least 12 weeks (not necessarily consecutive) out of the previous 12 months. In addition, the abdominal pain must meet at least two of the following three features: It is relieved by a bowel movement; there is a change in the frequency of bowel movements; or there is an alteration in the form and appearance of the stool.

With irritable bowel syndrome, the colon may have spasms or muscle contractions that are far stronger than normal. Food may be pushed through the intestine quickly, resulting in gas, bloating, and diarrhea. Also, the colon tends to leave too much fluid in the stool, resulting in diarrhea, or, conversely, remove too much fluid from the stool, causing constipation. In people with IBS, the colon responds strongly to foods and/or stresses that would not bother other people.

IBS is extremely common. It is one of the most frequent reasons people visit their doctors. As many as one in five Americans suffer from some degree of this medical disorder. Women are twice as likely as men to have IBS.

Causes and Risk Factors

Although the exact cause of irritable bowel syndrome is unknown, there is some evidence that the immune system is involved. There may be changes in the nerves that regulate sensation in the bowel, or the central nervous system may cause the colon to function abnormally. People with this disorder have a more reactive and sensitive colon, and the motility of their colons fails to function in the usual way.

Large numbers of those with IBS report that their symptoms began during times of

Some people with IBS actually have mild or hidden (occult) celiac disease, an autoimmune disorder in which there is an inability to digest gluten (found in wheat, oats, barley, and rye). When someone with celiac disease eats foods containing gluten, the small intestine is damaged. Ask your doctor for a blood test to rule out celiac disease.

major life stressors, such as the death of a loved one or a divorce. Others say that their first irritable bowel symptoms appeared following a gastrointestinal infection or abdominal surgery.

A number of foods seem to exacerbate IBS, including wheat, rye, barley, chocolate, milk products, foods with caffeine, and alcohol. Eating too much food at any one time has been associated with IBS, as have certain medications, such as antibiotics that disrupt normal bacteria in the bowel; stress; conflict; and emotional upset. An acute bout of infectious diarrhea (gastroenteritis) may cause IBS.

Irritable bowel syndrome tends to begin around the age of 20. In some instances, people have one bout, and the disease never reappears. However, many people experience a number of episodes and may even deal with it on a daily basis. The symptoms tend to worsen as people age.

IBS and Inflammatory Bowel Diseases

Don't confuse irritable bowel syndrome with inflammatory bowel diseases such as Crohn's disease or ulcerative colitis. IBS does not cause damage to the bowel, fever, bleeding, weight loss, inflammation, or cancer. Symptoms such as pain and the need to have a bowel movement do not disrupt sleep, as they may with inflammatory bowel disease. When the bowel is examined, there is no evidence of disease in IBS; the bowel simply does not work as it is supposed to work. On the other hand, irritable bowel syndrome is still a potentially life-altering medical problem. People who have the more serious forms of IBS often believe that the quality of their lives has been diminished. They may have problems holding a job and have higher rates of hospitalization.

Signs and Symptoms

The most frequent symptom of irritable bowel syndrome is abdominal pain or discomfort, usually in the lower abdomen area. Some people have diarrhea, often with an urgent need to move the bowels, while others have constipation. Many alternate between diarrhea and constipation. People with IBS may have bloating from gas that builds up in the intestines. It is not uncommon for those with IBS to have an urge to move their bowels but be unable to pass any stool. Most people have relatively mild symptoms. In some instances, however, symptoms are severe and quite debilitating. Approximately 40 to 60 percent of people with IBS experience psychological problems such as anxiety and depression.

Conventional Treatments
Dietary Modifications

Dietary changes are often a key element in the treatment of irritable bowel syndrome. Begin by keeping a journal of the food that you eat. Are you able to pinpoint any foods that tend to worsen your symptoms? If so, try avoiding them and see if you improve.

Many people with IBS are lactose intolerant—they have a problem digesting the lactose contained in dairy products. You might try reducing your intake of dairy products or taking a lactase enzyme, such as Lactaid, whenever you eat dairy foods. Often, people who are lactose intolerant are able to eat yogurt without problems.

Slowly increase the amount of soluble fiber in your diet. Soluble fiber may be found in oat bran, rice, potatoes, French or sourdough bread, soy, barley, pasta, and oatmeal.

You may benefit from eating smaller, more frequent meals, because larger meals tend to cause cramping and diarrhea. Lower-fat foods are better tolerated than foods higher in fat. Other foods that may cause IBS symptoms are chocolate, alcohol, caffeine, carbonated drinks, sorbitol (a sweetener), and gas-producing foods such as beans, broccoli, and cabbage. You may wish to limit your intake of these foods.

If you tend to be constipated, you should also increase your intake of fiber. Good sources of fiber include whole-grain breads, cereals, fruits, and vegetables. Also, drink lots of water—at least six to eight glasses a day.

A Quick Guide to Symptoms

- ☐ Abdominal pain or discomfort
- ☐ Diarrhea and/or constipation
- ☐ Bloating from gas
- ☐ An urge to move the bowels but an inability to pass any stool
- ☐ Anxiety and depression

Medications

Your doctor will probably begin by recommending a fiber supplement such as Metamucil (made from psyllium) or Citrucel (made of methylcellulose). Avoid the sugar-free forms of these products, which contain artificial sweeteners that may trigger attacks. To avoid constipation, be sure to drink lots of water.

If you have diarrhea, your doctor may recommend an over-the-counter medication such as loperamide (Imodium) or an anticholinergic prescription medication, such as Bentyl or Levsin, that relieves painful bowel spasms. Potential side effects of anticholinergic drugs include dry mouth, dizziness, and confusion.

The most controversial IBS medication is alosetron (Lotronex). It is approved only for women with severe cases of IBS with diarrhea. Side effects, which include severe constipation and ischemic colitis (reduced bloodflow to the colon), have the potential to be life-threatening.

If you have constipation as the predominant symptom for IBS, a laxative, such as lactulose or polyethylene glycol solution (Miralax), may be advised. Although a number of medications have been used to alleviate IBS symptoms, few have been rigorously tested with well-designed studies. So, at present, there is no way to know which medications are most effective.

If you have pain and depression, your doctor may advise a tricyclic antidepressant, such as imipramine (Tofranil) or amitriptyline (Elavil), or a selective serotonin reuptake inhibitor (SSRI), such as fluoxetine (Prozac) or paroxetine (Paxil). While relieving depression, these medications limit the activity of neurons that control the intestines. Tricyclic antidepressants may cause drowsiness and constipation, and SSRIs have negative side effects including nausea, agitation, insomnia, restlessness, weight gain, and sexual dysfunction. A rare but potentially life-threatening side effect with SSRIs is known as serotonin syndrome. This may occur when an SSRI reacts with another antidepressant, most commonly a monoamine oxidase inhibitor (MAOI), but it can also happen when an SSRI is mixed with a supplement that influences serotonin, such as St. John's wort. The symptoms of serotonin syndrome include blood pressure and heart rhythm fluctuations, confusion, hallucinations, fever, seizures, and coma. SSRIs usually require 2 to 4 weeks to be effective, or sometimes even longer.

Psychological Treatments

Dealing with irritable bowel syndrome on a daily basis, especially the more severe forms, takes a psychological toll. Psychological interventions may help you cope. In cognitive-behavioral therapy, people with IBS learn exercises, strategies, and new ways to think about their symptoms. Biofeedback and relaxation training aid in the awareness and control of physical and emotional responses. These are especially useful for dealing with the physiological consequences of stress. Hypnosis has also been used effectively for IBS. After you have entered a relaxed, hypnotic state, you imagine the intestinal muscles becoming smooth and calm.

Complementary Treatments

Changes in lifestyle and diet may be effective in providing relief from irritable bowel syndrome as well as helping to relieve the pain associated with IBS symptoms.

Aromatherapy

If a primary symptom of IBS is constipation, gas, abdominal cramping, or bloating, essential oils of orange and marjoram may be beneficial because of their relaxing and stimulating properties. You can prepare a therapeutic bath by adding 6 to 10 drops of either oil alone or 4 or 5 drops of each in combination. Orange oil aids in the regulation of the bowels, and marjoram promotes elimination and improves digestion. Since orange oil may increase the risk of sunburn and marjoram may cause drowsiness, it is best to have a bath with these oils relatively close to bedtime.

Herbal Medicine

During a bout of constipation, you can create your own natural laxative. Although it requires a day or two to begin working, this laxative will encourage your digestive system to work naturally, help soften stools, stimulate contraction, and facilitate the bowel movement process. Crush 1 teaspoon of flaxseed and 2 teaspoons of psyllium seed in a coffee bean grinder. When the seeds are reduced to a powder, stir them into an 8-ounce glass of water and drink once a day.

Chamomile and ginger. Chamomile, which has an antispasmodic effect, and ginger, a carminative (helps to relieve gas), may be taken as a tea three or four times a day between meals. Chamomile and ginger are readily available in prepared tea bags.

Curcumin. Curcumin, a substance derived from turmeric (a key ingredient in curry powder), is an antioxidant with anti-inflammatory properties. Recent studies have shown a decrease in abdominal pain and IBS prevalence in those taking curcumin. The dose used in the study was one or two 72-milligram tablets daily. Curcumin may also be incorporated into the diet by using curry powder in recipes.

Peppermint and fennel. Drinking peppermint tea throughout the day may be useful for relieving abdominal spasms. Fennel seeds help to prevent and relieve gas associated with IBS. Chew 1 tablespoon of fennel seeds slowly and thoroughly.

Naturopathy

Naturopathy is a system of holistic therapy that relies on natural remedies, such as homeopathy, hydrotherapy, diet, herbs, massage, acupuncture, and exercise. Naturopathic medicine has been found very effective in the treatment of digestive disorders. To find a naturopathic practitioner in your area, contact the American Association of Naturopathic Physicians at www.naturopathic.org.

Nutritional Counseling

Once a diagnosis of IBS has been established, you may find nutritional counseling beneficial. Nutritional counselors help individuals determine food hypersensitivities, allergies, or food intolerances through elimination diets. Nutritional counseling may help you design a specific diet that provides both variety and proper nutrition.

Nutritional Supplements

To increase your intake of fiber, ask your doctor if you should add a natural fiber supplement, such as Metamucil or Citrucel, to your diet. The added bulk stimulates contractions, softens stools, and encourages the digestive system to work better. If you do take such a supplement, be sure to drink extra water. If not, you may become constipated. Follow the directions on the product label.

It is necessary to add additional supplements to maintain proper levels of nutrients in the body, particularly during a flare-up.

- Multivitamin/mineral: Take as directed on the label. Should contain vitamins A, D, E, folic acid, magnesium, and zinc to ensure proper levels, especially during bouts of diarrhea.

- Bromelain: 1,500 milligrams daily in divided doses of 500 milligrams. Digestive enzyme that reduces inflammation. Take between meals.

- *Lactobacillus acidophilus*: 200 milligrams daily. (Bottle should state "live" or "active" cultures. Product should have 1 billion to 2 billion organisms per capsule.) Maintains the health of the intestine.

- Omega-3 fatty acids: 1 tablespoon flaxseed oil or 4,000 milligrams of fish oil capsules in divided doses of 2,000 milligrams daily. Aid in the regulation of pain and swelling, particularly effective in the digestive tract.

Therapeutic Massage

You can make your own massage oil and give yourself a gentle abdomen massage. Purchase a small plastic squirt bottle. To limit the exposure to light and increase the shelf life of the oil, select a dark-colored bottle. Fill the bottle with an oil such as canola, jojoba, or sesame, then place 4 or 5 drops each of marjoram and orange oil into the bottle and roll it gently between your fingers to mix the oils. Heat some water in a small pan just to boiling, and remove it from the heat. Place the container in the heated water.

After the massage oil is warmed, lie comfortably on your back. Place a small amount of the warmed oil in your hands and rub together. Then, massage the oil over your abdomen, particularly along the colon area. You'll be right over the colon if you follow this procedure: Begin on the right side of your body, next to your hipbone. Moving upward as you go, gently stimulate the area with your fingertips until you reach the bottom of your ribs. Continue straight along to the left side of your body, downward toward your left hip. You have just stimulated your ascending, transverse, and descending colon. Next, use both hands to massage the belly area, rhythmically and in a circular motion. This will relieve bloating and stimulate the bowels.

Lifestyle Recommendations

Add fiber and fluids to your diet. Begin by *gradually* eating more high-fiber foods such as fruits, vegetables, and whole-grain products. Increase your intake of high-fiber foods slowly so that your body can adjust. You should also increase your intake of fluids. Try to include about eight 8-ounce glasses of fluids that do not contain caffeine or alcohol in your daily diet.

Address the related psychological issues. Dealing with irritable bowel syndrome exacts a strong psychological toll. People with severe symptoms may fear leaving their homes, because they worry about the accessibility of bathrooms. Even those with milder symptoms may have some degree of reluctance, so it is easy for those with IBS to become isolated. Anxiety and depression go hand in hand with this disorder.

Consider joining a support group. Participating in a support group may enable you to cope better with your disease. You may benefit from the advice and suggestions offered by other members.

Manage the stress in your life. While stress does not cause irritable bowel syndrome, it may trigger flare-ups and increase the severity of your symptoms. When you are experiencing stress, the digestive area often becomes a holding place for tension-causing emotions, resulting in abdominal muscle tension and pain. Try to include stress-reducing techniques into your everyday life, such as exercise, biofeedback, yoga, meditation, massage, and deep breathing. Studies have shown that treating the mind with stress-reducing techniques such as these eases IBS.

Preventive Measures

There is no known way to prevent IBS. However, by making a few changes in your lifestyle, you may reduce your chances of a flare-up.

Consider an elimination diet. Attempting an elimination diet may help you determine which foods trigger your IBS. For the first 10 days, eliminate all citrus fruits and all foods containing corn, dairy, eggs, and gluten (wheat, oats, barley, and rye). After 7 to 10 days, if your symptoms remain unchanged, you are probably not sensitive to these foods. If your symptoms do improve, and you find that you have more energy and are in a better mood, then in order to determine the culprit or culprits, you need to start returning these food groups back into your diet, one at a time, every 3 to 4 days. To help you track your symptoms, keep a food journal.

Exercise. Regular exercise reduces the pressure inside the colon, moves food along faster, and promotes the normal functioning of the bowels. For improved bowel health, try to exercise at least 30 minutes a day as often as possible. One of the best exercises is a daily 20- to 30-minute walk. By including regular exercise in your daily lifestyle, you will help maintain your strength and reduce stress. If you have been leading a fairly sedentary lifestyle, before beginning an exercise regimen, you should consult with your doctor.

Kidney Stones

Kidney stones, also known as nephrolithiasis or urinary calculi, are hard masses of crystals that develop inside the kidneys. The most common types of stones are composed of calcium oxalate or calcium phosphate. A less common stone, called a struvite, contains magnesium ammonium phosphate. Uric acid stones are even less common, and cystine stones are rare.

If the crystals remain tiny, and they do in 70 to 90 percent of cases, they may pass through the urinary tract without being noticed. Problems may occur when a stone irritates the lining of the kidney or leaves the kidney and enters one of the two ureters that connect the kidneys to the bladder. The stone may become lodged in a ureter and prevent urine from flowing freely. The part of the ureter that is behind the blockage may dilate. As time passes, there may be injury to the kidney.

The kidneys filter a wide variety of substances, including calcium, oxalate, uric acid, and cystine. All four of these substances have a tendency to form crystals. Fortunately, when everything is working normally, citrate and magnesium, which are also in the kidneys, prevent crystal formation. Sometimes, however, the balance is upset. If your kidneys contain too much calcium, oxalate, uric acid, or cystine, or if they have too little citrate and magnesium, crystals may form. Crystal formation may also take place when the urine is too concentrated or is too acidic or alkaline. The key element in the development of kidney stones is supersaturation. That is, salts in the kidney become so concentrated that they are unable to dissolve, and they precipitate out and form crystals.

In the United States, more than 1 million cases of kidney stones are reported every year. During an average lifetime, an American has a 10 percent chance of developing a kidney stone. They are most common during the midlife years, and they occur three times more often in men than in women. Though it is not known why, over the past 20 years, the incidence has been rising.

Causes and Risk Factors

It is not always clear what triggers the imbalance that results in kidney stones. Family history is known to play an important role in the development of kidney stones. In those who are susceptible, diet may well play a role. And certain medical conditions have been associated with this disorder, including urinary tract infections, obesity, high blood pressure, gout, chronic diarrhea, kidney problems such as cystic kidney diseases, and metabolic problems such as hyperparathyroidism.

People who have chronic inflammation of the bowel or who have had an intestinal bypass operation or ostomy surgery are more likely to form calcium oxalate stones. Those who take the protease inhibitor indinavir, which is used to treat HIV and AIDS, are at higher risk for kidney stones. Other causes are high levels of uric acid in the urine, excess intake of vitamin D, and a urinary tract blockage. Some diuretics and calcium-based antacids add to the amount of calcium in the urine, thereby increasing the chance that you will have kidney stones. People who are confined to bed tend to reabsorb more calcium and are therefore at a greater risk.

White males have the highest risk for kidney stones. White people have a greater risk than African Americans. Being overweight also increases the possibility of kidney stones. Once you have had a kidney stone, you are more likely to have another. If you are not treated for your first bout with kidney stones, you have an 80 percent chance of having another episode within 10 years.

Signs and Symptoms

The most common first symptom of a kidney stone is excruciating pain, which may be referred to as renal colic by your doctor. At first, the sharp, cramping pain tends to be in the back and side—in the area of a kidney or the lower abdomen. There may also be nausea and vomiting. As time passes, the pain may spread to the groin. You may feel pain in the genitals, particularly the testicles in men and the labia in women.

There may be blood in the urine, which may be cloudy and foul-smelling. When the

A Quick Guide to Symptoms

☐ **Excruciating pain (renal colic)**
☐ **Nausea and vomiting**
☐ **Pain in the genitals**
☐ **Blood in the urine**
☐ **A burning sensation and the need to urinate often**
☐ **Fever and chills**

stone approaches the bladder, you may have a burning sensation and feel the need to urinate often. You may also have a fever and chills, usually indicating an infection and a medical emergency. If you are experiencing these symptoms, you need to contact your doctor immediately or visit an urgent care clinic or the emergency room of a hospital.

Conventional Treatments

In about 85 percent of individuals, kidney stones are sufficiently small—less than the width of a pencil eraser—that they are able to pass during normal urination. If there is no infection, watchful waiting is a perfectly acceptable option. To help the stone pass, you should drink 2 to 3 quarts of water each day.

The degree of pain that you feel from a kidney stone is not necessarily a function of the size of the stone. A small stone with sharp edges may cause more pain than a larger stone that is smooth.

Assessing the Stone

After your kidney stone attack, your doctor may want additional blood and urine tests. The blood tests help determine the levels of blood urea nitrogen, creatinine, calcium, phosphate, and uric acid in your blood. The urine test is used to detect the specific chemical and biological factors that play a role in the stone formation. You will probably be asked to collect your urine for 24 hours. The urine will be evaluated for levels of acidity, calcium, uric acid, oxalate, citrate, and creatinine. This information is used to establish the cause of the stone.

When collecting your 24-hour urine, be sure to discard the first urine of the first day and to include the first urine of the second day. This allows for accurate counting for the entire 24-hour period.

Your doctor will give you a collection kit that contains a filter for collecting the stone.

Medication

During the acute attack, while waiting for the stone to pass, you will be given painkilling medications such as nonsteroidal anti-inflammatory drugs (NSAIDs). In some instances, you may be given opioids such as meperidine (Demerol). If there is an infection, you may be admitted to the hospital, where you will receive intravenous antibiotics. Even if you are not admitted, if you have an infection, your doctor will prescribe an antibiotic.

A number of medications can help prevent the formation of calcium and uric acid stones. The diuretic hydrochlorothiazide reduces the amount of calcium that is excreted. Allopuri-nol lowers the amount of uric acid production. Potassium citrate attaches itself to calcium, allowing the calcium to be removed safely from the body. Sodium cellulose phosphate may be given to those with a condition known as absorptive hypercalciuria. This medication binds to calcium in the intestines, thereby preventing it from getting into the urine. Cystine stone formation may be treated with penicillamine or tiopronin, which facilitates the body's breakdown of cystine.

If you have struvite stones that can't be removed, your doctor may prescribe aetohydroamic acid (AHA), which is used in conjunction with antibiotic medications.

Some studies have attempted to determine if treatment with medications, including calcium-channel blockers or alpha-blockers, helps with the passage of the stones. Pooled results of a number of experimental trials suggest that, under certain conditions, these medications may be useful. Since this option may enable you to avoid surgery, you may wish to discuss medications with your clinician.

Surgery

Extracorporeal shock wave lithotripsy (ESWL). In this most common surgical procedure, shock waves are used to break the stones into small crystals that can be passed in the urine. The procedure is best for stones that are less than 1 centimeter in size. Usually, you will first be given some form of anesthesia, then either placed on a soft cushion or partially submerged in water. An ultrasound device generates shock waves that travel through your body and hit the stones. Though you won't feel the shock waves, they create a great deal of noise. To protect your hearing, you will be asked to wear earplugs or headphones.

As the shattered stones pass through the urinary tract, you may have some discomfort. It may take months for all the stones to pass. To aid the passage, your doctor may insert a stent or small tube through the bladder into the ureter. You may resume your regular schedule in a few days.

The most common complication of ESWL is blood in the urine, which may last for a few days. To reduce your risk, for 7 to 10 days before the procedure, you may be advised to stop taking aspirin or other NSAIDs. You may also have some bruising or minor discomfort in your back or abdomen. If the stone did not completely fragment, you may need another treatment. Success rates vary from 50 to 90 percent.

Percutaneous nephrolithotomy. If the stone is larger than 3 centimeters, or the ESWL was not successful, or there is evidence that your stone is blocking the flow of urine, damaging the kidney, or causing a urinary tract infection, your doctor may advise a percutaneous nephrolithotomy. In this procedure, your doctor makes a small incision in the back. Then, after a "tunnel" to the kidney is created, the stone is removed with an instrument known as a nephroscope. Sometimes, the stone must first be broken into smaller pieces.

Success rates with this surgery tend to be quite high—about 98 percent for stones in the kidney and 88 percent for stones in the ureters. About 3 percent of those who have this surgery have complications, which include scarring, blood loss, imbalances in the fluid used to irrigate the tunnel, collapsed lung, and injuries to the operative area.

Ureteroscopic stone removal. If your stone is stuck in the mid to low area of one of the ureters, your doctor may suggest a ureteroscopy. In this procedure, your doctor passes a ureteroscope, a small fiber-optic instrument, through the urethra and bladder into the ureter. After the stone is located, it will be held and removed by tiny forceps. Larger stones are generally shattered with an ultrasound. To help the ureter heal, a stent or small tube may be left in for a few days.

Treating Underlying Disorders

If the underlying cause of the kidney stones is determined, it is important that it be treated. Effective treatment of the underlying cause should significantly reduce the chances of another attack. For example, people with hyperparathyroidism have high amounts of calcium. As a result, they are at higher risk for kidney stones. Hyperparathyroidism is often caused by a tumor in one of the four parathyroid glands in the neck. When the tumor is removed, the condition is resolved.

Complementary Treatments

Complementary medicine treatments may be beneficial for pain relief of kidney stones. Herbs and dietary changes are useful in preventing further occurrences of kidney stones. Conventional medicine is the best course of action for this condition, especially when the stones are large and require immediate attention. Complementary medicine treatments should be used in conjunction with conventional medicine.

Diet

Diet plays a key role in the treatment and prevention of kidney stones, but before you make any changes in your diet, it is important to find out what type of stones you have. You may need to limit or eliminate foods containing calcium, salt, oxalate, protein, and potassium. While diet restrictions may vary, it is generally recommended that anyone with kidney stones avoid foods high in animal protein, fried foods, sugar, and processed foods.

Naturopathy

Since diet plays a key role in the treatment of kidney stones, visiting a naturopathic physician will be beneficial. A naturopath can also assist in nutritional supplement recommendations, if needed, along with other health and lifestyle changes to eliminate future stone attacks. To find a naturopathic practitioner in your area, contact the American Association of Naturopathic Physicians at www.naturopathic.org.

Nutritional Counseling

Contact a registered dietitian to help clear up any confusion associated with the type of stones you have and the foods to avoid. He or she will help you create a diet to reduce the incidence of future attacks.

Nutritional Supplements

A combination of nutritional supplements may be beneficial in preventing calcium kidney stones.

- B-complex vitamins: Take as directed on the label. B vitamins work best when taken together. B_6 in particular helps prevent crystallization and the reformation of calcium kidney stones. Take with magnesium.

- Magnesium: 500 milligrams daily. Take with B-complex vitamins. Do not take magnesium if you have kidney disease.

Lifestyle Recommendations

Apply heat. To provide relief while passing a kidney stone, apply moist heat to the lower back or soak in a hot tub.

Be careful of high-protein diets. Though it is not well understood, it is known that the incidence of kidney stones is associated with the amount of protein in the diet. Groups with higher intakes of dietary protein tend to have elevated rates of kidney stones. Since protein may aid stone production by increasing acidity of urine or facilitating the excretion of uric acid, phosphorus, and/or calcium, be careful with the amount of protein you consume.

Drink lemon juice. Fresh lemon juice may help reduce the pain of kidney stones and prevent future stone formation. For pain relief, add the juice of half a lemon to an 8-ounce glass of warm water. Drink a glass every hour. For the prevention of future stones, start your day with this same combination. Once a day is sufficient for prevention.

Preventive Measures

Avoid grapefruit juice. A number of studies have found that grapefruit juice increases the risk of kidney stones.

Use care when taking vitamin C. Because most stones will not form in acidic urine, increasing your intake of vitamin C may be useful. However, if you've been told that you have too much urinary oxalate, a condition known as hyperoxaluria, you should avoid vitamin C supplements. Vitamin C, also known as ascorbic acid, may convert to oxalates.

Drink lots of fluid. If you have already had a bout with kidney stones or if you have been told that you are at increased risk, you should drink at least 10 to 14 glasses of fluid each day. Of that, at least half should be water. If you have a tendency for cystine stones, you need to drink more than a gallon of fluids each day. If your urine is dark or yellow rather than watery, you are not drinking enough fluids. Remember, during the warmer months or if you live in a warm climate, you should drink even more. You goal is to drink a sufficient amount of fluids to produce at least 2 quarts of urine every day.

Water helps dilute the urine and pushes out concentrations of harmful chemicals. If you are prone to uric acid stones or calcium oxalate stones, you should avoid cranberry juice and any other products containing cranberries, as recent studies have shown that cranberry juice can actually raise the risk for these types of kidney stones. The study did show, however, that cranberry juice lowered the risk for brushite stones, which are rare. Orange juice may help prevent stone formation.

Exercise. Regular exercise may remove excess calcium from the blood and transport it to the bones, where it is better utilized. The lack of regular exercise may increase the level of calcium in the blood, which may lead to kidney stones. Get at least 40 minutes of exercise daily.

Limit soft drinks. Many soft drinks contain phosphoric acid, which increases your risk for kidney stones.

Lose weight. If you are carrying around excess weight, try to lose it. But drop the pounds slowly, as losing weight too quickly increases the risk for kidney stones.

Reduce your sugar intake. Consuming sugar promotes the release of insulin by the pancreas, which, in turn, causes calcium to be released into the urine.

Restrict your sodium intake. Salt increases the amount of calcium in the urine and may aid in the formation of kidney stones.

Take care with calcium supplementation. Although research has found that the dietary intake of calcium appears to be protective against calcium oxalate stones, calcium supplements may raise your risk for other types of kidney stones. Supplementation up to 1,200 milligrams per day is considered safe. Do not exceed 2,000 milligrams per day, as that level of supplementation is clearly associated with increased risk. If you are at risk for kidney stones, you should discuss calcium supplementation with your doctor.

Try to relax. People who are stressed tend to have more kidney stones than those who are less stressed. Find a way to incorporate relaxation techniques into your life.

Macular Degeneration

When your vision is impaired, as it is with age-related macular degeneration (AMD or ARMD), objects may appear unclear. You may have difficulty with everyday functions such as driving and reading. Faces of other people may become blurred, and you may be unable to differentiate one person from another. You may have a hard time determining the colors and fine points of items that appear within the center of your field of vision. And what you do see will tend to be in black and white, rather than in color. Fortunately, the peripheral vision of those dealing with AMD is normally spared.

The macula is a light-sensitive layer of tissues located in the back of the eye at the center of the retina. When light, which enters the eye via the cornea and lens, focuses on the macula, it is transformed into nerve signals. These nerve signals are, in turn, transmitted to the brain. This process enables you to see central vision (what is straight ahead) in sharp, fine details, and allows you to distinguish different colors.

Macular degeneration is a relatively common disease. Approximately 1.6 million Americans have the advanced form of the disease, which threatens vision. Another 6 million Americans are considered at risk for developing advanced macular degeneration in at least one eye. Macular degeneration is believed to be the leading cause of legal blindness in US residents over the age of 55.

There are two types of AMD, dry AMD (atrophic) and wet AMD (exudative). Approximately 90 percent of those affected by this illness have dry AMD. While the cause is not known, in dry AMD the light-sensitive cells in the macula stop working. As time passes, central vision is lost. Dry AMD typically begins by affecting one eye, but it may ultimately affect both eyes.

Wet AMD is the rapidly advancing form of this illness. Ninety percent of those who experience severe AMD-related vision loss have wet AMD. In wet AMD, new, fragile blood vessels behind the retina grow toward the macula, and, in the process, they leak blood and fluid. This damages the macula, which may cause a relatively swift loss of central vision. On occasion, people with dry AMD may also develop wet AMD.

Causes and Risk Factors

The risk of AMD increases with age. Those in their fifties have about a 2 percent risk of developing AMD, but that figure jumps to 30 percent in people over the age of 75. In addition to age, there are other risk factors. There is strong evidence of an association between smoking and AMD. Smoking reduces macular pigment up to 50 percent. The risk of AMD is about 2 to 4 times greater in smokers than nonsmokers. In smokers who have a certain genetic predisposition, the risk for AMD may be 34 times greater compared with nonsmokers without the genetic predisposition.

Some studies have found that women and whites are more likely to have AMD. Family history seems to play a role, as does elevated cholesterol, arteriosclerosis, high blood pressure, and smoking. Similarly, fair skin, light-colored eyes, extreme farsightedness, and prolonged exposure to sunlight add to the risk.

Signs and Symptoms

Neither form of macular degeneration triggers pain. The most frequent symptom of dry AMD is mildly blurred vision. For example, someone might notice that more light is needed for reading. Facial features and colors may appear harder to distinguish. Central vision colors will be difficult to determine, and objects will tend to be black or white. As the disease progresses, there may be a blurred spot at the center of vision. This spot may gradually grow larger and darker, thereby reducing still more of the central vision. When dry AMD occurs in only one eye, people usually do not notice any changes in their vision because they are still able to see fine details with the other eye. Often, dry AMD is first detected during a routine eye exam. Most people realize that there is a problem only when dry AMD affects both eyes.

Straight lines that look wavy are a frequent

A Quick Guide to Symptoms

☐ **Mildly blurred vision**
☐ **Colors are harder to distinguish**
☐ **Blurred spot at the center of vision**
☐ **Straight lines that look wavy (wet AMD)**
☐ **Rapid loss of central vision (wet AMD)**

first symptom of wet AMD. This indicator is caused by newly formed blood vessels that are leaking fluid under the macula. Another symptom of wet AMD is a rapid loss of central vision, and there may also be a blind spot.

If you are experiencing any of these symptoms, you should immediately contact an eye care professional, such as an ophthalmologist or optometrist. Describe your symptoms on the phone, and underscore your need to be evaluated quickly.

If you suspect that you may have AMD, you should seek emergency assistance from an eye care professional.

Conventional Treatments for Wet AMD

Thanks to the use of laser surgery, new types of medications, and combinations of lasers and light-sensitive drugs, people with wet AMD are retaining more of their sight.

Antiangiogenesis Drugs

It is well understood that cancer tumors obtain some of their blood supply by growing new blood vessels. A certain group of medications, known as antiangiogenesis drugs, is used to stop the growth of these vessels. In recent years, researchers have been examining whether they would be similarly useful for treating the vessels formed in wet AMD. They inject the antiangiogenesis drugs directly into the eye. The goal is to inhibit substances, such as the vascular endothelial growth factor (VEGF), that facilitate the growth of these new vessels. Another possibility is using the antiangiogenic steroid triamcinolone acetonide, not to destroy the blood vessels but to limit the amount of leaking fluid. Though still in the experimental stage, these drugs are showing enormous promise.

Laser Surgery

When laser surgery is appropriate, it involves a visit to a highly trained ophthalmologist. The physician will dilate your pupil and apply drops to numb the eye. It may also be necessary to numb the area behind the eye. During the laser treatment, the physician will aim a high-energy beam of light directly at the leaking blood vessels. You may see flashes of light. Do not defer or delay this treatment. It should be done as soon as possible, before the blood vessels have harmed the fovea (the central part of the macula).

Following treatment, you will be able to return home, but, since you will be unable to drive, prearrange a ride. Because the eye remains dilated for several hours, you should also wear sunglasses. Your vision will be blurry for most of the day, and there may be some localized pain, which should respond well to pain medication.

Using the Amsler Grid

If you are diagnosed with dry AMD, you should check your eyes daily with an Amsler grid, which is a grid with a pattern that looks like a checkerboard. In a small number of cases, dry AMD progresses to wet AMD, and you want to determine if that could be happening to you. The test allows you to see whether the disease is stable or progressing.

The Amsler grid has a black dot in the center. Be sure to place your grid in a convenient location, such as on the refrigerator. Stand 12 to 15 inches away from it. Cover your right eye when you look at the black dot with your left eye, and cover your left eye when you look at the black dot with your right eye. Keep a log, and record how the grid looks. One day, you may note that the straight lines in the pattern appear wavy, or they may simply be changed (appear blurry or distorted or discolored), or part of the grid may have disappeared.

If any of these events seems to be happening, make copies of the grid and use a new copy each day, and date it. Indicate the exact changes and their location on the grid. These symptoms may be a sign of wet AMD. If they occur, you need to visit your eye care professional quickly. Bring copies of the grid to your appointment. A picture of an Amsler grid is available on the Internet at www.nei.nih.gov/health/maculardegen/armd_facts.asp.

It is important to realize that laser surgery treats wet AMD, but it is not a cure. New vessels will probably develop, and they may require additional laser surgery. You will need relatively frequent evaluations by your physician.

An FDA-approved laser treatment uses photodynamic therapy (PDT). A drug in the form of a green dye, known as verteporfin or Visudyne, is injected into a vein in the arm. It takes about 10 to 20 minutes for the dye to make its way to the eye, where it tends to enter abnormal vessels. A physician then focuses a low-power laser beam on the back of the eye, which activates the drug to attack the abnormal vessels. The retina is spared. Obviously, the procedure requires extraordinary precision and, for now at least, is expensive. While the progression of the disease stops in about two-thirds of the people who have the surgery, only 10 percent witness an improvement in their vision. Further, photodynamic therapy works for only a somewhat brief period of time, so individuals may need to be retreated every few months.

Laser surgery comes with a degree of risk, though when carried out by a highly skilled practitioner, that likelihood should be minimal. While very small, there is the possibility that the laser beam will be aimed incorrectly. When that occurs, healthy retinal tissue may be destroyed. Further, bleeding and scar tissue may form on the retina. Also, the area that received the laser beam has an increased chance of a loss of vision.

Radiation

Researchers are studying a form of radiation known as proton-beam therapy to determine if it may be useful for wet AMD. Proton particles are directed precisely at the abnormal vessels and lesions. Although the abnormal vessels and lesions may be destroyed, the healthy cells appear to sustain little damage. Researchers believe that radiation may prove to be quite effective, particularly in the early stages of this disease.

Surgery

Some researchers are attempting to preserve central vision by removing abnormal blood vessels (submacular surgery). And surgeons are investigating retinal translocation in which part of the retina is detached and moved away from the problematic new blood vessels. This may improve vision. However, it is very risky. People having this surgery may run the risk of losing all vision.

Conventional Treatments for Dry AMD

Currently, there are no conventional treatments for dry AMD. So, what should you do if you are diagnosed with this disease? See an eye care professional at least once a year. Obtain an Amsler grid and, as previously noted, test your eyes every day. Then, you will be able to notice any sudden changes from dry AMD to wet AMD.

Complementary Treatments

A treatment plan will vary from person to person, since each individual has a unique constitution, as well as characteristic lifelong habits. However, there are basic lifestyle guidelines that aid in the treatment of AMD.

Diet

Many studies indicate that certain nutrients—carotenoids, specific vitamins, and essential fatty acids—are beneficial to treating AMD. Some of these nutrients concentrate in the part of the retina where macular degeneration strikes. Others work to strengthen capillaries carrying blood to the eye muscles. These powerful nutrients can be found in common foods, so increasing your intake of these foods may aid in reducing the effects of macular degeneration.

Lutein and zeaxanthin are antioxidants in the carotenoid family. They concentrate in the part of the retina where macular degeneration occurs and protect the delicate cells of the macula from the damaging effects of ultraviolet light. People with AMD have been found to have lower levels of these substances in their bodies. Good sources of lutein and zeaxanthin include green, leafy vegetables, such as spinach, kale, and collard greens.

Anthocyanosides are compounds with antioxidant properties found in blueberries, cherries, raspberries, red or purple grapes, and plums. The European species of blueberry, the bilberry, has the highest level of anthocyanosides. Anthocyanosides help improve capillary circulation, which is very important in the retina.

Avoid foods high in hydrogenated fats, such as solid shortening, margarine, and deep-fried foods. Many processed snack foods, such as cookies and cakes, are high in fat. In fact, try to stay away from as much processed food as you can. These foods contribute to elevated cholesterol, arteriosclerosis, and high blood pressure, all risk factors in macular degeneration. A diet with lots of whole grains, vegetables, fruits, and cold-water fish, such as bluefish, cod, herring, mackerel, salmon, and tuna, is healthier. New studies have found that a diet high in omega-3 fatty acids may reduce the risk of advanced age-related macular degeneration.

Herbal Medicine

Ginkgo biloba. Ginkgo, which has been shown to improve memory and enhance concentration, is also beneficial for macular degeneration. Since ginkgo contains a variety of bioflavonoids, it acts as an antioxidant, increases the oxygen supply to the eyes, and assists in improving circulation and reducing oxidative damage. The recommended daily dose is 120 milligrams twice a day of extract standardized to 24 percent of flavone glycosides and 6 percent terpene lactones. The flavone glycosides give ginkgo its antioxidant benefits, and terpene lactones increase circulation and have a protective effect on nerve cells. Ginkgo should not be used if you are presently taking a blood-thinning medication.

Proanthocyanidin bioflavonoids. Often referred to as PAC or grape seed extract, this antioxidant may suppress the progression of macular degeneration by allowing macular tissue to adjust to oxygen fluctuations. It also reduces sensitivity to glare and sunlight. The typical recommended dose is 150 to 250 milligrams per day.

Nutritional Supplements

Antioxidant nutrients protect against the damage of free radical cells. Some of these nutrients concentrate in the retina, and deficiency can lead to macular degeneration.

- Vitamin C: 2,000 milligrams daily in divided doses of 1,000 milligrams. Protects against oxidative damage from sunlight, thereby decreasing the symptoms of macular degeneration. Do not take with selenium.

- Vitamin E: 400 IU daily. Antioxidant that neutralizes free radicals. Take with selenium.

- Bilberry extract: 100 milligrams of extract three times a day. Improves capillary circulation, which is very important to the retina.

- Copper: 2 milligrams daily. Long-term use of zinc may interfere with copper absorption and supplementation may be necessary.

- Lutein: 10 milligrams daily. Protects cells of the macula from the damaging effects of ultraviolet light.

- Selenium: 200 micrograms daily. Antioxidant that neutralizes free radicals.

- Zeaxanthin: 0.6 milligram daily. Protects cells of the macula from the damaging effects of ultraviolet light.

- Zinc: 50 milligrams daily. Essential since zinc concentrates in the retina. Prevents AMD, prevents vision loss in those with AMD, and reduces symptoms of AMD.

Lifestyle Recommendations

Discuss related medications with your doctor. Elevated cholesterol levels increase the risk for AMD, so it's a good idea to have your cholesterol level checked. If it is high, revamp your diet and discuss with your doctor whether you are a candidate for a cholesterol-lowering drug. Similarly, high blood pressure has been correlated with higher risks for AMD. If your blood pressure tends to be high, you may wish to discuss medications with your physician.

Drink a glass of red wine. Red wine contains bioflavonoids such as quercetin, rutin, and resveratrol, which have antioxidant activity to prevent oxidative damage. This can help slow the progression of macular degeneration. It may also play a role in prevention.

Exercise. Exercising increases the delivery of nutrients to the eyes and facilitates the removal of waste products. In addition, maintaining a regular exercise program helps reduce many of the risk factors associated with macular degeneration. The most important exercise for eye health is aerobic—consider walking, running, or swimming on a regular basis.

Try microcurrent stimulation. In this procedure, a TENS (transcutaneous electrical nerve stimulation) unit is used to apply electrical stimulation to key nerves around the eyes. For the treatment of wet and dry macular degeneration, electrodes are placed on the skin over the nerve areas and a low-voltage electrical pulse is then applied. Supporters of this noninvasive procedure contend that it improves bloodflow to the macula, and there are patients who indicate that it has increased visual acuity and color perception.

Preventive Measures

Get your vitamin D. Getting 10 to 15 minutes of direct sunlight several times a week can ensure that your body absorbs sufficient vitamin D. New findings show that individuals with higher levels of vitamin D may reduce the risk of developing early-stage age-related macular degeneration by 40 percent. Remember to use sunscreen if you spend longer than the recommended 10 to 15 minutes in the sun. If you are unable to spend time in the sun, you can get vitamin D in your diet through eggs and fish such as cod, mackerel, sardines, salmon, and tuna. It is also available in supplement form. Take 400 IU daily or at least three times a week.

Stop smoking. The direct correlation between macular degeneration and smoking is well documented. It appears that smokers are $2\frac{1}{2}$ times more likely than nonsmokers to develop AMD. While the average age that a nonsmoker will become ill with AMD is 71, the average age that a smoker will develop AMD is 64.

Wear a hat and sunglasses. Most eye professionals believe that ongoing exposure to sunlight increases the risk of AMD. It is a good idea to wear a protective hat and sunglasses that block out 100 percent of ultraviolet (UVA and UVB) rays and filter out at least 85 percent of blue-violet sun rays. Some contend that brown to yellow lenses are better alternatives. Be aware that there are medications that make the skin and eyes even more sensitive to light. Ask your doctor if any of your medications has this potential. If you are taking such a medicine, you need to be extra vigilant with sun protection.

Male Menopause

Often referred to as andropause, male menopause consists of the physical and psychological changes men experience at midlife. As men age, their testes and adrenal gland produce less of the male hormone testosterone—a condition known as hypogonadism. While these changes may appear anytime between the ages of 30 and 70, they tend to occur when a man is in his forties and fifties. About 13 percent of men between the ages of 40 and 60 have lower than normal testosterone levels. An average 70-year-old man has 25 to 50 percent less testosterone than he had at the age of 20.

While the very existence of male menopause is controversial, those who believe that it is a real disorder also contend that it is somewhat common. It has been estimated that as many as 5 million men over the age of 40 in the United States have this condition.

With male menopause (also known as low testosterone syndrome, and climacteric), there is a decrease in the production of testosterone in the testicles, although this is more variable than the estrogen deficiency seen in women who have undergone menopause. Lower levels of testosterone may induce loss of muscle mass, weakness, and osteoporosis. The osteoporosis that is caused by andropause may result in higher risk of fracture. However, this usually occurs about 10 years later than it does in women.

The changes associated with male menopause may be divided into two main categories, urinary/sexual changes and more generalized physical and psychological changes. For example, a man with a lower level of testosterone may have a reduced interest in sexual relations and may have mood swings. But low levels of testosterone are not believed to have any effect on fertility.

Theoretically, all men at midlife are at risk for male menopause. Evidently, however, not all men experience the symptoms linked to this disorder.

Signs and Symptoms

Common symptoms of male menopause include increases in fat, decreases in muscle and bone mass, decreased beard growth, decrease in

A Quick Guide to Symptoms

- ☐ Increases in fat, decreases in muscle and bone mass
- ☐ Decrease in strength and endurance
- ☐ Irritability and mood swings
- ☐ Difficulty concentrating
- ☐ Hot flashes
- ☐ Sleep problems
- ☐ Lack of energy
- ☐ Depression
- ☐ Erectile dysfunction
- ☐ Problems with urination

strength and endurance, irritability, difficulty concentrating, hot flashes, sleep problems, lack of energy, decline in performance at work, depression, erectile dysfunction, mood swings, and problems with urination.

Conventional Treatments

If you have low levels of testosterone and your doctor believes this requires treatment, then you may be given a prescription for testosterone replacement therapy (TRT). This is available as injections, patches, or a rub-on gel. Men who receive TRT must be closely monitored for prostate cancer. Though there is no evidence that TRT causes prostate cancer, it may potentially accelerate the growth of any existing prostate cancer. Men who have been diagnosed with prostate cancer should not take TRT, and men taking TRT must be carefully watched. In addition, there is some evidence that TRT may increase bad cholesterol and decrease good cholesterol. Plus, TRT may potentially harm the liver, stimulate benign growth of the prostate, and aggravate sleep apnea.

Complementary Treatments

Whether andropause is part of the normal aging process or a condition unto itself, com-

plementary medicine offers numerous options to relieve and eliminate symptoms associated with male menopause.

Acupuncture

Due to its ability to produce a more controlled, higher level of continuous stimulus, electro-acupuncture for the treatment of erectile dysfunction has shown positive effects, according to numerous studies. In electro-acupuncture, needles are inserted at specific points on the body. After insertion, an electric current is passed through the needles.

Diet

Maintain a healthy weight by eating lots of whole grains, fruits, and vegetables. In addition to assisting with weight maintenance, eating foods high in nutrients keeps the body properly nourished. These foods help keep the vascular system healthy, thereby maintaining proper bloodflow to the penis, which is necessary for erections. Try to include a minimum of five servings of vegetables, four servings of fruit, and six servings of whole grains each day.

Eliminate foods that are high in fat and sugar. They not only have an adverse effect on weight, but they rob the body of essential nutrients and interfere with their absorption. Also, stay away from foods and supplements that contain caffeine. While caffeine is a stimulant, it relaxes muscles and may interfere with normal function of the genital area. Avoid alcohol, which robs the body of zinc. Studies have shown that zinc deficiency may lead to prostate problems. Zinc is found in pumpkin and sunflower seeds, so try to include these in your diet.

Exercise

Regular, moderate exercise is beneficial both for relieving the symptoms of male menopause and for slowing the male aging process. Regular exercise lowers your risk for diabetes, heart disease, and osteoporosis. It also increases the release of endorphins, brain chemicals that help regulate body temperature and decrease stress, mood swings, and depression.

Without exercise, bones diminish in size and strength. At any age, bones may be rebuilt with weight-bearing activity, such as walking. Weight-bearing exercise also helps normalize the flow of sugar from the blood into muscle tissue, where it may be properly metabolized, reducing the risk of diabetes. Exercise improves muscle mass, strength, and gait, while facilitating flexibility, balance, and coordination.

Regular exercise slows the loss of dopamine, a neurotransmitter that prevents shaking and stiffness. Dopamine also supports our ability to react, thereby reducing the risk of falling.

You should create an exercise routine that includes an overall body program. It should incorporate weight-bearing exercises, strength training for the arms and legs, and postural training to support the back. Any exercise is better than none, but try to exercise at least 40 minutes per day. Since they increase flexibility and strength, yard work and gardening are considered exercise. Simply walking a minimum of 20 minutes, three times a week, may enhance bloodflow.

Herbal Medicine

A number of herbs can help balance the hormones and are considered precursors to progesterone and testosterone.

Asian ginseng. Asian ginseng helps maintain an erection and is known to improve male potency. The recommended daily dose is 100 to 200 milligrams, standardized to 4 to 7 percent ginsenosides. However, do not use ginseng if you have high blood pressure, heart disorders, or hypoglycemia.

Damiana. Damiana may be more effective when combined with other, similar-acting herbs such as sarsaparilla. To make a tea, place 1 gram of dried leaves in 1 cup of water and steep for 10 minutes. Drink 2 to 3 cups per day. Damiana is also available in tincture and capsule form. Take 2 to 3 milliliters of the tincture, two or three times per day. In capsules, take 400 milligrams, twice a day.

Ginkgo biloba. Ginkgo has been shown to increase overall circulation as well as bloodflow to the penis. It is available in capsule form. The recommended daily dose is 120 milligrams, twice a day, of extract standardized to 24 percent flavone glycosides and 6 percent terpene lactones. The flavone glycosides give ginkgo its antioxidant benefits, and terpene lactones increase circulation and have a protective effect on nerve cells. However, if you are taking a prescription blood-thinning medication, be sure to consult your doctor before taking ginkgo supplements.

Maca. Maca is a perennial crop from Peru that has been used for centuries. It is grown at elevations of 12,000 feet and higher, is in the same family as turnips and radishes, and is a highly nutritious food. It has an overall nutritive effect that improves physical vitality, endurance, and stamina. Maca is also known for the treatment of male menopause because of its ability to increase sexual desire and performance. It is available in capsule form. The recommended daily dose is 550 milligrams twice a day.

Sarsaparilla. Sarsaparilla has long been regarded as a restorative for the male reproductive organs. It has been used for centuries in Central and South America for the treatment of impotency and as a general tonic for physical weakness. Take 1 cup of dried root tea 2 or 3 times daily. Sarsaparilla is available as packaged tea in natural health food or organic grocery stores. The powdered root is also available in capsules containing 1 to 2 grams of the root powder. In tincture form, take 2 to 3 milliliters of plant extract twice each day.

Hypnosis

Hypnosis has been successful for treating psychological symptoms of male menopause, particularly erectile dysfunction.

To learn more about hypnosis and to locate a qualified practitioner in your area, visit the Web site of the American Society of Clinical Hypnosis at www.asch.net. Schedule an introductory visit to determine his or her experience in treating your condition as well as your comfort level with this person.

Nutritional Supplements

Supplements can increase energy, reduce stress, and help restore normal sexual function.

- Multivitamin/mineral: Take as directed on the label. Ensures proper nutrient level for overall health and vitality.

- B-complex vitamins: Take as directed on the label. Reduce stress.

- L-arginine: 1,000 to 2,000 milligrams daily. Necessary for production of nitric oxide, which is needed to obtain a normal erection.

- Omega-3 fatty acid, like flaxseed oil or fish oil: 1 tablespoon of flaxseed oil daily or 4,000 milligrams daily of fish oil capsules. Beneficial for heart health and mood swings.

- Zinc: 30 milligrams daily. Necessary for normal sexual function in males.

Lifestyle Recommendations

Most men with sexual issues do not consult their physician. Consider bringing up the topic at the next office visit.

Improve your lifestyle. Find time to exercise more. Eat a healthier low-fat, high-fiber diet. Reduce your intake of caffeine and alcohol. Get the sleep that you require.

Lower your cholesterol. Studies have shown that high levels of cholesterol increase your risk for erectile dysfunction.

Reduce stress. Since stress speeds the aging process, find ways to relax, unwind, and reduce your stress. Every day, try to find at least 10 minutes to close your eyes, empty your mind, and breathe deeply.

Stop smoking. Men who smoke are at greater risk for erectile dysfunction than those who don't.

Memory Loss

Having problems remembering places, people, objects, or events? There are two main types of memory loss. Short-term memory loss is forgetfulness of a recent event. Were you just introduced to somebody? Have you already forgotten that person's name? That is short-term memory loss. Long-term memory loss is forgetfulness of something that took place a long time ago. There are three forms of long-term memory loss. Semantic memory involves recalling knowledge, such as an event of historical significance. Procedural memory relates to remembering how to do something, such as driving a car. Episodic memory concerns how you recollect everyday events, such as where you placed your keys. Aging is most likely to affect episodic memory.

There is also a profound form of memory loss known as amnesia, in which there is the partial or total loss of recall. Amnesia may be temporary or permanent.

As people reach midlife, some degree of memory loss is quite common. Fortunately, for most people, the degree of memory loss is mild. The vast majority of people do not develop a serious impairment that interferes with their daily lives.

Causes and Risk Factors

Though a certain amount of memory loss tends to occur with the aging process, memory loss may have other causes, including dementia, in which there are severe problems with memory and thinking. The two most common types of dementia are Alzheimer's disease, in which large numbers of brain cells die, and multi-infarct dementia, in which a series of small strokes or changes in the blood supply cause the death of brain tissue. Multi-infarct dementia is believed to be associated with high blood pressure.

Other causes of memory loss are thyroid disease, head injury, chronic alcohol abuse, use of hallucinogens, menopause, barbiturates, combinations of certain medications, vitamin B_{12} or B_3 (niacin) deficiency, strokes, seizures, infections, depression, atherosclerosis (hardening of the arteries), Parkinson's disease, Pick's disease, electroconvulsive therapy (ECT), and surgery in the temporal lobe of the brain.

Memory loss associated with a progressive illness such as dementia will tend to worsen. Over time, this kind of memory loss interferes with more and more of the activities of daily living.

Your risk for memory problems increases as you age. The simple act of aging places you at risk.

Signs and Symptoms

If you have memory loss, you forget things. Maybe you walk out of the grocery store without the item you most wanted to purchase. Or perhaps you fail to remember what you intended to retrieve when you entered your bedroom. You may have trouble immediately recalling the names of friends. You should realize that forgetfulness is ubiquitous. Everyone experiences some degree of memory loss, but, as you age, certain symptoms of memory loss tend to become more common. For example, it is more likely that you will have trouble learning new material. And you may require longer periods of time to remember already learned information, such as names.

If you have memory loss from a medical problem, you will probably have symptoms of that particular condition. Thus, if you have memory loss from hypothyroidism (low thyroid function), you may experience other symptoms such as fatigue; weight gain; brain fog; feeling cold; intolerance to cold; loss of hair; dry, scaly, itchy skin and scalp; leg cramps; and depression. Or if you have memory loss from depression, you may have a number of additional symptoms, such as depressed mood, agitation, irritability, sleep disturbances, a diminished energy level, reduced self-esteem, slowed movement, and thoughts of death or suicide.

While the early stages of memory loss from a serious progressive illness such as dementia may appear similar to other forms of memory loss, as the disease process continues, the symptoms become more troublesome. During the early stages, you may forget where you placed your keys. As dementia progresses, you may not be able to recall how to use your keys. Similarly, during the early stages, you may forget a phone number. As the disease worsens, you may forget how to use a phone.

It is not uncommon for people with dementia to fail to recall their own home address or other familiar locations. They may neglect personal hygiene and not remember to eat. Eventually, they fail to recognize family and friends. Alzheimer's disease tends to begin slowly, but as the disease continues, there is impairment in thinking, judgment, and the ability to perform everyday tasks. Multi-infarct dementia symptoms typically appear fairly quickly. People with this condition generally improve after a single stroke, and, if more strokes occur, become ill again. The symptoms of both Alzheimer's and multi-infarct dementia may appear together in the same person.

A Quick Guide to Symptoms

☐ **Forgetting everyday things such as where you put your keys**
☐ **Trouble immediately recalling the names of friends**
☐ **Failing to recall your own home address or other familiar locations (dementia)**
☐ **Neglect of personal hygiene and not remembering to eat (dementia)**
☐ **Impairment in thinking, judgment, and the ability to perform everyday tasks (Alzheimer's disease)**

Conventional Treatments

Most mild cases of age-related memory loss are not treated. However, to improve your memory, you may wish to use a number of coping mechanisms.

- Whenever possible, follow a routine. Keep lists of the things you need to do. Record future events on your calendar, and check the calendar often.

- When driving around your town, use landmarks to help you remember places.

- Always store certain items, such as keys, in the same place.

- When you meet new people, repeat their names or even write them down.

If your doctor determines that your memory loss has been caused by a medical disorder, then the underlying cause should be addressed. Thus, if you are found to have hypothyroidism, you will be told to take medication upon awakening every day. If you are found to be depressed, your doctor will likely prescribe medication and advise you to see a therapist. In both instances, when the primary medical problem is corrected, the degree of memory loss should lessen.

Medications

A few medications are helpful for those in the early and middle stages of Alzheimer's disease. By increasing the amount of acetylcholine in the body, they improve memory and delay the worsening of symptoms. These medications include tacrine (Cognex), donepezil (Aricept), rivastigmine (Exelon), and galantamine (Reminyl). Potential side effects include nausea, insomnia, vomiting, diarrhea, fatigue, muscle cramps, and liver damage. To monitor for possible liver damage, periodic liver function tests are ordered. People with multi-infarct dementia need to prevent future strokes

Self-Testing

While there are a number of informal memory tests available on the Internet, you will probably be aware if you have been experiencing trouble with your memory. You may wish to keep a diary of your memory loss to record the dates and times of your memory losses. What were you doing? Had you taken a certain medication or combination of medications?

by controlling their blood pressure, cholesterol, and diabetes. Since behavior problems are often seen in people with dementia, doctors may prescribe medications for agitation, anxiety, depression, and sleeping problems.

Complementary Treatments

Nutritional and lifestyle changes are often recommended to treat memory loss.

Diet

The old saying "You are what you eat" may easily be connected to memory loss. Your brain can function only as well as you feed it. So, it is extremely important to maintain a diet that is high in nutrient-rich foods and to avoid fried foods, hydrogenated fats, and processed foods containing artificial colors and other chemicals. Be sure to include lots of fresh fruits and vegetables and whole grains in your daily diet. Try to include a minimum of five servings of vegetables, four servings of fruit, and six servings of whole grains each day. Vitamin C and beta-carotene, found in many fruits and vegetables, have been shown to improve memory performance. Antioxidants, which are also found in fruits, vegetables, and soy products, may slow memory loss. Preliminary research has shown that monounsaturated fats, such as olive oil, may protect against memory loss and age-related cognitive decline (ARCD).

Herbal Medicine

A number of studies have shown that the antioxidant herb *Ginkgo biloba* improves mental clarity and memory, in addition to overall circulation to the brain. The typical recommended dose is 120 milligrams, twice daily, of extract standardized to 24 percent flavone glycosides and 6 percent terpene lactones. The flavone glycosides give ginkgo its antioxidant benefits, while terpene lactones increase circulation and have a protective effect on nerve cells. If you are also taking prescription blood-thinning medications, be sure to check with a doctor before using ginkgo supplements.

Melatonin

Melatonin, a hormone secreted by the pineal gland in the brain, has been shown to be useful for improving sleep, mood, and memory. As we age, our production of melatonin decreases. Since sleep and mood may affect our ability to remember and to maintain mental clarity, melatonin may be valuable. Take one 1-milligram tablet 30 minutes before going to bed if you have trouble falling asleep. You may need to increase the dose if you are having trouble staying asleep. Generally, 3 milligrams is the highest dose recommended. To ensure proper dosing and to prevent interactions with any other prescription or mood-enhancing medications, check with your doctor before supplementing with melatonin.

Nutritional Supplements

Nutritional deficiencies may lead to various forms of memory loss.

- Multivitamin/mineral: Take as directed on the label. Should include copper, zinc, calcium, and magnesium to help the brain retain memory.

- B-complex vitamins: Take as directed on the label. Essential in preventing and reversing memory loss. B_3 improves circulation to the brain while deficiency may produce dementia, B_1 can decrease effects of senility, and B_6 aids in long-term memory.

- Vitamin B_{12}: Injections. Deficiency may impair mental ability. Injections of B_{12} show improvement in memory.

- Vitamin C: 2,000 milligrams daily in divided doses of 1,000 milligrams. Antioxidant effects help reduce memory loss.

- Vitamin E: 400 IU daily. Antioxidant effects help reduce memory loss.

- Acetyl-L-carnitine: 1,000 milligrams daily in divided doses of 500 milligrams. Improves memory. Take with meals.

- Selenium: 400 micrograms daily, in divided doses of 200 micrograms. May protect the body against toxic effects of mercury.

Psychotherapy

Consider some form of psychotherapy. Internal pressures may lead to an increase in anxiety, anger, depression, and other dysfunctional behavior. When these pressures are addressed, the mind is able to concentrate more clearly and focus better.

Lifestyle Recommendations

Drink plenty of water. If your body lacks sufficient water, you may become dehydrated, feel tired, and have more trouble concentrating. Drink at least eight 8-ounce glasses a day.

Exercise. If you do not already exercise, begin a program of regular exercise. It will improve the flow of blood to your brain. Your exercise program should include some form of aerobic activity (brisk walking, bicycling, or swimming) at least 5 days a week, strength training (weight lifting) at least two or three times per week, and stretching every day.

Learn relaxation techniques. If you are nervous or anxious, you will have a harder time concentrating. Anxiety has been linked to poor memory performance. Studies show that individuals with chronic stress, anxiety, or anger throughout life have a greater chance of cognitive decline in later years. Find ways to reduce your stress.

Make associations. When trying to remember something, begin by thinking of associations. Gradually, the pieces may lead you to what you have forgotten. For example, when attempting to remember the name of a book, you may recall first that it was a mystery. Then, you might realize that it was a hardcover book, and you read it at the beach. Soon, you may be able to think of aspects of the story, even the author's name. Eventually, your mind will be refreshed and activate your memory to remember the title.

Rewrite notes. When trying to remember something, write it down. Then, within 5 hours, rewrite your notes. This will help to ensure that your brain files the information.

Preventive Measures

Avoid alcohol and recreational drugs. These may contribute to memory loss.

Get sufficient sleep. When you don't obtain adequate amounts of sleep, your mind feels foggy, and it is more difficult to concentrate, which contributes to memory loss.

Read labels. Some prescription medications, and even some over-the-counter medications such as antihistamines, may contribute to forgetfulness. Check the side effects of your medications or ask your doctor to determine if these may be contributing to your memory loss.

Stay intellectually challenged. Keep stimulating your mind.

- Enroll in a course at your local community college.
- Learn to play a new instrument.
- Join a study group.
- Attend political and cultural events.
- Do crossword puzzles or play Scrabble.
- Pick up a new hobby.
- Create an interesting part-time business.
- Volunteer.

Menopause

Menopause is a universal passage for all women. During their earlier, reproductive years, women's ovaries produce the hormones estrogen and progesterone, which regulate the monthly menstrual cycles. However, by the time women reach their late thirties, the ovaries are producing lower amounts of these hormones. During the forties, the levels continue to drop. These years are termed *perimenopause*. Eventually, the production of estrogen and progesterone stops, and menstruation ceases.

Though it may occur as early as age 40 or as late as the early sixties, most often this stoppage takes place around the age of 51 or 52. At that point, you are in menopause. When you have not had a period for 12 months, and you have symptoms of menopause, you are considered postmenopausal. With women living longer than in previous generations, it is possible that they may be postmenopausal for a considerable portion of their lives.

Even after the ovaries stop producing estrogen and progesterone, they may continue to make small amounts of the male hormone testosterone. In body fat, it may be converted to estrogen. And the adrenal glands make the male hormone androstenedione, which changes into estrogen-like substances in the body fat.

Several chronic medical conditions tend to appear in women after menopause. These include cardiovascular disease, osteoporosis, stress, urinary incontinence, and weight gain. Menopause has also been linked to gum and eye disorders, urinary tract infections, and colorectal cancer.

Risk Factors

For most women, menopause is a natural midlife process. However, in some cases, it is triggered by surgical or medical treatments. If you have had surgery to remove your uterus, but your ovaries have been left intact, you will begin menopause at your normal time. (Of course, after such surgery, you will not have periods.) On the other hand, if you have had surgery in which both the uterus and ovaries were removed, you will become suddenly menopausal. Also, chemotherapy and radiation therapy may hasten menopause.

Signs and Symptoms

A number of symptoms are associated with female menopause, including hot flashes (intense buildup of body heat that lasts an average of almost 3 minutes), night sweats, cessation of menstruation, pounding heart, difficulty sleeping, mood changes, decline in sexual responsiveness, forgetfulness, urine leakage, vaginal dryness, and joint stiffness. There is even a change in physical appearance. You will notice more fat in your waist and abdomen area and a loss of fullness in your breasts, and your skin will be thinner and more easily wrinkled. Since your body continues to produce small amounts of the male hormone testosterone, coarse hair may appear on your chin, upper lip, chest, or abdomen.

Conventional Treatments

Levels of follicle-stimulating hormone (FSH) increase with menopause. There is a menopause self-test that measures the level of FSH in urine. A separate test evaluates levels of FSH in saliva. However, these tests are considered somewhat unreliable.

If you are experiencing symptoms that may be related to menopause and believe that you may be entering menopause, you should visit your doctor. He or she may wish to determine the levels of FSH and estrogen (estradiol) in your blood. If your FSH level is above 30 and your estradiol level is less than 20, you have probably gone through menopause. If you are still taking birth control pills, then your FSH and estrogen tests should be scheduled at the end of your hormone-free week.

Hormone Replacement Therapy (HRT)

The most common treatment for menopause symptoms is hormone replacement therapy

A Quick Guide to Symptoms

- ☐ Hot flashes
- ☐ Night sweats
- ☐ Cessation of menstruation
- ☐ Pounding heart
- ☐ Difficulty sleeping
- ☐ Mood changes
- ☐ Decline in sexual responsiveness
- ☐ Forgetfulness
- ☐ Urine leakage
- ☐ Vaginal dryness
- ☐ Joint stiffness

(HRT), also known as hormone therapy (HT). If your uterus has been removed, you will take only low-dose estrogen. If your uterus is intact, your doctor will prescribe low-dose estrogen and progestin (any natural or synthetic agent that causes the effects of progesterone), which protects against uterine cancer. HRT is available in a number of forms, such as pills, patches, creams, and vaginal creams.

In addition to aiding with the symptoms of menopause, HRT is known to help prevent bone loss. It also raises the levels of high-density lipoprotein (HDL, the "good" cholesterol) and lowers the levels of low-density lipoprotein (LDL, the "bad" cholesterol). Still, there may be potential side effects such as nausea, bloating, breast tenderness, vaginal bleeding, headaches, dizziness, mood swings, fatigue, and increased risk for blood clots. The patches may cause skin irritation.

Research has also been showing a number of potentially negative health consequences of HRT, especially in those who take it for longer periods of time and at higher doses. HRT may be harmful for women with existing heart disease, and it probably increases the risk of breast cancer. HRT may also be linked to increased rates of stroke and dementia.

Medications

If you have experienced menopause-related bone loss, your doctor may advise taking alendronate (Fosamax) or risedronate (Actonel), which reduce bone loss and the risk of fractures. Alendronate may cause gastrointestinal problems and irritation of the esophagus. Your doctor may also suggest a group of medications known as selective estrogen-receptor modulators (SERMs), such as raloxifene (Evista). They help improve bone loss, but do not increase the risk of breast cancer or uterine bleeding. Unfortunately, they tend to cause hot flashes and increase the risk of blood clots and gallstones.

Complementary Treatments

Complementary medicine works to help a woman's body naturally adjust to the changes that take place during the menopausal years. It offers numerous choices to reduce and potentially eliminate the unpleasant symptoms of menopause. Dietary changes, nutritional supplementation, herbal medicine, exercise, and other lifestyle changes may make this transition process pass smoothly. Together with other complementary medicine therapies, these changes may reduce the risk of conditions associated with the postmenopausal period.

Acupuncture

Acupuncture has successfully treated menopausal symptoms. It can trigger the body to release endorphins, which have a positive effect on the nervous system and help to alleviate symptoms such as anxiety, depression, stress, and insomnia. It can rebalance the hormonal system and reduce the pain and headaches associated with menstruation. Studies have shown that acupuncture reduces hot flashes and night sweats.

Aromatherapy

Essential oils may be useful for many menopausal symptoms because of their sedating and stimulating effects on the nervous system. If you're experiencing menopausal depression, you may want to use oils that have calming and sedating effects, such as lavender, sandalwood, and chamomile. Or for a stimulating effect and to uplift, try clary sage, neroli, jasmine, rosemary, and peppermint. Clary sage, in particular, balances hormones and helps to eliminate night sweats. When your nervous system is fatigued from stress, a bath with oils of neroli, ylang-ylang, peppermint, and jasmine may be valuable.

You can use any of these oils as inhalants

on the edge of your pillow at night, on a tissue, or in a bowl of steaming water. You can also inhale the aroma directly from the bottle. They may be used individually or combined in a bath. If you prefer an individual oil, use 6 to 8 drops. When combining oils, use 2 or 3 drops of each. You can also add several drops of your favorite oils to a carrier oil, such as almond oil, to create a massage blend for daily use.

Ayurveda

Through the use of a special diet, herbs, oils, and incense, Ayurvedic medicine has been successful in treating various symptoms of menopause. To determine an individual's particular constitution and the types of symptoms that are experienced, and to create the appropriate approach to treatment, an assessment is made prior to treatment. There is no professional organization that offers membership to Ayurvedic practitioners. However, the Ayurvedic Institute may provide the names of appropriate professionals in your area. Contact the Institute through its Web site: www.ayurveda.com.

Diet

Diet plays an important role in reducing menopausal symptoms, such as hot flashes, night sweats, and vaginal dryness. A healthy diet may also prevent many conditions that may occur in menopausal women, such as osteoporosis, heart problems, elevated cholesterol levels, and breast cancer. Maintaining a low-fat, high-fiber diet that includes lots of fresh vegetables, fruits, and grains helps the body to adjust to hormonal changes and may reduce cholesterol levels.

To compensate for the body's low estrogen level, it may be useful to eat certain foods that are high in phytoestrogens, particularly soy. Soy contains a class of phytoestrogens (plant estrogens) known as isoflavones (genistein, daidzein, and glycitein). Isoflavones act as weak estrogen and decrease menopausal symptoms. Studies have shown that women who consume high amounts of soy products have a lower incidence of hot flashes. Soy also reduces night sweats and vaginal dryness. One cup of soy milk per day may reduce many menopausal symptoms. Consuming tofu, soybeans, tempeh, and miso is an excellent way to reap these benefits. (Since it contains very little phytoestrogen, soy sauce will not relieve menopausal symptoms.)

Other foods containing phytoestrogens include alfalfa, almonds, anise seeds, apples, barley, beans, beets, berries, carrots, cashews, cherries, clover, cucumbers, dates, eggplant, fennel, flaxseed, garlic, lentils, oats, olives, parsley, peanuts, peas, peppers, plums, pomegranates, rhubarb, sage, sesame seeds, sunflower seeds, tomatoes, yams, and whole grains.

Individuals consuming animal protein lose more calcium through urine excretion than those who get their protein from soy. Since calcium is essential in preventing osteoporosis, it's a good idea to cut back on animal protein and increase your consumption of soy protein. Other foods that contain calcium include dark green, leafy vegetables such as broccoli, collard greens, and kale; kelp; almonds; sesame seeds; and sardines.

Boron is a trace mineral that helps prevent osteoporosis by reducing the loss of calcium in the urine. Eating boron-rich foods will also raise estrogen levels. Boron is found in a number of fruits and vegetables such as apples, pears, grapes, peaches, peas, and beans. Almonds, peanuts, and raisins also contain boron.

Essential fatty acids (EFAs) are useful in maintaining hormonal balance and preventing vaginal dryness. EFAs may be found in salmon, bluefish, herring, mackerel, tuna, cod, almonds, peanuts, walnuts, and sunflower seeds. Flaxseed oil is also a good source of essential fatty acids.

It should be noted that there are some foods that trigger or aggravate menopausal symptoms. These include sugar, alcohol, caffeine, spicy foods, and refined foods. Caffeine, spicy foods, and alcohol cause the blood vessels to dilate, leading to hot flashes. Sugar and refined foods may cause mood swings. Alcohol, caffeine, soft drinks, refined foods, and animal protein rob the body of calcium and other minerals, increasing the risk of osteoporosis. Finally, there are a few foods that actually inhibit estrogen production, including onions, dill, and thyme. However, if you are eating the previously outlined diet, consuming these foods in moderation should not be a problem.

Exercise

There are numerous benefits to regular, moderate exercise. When estrogen levels decrease, the levels of endorphins released in the body also decline. Exercise increases the release of these endorphins, which are brain chemicals that help regulate body temperature and decrease stress, mood swings, and depression. Studies have shown that regular exercise—3 to 4 hours per week—may decrease the frequency and severity of hot flashes. Those who exercise are less likely to have mood swings than those who do not exercise. Further, they have quicker mental agility.

Regular exercise slows the loss of dopamine, a neurotransmitter that helps to prevent shaking and stiffness. Dopamine also supports our ability to react, thereby reducing the risk of falling.

During the 5 years that follow the cessation of menstruation, bone density decreases rapidly. Without exercise, bones diminish in size and strength. Exercise is even better for bones than estrogen replacement. While estrogen protects bones, exercise maintains and increases bone density. At any age, bones may be rebuilt with weight-bearing activity, such as walking. Weight-bearing exercise also helps normalize the flow of sugar from the blood into muscle tissue, where it may be properly metabolized, reducing the risk of diabetes. Exercise improves muscle mass, strength, gait, flexibility, balance, and coordination.

You should create an exercise routine that

includes an overall body program. It should incorporate weight-bearing exercises, strength training for the arms and legs, and postural training to support the back and posture. Otherwise, only the area being trained will receive adequate conditioning. For example, walking will increase bone density and muscle mass in the legs, but unless free weights are used to condition the arms during the walk, it will have no effect on the arms. In addition to walking, weight-bearing activities include running, jumping rope, step aerobics, and stair climbing. You may wish to use rubber exercise bands for your resistance training. The more resistance you use, the better the benefit. You may use light free weights with multiple repetitions for strength training.

It should be noted that almost any exercise is better than none. Since they increase flexibility and strength, housecleaning and gardening are considered exercise. Simply walking a minimum of 20 minutes, three times a week, may enhance bloodflow and stimulate the uptake of bone-building nutrients.

Herbal Medicine

Many herbal remedies may reduce the symptoms of menopause and assist in naturally replacing estrogen. However, each herb may not be for everyone. Choose an herb that addresses your individual symptoms, but make sure that it doesn't interact with any other medical problem you may have. For example, licorice decreases hot flashes, but it

Benefits of Exercise

The benefits of exercise for menopausal women include the following:

☐ **Better sleep**
☐ **Strengthening of bones and prevention of osteoporosis**
☐ **Prevention or elimination of constipation**
☐ **Weight control and reduction of body fat**
☐ **Diminished appetite with increased metabolism**
☐ **Decreased risk for heart disease, colon cancer, diabetes, and arthritis**
☐ **Decreased joint stiffness and muscular aches and pains**
☐ **Strengthening of muscles, ligaments, and tendons**
☐ **Boosting the immune system**

also increases blood pressure. So, if you are dealing with high blood pressure, you may want to consider another herb.

Black cohosh. Black cohosh, which is the natural alternative to hormone replacement therapy, may be taken in capsule form. The minimum recommended daily dose is 20 milligrams in the morning and 20 milligrams at night of standardized extract of 2.5 percent triterpene glycosides. Your doctor may advise a higher dose. Black cohosh relieves night sweats, hot flashes, cramping, ringing in the ears, heart palpitations, irritability, vaginal atrophy, profuse sweating, anxiety, and depression. Further, it lowers cholesterol levels and blood pressure. Expect to take black cohosh for about 4 weeks before you notice any improvement.

Chasteberry. Chasteberry contains estrogen- and progesterone-like compounds. Through its effect on the pituitary gland, chasteberry may balance hormones and alleviate depression. Look for products containing 0.5 percent agnuside, the active ingredient. Take 400 milligrams a day.

Dong quai and Asian ginseng. Dong quai and Asian ginseng are herbs with estrogenic properties that may be helpful for those with low estrogen levels. Dong quai relieves night sweats and hot flashes and also promotes relaxation and strengthens blood vessels. The recommended daily dose is 200 milligrams three times a day of extract standardized to 0.8 to 1.1 percent ligustilide. However, if you are taking a prescription blood-thinning medication, be sure to consult your doctor before taking dong quai supplements. Asian ginseng is effective for decreasing mental and physical fatigue and increasing energy. The recommended daily dose is 100 to 200 milligrams, standardized to 4 to 7 percent ginsenosides. However, do not use ginseng if you have high blood pressure, heart disorders, or hypoglycemia.

Maca. Maca is a perennial crop from Peru that has been used for centuries. It is grown at elevations of 12,000 feet and higher, is in the same family as turnips and radishes, and is a highly nutritious food. It has an overall nutritive effect that improves physical vitality, endurance, and stamina. Maca is also known for the treatment of menopause because of its ability to regulate hormones, reduce hot flashes and mood swings, and fuel

the endocrine system so that it can produce its own hormones. It is available in capsule form. The recommended daily dose is 550 milligrams twice a day.

Teas. Several herbal teas are beneficial for the symptoms of menopause. St. John's wort is good for anxiety or irritability. Sage is useful for night sweats. Valerian and chamomile are helpful for insomnia. And, as previously noted, licorice decreases hot flashes, while increasing blood pressure.

Naturopathy

A naturopathic physician is an excellent practitioner to guide you through the menopausal cycle. Naturopaths are trained in all facets of natural medicine and are able to offer advice about lifestyle changes. These may include how to develop a fitness regimen and suggestions for herbal and nutritional supplements and dietary changes. Contact the American Association of Naturopathic Physicians at www.naturopathic.org to find a practitioner in your area.

Nutritional Supplements

Nutritional supplements can help slow the aging process and alleviate symptoms associated with female menopause.

- Multivitamin/mineral: Take as directed on the label. Should include A, C, E, and selenium, which strengthen the immune system and slow the aging process.

- B-complex vitamins: Take as directed on the label. Maintain energy and reduce other menopausal symptoms such as anxiety, depression, insomnia, and loss of libido.

- Calcium: 1,500 milligrams daily in divided doses of 500 milligrams. Relieves muscle cramps and helps prevent bone density changes. Take with magnesium.

- Evening primrose oil: 3,000 milligrams daily in divided doses of 1,000 milligrams each to provide 240 milligrams of GLA (gamma-linolenic acid). May diminish the frequency and intensity of hot flashes.

- Magnesium: 750 milligrams daily in divided doses of 250 milligrams. Assists in calcium absorption and relieves anxiety.

- Omega-3 fatty acids: 1 tablespoon flaxseed oil or 2,000 milligrams fish oil in capsule form twice a day. Reduces vaginal dryness.

Relaxation/Meditation

Studies have shown that the frequency, intensity, and duration of hot flashes are associated with stress. As a result, any form of meditation or relaxation in which the mind is focused on a particular object, sound, visualization, breath, or activity is useful for reversing the body's fight-or-flight response to stress. Yoga and tai chi are considered meditation in movement and relax muscles, quiet the mind, and create inner peace. You can meditate while lying down or in a seated position. Be sure to sit properly—upright with your back straight, on a chair or the floor.

Yoga

Studies have shown yoga to be beneficial for alleviating menopausal symptoms such as insomnia, depression, hot flashes, mood swings, and vaginal and urinary problems. The postures increase flexibility and improve coordination and balance, while strengthening the muscles and increasing blood circulation. The deep breathing exercises that are part of a yoga session increase blood circulation and elevate the level of endorphins released in the brain.

Lifestyle Recommendations

Consider some of the following ways to help cope with the symptoms associated with menopause.

Avoid constipation. Be sure to maintain regular bowel movements. Women who are constipated and not on a regular elimination routine may reabsorb hormones that should be eliminated.

Be prepared for vaginal dryness. If you have been experiencing vaginal dryness, purchase some over-the-counter water-based vaginal lubricants such as Astroglide or moisturizers such as Replens. In addition, wheat germ oil, which contains vitamin E, may also be used as a lubricant. It may be combined with other soothing oils such as marigold, chamomile, or slippery elm.

Don't smoke. Women who smoke tend to have an earlier menopause and hot flashes that are more intense. Smoking significantly decreases a woman's total circulating estrogen. In addition, smoking is associated with heart disease, stroke, cancer, and other medical problems.

Drink water. Drinking lots of water throughout the day may help regulate body temperature and decrease hot flashes and vaginal dryness.

Exercise your pelvic floor. To strengthen your pelvic floor, practice Kegel exercises. Begin by identifying your pelvic muscles—this may be done by slowing or stopping the urine flow while you are urinating. These are the muscles you need to make stronger. Try to perform 5 to 15 contractions, three to five times daily. Hold each Kegel for a count of 5 to start, and gradually work your way to a count of 10. But don't do too many, as women who overexercise these muscles may make them too tight.

Get your vitamin D. Getting 10 to 15 minutes of direct sunlight several times a week can ensure that your body absorbs sufficient vitamin D. Vitamin D is essential for absorption of calcium, which is necessary for bone health. Remember to use sunscreen if you spend longer than the recommended 10 to 15 minutes in the sun. If you are unable to spend time in the sun, you can get vitamin D in your diet through eggs and fish such as cod, mackerel, sardines, salmon, and tuna. It is also available in supplement form. Take 400 IU daily or at least three times a week.

Help yourself sleep better. If you have trouble sleeping, don't exercise at night or drink caffeinated beverages after lunch. Learn some relaxation techniques such as deep breathing, progressive muscle relaxation, and guided imagery. If you have hot flashes, wear cool cotton clothing to bed.

Join or start a support group. To cope with the changes caused by menopause, you may benefit from talking to other women who are going through menopause.

Keep a hot flash diary. To help determine what triggers your hot flashes, keep a diary. If you are aware of the triggers, you may be able to take action to prevent them.

Wear breathable clothing. Cotton clothing is more absorbent and cooler for the body than clothing made from silk or synthetic fabrics. You may wish to dress in light layers, which may be easily removed during a hot flash.

Metabolic Syndrome

With metabolic syndrome, also known as insulin resistance syndrome, your fat, muscle, and liver cells are unable to respond appropriately to the hormone insulin. As a result, your pancreas keeps making high amounts of insulin. Metabolic syndrome also involves excess body fat, especially around the waist, abnormal blood lipid levels, and borderline or elevated blood pressure.

If your body is unable to regulate blood sugar levels, as is the case in about 25 percent of those affected by insulin resistance, you may develop type 2 diabetes. Type 2 diabetes is associated with a number of serious medical problems, such as heart disease, blindness, and kidney disease. In most instances, however, you will not develop type 2 diabetes. Instead, your body will simply keep producing increasing amounts of insulin, a condition known as hyperinsulinemia. Your glucose levels remain high, but within normal limits. Still, the high levels make you more vulnerable to a host of other medical problems, such as heart disease, stroke, and high blood pressure.

According to the National Cholesterol Education Program, if you have any three of the following medical problems, you probably have metabolic syndrome: blood pressure of at least 130 (systolic) or at least 85 (diastolic), fasting blood sugar of at least 110 (or greater than 140 at 2 hours into the glucose tolerance test), fasting triglycerides of at least 150, fasting HDL ("good") cholesterol of less than 40, or abdominal obesity. Abdominal obesity is defined as a waist size of greater than 40 inches in males and 35 inches in females.

Some believe that metabolic syndrome is responsible for as many as 50 percent of all heart attacks. Even when there is no evidence of diabetes or cardiovascular disease, men with metabolic syndrome are at increased risk for cardiovascular disease and mortality from any cause. In addition, since the presence of metabolic syndrome is a significant predictor for type 2 diabetes and cardiovascular disease, it may help identify those at high risk for these disorders.

Research has also linked insulin resistance to the formation of more dense LDL (bad) cholesterol, high levels of fat in the blood after eating, slow clearance of fat from the blood, a decreased ability to break up blood clots, and high blood levels of uric acid.

Metabolic syndrome is very common. The prevalence is around 6.7 percent for individuals between the ages of 20 and 29 to around 43.5 percent for people between the ages of 60 and 69. Mexican Americans have the highest prevalence. African American women have a 57 percent higher prevalence than African American men, and Mexican American women have 26 percent higher prevalence than Mexican American men. According to 2000 census data, about 47 million US residents have metabolic syndrome.

Causes and Risk Factors

While the exact cause of metabolic syndrome is unknown, it is quite apparent that family history plays a strong role. You are at increased risk if your family members tend to have type 2 diabetes, high blood pressure, or cardiovascular disease, or if you have a history of glucose intolerance, gestational diabetes, high blood pressure, elevated triglycerides and low HDL cholesterol, or cardiovascular disease. Women who have polycystic ovarian syndrome (PCOS), a leading cause of infertility in women, are at high risk for metabolic syndrome. Also, risk increases after the age of 40.

Nonwhites are at higher risk than whites. People with European ancestry have lower risks than those with non-European ancestry. Polynesian Islanders and Native Americans have an extremely high risk. But lifestyle factors appear to be equally important. Lack of physical exercise, obesity, a diet high in carbohydrates, and cigarette smoking all contribute to this disorder.

Signs and Symptoms

People with metabolic syndrome tend to gain weight, especially around the waist, have frequent cravings for sweets, breads, and other simple carbohydrates, and complain of fatigue, particularly after meals.

Conventional Treatments

Since insulin resistance grows worse as the pounds increase, treatment for metabolic syndrome generally begins with a weight loss program that includes exercise. To keep the glucose under control, your body has been producing more insulin. As your weight drops, your insulin resistance will improve. In many instances, weight loss and exercise are the only treatments needed.

Medications

When weight loss and exercise are unable to control metabolic syndrome, your doctor may prescribe medications to treat the problems associated with the disorder. Thus, if your lipids are high, you will probably be given a lipid-lowering medication, and if you have high blood pressure, you will probably be given a blood pressure–lowering prescription. On occasion, a medi-

A Quick Guide to Symptoms

☐ **Weight gain, especially around the waist**
☐ **Frequent cravings for sweets, breads, and other simple carbohydrates**
☐ **Fatigue, particularly after meals**

cation for diabetes, such as metformin, may be prescribed for someone with metabolic syndrome.

Complementary Treatments

The focus of complementary medicine is on examining lifestyle habits that may lead to conditions resulting in the metabolic syndrome. This includes a sedentary lifestyle and a diet high in nutrient-poor foods. Because the metabolic syndrome is a cluster of symptoms that are related, eliminating some of these may work toward improving the others.

Diet

Diet plays an important role in preventing and reversing metabolic syndrome. It is important to understand what foods to avoid and why you should avoid them. Simple carbohydrates such as breads, pasta, bagels, white flour, white rice, sweets, and other foods made with sugar and other concentrated sweeteners impair your ability to control blood sugar. These foods increase the risk for type 2 diabetes, increase triglycerides, and lower HDL. Complex carbohydrates such as whole grains, corn, and potatoes may also raise blood sugar levels. If you already have metabolic syndrome, these foods should be eliminated until your blood pressure, blood fats, and weight are normalized. Nonstarchy vegetables, such as salad greens, asparagus, green beans, spinach, and broccoli, may be eaten

freely. They raise the blood sugar only minimally and are filled with other nutrients and fiber.

Protein stimulates the production of a hormone called glucagon that opposes insulin. Because it helps to burn stored fat and prevents the urge to overeat carbohydrates, protein is useful when consumed in small amounts throughout the day. Good sources of protein are fish, poultry, and high-protein dairy foods such as eggs, cottage cheese, and tofu. However, beans, which also contain protein, are not good for individuals with metabolic syndrome, as they may raise blood sugar and insulin levels.

Omega-3 fatty acids lower blood pressure, reduce the risk of heart attack and stroke, and may help with weight gain—all issues associated with metabolic syndrome. Good sources of omega-3's are cold-water fish such as salmon, tuna, herring, and mackerel. In fact, eating cold-water fish once a week may reduce the risk of heart attack. Extra-virgin olive oil, grape seed oil, flaxseed oil, hempseed oil, and walnut oil should replace vegetable oils when cooking and preparing foods.

Fried foods, margarine, and any other foods that contain partially hydrogenated oils should be eliminated from the diet, as should sweetened fruit drinks, sodas, and alcohol.

Herbal Medicine

As it helps maintain normal liver function, milk thistle is extremely beneficial for preventing or reversing metabolic syndrome. The liver plays a role in maintaining blood sugar. Milk thistle is available in capsule form. The typical recommended daily dose is 300 milligrams per day. Look for capsules containing 80 percent silymarin.

Nutritional Supplements

Nutritional supplements play a role in proper insulin function.

- Vitamin C: 1,000 milligrams daily in divided doses of 500 milligrams. Helps normalize blood sugar and insulin function.

- Vitamin E: 400 IU daily. Helps normalize blood sugar and insulin function.

- Alpha-lipoic acid: 200 milligrams daily in divided doses of 100 milligrams. Helps normalize blood sugar and insulin function. Increases the potency of vitamins C and E.

- Calcium: 1,500 milligrams daily in divided doses of 500 milligrams. May improve insulin sensitivity in those with high blood pressure.

- Chromium picolinate: 200 micrograms daily. Deficiency disturbs normal insulin function. Necessary for preventing or reversing metabolic syndrome.

- Coenzyme Q_{10}: 200 milligrams daily. May reduce glucose and insulin blood levels.

- Glucomannan (bulk-forming dietary fiber derived from konjac root): dosage to be determined by your health-care provider. Drink at least 8 ounces of water with each dose. Stabilizes blood sugar in insulin-resistant individuals, reduces triglycerides and LDL cholesterol, and raises HDL cholesterol. Do not take if you have any esophageal disorder.

- L-carnitine: 1,000 milligrams daily in divided doses of 500 milligrams. May reduce glucose and insulin blood levels.

- Magnesium: 750 milligrams daily in divided doses of 250 milligrams. Deficiency disturbs normal insulin function. Necessary for preventing or reversing metabolic syndrome.

- Omega-3 fatty acids: 1 tablespoon of flaxseed oil daily. Lowers blood pressure and reduces risk of heart attack and stroke.

- Zinc: 30 milligrams daily. Deficiency disturbs normal insulin function. Necessary for preventing or reversing metabolic syndrome.

Lifestyle Recommendations

While obesity and physical inactivity do not cause metabolic syndrome, they do make the condition worse. Losing weight will help lower your insulin levels. Even a loss of only 10 to 15 pounds may significantly reduce insulin levels. And a loss of weight will make the body more insulin sensitive, so that less insulin is required for the same task of moving sugar from the bloodstream into various tissues.

Exercise will lower insulin and blood triglyceride levels while also raising HDL cholesterol. In the beginning, especially if you have been sedentary, you may be able to exercise for only 5 to 10 minutes. Try to build up to a minimum of 30 minutes of aerobic exercise at least three or four times each week. In people with insulin resistance, the combination of aerobic activity with strength training works best. In addition to the above benefits, regular exercise also reduces stress, lowers blood pressure, and strengthens the heart and blood vessels. Of course, before beginning an exercise program, you should check with your doctor.

Preventive Measures

Reduce stress. Studies have shown that stress may lead to decreased insulin sensitivity. Meditation, biofeedback, and relaxation techniques such as deep breathing are all good ways to reduce stress.

Stop smoking. Researchers have determined that smokers are more insulin resistant and have higher insulin levels than nonsmokers. Smokers also have higher levels of blood triglycerides and lower HDL cholesterol levels. By smoking, you increase your probability of developing metabolic syndrome. Secondhand smoke and nicotine patches have the same effect as smoking.

Watch salt intake. Salt should be used in moderation, whether you currently have metabolic syndrome or are trying to prevent it.

Muscle Cramps

During a cramp, a muscle involuntarily and painfully contracts. Muscles are bundles of fibers that produce movement by contracting and expanding. Muscle cramps, which are also called muscle spasms, may occur in part of a muscle group, over an entire muscle group, or in several muscle groups.

The most likely muscles to cramp are those that span two joints, such as the calves (gastrocnemius), the back of the thighs (hamstrings), and the front of the thighs (quadriceps). However, you may experience muscle cramps in other parts of the body, such as the arms, abdomen, hands, feet, and along the rib cage. If you spend a good deal of time writing with a pen or pencil, you may even have muscle cramps in your thumb and first two fingers.

Muscle Cramps May Signal a Serious Illness

While most muscle cramps are benign, sometimes they indicate a more serious condition. Some of the medical problems that may cause muscle cramps include narrowing of the spinal canal (stenosis), thyroid disease, chronic infections, cirrhosis of the liver, hardening of the arteries, spinal nerve irritation or compression (radiculopathy), and amyotrophic lateral sclerosis (ALS or Lou Gehrig's disease).

Muscle cramps may vary in intensity, ranging from a slight tic to severe pain. A badly cramped muscle may feel quite hard to the touch. It may appear distorted under your skin. And you may see it twitching. A muscle cramp may last a few seconds or more than 15 minutes, and it may recur.

Muscle cramps are extremely common. At some point, just about everyone has experienced them.

Causes and Risk Factors

Though the exact cause of muscle cramps is unknown, some contend that muscles that have not received adequate stretching or muscles that are fatigued are at increased risk for cramps. Other factors that may be associated with muscle cramps include exercising or working in intense heat, dehydration, and the depletion of salt and minerals known as electrolytes, such as calcium, magnesium, and potassium.

Muscle cramps and pain may also be associated with the use of statin drugs to lower cholesterol. Some studies report 1 to 5 percent incidence of these symptoms in statin users. In order to prevent muscle pain and cramps, you should use the lowest dosage of statin needed to lower cholesterol, and report any muscle pain immediately to your doctor.

Because of the normal muscle loss that comes with aging, we are at increased risk for muscle cramps as we age. Aging places us at particular risk for cramps that occur at night while we are sleeping. Inactivity only exacerbates the risk for muscle cramps. On the other hand, endurance athletes, such as those who run marathons, also have a greater risk for muscle cramps.

Signs and Symptoms

With muscle cramps, the most significant symptom is pain. You may also be able to feel the cramped muscle and to see it twitching under the skin.

Conventional Treatments

Muscle cramps may be treated in a number of ways. Begin by relaxing the cramped muscle and gently massaging the area. Then, slowly stretch the muscle.

For cramps in your calves, you may try standing about 3 feet from a wall. Keep your knees straight and your heels on the floor. While supporting yourself with your hands, lean into the wall; remain in that position for 1 minute. Repeat the exercise three times.

If you have muscle cramps that repeatedly disturb your sleep, your doctor may prescribe diazepam (Valium). It relaxes muscles and decreases stiffness. Other muscle relaxants include verapamil (Calan, Isoptin, Verelan), chloroquine (Aralen), and hydroxychloroquine (Plaquenil).

A Quick Guide to Symptoms

☐ **Pain**
☐ **Twitching**

Complementary Treatments

Complementary medicine works best when the cause of the muscle cramps has been determined. You can then make appropriate dietary and lifestyle adjustments. Treatments attempt both to reduce the severity of existing muscle cramps and to prevent future muscle cramps from occurring.

Aromatherapy

Peppermint oil relieves pain, eases muscle spasms, and reduces inflammation. The essential oils of eucalyptus, juniper, and rosemary relieve muscular aches and pains. To promote muscular relaxation, any of these oils may be used in a warm bath. When combining any of these oils, do not use more than 10 drops total. Eucalyptus and peppermint are very strong—even when used alone, you need only 2 or 3 drops in a tub full of water. You may also use these oils to massage a sore area. Place 10 drops in 1 ounce of oil, such as almond oil (if you do not want to purchase a special oil, you may use canola oil). To combine the oils, don't shake the bottle; gently roll it between your hands. Then, massage the sore area. When massaging calf muscles, massage from the ankles up toward the heart.

Diet

Many nutrients play an important role in preventing muscle cramps. As a nutritional deficiency may be the cause of your muscle cramps, don't overlook the following nutrients.

- Bioflavonoids: found in many fruits and vegetables
- Potassium: found in bananas, oranges, broccoli, dates, and raisins
- Magnesium: found in whole grains, beans, almonds, and brewer's yeast
- Calcium: found in dairy foods, tofu, figs, green leafy vegetables, and salmon

Iron and vitamin E are also helpful in preventing cramps. Iron may be found in brewer's yeast as well as in fortified cereals and dried fruit. Vitamin E is found in wheat germ, soybeans, whole grains, green leafy vegetables, and vegetable oils.

Exercise

Both the lack of exercise and excessive exercising may cause muscle cramps. Whether you have been exercising too little or too much, if you have been experiencing muscle cramps, start over with moderate, limited exercises. Gradually, over time, increase your routine. Don't use stretching as your warmup. Begin with a slow jog or walk to warm the body and supply oxygen and nutrients to the muscles, then stretch. Remember that the cooldown period is just as important as the warmup. After you cool down, end with some final stretches.

Homeopathy

Nux vomica 9C and *Cuprum metallicum* 9C are two homeopathic treatments commonly

Stretches for Your Muscles

Consider beginning and ending your exercise routine with the following stretches. These can also be practiced before going to bed. Hold each stretch for 30 to 45 seconds and repeat each one two or three times. Do not bounce when stretching. Bouncing activates the reflex that actually tightens the muscles. Also, the excess bouncing may cause muscles to rip.

☐ **Calf muscle stretch:** Stand 2½ to 3 feet from a wall. Lean forward and place your hands on the wall. Keeping your heels down, gradually move your hands up the wall as high as you can. Lean in toward the wall and hold the position for 45 seconds.

☐ **Hamstring muscle stretch:** Sit with one leg folded with the foot against the side of the other leg, which should be straight out with the foot upright. Lean forward and touch the foot of the straightened leg or come as close to touching the foot as you can without straining. Change leg positions and repeat.

☐ **Quadriceps muscle stretch:** While you are standing, bend your leg up behind you and hold the top of the foot with the opposite hand; pull the foot toward the buttocks. (Use your other hand on the wall or a chair to maintain your balance.) Repeat with the opposite leg.

used for muscle cramps. Alternate three pellets of each, three times per day. Another homeopathic treatment, arnica, is available as an ointment. Apply it to the affected area as directed. In order to obtain the best treatment for your particular muscle cramps, you may consider consulting with a homeopath, who will be able to individualize your treatment plan. To find a practitioner trained in homeopathy, visit the Web site of the National Center for Homeopathy at www.homeopathic.org.

Hydrotherapy

Alternating hot and cold compresses may bring relief to a muscle cramp. Wring out a washcloth soaked in hot water and apply it to the affected area for 2 minutes. Place the washcloth back in the hot water and wring out a washcloth soaked in cold water with ice. Place this over the affected area for 40 seconds. End by placing the hot cloth on the muscle again for 2 more minutes.

Nutritional Supplements

Certain supplements help improve circulation and prevent muscle cramps.

- Vitamin C: 2,000 milligrams daily in divided doses of 1,000 milligrams. Improves circulation.

- Vitamin E: 400 IU daily. Deficiency may cause muscle cramping in the legs.

- Calcium: 1,500 milligrams daily in divided doses of 500 milligrams. Works well with magnesium in preventing muscle cramps.

- Magnesium: 750 milligrams daily in divided doses of 250 milligrams. Prevents muscle cramps, promotes good night's sleep.

Therapeutic Massage

Regular massage therapy has been shown to relax muscles and increase circulation, providing oxygen and nutrients to tired, overworked muscles. For centuries, massage has been used as a preventive measure against muscular cramping as well as a therapeutic treatment to release muscle cramps.

Yoga

By stretching and increasing the circulation to the muscles, yoga has been shown to decrease the frequency of leg cramps.

Lifestyle Recommendations

Consider a medication change. If you are on a diuretic medication, check with your doctor. Often, because of dehydration from the diuretic, an adjustment in the dose will relieve muscle cramps.

Stop a cramp on the go. If you develop a cramp in your calf while walking, stop and shake the affected leg, then continue on your way. When you're able, stop and support yourself against a wall, a tree, a bench—whatever you can find. Then point your toes up toward your head to stretch your calf muscle.

Try tonic water. Quinine, found in tonic water, has been used for years as a remedy for muscle cramps.

Visit a physical therapist or personal trainer. Physical therapists and personal trainers are able to design special exercises to reduce your bouts with muscle cramps. By completing these exercises regularly, you may see considerable improvement in your condition.

When you exercise, drink extra fluid. If you can, about 2 hours before you begin physical activity or exercising, begin drinking fluid—at least 2 cups. For every 15 to 20 minutes of physical activity or exercise, try to drink another cup or more of fluid. Drink another cup of fluid upon completion of exercise.

Preventive Measures

Avoid overheating. Muscle cramps are one of the first signs of heat stroke. If you are exposed to warm temperatures for a prolonged period of time, the best prevention is to drink plenty of fluids, especially sports drinks with electrolytes.

Avoid tight clothing. In order to give your muscles room to move, avoid tight clothing. For those experiencing muscle cramps during sleep, this is particularly helpful at night. Make sure your pajamas are roomy.

Get your vitamin D. Getting 10 to 15 minutes of direct sunlight several times a week can ensure that your body absorbs sufficient vitamin D. Vitamin D is essential for absorption of calcium, which helps to prevent muscle cramps. Remember to use sunscreen if you spend longer than the recommended 10 to 15 minutes in the sun. If you are unable to spend time in the sun, you can get vitamin D in your diet through eggs and fish such as cod, mackerel, sardines, salmon, and tuna. It is also available in supplement form. Take 400 IU daily or at least three times a week.

Improve your posture. If you spend hours each day hunched before a computer, you increase your risk for neck and leg cramps due to a shortening of the muscles and poor circulation.

Loosen your bed covers. To reduce your risk for muscle cramps while you sleep, loosen your covers at the foot of the bed to prevent your feet from pointing down.

Participate in aquatic exercise. Regular exercise in water will stretch, lengthen, and strengthen your muscles, making them less likely to cramp.

Practice deep breathing. To help avoid side stitches (rib cage muscle spasms), practice slow, deep breathing exercises regularly.

Remain hydrated. To help avoid muscle cramps, it is recommended that every day you drink at least six to eight glasses of water or other fluids. If you are exercising or working in the heat, you may wish to drink a sports beverage that contains electrolytes to help prevent dehydration.

Stretch regularly. Throughout the day, periodically stretch your muscles, especially your calves. If you tend to have muscle cramps at night, before going to bed, you may wish to spend a few minutes stretching or riding a stationary bike.

Wear sensible shoes. Be realistic about your shoes. Be sure to pick comfortable styles that are appropriate for what you are doing. Improper shoes may leave you with muscle cramps in your legs and feet.

Nail Fungus

It's unsightly, it's aggravating, and it's persistent. Nail fungus, also known as onychomycosis or ringworm of the nail, is a parasitic infection in the nails of the fingers or toes. Most often, a nail fungal infection involves a group of fungi called dermatophytes, which include *Trichophyton rubrum* and *Trichophyton mentagrophytes*. They thrive on keratin, the protein in the nail. But a nail fungus may also thrive on yeasts (*Candida albicans* or *Candida parapsilosis*), mold, or even the acrylic nail bonding agent methyl methacrylate, which may be used by discount salons instead of the safer ethyl methacrylate. Toenails are more likely to be affected than fingernails. The big toes and little toes have the highest risk, probably because they are exposed to the most friction from shoes.

Nail fungus is a relatively common problem. Though many people are unaware of the condition, it has been estimated that 12 million Americans have this disorder. Men are twice as likely as women to have a nail fungus, and the incidence appears to increase with age.

Causes and Risk Factors

A nail fungal infection usually occurs when a nail is damaged or exposed over an extended period of time to a warm, moist environment. People who spend a good deal of time working with water, such as dishwashers and cleaning personnel, are at increased risk. Those with diabetes or HIV are also at greater risk, as are those who tend to perspire a lot from their feet and/or have a history of athlete's foot. Other factors that add to the risk include poor circulation and hot, humid weather.

Fungi are simple parasitic plant organisms. Since they lack chlorophyll, they do not need sunlight to grow.

Signs and Symptoms

A nail fungus usually begins with a small separation between the end of the nail and the skin under the nail (the nail bed). With time, a yellow material forms in this separation, and the nail becomes thick and yellow or brown. There may be white spots on the nail, and foul-smelling debris under the nail. Unless the area becomes infected or is so thick that it presses against the inside of your shoes, there should be little or no pain. But when a nail is infected, there may be a good deal of pain, and you may find it uncomfortable to walk or stand. However, in time, the nail separates, and you are left with a moderately destroyed yellow nail that may fall off. Even if the nail falls off, the new nail will grow in with the fungus.

Conventional Treatments

Unfortunately, without treatment, nail fungus persists. So, unless you are content to watch

A Quick Guide to Symptoms

- ☐ Separation between the end of the nail and the skin under the nail
- ☐ Nail becomes thick and yellow or brown
- ☐ White spots on the nail
- ☐ Foul-smelling debris under the nail

your nails deteriorate, see a doctor. Your treatment may begin with your doctor attempting to remove as much of the affected nail as possible. This may involve trimming the nail with clippers, filing it down, or dissolving it with a paste that contains urea and bifonazole.

If the affected area is relatively small, your doctor may prescribe a medicated nail polish that contains ciclopirox (Loprox). This should be applied to the nail daily until the fungus is completely gone. This treatment is more effective than placebo and appears to be safe. It may be useful for people who are unable to take oral antifungal drugs. Studies are needed to demonstrate how long the nail will remain free of the fungus.

Medications

Since nail fungus often involves a wider area or more than one nail, your doctor may prescribe an antifungal drug that is taken orally for several months, which is necessary because nails grow slowly. Terbinafine (Lamisil) and itraconazole (Sporanox) are each taken for up to 3 months and may be up to 70 percent effective. Griseofulvin (Fulvicin, Grisactin) is taken for 6 months and is up to 40 percent effective. The use of griseofulvin has been superseded by terbinafine and itraconazole.

These medications have potential side effects such as nausea, rash, vomiting, stomach upset, and headaches. Less common side effects are blood disorders and liver damage. Because of possible liver problems, itraconazole should not be used by people taking simvastatin, lovastatin, triazolam, or cisapride. Before beginning treatment, your doctor will test your liver enzymes, and again during the course of your treatment.

As an alternative, your doctor may recommend fluconazole (Diflucan). The recommended dose is one 150-milligram tablet a week for 26 weeks. While this drug's efficacy of 48 percent may not be as high as for the other medications, it has fewer side effects, and with only one pill per week, it is easier to take.

It should be noted that for all of these medications, the rate of relapse—where the fungus reappears—is high.

Surgery

If the nail fungus does not respond to treatment and is causing you pain, you may need permanent removal of the infected nail.

Complementary Treatments
Herbal Medicine

Chamomile, echinacea, goldenseal, rosemary, sage, and thyme. Chamomile, echinacea, and goldenseal have antiseptic properties. As a bonus, echinacea boosts the immune system, helping to fight off infections. Additional herbs that have antifungal properties are rosemary, sage, and thyme. Look for topical creams containing these herbs and use according to the directions on the label.

Garlic. Eating garlic has been shown to be effective against fungus.

Grapefruit seed extract. Provides antibacterial and antifungal protection while boosting the immune system. Grapefruit seed extract is available in capsule and tincture form. Take a 100-milligram capsule daily or add 10 drops of extract three times a day to a small glass of water.

Tea tree oil. A number of reliable studies have shown that tea tree oil may kill fungus and bacteria and is effective in treating fungal infection of the nails, even those that are resistant to some antibiotics. As it is toxic when swallowed, tea tree oil is always used topically and never taken internally. If used near the eyes, nose, and mouth, it could potentially cause burning. The oil is safe to use full strength on the nail, but it should be diluted when applied to the skin. In fact, it is best to use small amounts and to test for any sensitivity that may cause a rash or itching.

Lifestyle Recommendations

Be careful with artificial nails or nail polish. Normally, moisture that collects underneath a nail passes back out through the porous nail. If you are wearing artificial nails or nail polish, that process is unable to take place. The trapped moisture may become stagnant, creating an ideal environment for fungi. Always disinfect manicure and pedicure equipment. And if you think you may have a nail fungus, don't cover it with artificial nails or nail polish, which will only make the situation worse.

Drink plenty of fluids. Cracking nails may be a sign of fluid deficiency. Be sure to drink lots of fluids throughout the day to help prevent cracks where fungi can grow.

Preventive Measures

Get treatment for athlete's foot. If you have athlete's foot, be certain it is treated adequately. The fungus causing athlete's foot can cause a toenail infection, which is much more difficult to eradicate.

Care for your nails. Keep your nails short, dry, and clean. After bathing or showering, dry your toes and the area between your toes.

Change your socks. If your feet tend to swell or sweat, change your socks several times each day.

Don't pick at your nails. If you pick at the skin near the nail, you can create an entry point for fungi.

Use foot powder. A good-quality foot talcum (not cornstarch) will absorb excess perspiration.

Wear shoes, sandals, or flip-flops. Walking around a public pool, locker room, or shower without shoes places you at high risk for fungal infection. Also, wear comfortable shoes that have room for your feet to breathe.

Night Vision Problems

As people age, it becomes more likely that they will have difficulty seeing in dim light or darkness. For many, driving at night becomes challenging or even impossible. Vision that is impaired at night or in limited amounts of light is known as night blindness or nyctalopia.

Dealing with the lack of sufficient light could also be a problem during the day, for example, if you need to drive in a darkened area, such as a tunnel. In that type of situation, your eyes must quickly adapt to the darkened environment, and during the first few seconds in the tunnel, you may have trouble seeing. And if the lighting in the tunnel is inadequate, you could have problems similar to those you experience at night.

Night vision problems are believed to be quite common.

The word *nyctalopia* has Greek roots. *Nyct* means "night," *aloas* means "obscure or blind," and *opsis* means "vision." It was first referenced in the works of Hippocrates (circa 460–377 BC), the father of medicine.

more opaque. So, light that would normally go directly to the retina is scattered to other parts of the eye. When light is scattered in this way, contrasts are diminished, colors blur, and glare becomes stronger and harder to deal with. Between the ages of 20 and 60, the ability of the eye to detect contrasts declines about 2.5 times. After age 60, the decline continues, and it becomes progressively more difficult to see and drive at night.

In some cases, night blindness may be caused by other medical problems, such as cataracts and glaucoma. There is an ever-growing amount of evidence that some patients who have LASIK (laser in situ keratomileusis) or PRK (photorefractive keratectomy) surgeries to correct their vision problems are left with improved daytime vision but impaired nighttime vision. In some cases, this type of night blindness may not be correctable. There are also reports of postsurgical problems with nighttime glare, halos, and starbursts, which are especially common during the first months after surgery.

Night blindness may also be caused by a vitamin A deficiency, though this is rare in the United States.

Causes and Risk Factors

Night vision problems are a direct result of the process of aging. As the lens of the eye ages, it thickens, loses transparency, and becomes

Signs and Symptoms

Night vision problems tend to worsen over time. You will find driving at night to be progressively more difficult. It will be harder to distinguish contrasting colors. While you once barely noticed the glare from oncoming cars, that glare may soon make it very difficult for you to see. There may be halo images around lights. If you are not very careful, you may come close to hitting something.

Because of potential problems with LASIK, the American Society of Cataract and Refractive Surgery has noted that some people should not consider LASIK as a surgical option, particularly people with diseases such as cataracts, advanced glaucoma, and corneal thinning disorder.

Conventional Treatments

After noticing that you are having problems with your night vision, it is important to visit your eye care professional as soon as possible. In many instances, the solution is relatively easy. Your doctor may simply recommend a different prescription for nighttime driving. An antireflective coating on your glasses may also be a good idea to reduce the amount of glare you experience. If it is determined that you have cataracts or glaucoma, specific treatments will be offered.

Complementary Treatments

Night vision problems can be viewed as a deficiency of certain nutrients. The best course of treatment is careful monitoring of the diet. Certain nutritional supplements could also aid in the recovery of night vision.

Diet

While it is very rare in the developed world, vitamin A deficiency is known to cause night blindness. This deficiency is also seen in people who have trouble absorbing fat or who eat diets that are extremely low in fat. If your doctor has determined that you need more vitamin A, you will probably want to increase the amount of vitamin A in your diet. The main sources include sweet potatoes, carrots, mangoes, spinach, cantaloupe, kale, red peppers, dried apricots, fortified milk, eggs, and mozzarella and Cheddar cheese. Since the body converts the beta-carotene in fruits and vegetables to vitamin A, they are another good source.

Herbal Medicine

The European species of blueberry, the bilberry, has the highest level of an antioxidant compound called anthocyanosides. The rods

A Quick Guide to Symptoms

☐ **Driving at night is progressively more difficult**
☐ **Harder to distinguish contrasting colors**
☐ **Glare makes it difficult to see**
☐ **Halo images around lights**

in the eye use anthocyanosides for night vision. Therefore, bilberry is an important herb for those suffering from night vision problems. In fact, during World War II, pilots in the British Air Force reported improvements in their night vision after taking bilberry. The typical recommended dose of bilberry is 100 milligrams of extract standardized to 23 to 37 percent bilberry anthocyanosides three times a day.

Nutritional Supplements

The following nutrients guard against night vision problems.

- Vitamin A: 10,000 IU daily. Prevents night blindness.

- Zinc: 30 milligrams daily. Deficiency can decrease effectiveness of vitamin A in the retina.

Lifestyle Recommendations

Learn nighttime driving strategies. The following are a number of coping mechanisms that may be of assistance with your nighttime driving.

- Drive slowly. When you drive slower, you have more time to watch the road and more time to react.

- Don't wear sunglasses at night. While wearing sunglasses with UV protection is a good idea during the day, don't wear them at night.

- Try to drive on well-lit roads. When it is foggy or rainy, use the low-beam headlights.

- Do not look directly at oncoming headlights. You will have better vision if you look downward and a little to your right of the road.

- Whenever appropriate, use your high-beam headlights, which will add greatly to your vision.

- Give your eyes a few seconds to adjust before driving at night.

- Be sure to keep your windshields, mirrors, headlights, taillights, and glasses clean.

Try candle gazing. Candle gazing is also beneficial for eyestrain. Sit in a comfortable position, about 3 feet away from a lit candle. Stare at the candle for 10 seconds, without blinking, then "palm" your eyes for about 30 seconds. Then, repeat the candle gazing and palming using only one eye, followed by the other eye. Repeat them again with both eyes. Over a period of several weeks, you can gradually increase the amount of gazing time.

Palming allows the eyes to feel soothed from the warmth of the hands. Here is how to palm: After briskly rubbing your hands together until you feel heat, place your palms over your closed eyes in a cupping position. No pressure should be placed on the eyeballs. The warmth and darkness are a soothing end to the eye exercises.

Preventive Measures

Approach LASIK or PRK surgery with caution. People with diseases such as cataracts, advanced glaucoma, and corneal thinning disorder are generally advised not to have these surgeries, which may have the potential side effect of creating night vision problems. If you are considering LASIK or PRK surgery, be certain your eye surgeon is experienced and takes time to determine if you are a good candidate.

Begin exercising. Exercising increases the delivery of nutrients to the eyes and facilitates the removal of waste products. The most important type of exercise for eye health is aerobic, so consider walking on a regular basis.

Wear a hat and sunglasses. Exposure to sunlight may harm your eyes and trigger problems such as cataracts, which may interfere with night vision. So, it is best to protect your eyes from the sun. It is a good idea to wear a protective hat and sunglasses that block 100 percent of ultraviolet (UVA and UVB) rays and filter at least 85 percent of blue-violet sunrays. Some contend that brown to yellow lenses are better alternatives. Be aware that some medications make the skin and the eyes more sensitive to light. Ask your doctor if any of your medications have this potential. If you are taking such a medicine, you need to be extra vigilant about protecting yourself.

Obesity

Obesity is extremely common: About one in three Americans is considered to be obese, and among those between the ages of 50 and 60, that figure may be twice as high. Obesity in America appears to be growing among people of all ages and ethnic groups.

People who are obese are seriously overweight. In addition, they have an abnormally high proportion of body fat, often defined as a body mass index (BMI) of 30 or higher. If you are obese, you have a far greater risk for a host of other medical problems. These include high blood pressure (hypertension), type 2 diabetes, abnormal blood fats, coronary artery disease, stroke, osteoarthritis, sleep apnea and other sleep disorders, emotional problems, binge eating, gout, gallbladder disease, heart attack, gum disease, non-Hodgkin's lymphoma, multiple myeloma, and cancer (of the esophagus, colon, rectum, liver, gallbladder, pancreas, prostate, breast, uterus, cervix, ovary, and kidney). Since obesity takes a toll on the muscles and bones, people who are obese are more likely to have hernias, low back pain, and problems with arthritic conditions. It has been estimated that about 300,000 lives in the United States could be saved each year if people maintained a healthy weight.

Causes and Risk Factors

In general, obesity is caused by consuming far more calories than you are able to burn in your everyday life. Since calories that are not needed for energy are stored as fat, if you consistently eat excess amounts of food, you will gain weight. Eventually, you become obese. After the age of 25, there is a tendency to gain about a pound a year. Since muscle and bone mass decrease with age, the actual gain in fat per year is closer to $1\frac{1}{2}$ pounds. By midlife, many Americans weigh at least 30 pounds more than they did in their twenties.

Your risk for obesity increases if you regularly consume high-fat foods as well as sugary soft drinks, candy, and desserts. Some people eat to fill a psychological void, an unhealthy eating pattern that can lead to weight gain.

Genes, which help to determine the amount and location of body fat, also play a role. Ex-smokers have higher rates of obesity, as do people who work the late shift (between 4:00 p.m. and 8:00 a.m.).

Leading an inactive life also raises your risk. Since men have more calorie-burning muscle than women, women are at greater risk for obesity. As we age, our metabolism slows and we tend to have less muscle. Both of these factors raise the risk for obesity. Weight gain in men tends to plateau around age 50. In women, the plateau occurs around age 70.

A small number of medications may also cause weight gain. These include corticosteroids, some antipsychotic agents, and tricyclic antidepressants. And it is believed that less than 2 percent of obesity may be traced to a medical problem, such as a slow thyroid (hypothyroidism) or imbalanced hormones.

A Quick Guide to Symptoms

- ☐ Significantly overweight
- ☐ Body mass index (BMI) of 30 or higher
- ☐ Symptoms of weight-related medical problems such as high blood pressure

Signs and Symptoms

If you are obese, there is a good chance that you know it. You are significantly overweight, and your body mass index (BMI) is 30 or higher. You may have some of the symptoms of weight-related medical problems. For example, excess weight may have resulted in elevated blood pressure or type 2 diabetes.

Conventional Treatments

If you are obese, you have probably been advised to lose weight. Your weight loss program may include a number of different components. You should realize that if you have a medical problem that is related to your obesity, when you lose weight, it may improve. For example, as you lose weight, your total cholesterol may drop, and the osteoarthritis in your knees, ankles, and spine may improve.

Behavior Modification Therapy

With behavior modification, you change your daily patterns associated with eating. Begin by keeping a diary of everything you eat. Record when you eat and what you are doing while you eat. How long does each meal take? What is your emotional state? Then, review your diary with a therapist. If you always eat while watching TV, you may be advised to try eating in another room or to simply turn off the TV. Check with your local hospital for programs to treat obesity. You may want to enroll in a behavior modification program led by a psychologist.

Diet

Most weight loss begins with some form of calorie restriction. Normally, you need to reduce your daily caloric intake by 500 to 1,000 calories, and allow no more than 30 percent of your total calories to be from fat. Eliminate as much saturated fat as possible. Severely restrictive diets of less than 1,100 calories per day are typically not a good idea. You should never embark on such a program without proper medical monitoring.

Many people advise those who wish to lose

Self-Testing

Since a body mass index (BMI) of 30 or higher is an indicator of obesity, begin by determining your BMI. Multiply your weight in pounds by 703, then divide it by your height in inches squared. For example, if you are 5'10" (70 inches) tall and weigh 200 pounds, 200 multiplied by 703 equals 140,600; then 140,600 divided by 70 squared (4,900) is 28.69, rounded off to a BMI of 29. (To square a number, you simply multiply it by itself; 4 squared is 4 times 4, which equals 16.) You can also calculate your BMI on the Internet at www.nhlbisupport.com/bmi/.

Another frequent self-test involves measuring your waist. If you are a woman whose waist is larger than 35 inches or a man whose waist is larger than 40 inches, you may be obese. You may also want to determine the distribution of body fat around the abdomen and hips. To do this, divide your waist size by your hip size. So, a woman with a 28-inch waist and 35-inch hips has a ratio of 0.8. Lower ratios are preferable—the risk of heart disease increases when a woman's ratio is above 0.8 and a man's is above 1.0. Discuss your results with your doctor.

weight to replace higher-fat foods with lower-fat, higher-fiber alternatives. While 1 gram of fat has nine calories, 1 gram of carbohydrates or protein has only four calories. Moreover, dietary fat converts more easily than carbohydrates and proteins to body fat.

Fat substitutes have become popular additions to many foods. A number of these have been used for decades and are considered safe. These include carrageenan (made from seaweed), guar gum, gum arabic, and the cellulose gel Avicel. Olestra, a more recently created fat substitute, leaves some people with cramps and diarrhea, and there is concern that it may deplete the body of some vitamins. If you plan to eat foods containing olestra on a regular basis, you should discuss vitamin supplementation with your doctor or nutritionist.

Insoluble fiber is especially useful for weight loss. It is found in whole grains, seeds, wheat bran, fruit, and vegetable peels. Pectin, a soluble fiber found in apples, provides a sense of fullness, so you may potentially eat less.

Although consuming sugar does not appear to be a key factor in the development of obesity, you should limit your sugar intake. In some instances, you may wish to use a sugar substitute, such as aspartame (NutraSweet, Equal), acesulfame K (Sweet One), or sucralose (Splenda).

High-protein diets have been around for decades and periodically reemerge in a variety of formats. Though they may lead to quick weight loss, one by-product of this diet is the release of ketones, which may cause bad breath, nausea, and lightheadedness. To ensure that you are a good candidate for a high-protein diet, you should check with your doctor.

Exercise

A key element of any weight loss program is exercise. If you are obese, before starting an exercise program, you should visit your doctor. Generally, you will be advised to work up to about 45 to 60 minutes of daily aerobic exercise, such as walking, dancing, or hiking. But you may need to begin with only 5 to 10 minutes per day. Don't forget to include resistance or strength training at least two or three times each week. But you should realize that exercise alone tends to lead to only minimal weight loss—although it may result in greater total body fat loss compared to a restricted calorie intake without the exercise component.

Medications

Due to issues surrounding efficacy, potential abuse, and possible side effects, the role of medication in weight loss programs is frequently questioned. Still, there are a number of over-the-counter natural and prescriptive medications used for weight loss. Collectively, these are known as anorexiants. Acutrim and Dexatrim are over-the-counter medications that contain phenylpropanolamine. While these suppress the appetite, when taken in doses of 75 milligrams or higher in the immediate-release form, they may cause high blood pressure or stroke.

A number of over-the-counter weight loss products contain ephedrine, a component in adrenaline. Ephedrine may trigger high blood pressure, rapid heartbeat, insomnia, heart rate irregularities, nervousness, tremors, strokes, psychosis, seizures, and death. Pseudoephedrine, which is found in many antihistamines and is sometimes used by dieters, may have similar side effects. Benzocaine is a local anesthetic that is sold as a gum; when chewed, it numbs the mouth and alters taste, which may make food seem less appetizing.

The appetite suppressant phentermine was previously prescribed in conjunction with fenfluramine ("fen-phen"), which was found to have some serious side effects and is no longer available. Potential side effects of phentermine include dizziness, drowsiness, and lightheadedness. This drug should not be mixed with certain medications, and it may alter the way some medications react in your body. Be sure to tell your doctor about every medicine you are taking. Also, this drug should be used for no more than a few months.

Sibutramine (Meridia) improves mood and energy levels while it increases metabolism and the feeling of fullness. Obese people do lose weight on this prescription medication, but when the medication is stopped, the weight may return. Frequent side effects include constipation, insomnia, and dry mouth. There are also reports of increases in blood pressure and heart rates. It should not be taken by people who have high blood pressure or a history of stroke or arrhythmias. Other people who should avoid sibutramine are those taking a decongestant, a monoamine oxidase inhibitor (MAOI), or a selective serotonin reuptake inhibitor (SSRI), or those using a bronchodilator.

Orlistat (Xenical) is a prescription medication that reduces the body's absorption of fat. After 1 year of use, expect to achieve a 5 to 10 percent drop in weight. But there may be gastrointestinal side effects, and orlistat may interfere with the absorption of the fat-soluble vitamins A, D, E, and K and other nutrients. Adhering to a low-fat diet tends to lessen the side effects.

In one study, researchers attempted to determine if topiramate (Topamax), an anti-seizure medication, would help obese patients with type 2 diabetes lose weight. For 40 weeks, people in the study were divided into three treatment groups. The first group received a placebo, the second group received 96 milligrams of topiramate each day, and the third group received 192 milligrams of topiramate each day. At the end of the study, the placebo group averaged a 2.5 percent weight loss, the low topiramate group averaged a 6.6 percent weight loss, and the high topiramate group averaged a 9.1 percent weight loss. Still, it is important to note that the FDA has not approved topiramate for weight loss management.

Surgery

Surgery is generally reserved for those who are dangerously obese. Typically, your BMI should be more than 40, and you should be at least 180 percent more than your ideal weight. There are two main types of surgery. Both should be considered only after more conservative weight loss efforts have failed. In a study published in the *New England Journal of Medicine*, surgery for severe obesity was associated with weight loss over the long term and a decreased overall mortality compared to those individuals who did not have surgery.

Gastric bypass. In this procedure, most of the stomach is blocked off. In a Roux-en-Y gastric bypass, a small stomach pouch is created and connected to the small intestine. Potential complications include obstruction, problems with the staple line, and overexpansion of the pouch. In about 10 to 20 percent of cases, these complications result in additional surgery. Weight loss occurs because the stomach is much smaller. In addition, the connection to the small intestine may cause some malabsorption of calories; only a portion of consumed calories are actually absorbed.

Normally, within about 2 years of the procedure, you will lose about two-thirds of your excess weight, and your weight-related health problems should improve. The most common side effect is vomiting. Another frequent problem is "dumping syndrome," which occurs when food moves too quickly through the intestine. It may cause weakness, nausea, and faintness, especially after eating sweets. You may develop anemia and require supplements of folic acid and vitamin B_{12}. In addition, the surgery increases your risk for bone loss and osteoporosis.

The lap-band. In this procedure, which is also known as laparoscopic gastric banding, tiny incisions are made in the abdomen. A surgeon then uses special laparoscopic instruments to place a silicone band around the upper portion of the stomach. This limits the amount of food that you are able to eat and leaves a feeling of fullness. Attached to the band is a small balloonlike reservoir that contains saline, which may be added to tighten the band or removed to loosen it. Weight loss tends to be significant. But there are potential complications, including infection, bleeding, and slippage or rupture of the band. In rare instances, there may be blood clots, pneumonia, or perforation of the stomach. If the band needs to be removed, the intestinal tract returns to normal.

Weight Loss Programs

There are many commercial weight loss programs. Some provide a good deal of personal attention, while others emphasize group support. Most programs have prepared foods that you can purchase. Examples of these commercial programs are Jenny Craig, Nutri-System, and Weight Watchers.

There are two well-known nonprofit sources for weight loss support as well. TOPS Club Inc. (Take Off Pounds Sensibly) consists of weekly group meetings, confidential weigh-ins, talks by various professionals from the community, and support from other members and volunteers. Before beginning the program, you are encouraged to see your doctor. If you believe that you are a compulsive overeater or one who is recovering from this problem, you may wish to consider Overeaters Anonymous (OA), which is based on the same 12-step program used by Alcoholics Anonymous.

Complementary Treatments

Through appropriate dietary and lifestyle changes, obesity may be decreased and the many symptoms associated with this condition may be lessened or eliminated.

Acupuncture

Auricular (ear) acupuncture may be useful in regulating your appetite. To locate an acupuncturist in your area, visit the Web site of the National Certification Commission for Acupuncture and Oriental Medicine (NCCAOM) at www.nccaom.org.

Ayurveda

An Ayurvedic medicine practitioner may help you eliminate foods that are not appropriate for your body's constitution. These foods may be contributing to your weight gain. There is no professional organization that offers membership to Ayurvedic practitioners. However, the Ayurvedic Institute may provide the names of appropriate professionals in your area. The Institute may be contacted through its Web site: www.ayurveda.com.

Diet

Start by eating a healthy diet that includes lots of fresh fruits, vegetables, and whole grains. Try to include a minimum of five servings of vegetables, four servings of fruit, and six servings of whole grains each day.

Eliminate from your diet foods high in fat, such as fried foods and fatty meats, as well as highly processed foods, fast foods, and foods high in sugar. In addition to increasing weight, these may contribute to many other health problems, including high cholesterol and high blood pressure. Also, it has been shown that eating foods such as white rice, white flour products, and potatoes may increase your hunger after they are consumed, thereby encouraging the intake of more food. Try substituting with brown rice, bran, whole grains, and cereals.

Studies have shown that sensitivity to certain foods may lead to overeating, causing obesity. To assist in eliminating certain foods from your diet, it may be useful to consult with a nutritionist or doctor who specializes in food intolerances.

Herbal Medicine

Cayenne pepper. Studies have shown that 10 grams of cayenne pepper consumed with meals may increase the metabolism of dietary fats and reduce appetite. Capsaicin, a main component of cayenne peppers, may also suppress the appetite. A study found that individuals eating a meal containing capsaicin reduced food intake by 200 calories.

Hoodia. Hoodia, a plant indigenous to the Kalahari Desert in South Africa, has been getting widespread attention as an appetite suppressant for its ability to fool the brain into thinking the stomach is full. It has been used for centuries by South African Bushmen. It took 30 years of researching the plant by the South African national laboratory to find the appetite-suppressing ingredient. Once the ingredient was found, the laboratory applied for a patent and licensed it to a company called Phytopharm, which is working to farm enough Hoodia in South Africa to make products such as shakes and bars containing the plant. For now, these products are not available in the United States, as clinical trials of Phytopharm's patented ingredient are ongoing. Many products currently on the market claim to contain Hoodia, but their quality is questionable.

Naturopathy

Naturopathy is a system of holistic therapy that relies on natural remedies, such as homeopathy, hydrotherapy, diet, herbs, massage, acupuncture, and exercise. A naturopath may investigate your lifestyle and potential food intolerances and recommend an appropriate diet and exercise program for your obesity. Contact the American Association of Naturopathic Physicians at www.naturopathic.org to find a naturopathic practitioner in your area.

Nutritional Counseling

What we should eat and what we do eat are rarely the same. Many factors, from lifestyle and time constraints to culturally learned eating habits, determine our diets. Nutritionists offer education on numerous subjects, including facts about nutrition, eating patterns, and vitamins/minerals while also providing motivational support. Nutritionists will help individuals design specific diets that provide both variety and proper nutrition.

Nutritional Supplements

Nutritional supplements are beneficial for fat burning and providing additional nutrients when on a low-calorie diet.

- Multivitamin/mineral: Take as directed on the label. Can help make up for any nutritional shortfalls on a low-calorie diet.
- Chromium: 150 micrograms daily. Trace mineral that metabolizes carbohydrates and fats.
- L-carnitine: 500 milligrams daily. Amino acid that helps burn fat and lowers the fat level in the blood.

Psychotherapy

Since it can aid in the resolution of emotional problems that may be causing you to overeat, psychotherapy may be useful for obesity. Psychotherapy focuses on the healing of the mind and the emotions. It provides a good listener and comfortable, safe surroundings, giving the individual an opportunity to identify conflicts, release emotions, and find useful coping strategies.

Lifestyle Recommendations

Beware of natural weight loss products. Natural weight loss products come in a variety of forms. Some are teas that contain laxatives such as rhubarb root, aloe, buckthorn, senna, cascara, and castor oil. These may result in gastrointestinal distress. Neither chitosan, a dietary fiber made from shellfish, nor garcinia (mangosteen), a tropical fruit that contains hydroxycitric acid, has been proven to result in weight loss.

Don't get discouraged. When you have a great deal of weight to lose, it is easy to become disheartened, especially when the pounds drop slowly. Maintain your routine of healthy eating and other therapies. You will ultimately be rewarded. Remember, it took a long time to become obese, so now you need time to lose the weight.

Don't starve yourself. Maintaining a high metabolism should be the ultimate goal in losing weight. By eating several smaller meals throughout the day along with daily exercise, you can increase your metabolism. By doing this, your body becomes accustomed to burning energy through exercise and using food properly. Food is used as energy, and what is not used is stored for later use. Many individuals starve themselves thinking it is the fastest way to lose unwanted pounds. What they don't realize is that they end up slowing down their metabolism because the body panics and takes whatever food is eaten and immediately stores it as fat.

Forgive your setbacks. Adhering to your new routine will not be easy, and you may have an occasional setback. Learn to forgive yourself.

Increase your physical activity. Add more

physical activity to your daily life. Rather than taking the elevator, walk up and down the stairs. Select a parking space that is far from the store or walk to the store. Wash your car manually. Use a push mower. Regularly use an exercise bike or a treadmill. Go for an after-dinner walk. Be active 60 minutes per day. When beginning an exercise program, remember to choose low weight-bearing activities such as walking, bicycling, or swimming. Be sure to include strength training, too.

Hire a personal trainer. A personal trainer will provide a combination of fitness assessment, fitness instruction, and motivational techniques that can help you achieve physical conditioning goals. Special benefits to your weight loss program come from positive reinforcement and help with staying motivated.

Join a support group. Studies have shown that overweight people have greater success with weight loss if they have the support of others. Making lifestyle and dietary changes may be easier if you join some form of support group. Others may share their exercise patterns, how and where to shop, and better ways to cook and store foods.

Keep a food diary. Record when and what you are eating. Also, keep a record of your exercise activities. This will help ensure that you are following a reasonable program.

Preventive Measures

Consume smaller portions. Americans tend to eat far too much. Reduce the amount of food that you eat at each meal. When eating in a restaurant, consume half of the meal and take the rest home. You will be less likely to gain weight. Avoid all-you-can-eat buffets.

Eat a healthier diet. Eat lots of fruits and vegetables as well as low-fat, protein-rich foods such as fish and skinned chicken. Eat far fewer higher-fat foods such as red meat, and eliminate your consumption of processed foods, saturated fats, and refined sugar.

Fill your kitchen with healthier choices. If you buy doughnuts, you will eat them. If you don't store higher-fat foods in your kitchen, you are less likely to be tempted. Fill your refrigerator and pantry with lots of healthy alternatives. Fruits, such as apples, oranges, and pears, are far better for you.

Start to exercise. If you want to prevent obesity, it is important to exercise. Try to find time for at least 30 minutes of daily aerobic exercise. And don't forget to add some form of resistance or weight-bearing exercise several times a week.

Osteoarthritis

Osteoarthritis causes pain, swelling, and loss of motion in joints. It's easy to understand the symptoms when you understand what's taking place inside the joints: With osteoarthritis there is a deterioration of the cartilage that cushions the ends of the bones in the joints. As this occurs, the smooth surface of the cartilage roughens. In time, the cartilage may become completely worn and you may be left with bone rubbing against bone.

While the body tries to repair the damage from osteoarthritis, bone spurs (small growths known as ostephytes) may grow at the edge of the joint and small amounts of bone or cartilage may separate and drift in the joint. This triggers more pain.

Osteoarthritis (also called degenerative arthritis, degenerative joint disease, or osteoarthrosis) is a very common medical disorder. In the United States, it affects about 20 million people and accounts for about half of all cases of arthritis. Before midlife, it affects more men; after midlife, women are at far greater risk. Most often, osteoarthritis develops after the age of 45. Just about everyone over the age of 60 has some evidence of the disease.

Unlike some other forms of arthritis which spread throughout the body, osteoarthritis affects only the joints. Depending upon the location in the body, osteoarthritis acts in different ways. It is frequently found in joints in the fingers, knees, hips, and spine, and is rarely seen in joints in the shoulders, elbows, wrists, and jaw.

- Fingers: Osteoarthritis in fingers is more often seen in older women, and it is believed to have a genetic component. Bony knobs appear on the ends of joints. It commonly affects the first joint beyond the fingertips (Heberden's nodes), and it less often affects the second joint (Bouchard's nodes). Fingers become enlarged and gnarled. They tend to be stiff and ache, and sometimes they are numb. Osteoarthritis also often damages the base of the thumb.

- Knees: Osteoarthritic knees tend to become stiff, swollen, and painful. It may be hard to walk or climb stairs. When sitting down or standing, you may need to hold onto a support.

- Hips: Hips are a frequent target for osteoarthritis. Pain tends to develop slowly in the groin, on the outside of the hips, or in the buttocks. Sometimes, the pain spreads to the knee. If you have this disorder, you may rotate your leg to avoid pain, which will cause you to walk with a limp.

- Spine: Osteoarthritis may affect the cartilage in the disks that serve as cushioning between the bones in the spine. Or, it may affect the spine's moving joints. Sometimes, it affects both. There may be pain, muscle spasms, and reduced mobility. If nerves become pinched, there will be added pain. When osteoarthritis in the spine is advanced, there may be numbness and muscle weakness.

Causes and Risk Factors

Osteoarthritis is more likely to occur in older people. However, since osteoarthritic cartilage is chemically different from normal aged cartilage, osteoarthritis is not believed to be caused by aging. Instead, a number of other factors have been suggested. Osteoarthritis has a strong genetic component, so having close relatives with this disease places you at higher risk.

Have you injured a joint? Do you do physical work that involves repetitive stressful motions? These two factors increase risk. Also, excess weight places extra stress on weight-bearing joints. If you are obese, you are adding to your risk for osteoarthritis. Certain medications, such as corticosteroids, are associated with higher rates of osteoarthritis.

While most older people are at risk for osteoarthritis, there is some variability between ethnic groups. Whites are more likely than Asians to have osteoarthritis. Still, Asians have a higher incidence of osteoarthritis in the knee, and whites and Asians have an equal risk for osteoarthritis in the spine. African Americans have the highest overall risk for osteoarthritis.

Signs and Symptoms

Symptoms associated with osteoarthritis include aching pain in a joint or joints made worse by humid weather and excessive use of the joint, and stiffness after periods of inactivity, such as sleeping. The pain may come and go, and there may or may not be inflammation. When you move your knees, there may be a cracking noise.

A Quick Guide to Symptoms

☐ **Aching pain in a joint made worse by humid weather or excessive use**
☐ **Stiffness after periods of inactivity**
☐ **Pain that comes and goes**
☐ **Inflammation**
☐ **A cracking noise when you move your knees**

Conventional Treatments
Exercise

Exercise is now viewed as a conventional treatment for osteoarthritis. It reduces pain and stiffness and increases muscle strength and flexibility. Without exercise, your joints will further stiffen. Consult with your doctor before beginning an exercise program. In general, you should include range-of-motion, strengthening, and aerobic exercises. If your doctor agrees, you may wish to meet with a physical therapist or personal trainer, who can design an exercise program that will meet your particular needs.

Heat and Ice

Applying ice to an inflamed joint may bring a good deal of relief. Keep the ice on for about 20 to 30 minutes. If you don't have an ice pack, use a bag of frozen peas, which works equally well. If you have osteoarthritis in your hands, try hot soaks and warm paraffin applications.

Lifestyle Changes

If stress to your joints caused your osteoarthritis, you need to eliminate or reduce the stress. Continued stress on the joints will only increase the rate of degeneration. Find alternative ways to complete necessary tasks. If extra assistance is needed, consider consulting with an occupational therapist.

Medications

Capsaicin. Made from the seeds of hot chili peppers, capsaicin (Zostrix, Capzasin-P) is a cream that reduces levels of substance P, an element in the nerve fibers that fosters the delivery of pain impulses to the brain. When using capsaicin, rub a small amount of cream on the affected area four times a day. During the first few days of use, you may have a localized feeling of warmth and stinging. That passes, and pain relief begins within 1 to 2 weeks.

COX-2 inhibitors. COX-2 inhibitors are often effective. Examples are celecoxib (Celebrex) and meloxicam (Mobic). They suppress the enzyme cyclooxygenase-2, or COX-2, that causes joint inflammation and pain, while preserving the COX-1 enzyme, which protects the stomach lining. Patients taking COX-2 inhibitors tend to have fewer gastrointestinal concerns than those taking nonsteroidal anti-inflammatory drugs (NSAIDs). Nevertheless, many of those who take these medications do have gastrointestinal problems, and they may also experience other potential side effects such as headache, dizziness, and kidney problems. Those on anticoagulant drugs may be at greater risk for bleeding. And, in a small number of cases, higher doses of COX-2 have been related to hallucinations, a buildup of fluid, high blood pressure, and excess potassium in the blood.

Hyaluronic acid. If you have osteoarthritis in your knee, your doctor may try injecting hyaluronic acid, a natural substance found in the body. It makes the joint better able to absorb shock. Generally, it is given in a series of three to five injections.

Pain relievers. About 20 to 30 percent of people with osteoarthritis are helped by the pain reliever acetaminophen (Tylenol). Be aware that taking higher doses over an extended period of time increases your risk for kidney and liver damage. Heavy alcohol drinkers, people taking blood-thinning medications, and those with liver disease must use acetaminophen with caution.

Doctors commonly advise their patients with osteoarthritis to take NSAIDs. These include aspirin, ibuprofen (Motrin, Advil), and naproxen (Aleve, Naprosyn). It may take a week or two before you experience significant amounts of pain relief. While NSAIDs are quite effective in treating osteoarthritis, they frequently cause gastrointestinal problems such as ulcers, upset stomachs, and internal bleeding. This occurs even when these medications are injected intravenously. NSAIDs may also increase blood pressure, especially among those who already have hypertension. Other potential side effects include headaches, skin rashes, ringing in the

If you have high blood pressure, a severe circulation disorder, or kidney or liver problems, or if you are taking diuretics or oral hypoglycemics, and your doctor places you on NSAIDs for an extended period of time, then you need to be monitored carefully. Also, since NSAIDs reduce blood clotting, stop taking them a week before any scheduled surgery.

ears, dizziness, and depression. There is some evidence that NSAIDs may damage cartilage and/or cause kidney damage. These medications should be used with caution—the longer they are used, the more likely they are to cause side effects.

For some people with severe osteoarthritic pain, narcotics may be an option. There are two types. Opiates (such as morphine and codeine) are derived from natural opium, while opioids such as oxycodone are synthetic drugs. Since these are highly addictive medications, those taking narcotics should be monitored carefully.

Another choice for severe pain is the use of corticosteroid injections to the affected area. These are used when pain is accompanied by inflammation. But they work only for relatively short periods of time, and no more than two or three injections should be given each year.

Surgery

Arthrodesis (joint fusion). If a joint needs to be stabilized but cannot be replaced, arthrodesis may be advised. During the procedure, bones are fused together. After healing, the joint may bear weight, but it is inflexible. The most common sites for this surgery are the wrist and ankle.

Arthroplasty (joint replacement). In this procedure, a surgeon reconstructs the joint with artificial or prosthetic implants. It may be advised when pain and immobility from an osteoarthritic joint have made normal functioning impossible. The most commonly replaced joints are the hip and knee, accounting for about 80 percent of such surgeries in the United States. But joints in the ankles, shoulders, elbows, and knuckles are also successfully replaced.

During the surgery, which is done under general anesthesia, the surgeon will open the joint and separate the tendons and ligaments. The surgeon removes the damaged portions of the joint and replaces them with plastic and/or metal prostheses. Sometimes, the prostheses are cemented into place. Then, the remainder of the joint parts, as well as the ligaments and tendons, are reattached. Since some blood loss is associated with arthroplasty, a month or two before your surgery, you may wish to donate one to three units of your own blood. If you require a transfusion, your blood may be used.

Depending on the type of surgery, expect to spend 3 to 7 days in the hospital, then a week or two in a rehabilitation facility. This will be followed by outpatient therapy.

The majority of people who have undergone joint replacements are thrilled with the pain relief and newfound independence. As with all surgeries, there are risks for complications. Infections, which occur in about 1 percent of all joint replacements, may require the removal of the implant. You may experience blood clots and damage to the nerves near the joint. A prosthesis may loosen or a joint may dislocate, and the replacement parts of weight-bearing joints may wear out and fail. Hips tend to last between 10 and 15 years, while you may have as many as 20 years with new knees.

Arthroscopic debridement. In general, arthroscopic surgery is performed to remove the bone and cartilage fragments in the knee that are causing pain and inflammation. The surgeon begins by making a small incision into which a sterile solution is injected. Since that makes the joint swell, it is easier for the surgeon to see. A lighted tube called an arthroscope is inserted into a second small incision. Entering through a third incision, the surgeon trims or stitches the damaged

Treating an NSAID-Induced Ulcer

If your doctor determines that you are at risk for developing an ulcer from NSAIDs, or if you actually develop one, there are a number of medications that may be used to treat it. Generally, proton-pump inhibitors are useful in preventing ulcers in those who are at high risk. Examples are omeprazole (Prilosec), lansoprazole (Prevacid), rabeprazole (Aciphex), and pantoprazole (Protonix). When compared to no treatment, these medications reduce the rate of ulcers by up to 80 percent. Misoprostol has been found valuable in preventing, but not treating, NSAID-induced ulcers. The medication Arthrotec is a combination of misoprostol and the NSAID diclofenac. In one study, individuals who took Arthrotec had between 65 percent and 80 percent fewer ulcers than those who took NSAIDs alone.

tissue. Typically, this procedure is done under local anesthetic. Recovery rarely takes more than a few weeks.

Joint lavage. In this procedure, which is also known as tidal irrigation, your physician uses a trocar or large-bore needle to infuse a joint with a salt-and-water combination. Joint fluid is then drained, which removes particles of cartilage debris and other substances. Improvements may last from months to years.

Osteotomy. If your osteoarthritis has

caused a deformity in your knee or hip joints, your doctor may recommend an osteotomy. In this surgery, the physician opens the knee or hip and reshapes a wedge of bone, thereby correcting the weight-bearing problems you have been experiencing. This procedure is advised for heavier adults who are under the age of 60. It may provide pain relief, increased joint stability, and better range of motion.

Complementary Treatments

With proper care and attention, osteoarthritis may be controlled or even reversed. Approaches that allow the body to heal itself by assisting in the normal function of the cartilage and repairing the damage already done are beneficial. Practitioners will also address the underlying cause of the joint degeneration and try to relieve the pain and inflammation. Dietary changes are a significant factor in the healing process.

Acupuncture

Recent studies have shown acupuncture to be very effective in reducing the pain and inflammation associated with osteoarthritis. To locate an acupuncturist in your area, visit the Web site of the National Certification Commission for Acupuncture and Oriental Medicine (NCCAOM)at www.nccaom.org.

Aromatherapy

A number of oils may be used to relieve symptoms of osteoarthritis, such as stiff joints, inflammation, and pain. Fennel prevents the buildup of toxins in the joints. Coriander releases toxins in the body and relieves pain. Rosemary, pine, and vetiver ease joint pain and stiffness. Benzoin increases circulation and eases arthritis pain. Chamomile reduces any type of inflammation and arthritis pain, as do cedarwood, eucalyptus, and helichrysum. Any of these oils may be added to a bath. In combination or alone, be sure not to exceed 10 drops total. Or add 2 or 3 drops to an unscented oil and massage over the affected joint.

Ayurveda

Ayurvedic treatments vary according to physical constitution, emotional makeup, specific symptoms, dietary habits and preferences, present lifestyle, and sleeping habits. However, practitioners of Ayurvedic medicine believe that osteoarthritis is due to poor digestion, and will design a treatment to improve the digestive process. There is no professional organization that offers membership to Ayurvedic practitioners. However, the Ayurvedic Institute may provide the names of appropriate professionals in your area. The Institute may be contacted through its Web site: www.ayurveda.com.

Diet

The process of healing osteoarthritis begins on the cellular level. It is important to eat foods that aid in the destruction of damaging free radicals—molecules that bind to and kill healthy cells, damage the joints, and deplete the antioxidant nutrients necessary for the body to heal itself. The diet should be rich in fruits and vegetables, which contain the antioxidants beta-carotene, flavonoids, and vitamin C. Foods rich in vitamin E and selenium are also recommended, because these nutrients block the damaging effects of free radicals.

Vitamin C and beta-carotene are found in almost all fruits and vegetables, including dark green, leafy vegetables. Fruits rich in flavonoids are cherries, blackberries, and blueberries. Vitamin E may be found in vegetable oils, nuts, seeds, and wheat germ; smaller amounts are found in leafy vegetables and whole grains. Selenium is available in whole grains, red meat, chicken, broccoli, asparagus, egg yolks, milk, and onions. Juicing fresh fruits and vegetables is an excellent way to obtain these nutrients and to have them better absorbed by the body.

It is also useful to eat foods that have anti-inflammatory properties, such as wheat grass and barley, and sulfur-containing foods, such as onions, garlic, brussels sprouts, and cabbage. Sulfur repairs and rebuilds bones, cartilage, and connective tissues and assists in calcium absorption.

In people who are genetically susceptible to arthritis, nightshade vegetables (potatoes, eggplant, peppers, and tomatoes) have been known to increase inflammation and inhibit the repair of cartilage. It may be necessary to see a doctor who will test for allergies to these and other foods that may be causing or aggravating this condition.

Avoid fried foods and other foods high in trans fats, saturated fat, refined sugar products, and excess salt. Aside from having no nutritional benefit and increasing body weight, these foods contribute to osteoarthritis.

Feldenkrais Method

Sandra Bradshaw.com
250 862 8489

Practitioners teach individuals to become aware of their movement patterns. This improves body motion and corrects poor postural habits. It may relieve stiffness and inflammation, which may decrease pain. Feldenkrais practitioners may be found at the Web site www.feldenkrais.com.

Flower Essences

Rescue Remedy cream rubbed over the affected joints three or four times a day may reduce osteoarthritis pain. Emotional conditions such as repressed anger, frustration, and an inflexible attitude may further exacerbate osteoarthritis pain. Various flower essences address these emotional states and personality patterns. Rescue Remedy is available as a cream or as a tincture. Other flower essences are available in tincture form and may be purchased at health food stores. Follow the directions on the label.

Herbal Medicine

Because of their anti-inflammatory properties and their ability to relieve pain and rebuild bones, many herbal remedies have been used in the treatment of osteoarthritis.

Boswellia serrata. Boswellia is an anti-inflammatory herb that improves blood supply to the joint tissue. Boswellia is available in capsule, tincture, and ointment form. The recommended dose in capsule form is 400 milligrams three times a day. Look for products containing 60 percent boswellic acids.

Capsaicin. Since capsaicin interferes with pain messages, it is good for pain relief. It is available in cream form. Rub a small amount on the affected area.

Ginger. Ginger is an anti-inflammatory herb. Fresh ginger is best and may be taken as a tea or applied directly to the joint as a warm compress.

Proanthocyanidin bioflavonoids. Proanthocyanidin bioflavonoids, often referred to as PAC or grape seed extract, are antioxidants and free-radical scavengers that reduce inflammation. The typical recommended dose is a 100-milligram capsule three times a day of extract standardized to contain 92 to 95 percent PCOs.

Hydrotherapy

Warm water is an ideal medium for the treatment of the pain and stiffness associated with osteoarthritis. The gentle, rhythmic movements in the water may release toxins that build up in joints and may increase flexibility, coordination, balance, and circulation. This will improve joint mobility, strengthen muscles, and decrease pain and stiffness.

Electric heating pads and dry heat applications are not recommended for osteoarthritis. Moist heat packs applied over or near the affected area for 20 minutes will penetrate deeper and lessen stiffness and pain much better than dry heat.

Nutritional Supplements

Many nutritional supplements have anti-inflammatory properties and support healthy cellular structure.

- Multivitamin/mineral: Take as directed on the label. Should include A, C, E, beta-carotene, calcium, copper, magnesium, selenium, and zinc to aid in healthy cell structure and provide anti-inflammatory properties.

- B-complex vitamins: Take as directed on the label. B_5 levels may be low in people with osteoarthritis. B vitamins work best when taken together.

- Boron: 3 milligrams twice a day. Aids in the regulation of calcium.

- Bromelain: 500 milligrams daily. Enzyme found in pineapple with anti-inflammatory properties.

- Vitamin D: 400 IU daily. Essential for cartilage health, needed for absorption of calcium; deficiency linked to osteoarthritis.

- DLPA (DL-phenylalanine): 750 milligrams daily. Enhances body's ability to deal with pain. Requires 1 to 2 weeks to become effective. May raise blood pressure.

- Essential fatty acids—omega-3 (flaxseed and fish oil) and omega-6 (borage, evening primrose, and black currant seed oils): Available in oil and capsule form. Take as directed on the labels. Increase anti-inflammatory agents in the body.

- Glucosamine sulfate: 500 milligrams daily. Slows the breakdown, aids in the repair, and stimulates the growth of new cartilage. Pain relief may be initially slow, but results are extremely promising.

- MSM (methylsulfonylmethane): 1,000

milligrams daily. Effective against arthritis pain and inflammation.

- SAMe (S-adenosyl-methionine): Dose varies depending on symptoms. See your doctor for a starting point. Amino acid that helps lubricate joints and relieve pain and stiffness.

Shiatsu

The deep finger pressure of shiatsu massage may help release obstructions in the muscles and vital energy system. Shiatsu may be stimulating and relaxing, aiding in the relief of pain. To find a practitioner trained in shiatsu, visit the following Web sites: www.aobta.org (American Organization for Bodywork Therapies of Asia) and www.ncbtmb.org (National Certification Board for Therapeutic Massage and Bodywork).

Therapeutic Massage

Massage treatments may remove toxins that build up in the joints, causing inflammation and pain. Massage reduces muscular tension, which places added stress on joints that are already stiff. It has an overall calming effect on the body and mind.

Lifestyle Recommendations

Begin exercising. Probably your best coping mechanism for osteoarthritis is regular exercise. A physical therapist or personal trainer can help you design a program that will work best for your individual needs. Exercising and stretching regularly will aid mobility and flexibility. Any type of exercise that does not overly stress the joints—such as swimming, walking, and bicycling—is beneficial. Because it increases bone density, walking is an excellent form of exercise for people with osteoarthritis. Tai chi, yoga, and qigong are other forms of exercise that are gentle and may increase balance, thereby reducing the risk of falls. They also improve coordination, muscular strength, and flexibility.

Consider magnet therapy. Preliminary studies have shown a reduction in pain when magnets are applied directly over the affected area for several hours. It is also thought that low-energy AC and DC fields may help stimulate the production of cartilage-building cells.

Lose weight. If your doctor has indicated that excess weight is contributing to your osteoarthritis, you will need to drop some of the pounds. Ask your doctor for some suggestions or a referral to a weight loss program.

Reduce stress. Stress and tension may aggravate and increase the severity of pain. Every day, find a way to reduce stress and relax your body and mind. Even 15 minutes of deep breathing exercises while listening to quiet music may have a healthy effect on the physical body and help reduce pain.

Preventive Measures

Both serious injury and repeated minor injuries may place your joints at greater risk. Try to avoid actions that may be injurious to your joints.

Osteoporosis

Osteoporosis is a skeletal disease that leads to porous, fragile, easily broken bones. In someone with this disease, the amount of calcium contained in the bones gradually decreases. As the bones become more and more brittle over time, they are at ever increasing risk for fractures. Until the early midlife years, the osteoblasts (cells that build bone) produce about the same amount as the osteoclasts (cells that break down bone). This is a process known as remodeling. Around the age of 40, however, the cells break down more bone than they make.

A diagnosis of osteoporosis is made when the bone density has so diminished that even mild stress may result in fractures. This is known as the fracture threshold. You are diagnosed with osteoporosis when your bone mineral density (BMD) is 2.5 standard deviations (SD) or more below the average BMD for young healthy adults of the same sex. If your BMD is between 1 and 2.5 SD below normal, you get a diagnosis of osteopenia. Bones that are osteopenic are weak and thin; osteoporotic bones are even thinner and weaker.

An estimated 44 million adults in the United States either have osteoporosis or are at risk for developing it. Ten million people already have the disease, and another 34 million have low bone mass, which places them at increased risk. Eighty percent of those who are affected are women, and 30 percent of women over the age of 65 have osteoporosis. A striking 93 percent do not know they have this condition. With their higher bone density and slower rate of calcium loss, men are far less likely to have osteoporosis. Nevertheless, about 3 million men are at risk, and almost 1.5 million men over the age of 65 have osteoporosis. Low levels of testosterone place some men at increased risk.

There are two primary types of osteoporosis. Type I (high-turnover osteoporosis) is caused by the relatively rapid reduction in the hormone estrogen that takes place during menopause. It is seen in women between the ages of 50 and 75 and is associated with the fractures that occur as vertebrae compress together and collapse the spine. In addition, fractures may occur in the forearm, hip, and wrist from a fall. Type II (low-turnover osteoporosis) takes place when bone mass is breaking down far faster than it is building. It affects midlife men and women, as well as older women.

Whether or not you develop osteoporosis is a function of how much calcium remains in your skeleton. If you have very dense bones, you may never lose a sufficient amount of calcium to have osteoporosis. If you have relatively low bone density, it may not require very much calcium loss to give you the disease.

Often, an osteoporosis diagnosis is made only after someone has already broken a porous bone, either from a minor incident or a fall. Every year in the United States, there are an estimated 1 to 3 million osteoporotic fractures, most often in the vertebrae, wrists, and hips. Hip fractures, which may be particularly debilitating, account for 300,000 of these fractures. About 24 percent of those who experience a hip fracture die within a year of their injury, often due to a complication from the fracture, such as pneumonia or blood clots; 50 percent never regain their previous quality of life.

Causes and Risk Factors

A number of factors play a role in the development of osteoporosis. In addition to the rapid reduction of estrogen during menopause, genetics is known to be an important factor. If either or both of your parents have osteoporosis, you are at higher risk. Consider yourself at an even higher risk if a close relative developed osteoporosis at a young age. The lighter your skin, the greater your risk. Whites and Asians have a higher risk than Hispanics. As many as half of today's 50-year-old white women will develop osteoporosis. Hispanics have a higher risk than African Americans. Yet, just because you may be Hispanic or African American, do not assume that you will never suffer serious bone loss. Approximately 10 percent of Hispanic women age 50 or older have osteoporosis.

Women who begin menstruating at age 15 or later are at higher risk, as are women who experience menopause before the age of 45 or who have a history of anorexia nervosa. Women who are slender have less bone mass than heavier women. Additionally, many postmenopausal women with hip fractures apparently have lower levels of vitamin D and higher levels of parathyroid hormone. Chronic calcium and vitamin D deficiency causes an increase in parathyroid hormone, which in turn causes calcium to leach from the bone into the bloodstream.

Some factors increase the risk of osteoporosis in both men and women. These include lack of exercise, thinness, a history of yo-yo dieting, weak thigh muscles, poor balance, inadequate exposure to sunlight, smoking, and high consumption of coffee, tea, or alcohol. People who have a malabsorption problem, such as celiac disease, are at greater risk. There is even a relationship between gray hair and thinning bones. If your hair turns gray in your twenties or is half gray by the age of 40, your incidence of bone thinning is four times higher than someone who turns gray later in life.

Certain medications have been correlated with bone loss. For example, the use of corticosteroids, such as prednisone, for 3 to 6 months is associated with calcium loss. Anyone taking a corticosteroid should be diligent about getting enough calcium. Excessive doses of thyroid medication have similar effects. Other medications that cause calcium loss include antiseizure medications such as phenytoin and antacids that contain aluminum.

Signs and Symptoms

Many people have osteoporosis for years before they exhibit symptoms. Frequently, people learn that they have osteoporosis only after experiencing a minor trauma that results in a broken hip, vertebra, forearm, or other bone. In the more advanced stages of the disease, there may be pain and disfigurement or loss of stature. Collapsing vertebrae in the spine may cause a stooped position (kyphosis), which is commonly referred to as a dowager's hump. As height is lost, the stomach will protrude forward. With the abnormal posture comes pain.

Conventional Treatments
Medications

Currently available medications slow the rate of bone remodeling, but none actually rebuilds bones. The list includes alendronate and other bisphosphonates, calcitonin, hormone replacement therapy, and raloxifene.

Alendronate. Alendronate and other bisphosphonates have the potential to sig-

nificantly increase bone density. In a study published in the *New England Journal of Medicine*, postmenopausal women who took alendronate daily were studied for 10 years. Increases in bone mineral density were noted at the spine, trochanter, and femoral neck (parts of the hip). The medication appeared to have sustained and well-tolerated effects over the 10-year study period.

Alendronate is also useful for treating osteoporosis in men. Researchers studied males between the ages of 31 and 87 who had osteoporosis for 2 years. Some took 10 milligrams of alendronate every day; others were given a placebo. The men who received alendronate had a significantly increased bone mineral density at the lumbar spine and femoral neck compared to those who received the placebo. Alendronate also helps to prevent vertebral fractures and decreases in height.

Because they may cause gastrointestinal side effects, alendronate and bisphosphonates may not be prescribed for people who have heartburn, ulcers, or other gastrointestinal disorders. They must be taken on an empty stomach in the morning with at least 8 ounces of water. After taking the medicine, you may sit but you may not eat or lie down for at least 30 minutes. Other potential side effects include nausea, diarrhea, and abdominal pain.

Calcitonin. Calcitonin improves bone density and reduces fractures, especially those of the spine. Unlike the other medications, calcitonin relieves the pain of recent vertebral fractures, and it does so in a relatively brief period of time—only 2 to 4 weeks, a

A Quick Guide to Symptoms

- ☐ **A minor trauma that results in a broken hip, vertebra, forearm, or other bone**
- ☐ **Pain and disfigurement**
- ☐ **Loss of stature**
- ☐ **A stooped position (kyphosis)**

short-term benefit. However, calcitonin has marginal benefits for the long-term treatment of osteoporosis. Since calcitonin is a protein, it may cause allergic reactions. Also, because it is administered as a nasal spray, some people report nasal irritation, itchiness, nosebleeds, or redness. Calcitonin is also available in an injected form. When injected, it may potentially cause flushing, skin rash, and nausea.

Strontium ranelate. A study published in the *New England Journal of Medicine* found that when postmenopausal women with osteoporosis who had at least one vertebral fracture were treated with strontium ranelate, their risk for future vertebral fractures dropped considerably. In fact, over 3 years, they showed a 41 percent risk reduction compared to women who were not treated with the medication. The improvements are about the same as those produced by raloxifene but less than those obtained with hormone replacement therapy or alendronate. Strontium ranelate is available in Europe as an oral preparation.

Hormone replacement therapy. Hormone replacement therapy, such as estrogen, increases bone density and reduces fractures. It may also protect against colon cancer and positively affect mental functioning. But it has the potential to increase the risk of blood clots and heart attacks and foster vaginal bleeding and breast pain.

Raloxifene. Raloxifene, a "designer estrogen," increases bone density and reduces fractures. It also appears to reduce the risk of

Dual-Energy X-ray Absorptiometry (DEXA)

This is an easy, quick, and painless test that will enable your doctor to determine if you have experienced significant amounts of bone loss. Dual-energy x-ray absorptiometry (DEXA) takes only a few minutes to measure bone density of the spine, hip, or wrist. DEXA generates very low-level x-rays. The results are calculated to determine if bone density has dropped to the fracture threshold. If bone mineral density (BMD) is found to be 2.5 standard deviations (SD) or more below the average BMD for young healthy adults of the same sex, you have an osteoporosis diagnosis.

On the day of a DEXA test, wait until the test is over to take any calcium supplements. The intestinal tract is located near the spine, and an undigested calcium pill might be measured with the calcium in the bones.

Also, wear pants with an elastic waist band. If you wear clothing with metal zippers, dense plastic buttons, or any metal ornaments, you will probably be asked to change into a hospital gown.

breast cancer and lower cholesterol levels. But it increases the risk of blood clots, and it tends to trigger menopausal symptoms such as hot flashes.

Complementary Treatments

A combination of a healthy diet, nutritional supplements, movement therapies, and exercise is effective in preventing and treating osteoporosis.

Aquatic Therapy

Because it doesn't place stress on muscles, bones, and joints, exercising in a heated pool, with the buoyancy and resistance of water, is an ideal way to develop strength, flexibility, and endurance. In addition, by calming the nerves, increasing circulation, and decreasing muscle stiffness, aquatic therapy exercises help to reduce the pain often associated with osteoporosis.

Diet

A low-fat, well-balanced diet that contains plenty of whole grains, fresh fruits, and calcium-rich foods is useful for keeping your body strong and healthy. Since vitamin D and the mineral magnesium play a role in the body's absorption and metabolism of calcium, your diet should include foods rich in these nutrients. Milk that is fortified with vitamin D is a very good source of calcium. However, since whole milk is high in fat, you should select a low-fat or skim alternative. Other foods that are high in calcium include shrimp, blackstrap molasses, calcium-fortified tofu, almonds, sardines, green leafy vegetables such as kale and broccoli, beans, oranges, and raisins.

Relatively few foods contain significant amounts of vitamin D. The best sources are seafood such as salmon, tuna, Atlantic mackerel, oysters, shrimp, herring, and halibut. The liver and oil from these fish have high amounts of vitamin D. Other sources include milk, eggs, and Cheddar and Swiss cheeses.

On the other hand, because magnesium is in a host of healthful foods, including dairy products and seafood, it is easy to consume an adequate amount of it. Other good sources are whole grains, legumes, nuts, potatoes, seeds, dark green vegetables, bananas, oranges, and tomatoes.

Soy products, which contain plant estrogens known as isoflavones, are believed to support bone density. Calcium-fortified tofu is considered a good source for this nutrient; 3 ounces of tofu contain 60 percent of the daily calcium requirement.

By helping you hold on to the calcium in your bones, vitamin K may be another important bone-supporting part of the diet. There is some evidence that women who consume higher amounts of vitamin K have fewer hip fractures. Eating fruits and vegetables will give you the extra vitamin K that you may require. Especially good sources are strawberries, broccoli, spinach, cauliflower, brussels sprouts, blackstrap molasses, and collard greens.

Herbal Medicine

Black cohosh contains estrogen-like properties that can help protect against bone loss. The minimum recommended daily dose is 20 milligrams in the morning and 20 milligrams at night of standardized extract of 2.5 percent triterpene glycosides.

Nutritional Supplements

The combination of these nutrients helps maintain bone density and reduce the risk of fractures.

- Vitamin D: 400 IU daily. Promotes healthy bones; deficiency causes bone weakening. Regulates absorption of calcium.

- Boron: 750 micrograms daily. Aids in metabolism of calcium and magnesium. Especially effective with vitamin D deficiency or calcium absorption problems.

- Calcium: 1,500 milligrams daily in divided doses of 500 milligrams. Essential for healthy bones.

- Magnesium: 750 milligrams daily in divided doses of 250 milligrams. Works well with calcium.

- Evening primrose oil: 3,000 milligrams daily in divided doses of 1,000 milligrams each to provide 240 milligrams of GLA (gamma-linolenic acid). Deficiency may lead to bone loss.

- Omega-3 fatty acids: 1 tablespoon flaxseed oil or 2,000 milligrams of fish oil in capsule form twice a day. Deficiency may lead to bone loss.

Lifestyle Recommendations

Begin exercising. Bone health usually requires exercising several times a week. Include aerobic weight-bearing exercises such as walking in your routine, as well as strength or resistance training. Use light weight when doing arm exercises; do not go over 20 pounds. An optimal exercise program includes 30 minutes of walking daily. If you have been relatively inactive, you should check with your doctor before beginning an exercise program.

> **If you would like to test the absorbability** of your calcium supplement, place it in a glass of white vinegar. Does it break up within 30 minutes? If not, you may wish to try another form of calcium supplementation.

Also, if you already have osteoporosis, there are certain exercises that you should not do. Do not do exercises that may hurt the spine, such as jumping, jogging, or running. And don't do any exercise in which you must bend forward from the waist with a rounded back, such as abdominal crunches, situps, toe touches, or bringing the knees to the chest. When you're exercising, your back should be supported and stable. Strong abdominal muscles are necessary for maintaining back stability. Since situps are contraindicated, isometric exercises (using elastic stretch bands) work best.

Don't participate in any exercise in which you could easily fall, such as step aerobics, and don't do any exercise in which you need to move your leg sideways against resistance. This would occur with some resistance exercise machines. Under pressure, a weakened hip could break.

Movement therapies that improve balance, coordination, muscle strength, and joint range of motion are useful for those who have osteoporosis or are interested in prevention. Examples of movement therapies are yoga, tai chi, and qigong. Because the slow, graceful movements of these therapies focus on balance, coordination, and flexibility, they may help prevent falls. Exercise improves posture, which can help reduce the slumping posture associated with osteoporosis.

Control your weight. In both men and women, excessive weight loss has been correlated with hip fractures.

Maintain good posture. Good posture will help avoid stress to the spine and reduce the risk of falling.

Preventive Measures

Add supplemental calcium and vitamin D to your self-care regimen. A report in the *New England Journal of Medicine* concluded that evidence supported the use of calcium or calcium in combination with vitamin D supplementation to prevent osteoporosis in people 50 years or older. The report recommended at least 1,200 milligrams of calcium with 800 IU of vitamin D daily for the best therapeutic effect.

Limit your intake of alcohol. Alcohol not only interferes with the absorption of calcium in your body, but it also robs your body of this necessary nutrient.

Reduce coffee consumption. Women who drink 4 cups of coffee each day have double the risk of hip fractures. The caffeine in the coffee has a diuretic effect, and more calcium will be excreted in the urine. If you are a woman who has been drinking large amounts of coffee, consider reducing your consumption or switching to another beverage.

Spend a little time in the sun. Your body uses sunlight to produce vitamin D, a vitamin that is critical to bone production. Spending only a little time (10 to 15 minutes) in the sun several times a week will help prevent bone loss. During this time, you should use sunscreen on your face but not on your arms and legs. Exposure should be direct, not filtered through a window. This is most effective in the spring and summer and least useful in the winter. After this brief period in the sun, you should also cover your arms and legs with sunscreen.

Stop smoking. It is well known that there is a direct relationship between smoking and decreased bone density. All women who smoke have higher rates of spine and hip fractures than women who do not smoke. This is particularly true for postmenopausal women. Moreover, if women who take hormone replacement therapy also smoke, they lose the bone-protective effect of the therapy. Male smokers also have lower levels of bone density. On the positive side, when people stop smoking, even later in life, they help to limit the loss of bone.

Overactive Bladder

Overactive bladder is the need to urinate more than eight times during the course of a typical day. It is not uncommon to also awaken at night to urinate. You may experience the sudden, immediate need to urinate. And if you are unable to reach a bathroom in time, the urine may leak. In some instances, the entire bladder may empty, soaking your clothes. This loss of control is known as urge incontinence. It affects about one-third of those who also have problems with urgency and frequency.

Overactive bladder is a very common problem. In the United States, 17 million to 20 million people have this disorder. At least 16 percent of those over the age of 40 are affected.

Causes and Risk Factors

Overactive bladder is caused by overactivity in the detrusor muscle, which plays an important role in controlling the bladder. If you have an overactive bladder, the detrusor muscle contracts often and inappropriately. It is unknown what triggers the detrusor muscle's actions, but there may be a neurological problem that confuses the signals from the brain to the bladder. In men, this action may be related to prostate problems.

While men and women are equally at risk for overactive bladder, women are at far greater risk for urge incontinence. This may be due in part to movement of the pelvic organs (such as the uterus and vagina) during childbirth or menopause or because of weight problems or prior pelvic or abdominal surgery.

Signs and Symptoms

With overactive bladder, you urinate frequently. You might feel the need to urinate shortly after you have urinated. In addition, there is the feeling that you must urinate urgently. Sometimes, you are unable to hold your urine, and it leaks onto your clothing.

Conventional Treatments
Bladder Retraining

In general, bladder retraining is the first treatment for overactive bladder. Safe and free, it improves symptoms in about two-thirds of the women who have this disorder. Begin by recording the times that you void and leak. Then, make a point of urinating before the time that you would usually void. Gradually,

A Quick Guide to Symptoms

- ☐ Frequent urination
- ☐ Feeling that you must urinate urgently
- ☐ Inability to hold your urine

lengthen the times between voiding by 15 minutes. As an alternative, you can start voiding on the hour, every hour. After about 2 weeks, increase the times between voiding by 30 minutes. When that becomes comfortable, increase the times again. Try to work up to 3 to 4 hours between each voiding.

Devices

InterStim. InterStim is an electronic device that is used to help severe urge incontinence that has not responded to other treatments and behavior modifications. InterStim, which is surgically implanted, employs mild electrical stimulation of the sacral nerves to control the actions of the bladder, sphincter, and pelvic floor muscles.

Pessary. In some instances, your doctor may recommend a pessary, a plastic device that fits in the vagina. When properly inserted, a pessary returns the pelvic organs to the correct position. However, a pessary may cause complications, such as open sores in the vaginal wall and bleeding. If the pessary fits well, the chance for complications is reduced. Follow your doctor's instructions on how and when to clean and reinsert the pessary.

Medications

A few medications are approved for treating overactive bladder. They prevent bladder contractions and tighten the muscles at the neck of the bladder and urethra, thereby stopping leakages. Some examples of well-known oral medications are tolterodine (Detrol, Detrol LA) and oxybutynin (Ditropan). There is evidence from controlled clinical trials that these medications are useful for overactive bladder.

Though some people experience a fairly quick response to the medications, in many others it may take as long as 4 weeks. Potential side effects include dry mouth and constipation. A patch containing oxybutynin (Oxytrol) is also available, and there appears to be a lower incidence of side effects with the patch.

Hormone replacement therapy is also useful for strengthening pelvic muscles and nerves. It is available in a number of forms, such as pill, patch, and cream. Still, the evidence is not as strong that estrogen therapy is useful for overactive bladder.

According to an article in the *New England Journal of Medicine*, future treatments for an overactive bladder may include designing drugs that affect the sensory nerves of the lower urinary tract, drugs that are more specific for bladder control, and alternative drug delivery systems.

Pelvic Floor Muscle (Kegel) Exercises

Kegel exercises, which help to strengthen the muscles of the pelvic floor that support the bladder and close the sphincter, were originally designed to assist women before and after childbirth. However, they have been found quite useful for overactive bladder.

Begin by identifying your pelvic muscles. This may be done by slowing or stopping the urine flow while you are urinating. These are the muscles you need to make stronger. Try to perform 5 to 15 contractions, three to five times daily. Hold each Kegel for a count of 5 to start, and gradually work your way to a count of 10. But don't do too many, as women who overexercise these muscles may make them too tight. Once you learn to do Kegel exercises, try to avoid them when you are urinating, because this practice has the tendency to weaken muscles.

You will need to commit to Kegel exercises for your lifetime. If you discontinue, any benefits you have achieved will disappear. Also, it may take several months of Kegel exercises before you see any improvements.

Surgery

If a severe case of overactive bladder does not respond to any other treatments, you might want to opt for surgery. In an enterocystoplasty, a portion of the bowel is removed and attached to the top of the bladder, thereby enlarging the bladder. An enlarged bladder is able to hold more urine. Potential complications from this procedure include electrolyte problems, blood clots, pneumonia, bowel obstruction, an inability to empty the bladder completely, and a higher risk of cancer.

In auto-augmentation, part of the bladder muscle is removed. When filled with urine, the bladder forms a "pouch" in the bladder wall. Since the pouch gives more room, the urge to urinate is delayed. However, this surgery is not believed to be as effective as the enterocystoplasty.

Complementary Treatments

Practitioners of complementary medicine attempt to reduce the symptoms of an overactive bladder by recommending lifestyle changes, adjusting dietary habits, and strengthening the pelvic muscles and urinary system.

Biofeedback

Biofeedback has been effective in teaching people how to control muscle contraction and relaxation to avoid leakage during coughing or other unexpected triggering activity.

Combined with biofeedback, the effectiveness of Kegel exercises may be enhanced. In the privacy of your home, you insert a vaginal or rectal probe that transmits information to the monitoring equipment. You isolate the pelvic floor and bladder muscles and perform Kegel exercises. The monitor will indicate how strongly you are contracting the pelvic floor muscles and how successfully the bladder muscles are released.

To try biofeedback, seek a health care practitioner who has been certified through the Biofeedback Certification Institute of America (BCIA). To locate a practitioner in your area, look on the BCIA Web site at www.bcia.org, check your local hospitals or medical clinics, or look in the Yellow Pages.

Herbal Medicine

Uva ursi strengthens the sphincter muscles and prevents the loss of bladder control. It is also a good herb for any bladder or kidney problem. Drink 1 cup of tea every morning. The tea is readily available in health food stores.

Lifestyle Recommendations

Be vigilant about hygiene. After a urinary accident, you can reduce the chances of skin irritation by thoroughly cleansing the area and applying both a moisturizer and an occlusive cream, which acts as a barrier on the skin. An occlusive cream usually contains petrolatum, zinc oxide, or lanolin. Take care not to apply the cream inside the urethra.

For yeast infections, you should use an antifungal cream that contains miconazole nitrate or another approved topical antifungal agent.

Check your medications. Certain medications have the potential to exacerbate an overactive bladder. These include antidepressants, diuretics, sedatives, antihistamines, narcotics, calcium-channel blockers, and alpha-blockers.

Preventive Measures

Avoid constipation. Constipation may be a contributing factor to overactive bladder. The accumulation of stool pressed against the bladder and urethra, as well as the straining movements, may put undue force on the bladder, triggering leakage. Eating a high-fiber diet with plenty of fresh fruits and vegetables may be beneficial.

Drink more fluids. While you may believe that reducing your fluid intake will lower your risk for overactive bladder, the opposite is true. If you reduce your fluid intake, the lining of the urethra and bladder may become irritated, which may increase leakage. Also, drink some cranberry juice, which will reduce your risk for urinary tract infection. However, stop drinking fluids at least a few hours before you go to bed.

Eliminate certain foods from your diet. The following foods are believed to be associated with overactive bladder. You may wish to try to eliminate them from your diet, at least for a brief period of time.

- Caffeinated beverages and medications that contain caffeine
- All types of coffee and tea
- Carbonated beverages
- Citrus fruits and juices
- Chocolate
- Sugars and honey
- Artificial sweeteners
- Milk and milk products
- Spicy foods
- Tomatoes and tomato-based foods
- Alcoholic beverages
- Corn syrup

Empty the bladder completely. A good technique to empty the bladder completely is called double voiding. Begin voiding and go until you feel that you are done. Wait a moment, relax, then lean forward and void some more. Often, there is a little left that needs to be released. This technique helps to avoid leakage.

Lose weight. Excess weight may aggravate and weaken bladder muscles.

Stop smoking. The persistent cough that many smokers have may cause urinary leakage. In addition, it has been shown that nicotine causes irritation to the bladder.

Paget's Disease

In healthy adults, bones go through a constant natural cycle of breaking down and reforming. With Paget's disease, this breaking down and reforming process is abnormal. Bone breakdown and formation are accelerated and out of balance, leading to an excess of new bone formation and areas of weakened (osteolytic) bone. As a result, bone is fragile, dense, and structurally unsound. Paget's disease, which is a metabolic disorder, may affect only one or two bones or be quite widespread. The weakening of the bone may result in bone pain, deformities, arthritis, and fractures. The cartilage in the joints may also be damaged. Paget's disease (also called osteitis deformans) is most often seen in the bones of the skull, collarbone, pelvis, spine, upper arms, thighs, and lower legs.

Though many people have never heard of Paget's disease, it affects significant numbers of Americans. Paget's disease is the second most common bone disease, and it has been estimated that 3 to 4 percent of those over the age of 40 have this disorder. In the United States, it is more often seen in the northern parts of the country. Men and women are equally affected, and the incidence increases with age.

People with Paget's disease are at greater risk for a number of other medical problems. If the long bones of the leg bow or if a bone enlarges, extra pressure may be placed on joints, resulting in osteoarthritis. When Paget's disease affects facial bones, teeth may loosen, and chewing may become difficult. The heart may experience strain if it must work harder to pump blood to the affected bones. Kidney stones are more common in people with Paget's disease, as is primary bone cancer, especially osteosarcoma. Giant cell tumors, which are benign, are also associated with Paget's disease. They are most often seen in people with Paget's who are of Italian descent.

Causes and Risk Factors

Though the cause of Paget's disease is unknown, it may be the result of a slow-acting viral infection. The risk for Paget's disease increases with age. It most often occurs between the ages of 50 and 70. In addition, there is a hereditary component to this disease. Frequently, more than one family member is affected. Studies indicate that first-degree relatives of people with Paget's disease have a sevenfold increase in the risk of developing this condition.

Signs and Symptoms

People with mild cases of Paget's disease may experience no symptoms. The most common symptom is bone pain. Pain may

A Quick Guide to Symptoms

☐ Bone pain
☐ Nerve pressure, resulting in neck pain, hearing loss, headaches, or loss of vision
☐ The skin area over an affected area of bone may feel hot
☐ Increase in head size, skeletal deformities, bowing of the legs, or curvature of the spine (in advanced cases)
☐ Bones may break easily

be most acute near joints and at night. If Paget's disease has affected your skull or spine, there may be pressure on the nerves, which may result in neck pain, hearing loss, headaches, or loss of vision. If the disease appears in your pelvis or hipbone, there may be hip pain. The skin area over an affected area of bone may feel hot. In advanced cases of Paget's disease, there may be an increase

If you are taking a bisphosphonate medication as well as calcium, don't take them at the same time. It is best to allow several hours to elapse between taking the two medications. When taken too close together, they will not be adequately absorbed.

in head size, skeletal deformities, a bowing of the legs, or a curvature of the spine. Bones may break easily.

Conventional Treatments

In Paget's disease, the goal of treatment is to control pain, prevent deformation of bones, avoid complications, and relieve nerve compression. Though Paget's disease is a chronic illness that has no cure, it may be effectively managed. Treatment is best started when an individual has symptoms, but before there are major bone changes. Clinical trials have shown that medications may reduce pain and help to heal osteolytic areas.

Medications

Bisphosphonates. To alter the rate of bone turnover, your doctor may recommend a bisphosphonate medication such as risedronate (Actonel), alendronate (Fosamax), tiludronate (Skelid), or etidronate (Didronel). These are taken first thing in the morning, on an empty stomach, with a large glass of water. After taking these medications, you may sit, but you may not eat or lie down for at least 30 minutes. Because they may cause gastrointestinal side effects, these medications may not be prescribed for people who have heartburn, ulcers, or other gastrointestinal disorders. They should also not be used by people with severe kidney disease. Potential side effects include nausea, diarrhea, increased bone pain, mild musculoskeletal pain, and abdominal pain. If there are osteolytic lesions in weight-bearing bones, etidronate is not recommended.

There is also an intravenous bisphosphonate known as pamidronate (Aredia). Potential side effects are abdominal cramps, nausea, chills, confusion, fever, muscle spasms, pain at the location of the injection, and sore throat.

Calcitonin. If you do not respond to bisphosphonate medications, your doctor may recommend injections of calcitonin (Miacalcin). Calcitonin injections have been shown to reduce the rate of bone turnover by 50 percent as well as decrease bone pain and promote healing. Calcitonin is also available in a nasal spray, although some people report nasal irritation, itchiness, nosebleeds, or redness.

Pain relievers. Your doctor will probably recommend different types of pain medication. One of these is acetaminophen (Tylenol). If you are taking acetaminophen, you should realize that the consumption of higher amounts over an extended period of time increases your risk for kidney and/or liver damage. This medication needs to be used with caution by heavy alcohol drinkers, people taking blood-thinning medications, and those with liver disease.

Doctors also commonly advise their Paget's disease patients to take nonsteroidal anti-inflammatory drugs (NSAIDs). These include aspirin, ibuprofen (Motrin, Advil), and naproxen (Aleve, Naprosyn). It may take a week or two before you experience significant amounts of pain relief. While NSAIDs are quite effective in treating pain, they frequently cause gastrointestinal problems, such as ulcers, upset stomach, and internal bleeding. These problems can occur even when the medications are injected intravenously. NSAIDs may also raise blood pressure, espe-

cially among those who already have this disorder. Other potential side effects include headaches, skin rashes, ringing in the ears,

If you have high blood pressure, a severe circulation disorder, or kidney or liver problems, or if you are taking diuretics or oral hypoglycemics, and your doctor places you on NSAIDs for an extended period of time, then you need to be monitored carefully. Also, since NSAIDs reduce blood clotting, stop taking them a week before having surgery.

dizziness, and depression. There is some evidence that NSAIDs may damage cartilage and/or cause kidney damage. These medications should be used with caution. The longer they are used, the more likely they are to cause side effects.

Physical Therapy

Your treatment will probably include a few visits with a physical therapist, who can teach you specific exercises to help you manage the symptoms of the illness. If you do these exercises regularly, you should notice some improvement.

Surgery

Sometimes, treatment is unable to curtail the progression of Paget's disease. If you have become disabled, your doctor may recommend joint replacement of the hips or knees. Surgery is also used to help fractures heal. And in a procedure known as an osteotomy,

NSAIDs and Ulcers

If your doctor determines that you are at risk for developing an ulcer from your NSAID or if you actually develop one, there are a number of medications that may be used to treat it. Generally, proton-pump inhibitors are useful in preventing ulcers in those who are at high risk. Examples are omeprazole (Prilosec), lansoprazole (Prevacid), rabeprazole (Aciphex), and pantoprazole (Protonix). When compared to no treatment, they reduce the rate of ulcers by up to 80 percent. Misoprostol has been found valuable in preventing, but not treating, NSAID-induced ulcers. The medication Arthrotec is a combination of misoprostol and the NSAID diclofenac. In one study, people who took Arthrotec had up to 80 percent fewer ulcers than those who took NSAIDs alone.

Pagetic bone is cut and realigned. This procedure is used for painful weight-bearing joints, particularly the knees.

Complementary Treatments

Complementary treatments that help to strengthen the bones and decrease pain are the most effective in lessening the symptoms of Paget's disease.

Aquatic Therapy

The buoyancy and resistance of water in a heated pool create an ideal environment to develop strength, flexibility, and endurance without placing stress on muscles, bones, and joints. In addition, by calming the nerves, increasing circulation, and decreasing muscle stiffness, aquatic therapy helps to reduce the pain often associated with Paget's disease.

Diet

Since vitamin D and the mineral magnesium play a role in the body's absorption and metabolism of calcium, your diet should include foods that are rich in these nutrients. Milk that is fortified with vitamin D is a good source of calcium. However, since milk is high in fat, you should select a low-fat or skim alternative. Other foods that are high in calcium include dark green, leafy vegetables such as broccoli, kale, collard greens, and turnip and beet greens; calcium-fortified tofu; canned sardines and salmon (with bones); blackstrap molasses; and dried beans. Many breakfast cereals, including oatmeal, are fortified with calcium, as are some brands of orange juice.

Relatively few foods contain significant amounts of vitamin D. The best sources are seafood such as salmon, tuna, Atlantic mackerel, oysters, shrimp, herring, and halibut. The liver and oil from these fish have high amounts of vitamin D. Other sources of vitamin D include fortified eggs and Cheddar cheese.

Magnesium is found in a host of different healthful foods, including dairy products and seafood, so it is easy to consume an adequate amount of this nutrient. Other good sources are whole grains, legumes, nuts, potatoes, seeds, and dark green vegetables.

Soy products, which contain plant estrogens known as isoflavones, are believed to support bone density. Calcium-fortified tofu is considered a good source. Three ounces of tofu has 60 percent of the daily calcium requirement.

By helping retain the calcium in your bones, vitamin K is another important bone-supporting nutrient in the diet. Eating fruits and vegetables will give you extra vitamin K. Especially good sources are strawberries, broccoli, cauliflower, brussels sprouts, collard greens, asparagus, and blackstrap molasses.

Nightshade vegetables, such as potatoes, eggplant, peppers, and tomatoes, contain high amount of alkaloids, which interfere with the proper metabolism of calcium. By harmfully distributing calcium to the joints and kidneys, they have been known to increase inflammation and inhibit the repair of cartilage. You might want to limit consumption of these vegetables or avoid them altogether.

Exercise

Bone health usually requires exercising several times a week. Include in your routine aerobic weight-bearing exercises, such as walking, as well as mild strength or resistance training. This will help maintain joint mobility. If you have been relatively inactive,

before beginning an exercise program, you should check with your doctor.

If you have Paget's disease, there are certain exercises that you should not do and some that must be done with extra care. Do not do exercises that may hurt the spine, such as jumping, jogging, or running. Use caution when doing exercises in which you bend forward from the waist with a rounded back, such as abdominal crunches, situps, toe touches, or bringing the knees up to the chest. When you are exercising, your back should be supported and stable. Strong abdominal muscles are necessary for maintaining back stability. Don't participate in any exercise in which you could easily fall, such as step aerobics. And don't do any exercise in which you need to move your leg sideways against resistance, as with some exercise machines—under pressure, a weakened hip could break.

Movement therapies that improve balance and coordination and increase muscle strength and joint range of motion, such as tai chi and qigong, are beneficial. Because the slow, graceful movements of these therapies focus on balance, coordination, and flexibility, they may help prevent falls.

Nutritional Supplements

The combination of these nutrients helps maintain bone density and reduce the risk of fractures.

- Multivitamin/mineral: Take as directed on the label. Helps maintain bone health.

- Vitamin D: 400 IU daily. Promotes healthy bones; deficiency causes bone weakening. Regulates absorption of calcium.

- Boron: 750 micrograms daily. Aids in metabolism of calcium and magnesium. Especially effective with vitamin D deficiency or calcium absorption problems.

- Calcium: 1,500 milligrams daily in divided doses of 500 milligrams. Essential for healthy bones.

- Magnesium: 750 milligrams daily in divided doses of 250 milligrams. Works well with calcium.

Preventive Measures

Limit your intake of alcohol. Alcohol not only interferes with the absorption of calcium in your body, it also robs your body of this necessary nutrient.

Reduce coffee consumption. The caffeine in the coffee has a diuretic effect, and more calcium will be excreted in the urine.

Stop smoking. There is a direct relationship between smoking and decreased bone density. This affects both men and women. On the positive side, when people stop smoking, even later in life, they help to limit the loss of bone.

Take a blood test. Though there is no known prevention for Paget's disease, in order to control the symptoms, early diagnosis and treatment are important. If someone in your family has been diagnosed with Paget's, you should have a blood test every few years after you turn 40 to monitor your alkaline phosphatase levels. Alkaline phosphatase may be a marker for the presence of, or a rise in risk of, Paget's disease.

Parkinson's Disease

People with Parkinson's disease often have tremors and difficulty with walking. This happens because the disease causes a significant loss of the brain cells that produce the muscle-directing chemical known as dopamine. As a result, there is a slow, but progressive, loss of muscle control, coordination, and balance. The disease may also harm nerve endings that control the release of norepinephrine, a hormone that regulates pulse rate, perspiration, blood pressure, and other automatic responses to stress.

Parkinson's disease is far more common than most people realize. Though the exact figures are hard to determine, it is believed that at least 1 million Americans are living with this disorder. Each year, about 50,000 new cases are diagnosed.

Causes and Risk Factors

Parkinson's disease is frequently referred to as an idiopathic disorder, which means that the cause is unknown. No one has been able to determine the exact reason for the loss of dopamine. Parkinson's disease has, however, been linked to a number of genetic and environmental factors. Those who have a first-degree relative (parent, sibling, or child) with Parkinson's are three times more likely to develop the disorder. In addition, some people who have been exposed to herbicides and pesticides may have three times the risk. Exposure to other environmental toxins, such as manganese dust or the chemical MPTP, or to infectious agents may also place people at increased risk.

Lowered amounts of estrogen in the body, which occurs in menopausal women who do not take hormone replacement therapy, have also been associated with Parkinson's disease. And it is believed that low levels of folate (folic acid), a B vitamin, may increase susceptibility.

When taken in excessive doses or consumed over an extended period of time, a number of medications may cause Parkinson's-type symptoms. These include metoclopramide (Reglan) and prochlorperazine (Compazine, Compro), which are used for nausea; haloperidol (Haldol, Halperon) and chlorpromazine (Thorazine, Sonazine), which are used for some psychiatric disorders; and valproate (Depakote), a medication for epilepsy.

The vast majority of cases of Parkinson's disease appear in people over the age of 50—the average age of onset is 55. But about 10 percent of cases are in people under the age of 40. After the age of 75, the incidence appears to decline and the very elderly are at low risk.

Genes seem to play a crucial role. So, those with a close relative who has been diagnosed with this disorder should be aware of their increased risk and watch for symptoms. Men may face up to twice the risk of women. Americans of European descent have a higher risk than those of African or Asian descent. Interestingly, people who smoke and/or drink coffee have lower rates of the disease.

Signs and Symptoms

During the earliest stages of Parkinson's disease, the symptoms may be rather subtle. When you walk, one of your arms may not swing. You may have trouble getting out of a chair, and you may feel shaky. You may speak softly, or your handwriting may be cramped or spidery. There may be mild tremors in the fingers of one hand or speech may be slightly mumbled. You may be tired, irritable, depressed, and have trouble sleeping. It may take you a little longer to complete routine tasks.

As the disease progresses, the symptoms become more obvious. Tremors that began in a finger spread to the entire arm. Hand tremors sometimes involve the back-and-forth rubbing of the thumb and forefinger, which is known as pill rolling. Tremors may also develop in other parts of the body, such as the head, lips, and feet. They tend to be more noticeable when you are under stress and disappear during sleep.

Many people with Parkinson's move more slowly, a condition known as bradykinesia. They may have a shuffling walk, an unsteady gait, and a stooped posture. There may be postural instability or impaired balance and coordination. On occasion, muscles may freeze. The digestive system may slow, resulting in problems with chewing, swallowing (dysphagia), and constipation. Bladder control and incontinence are frequent medical concerns,

as are insomnia and sexual dysfunction.

Still other symptoms of Parkinson's disease include rigid muscles (akinesia), often in the limbs and neck, the loss of automatic movements such as blinking and smiling, and impaired speech. There may also be changes in temperature response, hot flashes, excessive sweating, and a sudden drop in blood pressure when standing (orthostatic hypotension), which results in dizziness and fainting. Many people with Parkinson's disease have an impairment of their sense of smell and/or vision loss, and the skin on the forehead and the sides of the nose tends to become quite oily. Some have a problem with drooling.

About 40 percent of those with Parkinson's disease experience depression. In approximately 25 percent of these people, the depression precedes the Parkinson's diagnosis by months or years. People with Parkinson's disease are also prone to other emotional changes, such as fear, insecurity, and a loss of motivation. There may be memory loss and slow thinking. Moreover, as many as one-third of those who have Parkinson's disease become demented—they experience memory loss, impaired judgment, and changes in their personality.

Conventional Treatments

Most treatments for Parkinson's disease begin with dietary changes, exercise, and physical therapy. Though these do not stop the progression of the disease, they will help build muscle strength and improve gait and balance. If you have speech problems, you may want to work with a speech therapist. When lifestyle changes provide insufficient relief, other treatments may be advised.

Medications

A number of medications that increase the brain's supply of dopamine are used to treat Parkinson's disease. (Unfortunately, since dopamine does not cross the body's blood-brain barrier, treatment with dopamine itself is ineffective.) Though they may have uncomfortable side effects, none of these medications should be discontinued without consulting your doctor.

Amantadine. Amantadine is an antiviral medication that is effective in reducing the symptoms of Parkinson's disease. Often used in the early stages of the disease, this medication's effectiveness wanes within a few months in about one-third to one-half of all people taking it. Potential side effects include blurred vision, confusion, swollen ankles, mottled skin, edema, and depression. Overdoses may result in life-threatening toxicity.

Anticholinergics. Anticholinergics, the main treatment for Parkinson's disease before the introduction of levodopa, are useful in controlling tremors in the early stages of the disease. Examples are trihexyphenidyl (Artane, Trihexy), benztropine (Cogentin), biperiden (Akineton), and procyclidine (Kemadrin). Potential side effects of anticholinergics are dryness of the mouth, nausea, urinary retention, constipation, and blurred vision. They may also cause mental problems such as memory loss, confusion, and hallucinations, and those who

have glaucoma should use them with care.

Catechol-O-methyltransferase inhibitors. Catechol-O-methyltransferase (COMT) inhibitors block an enzyme that breaks down dopamine. In so doing, they prolong the effect of levodopa therapy. An example is tolcapone (Tasmar). Nevertheless, because they have been associated with liver damage and liver failure, these medications are usually given only to those who have not responded to other therapies. Other potential side effects include involuntary muscle movements, cramps, headache, nausea and vomiting, mental confusion and hallucinations, urine discoloration, diarrhea, constipation, sweating, susceptibility to respiratory infection, and dry mouth.

Dopamine agonists. Dopamine agonists are medications that imitate the effects of dopamine in the brain. They cause the cells to react

A Quick Guide to Symptoms

- ☐ Tremors in the fingers of one hand
- ☐ Slightly mumbled speech
- ☐ Bradykinesia (slow movements)
- ☐ Impaired balance and coordination
- ☐ Slowed digestive system
- ☐ Insomnia
- ☐ Rigid muscles (akinesia)
- ☐ Changes in temperature response
- ☐ Impairment of sense of smell and/or vision loss
- ☐ Drooling
- ☐ Depression and other emotional changes
- ☐ Dementia

as if there were sufficient amounts of dopamine. The potential side effects include sudden drop in blood pressure upon standing (orthostatic hypotension), headache, nausea and constipation, nightmares, hallucinations, psychosis, sudden sleep attacks, and nasal congestion. They should be avoided by anyone who has experienced hallucinations or confusion. Examples of dopamine agonists are bromocriptine (Parlodel), pergolide (Permax), pramipexole (Mirapex), and ropinirole (Requip).

Levodopa. The most common medication for Parkinson's disease is levodopa (L-dopa), which is able to cross the blood-brain barrier. When levodopa is combined with the antinausea medication known as carbidopa (Sinemet), it is even better able to cross the blood-brain barrier, making it more effective.

Treating the Complications of Parkinson's

Many people with Parkinson's disease suffer from depression and/or insomnia. Your doctor may recommend treating these problems. Similarly, if your medications have triggered psychotic symptoms, your doctor may recommend the drugs clozapine (Clozaril) and quetiapine (Seroquel). To combat daytime sleepiness, you may be placed on modafinil (Provigil), and to improve your voice loss, you may be given collagen injections in the neck. Shots of botulism toxin (Botox) have been found to be useful for drooling.

Levodopa tends to work best for rigidity and slowness. Less benefit may be obtained for problems with tremor, balance, and gait.

During the earlier stages of Parkinson's disease, the side effects of levodopa treatment are usually minimal. But as the medication is used for longer periods of time, potential side effects that may appear include a drop in blood pressure (especially when standing), abnormal heart rhythms (arrhythmia), nausea and gastrointestinal bleeding, hair loss, confusion, anxiety, vivid dreams, sleepiness and sleep attacks, and hallucinations. As the disease progresses, this therapy may be less effective, a process called the "wearing-off effect," and you may experience involuntary movements (dyskinesia). Moreover, each dose of the medication controls symptoms for shorter periods of time.

Selegiline. An adjunct to levodopa therapy, selegiline (Atapryl, Carbex, Eldepryl) helps stop the breakdown of dopamine. Potential side effects of selegiline include nausea, vomiting, diarrhea, insomnia, vivid dreams, confusion, and agitation. People taking this medication and other monoamine oxidase (MAO) inhibitors should not consume foods or beverages that contain tyramine, such as aged cheese, red wines, vermouth, dried meats and fish, canned figs, fava beans, and concentrated yeast products. Consuming such foods could seriously raise blood pressure. Some people who have taken this drug with meperidine (Demerol, Pethadol) have had toxic reactions.

Surgery

When medications fail to improve the symptoms of Parkinson's, surgery may be an option. There are several potential procedures. Though they may relieve symptoms, they are not a cure.

Deep-brain stimulation (DBS). With this procedure, a device known as a thalamic stimulator is implanted in a region of the brain known as the subthalamic nucleus. Then, through a wire, a pacemaker-like chest unit sends electrical pulses to the implant. These pulses stop the signals that cause tremors. The pulse generator may be controlled by passing a magnet over the chest. Because it may be used in both sides of the thalamus, tremors in both sides of the body may be controlled. The device may also be placed in the thalamus or globus pallidus. About every 3 to 5 years, the generator must be replaced. Potential complications include bleeding in the brain, infection, and decrease in verbal memory and the ability to work on mental tasks involving visual-spatial functions.

In one study, 156 people with Parkinson's were divided into two treatment groups. One group was given deep-brain stimulation, and the other group was given medication. After 6 months, researchers determined that people with advanced Parkinson's disease who received deep-brain stimulation had better outcomes than those who received medication.

Pallidotomy. During a pallidotomy, which requires about 6 hours, an electric current kills a small amount of tissue in the pallidum (globus pallidus), the location in the brain that causes many of the Parkinson's symptoms. The procedure may result in an improvement in many symptoms, including tremors, rigidity, and slowed movement, as well as the involuntary movements caused by drug therapy. But the benefits may not last. The surgery has potential risks, such as disabling weakness, slurred speech, stroke, decline in memory capacity and verbal fluency, apathy, and vision problems. Individuals with dyskinesia (uncontrolled movements), rigidity, and tremor are considered the best candidates for this procedure.

Thalamotomy. In a thalamotomy, a small section on one side of the thalamus, a portion of the brain, is destroyed. If the surgery is effective, it will relieve tremors on the opposite side of the body. Since operating on both sides of the thalamus poses a risk of speech loss and other complications, surgeons normally operate on only one side.

Complementary Treatments

Complementary medicine addresses the symptoms associated with Parkinson's disease through nutritional and dietary changes and by using approaches that help to increase coordination, balance, and muscle control.

Acupuncture

Acupuncture may alleviate muscle stiffness and soreness as well as address the tremors associated with Parkinson's disease. To locate an acupuncturist in your area, visit the Web site of the National Certification Commission for Acupuncture and Oriental Medicine (NCCAOM) at www.nccaom.org.

Aquatic Therapy

Resistive exercises in the water may increase strength and improve balance and flexibility.

A heated pool provides a safe environment to do exercises for improving the symptoms of Parkinson's disease.

Craniosacral Therapy

Craniosacral therapy (CST) is the hands-on gentle manipulation of the craniosacral system—the brain, spinal cord, cerebrospinal fluid, dural membrane, cranial bones, and sacrum. Craniosacral therapy balances the cerebrospinal fluid, which may help to alleviate tremors. To search for a qualified therapist in your area, visit the Web site of the International Association of Healthcare Practitioners at www.iahp.com.

Diet

Many foods may interfere with the effectiveness and absorption of medications for Parkinson's disease. For this reason, you may need a specific diet that is closely watched. To create the best diet for your needs, consult with a registered or licensed dietitian or certified nutritional consultant. As studies have shown that individuals with Parkinson's disease are low in certain vitamins and minerals, you may also want to discuss nutritional supplementation. However, when taking prescription medications, caution must be used before embarking on a nutritional supplement regimen.

Feldenkrais Method

Since it helps to support the neuromuscular system and improves the autonomic motor response, Feldenkrais is an especially useful technique for people with Parkinson's disease. Practitioners teach individuals to become aware of their movement patterns.

This improves body motion and corrects poor postural habits. It may relieve stiffness and inflammation, which may decrease pain. To locate a practitioner, visit the Web site of the Feldenkrais Educational Foundation of North America (FEFNA) at www.feldenkrais.com.

Nutritional Supplements

While studies have found that some individuals with Parkinson's disease have low levels of vitamin B_6, it is important to not supplement with B_6 if you are taking the medication L-dopa alone. Outside the brain, B_6 converts L-dopa to dopamine, thereby lowering the level of dopamine delivered to the brain. This does not happen when L-dopa is combined with carbidopa (Sinemet).

Because people with Parkinson's disease are usually deficient in essential fatty acids, it is recommended that evening primrose oil and flaxseed oil be taken daily. The recommended dose is 1 tablespoon, twice a day.

Tai Chi and Qigong

The gentle movement therapies of tai chi and qigong help improve balance, coordination, and flexibility and reduce anxiety.

Therapeutic Massage

Therapeutic massage, particularly deep muscle work, may stretch the connective tissue, relieve tension in tight muscles, and alleviate cramping. This may lead to an increase in joint range of motion, balance, and coordination. Massage also stimulates the lymphatic system. Because of the lack of mobility, a sluggish lymphatic system may be found in people with Parkinson's disease.

Trager Approach

The Trager Approach reeducates the nerves to control muscle movement and releases patterns of muscle tension and restriction, making it beneficial for people with Parkinson's disease. As it is a passive treatment, it is especially useful for people with limited mobility. Over time, the body's nervous system is reeducated to respond in the proper manner to relieve pain and discomfort. To locate a Trager therapist, visit www.trager-us.org (the Web site of the United States Trager Association) or www.ncbtmb.org (the Web site for the National Certification Board for Therapeutic Massage and Bodywork).

Lifestyle Recommendations

Be sure to get enough sun. Fifteen minutes of sunshine a day may provide an adequate amount of vitamin D. Since all people with Parkinson's disease are prone to osteoporosis, this is particularly important as vitamin D helps protect against this disorder.

Exercise. To improve the quality of your life and maintain productivity, you should exercise. You need exercises that will help retain your balance and reduce muscle freezing. Include exercises such as stretching, walking, and marching in place. A physical therapist or personal trainer may help create an exercise program designed for your particular needs and in keeping with your limitations.

Join a support group. You may benefit from talking to others who are also dealing with Parkinson's disease. You will derive psychological benefits and may learn additional coping mechanisms.

Limit protein. In the advanced stages of Parkinson's, higher levels of protein in the diet reduce the effectiveness of levodopa. Though you should not avoid protein, try to keep protein to about 12 percent of your total daily calories.

Prevent constipation. Since constipation is an ongoing problem for many people with Parkinson's disease, eat a diet that is high in fiber and water. You may wish to take a soluble-fiber supplement such as Metamucil. Psyllium seed husks have also been very effective in improving bowel function and eliminating constipation. It is important to maintain gastrointestinal health. Taking acidophilus, which are friendly bacteria, may be useful in preventing constipation and ensuring a healthy gastrointestinal tract.

Remain mentally active. Using your mind will help you retain the brain's dopamine. Learn a new hobby, especially one that requires finger and hand mobility. Or study a new language and keep up with the daily news.

Take a digestive enzyme. Since people with Parkinson's disease may not be able to utilize nutrients effectively, a digestive enzyme should be taken after each meal.

Preventive Measures

There is a direct link between pesticides and the development of Parkinson's disease. If you are going to continue to use pesticides, take precautions and wear protective clothing, gloves, and a mask.

Peripheral Neuropathy

People with peripheral neuropathy can experience anything from mild tingling to loss of feeling to intense pain. *Peripheral neuropathy* is a general term used to describe disorders of the peripheral nervous system, the complex network of nerves that link the spinal column to the other parts of the body. With this disorder, there is some form of damage to the nerves that communicate between your brain and your muscles, internal organs, skin, and blood vessels. When only one nerve is affected, it is called mononeuropathy. Yet, often many peripheral nerves are involved, and then it is called polyneuropathy.

Peripheral neuropathy is very common. It is believed that more than 2 million Americans have some form of this disorder.

Causes and Risk Factors

Damage to the peripheral nerves may occur in a number of ways. With mononeuropathy, the cause is normally trauma or some form of repetitive use. Thus, it may be the result of using crutches or typing at a computer keyboard. One such example is carpal tunnel syndrome. On the other hand, polyneuropathy is more often the result of a medical problem, such as diabetes, a condition called diabetic neuropathy. For some unknown reason, high levels of sugar in the blood appear to inhibit the ability of your nerves to transmit signals.

Peripheral neuropathy is also more frequently seen in those with autoimmune diseases, such as rheumatoid arthritis; in alcoholics; in people with compromised immune systems; and in people who take certain medications or who have specific vitamin deficiencies, such as low levels of vitamin B_{12}. Further, those who are dealing with liver and kidney disease and hypothyroidism are more likely to have peripheral neuropathy. It is believed that exposure to toxic substances, such as lead and mercury, may result in peripheral neuropathy. And an attack of acute Guillain-Barré syndrome may destroy the myelin sheath that covers nerve fibers, leaving an individual with a case of peripheral neuropathy.

Signs and Symptoms

People with peripheral neuropathy have a wide range of symptoms, which may vary dramatically in intensity. Sometimes, you may be hardly aware of your symptoms, while at other times you may find them unbearable. Symptoms from peripheral neuropathy include tingling, pain, numbness, burning, and a loss of feeling. These often begin gradually and then intensify. For example, you may have pain in your hands that travels up your arms or pain in your feet that extends up your legs. On occasion, the pain can be so intense that you may feel pain even from the light touch of a sheet that covers you at night. Often, there is numbness or a lack of feeling in your hands or feet. Because people with diabetic neuropathy are prone to nerve damage and poor circulation in their feet and other parts of their bodies, they may develop ulcers or gangrene.

If your peripheral neuropathy has affected your motor nerves (such as in Guillain-Barré syndrome), you may have problems with the muscles controlled by those nerves. You may have weakness or even paralysis. If your condition has damaged nerves that control some autonomic nerve system functions, you may have reduced ability to sweat, frequent constipation or diarrhea, bladder problems, or impotence. Your stomach may empty too slowly, resulting in nausea, vomiting, and bloating. In some cases, when you stand after sitting or lying down, your blood pressure may drop and you may become lightheaded or faint. People with peripheral neuropathy may also have problems with insomnia, depression, weight loss, or difficulty breathing or swallowing.

Conventional Treatments

Treatments vary according to the underlying cause of your neuropathy. The goal of treatment is to manage the condition that is causing the neuropathy, thereby providing symptom relief. So, if your peripheral neu-

A Quick Guide to Symptoms

- ☐ **Tingling or burning**
- ☐ **Pain**
- ☐ **Numbness, loss of feeling**
- ☐ **Weakness or even paralysis**
- ☐ **Reduced ability to sweat, frequent constipation or diarrhea, bladder problems, or impotence**
- ☐ **Insomnia, depression, weight loss, or difficulty breathing or swallowing**

ropathy is a result of high blood sugar levels, for example, then your doctor will want you to work to control them. If your symptoms are triggered by a vitamin B_{12} deficiency, you will receive injections of the vitamin. If you have pressure on a nerve, then treatment will center on ways to eliminate the pressure. Thus, if your keyboard is causing pain in your wrists, then you will be advised to use an ergonomically correct keyboard.

However, when there is no obvious cause of your peripheral neuropathy, you will be offered a number of pain-relieving alternatives.

Medications

Numerous over-the-counter pain medications may provide some relief. These include acetaminophen (Tylenol) and nonsteroidal anti-inflammatory drugs (NSAIDs) such as aspirin and ibuprofen (Advil, Motrin). If your pain is more severe, your doctor may prescribe stronger NSAIDs. NSAIDs taken in higher doses or over a long period of time may cause stomach pain and bleeding, nausea, and ulcers. Large doses may also result in kidney problems and heart failure.

Since they interfere with the chemical processes in the brain that cause you to feel pain, tricyclic antidepressants are often used for pain from peripheral neuropathy. Examples are amitriptyline (Elavil), nortriptyline (Pamelor), imipramine (Tofranil), and desipramine (Norpramin). These medications have potential side effects, including nausea, tiredness, dry mouth, dizziness, weight gain, and weakness. To reduce the chance that you will be forced to deal with these side effects, your doctor will probably start you on a low dose. If you have a good tolerance of the medication, then the dose may be increased.

If you are dealing with bouts of jabbing pain, your doctor may suggest an antiseizure medication, originally developed for those with epilepsy. Examples are gabapentin (Neurontin), phenytoin (Dilantin), and carbamazepine (Tegretol). Potential side effects include confusion and drowsiness. In a clinical trial, lamotrigine, an anticonvulsant, has been shown to be effective against moderate pain from peripheral neuropathy caused by diabetes or HIV. Minimal side effects were reported.

Still another medication is mexiletine (Mexitil), more commonly used for irregular heart rhythms. Potential side effects include nausea, lightheadedness, vomiting, shaking

hands, or difficulty walking. If you have diabetes-related peripheral neuropathy, you may wish to try the topical ointment capsaicin (Capzasin-P, Zostrix). You may see results in a week or two. Potential side effects include mild skin irritation, tingling, or burning at the point of application.

Transcutaneous Electrical Nerve Stimulation (TENS)

Transcutaneous electrical nerve stimulation (TENS) uses low-level electrical pulses to reduce pain. Typically, 80 to 100 pulses per second are given for 45 minutes, three times per day. The sensations are barely felt. In a similar procedure, known as percutaneous electrical nerve stimulation (PENS), the pulses are applied in small needles to acupuncture points. While this approach appears to provide some relief for most people with pain, it tends to work better in men than in women.

Complementary Treatments

To determine the best treatment plan, complementary medicine practitioners seek to find the underlying cause of peripheral neuropathy. However, the symptoms of peripheral neuropathy may also be treated individually by various complementary medicine treatments.

Acupuncture

Acupuncture can help reduce the pain associated with peripheral neuropathy. To locate an acupuncturist in your area, visit the Web site of the National Certification Commission for Acupuncture and Oriental Medicine (NCCAOM) at www.nccaom.org.

Biofeedback

Biofeedback uses an electric monitoring device to obtain data on vital body functions. During a session, you will be taught ways to use relaxation techniques to alter or slow the body's signals. Biofeedback can help teach individuals how to control the bodily responses that can help reduce pain. Various health care professionals incorporate biofeedback into their practice, including psychiatrists, psychologists, social workers, nurses, physical therapists, occupational therapists, speech therapists, respiratory therapists, exercise physiologists, and chiropractors.

Seek a health care practitioner who has been certified through the Biofeedback Certification Institute of America (BCIA). To locate a practitioner in your area, look on the BCIA Web site at www.bcia.org, check your local hospitals or medical clinics, or look in the Yellow Pages under the practitioners mentioned above.

Diet

Following a healthy, low-fat diet that includes lots of whole grains, fresh fruits, vegetables, and essential fatty acids may help reduce your risk of developing some forms of neuropathy. These foods are high in essential nutrients that feed the nerves and the brain and ensure proper communication between the two. They also support the immune system, which keeps the body healthy and fights viruses. If you have neuropathy that is caused by a particular medical condition, to ensure that the foods you are eating do not aggravate your condition, you should consult with your doctor.

Nutritional Supplements

To guarantee that you are receiving proper nutritional support, take a high-quality multivitamin/mineral supplement. Additional supplementation of vitamin B_{12} injections may also be a good idea. If injections are not available, take a 1,000-microgram tablet sublingually (under the tongue) daily.

Relaxation/Meditation

Relaxation/meditation techniques can help release the muscular tension that often leads to an increase in pain. A regular routine of guided imagery, meditation, yoga, or deep breathing exercises will promote relaxation, thus allowing the release of physical and emotional tension.

To practice deep breathing, lie flat on your back and place both hands on your abdomen. Slowly inhale through your nose, pushing your abdomen up as if you were blowing up a balloon. Then, exhale slowly through the mouth, and feel your abdomen deflate. Repeat this process 8 to 10 times, and practice this breathing process as often as possible.

Lifestyle Recommendations

Calm your burning hands and feet. Try soaking your hands and feet in cool water for 15 minutes, twice each day. After you finish, rub your hands and feet with petroleum jelly.

Exercise. Following an exercise program will help you deal with your symptoms. Ask your doctor to suggest an exercise routine. A referral to a physical therapist who has special training in dealing with the symptoms of peripheral neuropathy is also a good idea.

Limit caffeine and alcohol. Caffeine and alcohol exacerbate peripheral neuropathy symptoms, so limit your intake.

Regularly massage your hands and feet. By massaging your hands and feet, you will improve circulation and stimulate the nerves, which may also relieve the pain.

Stop smoking. Smoking will only aggravate your peripheral neuropathy.

Take care of your feet. Don't wear tight shoes or socks. This is particularly important if you have diabetes. If your bedcovers are bothering your sensitive feet, purchase a semicircular hoop that holds the covers over your body. You can find this device in a medical supply store.

Preventive Measures

Avoid repetitive motions. People who engage in repetitive motions are more likely to suffer from peripheral neuropathy. Try to be proactive in avoiding repetitive motions, such as typing or other job-related activities.

Be careful with chemicals. Toxic chemicals may harm your nerves. Try to avoid using them, or if you must use them, wear protective clothing.

Manage your medical condition. If you have a medical condition, such as diabetes, that places you at increased risk for peripheral neuropathy, then you need to control it. In the case of diabetes, you need to manage your sugar levels.

Peripheral Vascular Disease

With peripheral vascular disease (PVD), the arteries that carry blood to the arms or legs become narrowed or clogged. Blood is unable to flow normally.

Also known as peripheral artery disease (PAD) or occlusive arterial disease, peripheral vascular disease is very common. Over the age of 50, about one out of every 20 people has this disorder. About 10 million Americans are affected, yet 2.5 million are undiagnosed.

Causes and Risk Factors

Most often, peripheral vascular disease is caused by atherosclerosis, which is also called hardening of the arteries. With atherosclerosis, cholesterol and scar tissue (plaque) build up inside the blood vessels, which become narrowed or clogged. However, blood clots in the arteries may also cause PVD.

Men are more likely than women to have PVD. People over the age of 50 have an increased risk, as do smokers, people with diabetes, and people who are overweight and do not exercise. High blood pressure, high cholesterol, and a family history of heart or vascular disease all raise the risk.

Signs and Symptoms

The most frequent symptom associated with peripheral vascular disease is painful cramping in the legs, calves, hips, or feet, especially when walking. This painful cramping, which is called intermittent claudication, is a result of inadequate bloodflow in the leg muscles. While the pain tends to disappear when you stop walking, as soon as you start walking again, it will likely reappear. Men may experience erectile dysfunction. Other common symptoms include numbness, tingling, or weakness in the affected legs. The skin of the

A Quick Guide to Symptoms

- ☐ Painful cramping in the legs, calves, hips, or feet, especially when walking
- ☐ Erectile dysfunction
- ☐ Numbness, tingling, or weakness in the affected leg
- ☐ The skin of the affected legs and feet may seem cooler and change color
- ☐ Loss of hair on the legs
- ☐ Feet and toes may burn and ache
- ☐ Leg or foot sores that do not heal

affected legs and feet may seem cooler and change color. There may be a loss of hair on the legs. In the worst cases, your feet and toes may burn and ache, even when resting, and you may have leg or foot sores that do not heal. Sometimes, untreated PVD may lead to gangrene.

Conventional Treatments

Your treatment will probably begin with a review of your lifestyle. If you smoke, you will be told to stop. If you have diabetes, you'll need to maintain better control of your blood sugar. Do you have high blood pressure? If so, you need to lower it. Is your cholesterol too high? You must find ways to lower it.

Angioplasty

During an angioplasty, a surgeon places a tiny balloon in a blood vessel at the site of the blockage. When the balloon is inflated, the blockage opens. Sometimes, to keep a vessel open, a metal cylinder called a stent may be inserted.

Exercise

Regular exercise appears to be the most consistently effective treatment for peripheral vascular disease. If you participate in a regular exercise program, you will gradually be able to reduce your level of pain. Begin with brief walks, then slowly increase the amount of time that you walk.

Interventional Radiology Treatments

A number of interventional radiology treatments are available for PVD. These use catheters or tiny tubes and other miniaturized tools as well as x-rays.

Medications

A variety of medications may be prescribed for people with PVD. If you have high blood pressure or high cholesterol, you may get a prescription to treat those conditions. You might get a prescription for ticlopidine

Self-Testing

The following is a self-test for peripheral vascular disease. The more "yes" answers that you have, the more likely it is that you have this disorder.

☐ Do you have a history of cardiovascular (heart) problems, such as high blood pressure, heart attack, or stroke?

☐ Do you have diabetes?

☐ Do you have a family history of diabetes or cardiovascular problems with immediate family members (mother, father, sister, or brother)?

☐ Do you have aching or cramping in your legs when you walk or exercise? Does the pain stop when you rest?

☐ Do your feet and toes hurt at night?

☐ Do ulcers or sores on your feet heal slowly?

☐ Do you smoke?

☐ Did you previously smoke?

☐ Are you more than 25 pounds overweight?

☐ Do you eat fatty foods at least three times each week?

☐ Are you inactive?

(Ticlid), which helps some people with PVD to walk longer distances. Still, the pharmacologic management of PVD has not been as successful as the pharmacologic treatment of coronary artery disease. Pentoxifylline (Trental) has been shown to increase the duration of exercise in individuals with claudication, but its efficacy has not been demonstrated consistently in clinical trials.

Surgery

In severe cases of PVD, surgery may be required. These procedures should be performed by a vascular surgeon.

Amputation. Without bloodflow, tissue dies and poses an extremely high risk for serious infection. An amputation is done only as a last resort, when there is little or no bloodflow to the foot or leg, and when there are no other options.

Bypass grafts. In a bypass graft, a portion of vein is removed from another part of the body. It is then grafted onto the affected area, creating a detour around the blockage. Sometimes, rather than taking a vein from another part of the body, the surgeon uses a synthetic graft.

Thrombectomy. A thrombectomy is done only when PVD symptoms develop suddenly from a blood clot. During this procedure, the surgeon inserts a balloon into the artery beyond the blood clot. The balloon is inflated and pulled back, thereby removing the clot.

Thrombolytic Therapy

If a clot is causing the blockage in an artery, an interventional radiologist may use a catheter to administer a clot-busting drug. Thrombolytic therapy is often combined with another treatment, such as an angioplasty.

> # Legs for Life
>
> The Society of Interventional Radiology has created Legs for Life, a community screening program for PVD. People who are believed to have PVD are referred to their primary care physician for additional diagnosis. To determine when and where the screenings will be held, log on to the program's Web site at www.legsforlife.org.

Complementary Treatments

The best complementary medicine treatment approach is prevention through dietary modification, nutritional supplementation, herbal therapies, and lifestyle changes.

> **In some uncommon instances,** your doctor will advise against exercising. Before beginning any exercise program, check with your doctor.

Aquatic Therapy

Aquatic therapy is a gentle way to begin an exercise program. Water is an ideal environment to promote relaxation. The rhythmic movements and simple stretches help the mind and body to unwind and reduce stress. Aerobic exercise and relaxation techniques have been shown to lower blood pressure.

Diet

Eating a balanced and healthy diet is most beneficial for maintaining a healthy cardiovascular system. Your diet should include lots of vegetables, fruits, whole grains, and nuts and seeds (walnuts, almonds, and sesame seeds). Try to include a minimum of five servings of vegetables, four servings of fruit, and six servings of whole grains each day.

You should avoid trans fatty acids, fried foods, sugar, and other processed foods. Since the regular consumption of animal products increases the risk of cardiovascular problems, saturated fats and cholesterol-rich foods, such as fatty meats, egg yolks, milk fat, and margarine, should be eliminated from the diet.

Increase your intake of water-soluble fiber. By removing fat that has accumulated in the intestines and by decreasing the absorption of this fat, water-soluble fiber, which is contained in many healthy foods, may lower cholesterol and blood pressure. Also, reduce your intake of dairy products, as dairy has been linked to an increased risk of developing cardiovascular disease.

Foods rich in essential fatty acids and the antioxidants beta-carotene, the B vitamins, and vitamins C and E; magnesium; and selenium are all useful for heart health. Essential fatty acids are found in flaxseed oil, salmon, and other cold-water fish. Beta-carotene is contained in almost all fruits and vegetables. It is the substance that provides their color. Good sources of vitamin C also include almost all fruits and green vegetables, especially strawberries, cranberries, melons, oranges, mangoes, papayas, peppers, spinach, kale, broccoli, tomatoes, and potatoes.

Vitamin E may be found in vegetable oils, nuts, seeds, and wheat germ. Smaller amounts of vitamin E are in leafy vegetables and whole grains. The B vitamins are found in dark green, leafy vegetables; whole grains; oranges; avocados; beets; bananas; potatoes; dairy products; nuts; beans; fish; and chicken. Magnesium is found in green, leafy vegetables such as spinach, parsley, broccoli, chard, kale, and mustard and turnip greens. It is also in raw almonds, wheat germ, potatoes, and tofu. Selenium is contained in seafood, chicken, whole-grain cereals, and garlic.

Anthocyanosides are compounds that have antioxidant properties and are found in blueberries, cherries, raspberries, red or purple grapes, and plums. The European species of blueberry, the bilberry, has the highest level of anthocyanosides. Anthocyanosides help improve capillary circulation.

Garlic, onions, cayenne pepper, ginger, turmeric, and alfalfa all reduce cholesterol, thus aiding in the health of the heart. Garlic, onions, and cayenne pepper also thin the blood, thereby preventing clotting. And foods containing soy have been shown to drop elevated cholesterol levels.

To ensure that there is no interaction between medicines and the nutrients found in food, if you are taking any prescription medication for your heart, you should consult with your doctor.

Herbal Medicine

Garlic. Garlic, an antioxidant that lowers cholesterol, may also reduce high blood pressure and improve the elasticity of blood vessel walls. The daily dose of fresh garlic is two to three cloves per day, while the supplement dose is 500 milligrams. If you have a choice, select fresh garlic over supplements. The supplements contain concentrated extracts, which may increase the risk of excessive bleeding.

Ginkgo biloba. Ginkgo is an antioxidant that supports circulation; it is available in capsule form. The recommended daily dose is 120 milligrams, twice a day, of an extract standardized to 24 percent of flavone glycosides and 6 percent terpene lactones. The flavone glycosides give ginkgo its antioxidant benefits, while terpene lactones increase circulation and have a protective effect on nerve cells. If you are also taking prescription blood-thinning medications, be sure to check with a doctor before using ginkgo supplements.

Green tea. Green tea is a powerful antioxidant that helps to decrease cholesterol, lower blood pressure, and prevent the clogging of arteries. Green tea can be taken as a tea or in capsules. Drinking 3 cups of green tea per day provides 240 to 320 milligrams of polyphenols. In capsule form, standardized extract of EGCG (a polyphenol) may provide 97 percent polyphenol content, which is the equivalent of drinking 4 cups of tea per day.

Hawthorn. Like green tea, hawthorn works to decrease cholesterol and lower blood pressure. In addition, hawthorn helps to strengthen heart muscles, improve circulation, and rid the body of unnecessary fluid and salt. Hawthorn is available in capsule or tincture form, standardized to 2.2 percent total bioflavonoid content. It may take up to 2 months before you see the effects of this herb on your health. The recommended daily dose of hawthorn capsules varies widely, ranging from 100 to 300 milligrams, two to three times per day. Be aware that higher doses may significantly lower blood pressure, which may cause you to feel faint. When using the tincture, the recommended dose is 4 to 5 milliliters, three times per day.

Nutritional Supplements

The following nutritional supplements are very beneficial to maintaining a healthy vascular system.

- B-complex vitamins: Take as directed on the label. Help prevent the arteries from getting clogged and prevent inappropriate blood clot formation.

- Vitamin B_6: 50 milligrams daily in divided doses of 25 milligrams. Helps with absorption of calcium, magnesium, and vitamin C.

- Vitamin C: 1,000 milligrams daily in divided doses of 500 milligrams. Essential for heart health. Vitamin C converts cholesterol into bile, strengthens the arterial walls, and stops the buildup of cholesterol.

- Calcium: 1,500 milligrams daily in divided doses of 750 milligrams. Lowers total cholesterol and increases HDL cholesterol.

- Chromium: 200 micrograms daily. Aids in the prevention of the buildup of cholesterol and increases HDL.

- Coenzyme Q_{10}: 200 milligrams daily in divided doses of 100 milligrams. Increases oxygen to the heart tissue and may help lower blood pressure and prevent oxidation of LDL ("bad") cholesterol.

- Vitamin E: 400 IU daily. Stops the oxidation of LDL cholesterol, prevents damage to the arterial lining, improves circulation, and fortifies the immune system. Vitamin E may thin the blood. If you are taking blood-thinning medication, consult your doctor before taking this supplement. If there are no contraindications, take vitamin E with selenium for best absorption.

- L-carnitine: 500 milligrams daily in divided doses of 250 milligrams. Effective for intermittent claudication (leg cramps). Lowers total cholesterol and increases HDL cholesterol.

- Magnesium: 800 milligrams daily in divided doses of 400 milligrams. Helps to lower total cholesterol and increases HDL cholesterol.

- Selenium: 400 micrograms daily in divided doses of 200 micrograms. Helps prevent heart disease and future heart attacks by thinning the blood. However, if you are taking blood-thinning medication, consult your doctor before taking this supplement. Selenium should not be taken at the same time as vitamin C as they interfere with each other's absorption.

Relaxation/Meditation

Many practitioners recommend relaxation/meditation techniques to help people reduce stress, control their emotions, and lower blood pressure. Clinical trials have shown that by combining biofeedback, yoga, and meditation, you will improve your ability to lower blood pressure. A 2006 study showed that practicing mental relaxation or slow breathing can reduce blood pressure and heart rate. Other effective techniques for reducing stress include qigong, tai chi, yoga, deep breathing exercises, and visualization.

Lifestyle Recommendations

If you have peripheral vascular disease, you may be tempted to stop exercising. Work together with your doctor to develop an exercise plan. In general, you should start with something as brief as a 5-minute walk, then gradually increase the length of your exercise routine. By reducing blood pressure and decreasing resting heart rate, exercise improves the bloodflow in the arteries. Further, exercise helps you lose weight and manage stress. So, over time, it reduces the symptoms of PVD.

Preventive Measures

A healthy weight, lipid profile, and blood pressure are a good start to preventing peripheral vascular disease.

Avoid excess salt consumption. Sodium causes the body to retain fluid, creating more work for the heart.

Control the stress in your life. Find some means to reduce the stress in your life. Consider meditating or some other way to calm yourself.

Decrease coffee consumption. Coffee increases stress hormones, which puts coffee drinkers at greater risk for heart problems. However, studies have failed to prove a link between atherosclerosis and caffeine intake.

Reduce alcohol consumption. Alcohol may raise blood pressure and overtax the liver, interfering with the liver's ability to detoxify foods. This may result in a buildup of cholesterol. Studies have shown that red wine may be beneficial for the cardiovascular system, as the flavonoids in the wine help stop the buildup of fatty deposits in blood vessels. The recommended daily intake is one 5-ounce glass for women, and no more than two 5-ounce glasses for men.

Stop smoking. Smoking is a major risk factor in the development of PVD. Smoking can also interfere with the treatment of the disease. The carbon monoxide produced from cigarette smoking decreases the oxygen in the blood, causing the heart to work harder. Smoking also causes blood platelets to stick together, which blocks the arteries. In some instances, smoking may interfere with your prescription medications.

Pick's Disease

Pick's disease is one of a group of brain disorders collectively termed frontotemporal dementia (FTD). These disorders involve the shrinking or atrophying of the brain's frontal and temporal lobes, which control speech and personality. With Pick's disease, abnormal brain cells (Pick's bodies) may be found in these lobes and other areas of the brain. Affecting about one out of every 100,000 people, Pick's disease is relatively rare.

People with Pick's disease may exhibit significant changes in personality that affect all aspects of their lives. They may be apathetic and disinterested in daily activities, and they may disregard social decorum and the feelings of other people. Sometimes, they may act out with antisocial behavior. In addition, though mathematical skills tend to be well

Unlike with Alzheimer's disease, during the early stages of Pick's disease, the memory is not impaired. And while Alzheimer's most often is seen in those over the age of 65, Pick's disease tends to appear in people who are in their prime of life.

preserved, people with Pick's disease may lose the ability to initiate and complete even simple functions. As the illness progresses, there may be problems with language and communication, and memory and attention span may be poor. In the final stage of the disease, there is a generalized dementia. While the disease may last for up to 15 years, eventually the individual enters a terminal vegetative state. Death is usually the result of an infection.

A definitive diagnosis of Pick's disease may be made only after death, when a brain biopsy is performed. A doctor may be able to reach a working diagnosis through evaluation of the patient and the results of various tests.

Causes and Risk Factors

The cause of Pick's disease is unknown. While the age of onset may range from 20 to 80, the disease most often occurs in people between the ages of 40 and 64. The average age of onset is 54. There is evidence of a genetic link. People of Scandinavian origin/descent may have an increased risk. The disease equally affects both sexes. Up to 40 percent of people who have Pick's disease have a family history of the disease.

Signs and Symptoms

There are two main types of Pick's disease. In the first, there are gradual and progressive changes in behavior. These may include socially and sexually inappropriate behavior, apathy and loss of initiative, compulsive eating and a tendency to gain weight, oral fixation, incontinence, emotional dullness, and lack of concern for others. In the second type, there are gradual and progressive speech and language problems. As the disease progresses, there is a loss of memory.

Conventional Treatments

There are no proven treatments for Pick's disease and no ways to slow the progression of the disease. In general, treatments help manage the various symptoms. Your doctor may prescribe antidepressants or antipsychotic medications. In some instances, medications may be needed to control agitated or aggressive behaviors.

Complementary Treatments

It is best to treat the symptoms associated with Pick's disease. Dietary changes and nutritional supplements may be useful in stimulating brain function.

Diet

Although food is unable to cure Pick's disease, eating foods high in nutrients may help address symptoms such as memory loss, short attention span, and dementia. As your brain may function only as well as you feed it, the old saying "you are what you eat" may be appropriate. It is extremely important to maintain a diet high in nutrient-rich foods.

A Quick Guide to Symptoms

- ☐ Socially and sexually inappropriate behavior
- ☐ Apathy and loss of initiative
- ☐ Compulsive eating and a tendency to gain weight
- ☐ Oral fixation
- ☐ Incontinence
- ☐ Emotional dullness
- ☐ Lack of concern for others
- ☐ Speech and language problems

Be sure to include lots of fresh fruits and vegetables and whole grains. Try to include a minimum of five servings of vegetables, four servings of fruit, and six servings of whole grains each day.

Vitamin C, which is found in many fruits and vegetables, has been shown to improve memory performance. Antioxidants, found in fruits, vegetables, and soy products, may slow memory loss. Preliminary research has shown that monounsaturated fats, such as olive oil, may protect against memory loss and age-related cognitive decline (ARCD). Avoid fried foods and other hydrogenated fats as well as processed foods containing artificial colors and other chemicals.

Herbal Medicine

A number of studies have found that ginkgo improves mental clarity, memory, and overall circulation to the brain. To see noticeable change in as soon as 4 weeks, the typical recommended daily dose of ginkgo is 80 milligrams, three times a day, of extract standardized to 24 percent of flavone glycosides and 6 percent terpene lactones.

Nutritional Supplements

Nutritional deficiencies may lead to various forms of memory loss.

- Multivitamin/mineral: Take as directed on the label. Should include copper, zinc, calcium, and magnesium to help the brain retain memory.

- B-complex vitamins: Take as directed on the label. Essential in preventing and reversing memory loss. B_3 improves circulation to the brain, while deficiency may produce dementia. Vitamin B_1 can decrease effects of senility, and B_6 aids in long-term memory.

- Vitamin B_{12}: Injections. Deficiency may impair mental ability. Injections of B_{12} show improvement in memory.

- Vitamin C: 2,000 milligrams daily in divided doses of 1,000 milligrams. Antioxidant effects help reduce memory loss.

- Vitamin E: 400 IU daily. Antioxidant effects help reduce memory loss.

- Acetyl-L-carnitine: 1,000 milligrams daily in divided doses of 500 milligrams. Improves memory. Take with meals.

Lifestyle Recommendations

Check water temperature. To prevent accidental scalding, set your hot water heater so that it is no higher than 120°F.

Exercise. Engaging in physical activity as simple as a daily walk can help maintain a healthy weight, increase circulation, and encourage social interaction.

Make room modifications. You may wish to make modifications to meet the needs of an individual with Pick's disease. For example, positioning the bed toward the bathroom may reduce incidents of incontinence. Placing familiar objects and photographs nearby may reinforce memory.

Make safety modifications. To prevent accidents, you may need to place sharp objects, tools, and toxic chemicals in a locked area. You may also want to use childproof locks on doors and cabinets.

Obtain help and support. Because Pick's disease generally strikes so profoundly in the prime of life and because the prognosis is so dismal, a diagnosis of Pick's disease is devastating for both the patient and caregiver. If you are the caregiver of someone with Pick's disease, you need to reach out to your community and obtain the assistance you require. Because of the behavioral problems, caring for someone with Pick's is particularly difficult. Eventually, many of those with Pick's disease need to reside in an institutional setting.

Prostate Enlargement

Prostate enlargement shows up in men as they age. The older they are, it seems, the more likely they'll be dealing with problems of the prostate gland. Located in front of the rectum and just below the bladder, the walnut-size prostate gland squeezes fluid into the urethra as sperm move through during ejaculation. When the prostate first begins to enlarge, a condition also called benign prostatic hyperplasia (BPH) or benign prostatic hypertrophy, it rarely causes any problems. However, eventually, it presses against the urethra, resulting in the bladder becoming thicker and irritated. The bladder may contract when it contains only a small amount of urine. More frequent urination becomes necessary, but since the bladder may be unable to empty itself fully, urine may remain in the bladder after urination.

Prostate enlargement is a common disorder. Though rare before the age of 40, more than half of all men who are in their sixties have prostate enlargement. Almost all men in their seventies and eighties have evidence of this problem.

Causes and Risk Factors

Though there is no clear cause for prostate enlargement, it is known that married men develop the disorder more often than single men. It is more common in American and European men than Asian men. And genetics appears to play a role. If members of your family tend to have prostate enlargement, then you are at increased risk.

> **If you find that you are unable to pass** any urine, you may have a serious medical problem known as acute urinary retention. You need to seek emergency medical assistance.

Signs and Symptoms

Only about half of the men with prostate enlargement are so significantly bothered by their symptoms that they seek medical care. Symptoms associated with prostate enlargement include difficulty starting urination, stopping and starting while urinating,

A Quick Guide to Symptoms

- [ ] Difficulty starting urination
- [ ] Stopping and starting while urinating
- [ ] Dribbling at the end of urination
- [ ] Urgent need to urinate
- [ ] Frequent need to urinate
- [ ] Weak urine stream
- [ ] Increased rate of nighttime urination (nocturia)

dribbling at the end of urination, urgent need to urinate, frequent need to urinate, weak urine stream, and increased rate of nighttime urination (nocturia).

Conventional Treatments

If an enlarged prostate has caused no symptoms, then no treatment will be recommended. However, if you do have symptoms, a number of treatments are available. The recommended treatment will depend upon the type of symptoms you are experiencing.

Medications

If you have moderate symptoms, there is a good chance that your treatment will begin with medication. There are two types of medications used for prostate enlargement, alpha-blockers and finasteride.

Alpha-blockers. Although originally developed to treat high blood pressure, alpha-blockers have been found useful for other medical problems, including an enlarged prostate. They relax the muscles at the neck of the bladder, thereby making it easier to urinate. Examples of alpha-blockers approved for prostate enlargement are tamsulosin (Flomax), terazosin (Hytrin), and doxazosin (Cardura). Effective in about 75 percent of the men who take them, alpha-blockers begin working in a day or two. Men will note that they need to urinate less often, and that there is an increase in the urinary flow. Potential side effects include headaches, dizziness, lightheadedness, and tired-

ness. It is recommended that you take the medication before bedtime. In some instances, the medication may cause low blood pressure when standing, as well as erectile dysfunction (impotence). Tamsulosin, which is the newest of these medications, tends to cause less dizziness, but it may result in abnormal ejaculation.

Finasteride. Finasteride, which actually shrinks the prostate, works best for men with large prostate glands. It is not as effective for those with moderately enlarged prostate glands, in which it may result in an obstruction. Examples are Proscar and Propecia. Unfortunately, finasteride takes a while to work. While you may have some improvement within 3 months, it often requires up to a year. In addition, finasteride lowers your baseline PSA level, which could interfere with a proper determination of your risk for prostate cancer. (PSA, or prostate-specific antigen, is a protein made by cells in the prostate gland. High levels are considered a marker for prostate cancer.)

Nonsurgical Therapies

Nonsurgical therapies for prostate enlargement focus on widening the urethra, thus making it easier to urinate.

Heat therapy. With heat therapy, heat energy, which is delivered via the urethra, is used to destroy excess prostate tissue. It is better than medications for prostate enlargement that is causing moderate to severe symptoms, and it has fewer side effects than surgery. Though heat therapy is usually performed on an outpatient basis, you may need to spend the night at the hospital.

Microwave therapy. Transurethral microwave therapy (TUMT) uses computer-controlled heat in the form of microwave energy to destroy excess tissue in the enlarged gland. During the procedure, you will be given a local anesthetic. Then, a urinary catheter (a tube that has a tiny microwave device) will be used to heat enlarged prostate cells and destroy them. You will probably feel some heat in the prostate and bladder area, and you will have a strong desire to urinate. You may also have bladder spasms. Most likely, you will need to wear a urinary catheter for a few days. As you recover, you may have periods when you have urgent, frequent urination and blood in your urine, and there may be changes in the semen you ejaculate. You should not have TUMT if you have a pacemaker or any metal implants.

Radiofrequency therapy. With transurethral needle ablation (TUNA), radio waves are sent through needles inserted into the prostate gland. This heats and destroys the tissue. TUNA tends to be less effective than surgery in reducing symptoms and improving the flow of urine, and it is not as useful for men with large prostates. Among the potential side effects are painful urination, blood in the urine, urine retention, and a slight risk for retrograde ejaculation, a condition in which part of the semen goes backward into the bladder.

Electrovaporization. During a transurethral electrovaporization of the prostate (TVP), a metal instrument that emits a high-frequency electrical current is used to cut and vaporize excess prostate tissue. To prevent bleeding, tissue is sealed. This procedure is particularly useful for men at higher risk for bleeding, such as those who take blood-thinning medications.

Laser therapy. With laser therapy, heat from lasers is used to destroy prostate tissue. Transurethral evaporation of the prostate (TUEP) is similar to electrovaporization. It is considered quite safe and results in only a small amount of bleeding. Urine flow tends to improve fairly quickly. Noncontact visual laser ablation (VLAP) uses laser energy to damage excess prostate cells, which are eliminated over an extended period of time. As a result of the swelling and slow wearing away of the tissue, urine is often retained, and you will probably need to wear a catheter for several days. You may also have burning during urination for days or even weeks. Interstitial laser therapy sends laser energy inside prostate growths, resulting in moderate reductions in the size of the prostate and moderate improvements in urine flow. It appears to be useful for men with large prostates, but there tends to be a lot of postsurgical inflammation, so you may require a catheter for up to 3 weeks, and infections are fairly common.

Surgery

Years ago, surgery was frequently used for an enlarged prostate. Because of the other available options, it is now used most often for those who have the most severe symptoms or complicating factors such as bleeding through the urethra, kidney damage from urinary retention, frequent urinary tract infections, and stones in the bladder. Unless no other therapy is effective, it tends not to be used for men with serious lung, kidney, or heart conditions; uncontrolled diabetes; cirrhosis of the liver; or major psychiatric disorder.

Transurethral resection of the prostate (TURP). With TURP, while you are either under general anesthesia or anesthetized from the waist down, part of the prostate is removed. The surgeon inserts a narrow instrument known as a resectoscope into the urethra. The resectoscope has an electrical loop that may be used to remove prostate tissue and seal blood vessels. Potential complications from TURP surgery include blood in the urine, a sense of urgency to urinate,

short-term difficulty controlling urine, and problems with sexual function. Some men develop retrograde or dry ejaculation—in this condition, part of the semen goes backward into the bladder. In up to 10 percent of cases, prostate tissue grows back, and a second surgery may be required.

Transurethral incision of the prostate (TUIP). If you are not considered a good candidate for TURP, your doctor may recommend TUIP. As with TURP, several instruments are inserted through the urethra. However, rather than remove prostate tissue, the urethra is enlarged. While there are fewer side effects from this procedure, it is not as effective and it frequently must be repeated.

Open prostatectomy. If you have extreme prostate enlargement or a complicating factor such as bladder damage, bladder stones, or urethral strictures, your doctor may advise an open prostatectomy, the removal of the inner portion of your prostate via an incision in your lower abdomen. Potential complications tend to be the same as with TURP, though they are often more severe.

Recovering from Surgery

During your surgical procedure, a catheter will be inserted through the penis into the bladder. It will enable urine to be collected into a collection bag. You will probably be required to wear this catheter for several days. In some instances, it may cause painful bladder spasms. These should go away fairly quickly. Most likely, there will be blood in your urine. Be sure to drink lots of water, which helps flush the bladder and aids in healing. After surgery, you should not do any heavy lifting for several weeks.

Complementary Treatments

Dietary changes and nutritional and herbal supplementation have been shown to be effective in reducing and eliminating prostate enlargement.

Diet

To avoid prostate enlargement, it is extremely beneficial to maintain a healthy diet low in saturated fats. By substituting soy protein for animal protein, you may quickly and effectively reduce cholesterol. Essential fatty acids have also been shown to be useful to prevent prostate enlargement. Good food sources are seafood (particularly bluefish, herring, salmon, and tuna), almonds, peanuts, walnuts, and sunflower seeds. Although seafood is, in fact, animal protein, the essential fatty acid content is so beneficial that including it in your diet is a good thing.

Herbal Medicine

Pygeum and stinging nettle. Along with saw palmetto, pygeum and stinging nettle are diuretics, which increase the secretion and flow of urine and reduce irritation of the bladder and urethra. Both are available in tincture form. Pygeum, in particular, has been shown to aid males who have trouble initiating urination, and it also supports the complete emptying of the bladder. The typical recommended daily dose for pygeum is 50 milligrams twice a day of extract standardized to 13 percent total sterols; for stinging nettle, the recommended daily dose is 250 milligrams of nettle root twice a day.

Saw palmetto. Clinical studies have shown saw palmetto to be useful for the relief of symptoms of an enlarged prostate. Saw palmetto is available in capsules containing 160 milligrams of extract standardized to 85 to 95 percent fatty acids and sterols. The typical recommended daily dose is 320 milligrams. Though you may notice symptom relief

within 30 days, you should continue to take the supplement.

Naturopathy

There is a link between food sensitivity and prostate problems. A naturopathic physician may test for food allergies or sensitivities that could be causing enlargement of the prostate. To find a naturopathic practitioner in your area, contact the American Association of Naturopathic Physicians at www.naturopathic.org.

Nutritional Supplements

Nutritional supplements are beneficial in shrinking an enlarged prostate.

- Omega-3 fatty acids: 1 tablespoon of flaxseed oil or fish oil capsules as directed on the label. May prevent the prostate from swelling.

- Zinc: 30 milligrams daily. Effective in shrinking an enlarged prostate and enhancing the immune system.

Lifestyle Recommendations

Empty your bladder. When you void, try to urinate as much as possible. Some men void more effectively when they sit on the toilet.

Keep warm. You are more likely to retain urine when you are cold. And you are also more likely to experience an urgency to urinate when you are cold.

Limit alcohol intake. Alcohol irritates the bladder and increases urine production.

Limit your evening beverage intake. While you should drink a good deal of water during the day, reduce the amount of water you drink in the evening to lessen your need to urinate while you sleep.

Stay active. Inactivity may trigger urine retention.

Take care with over-the-counter decongestants. In some instances, decongestants may cause the urethral sphincter (the band of muscles that controls urine flow) to tighten, making urination more difficult.

Preventive Measures

Eat a healthy diet. Eating excess amounts of protein and fat, especially from junk food, has been associated with prostate enlargement. It is always advisable to remove junk food from your diet. Beans and legumes contain pectin, a water-soluble fiber that helps move cholesterol out of the body. It is recommended to eat one serving of beans (1½ cups) each day. Especially good choices are soybeans, lima beans, kidney beans, navy beans, pinto beans, black-eyed peas, and lentils. Fruits also contain pectin and should be eaten regularly. Carrots, cabbage, broccoli, and onions have pectin in the form of calcium pectate, which also helps move cholesterol. Starting your day with half a grapefruit and eating two raw carrots at lunch is an ideal way to begin lowering your cholesterol. A compound found in skim milk may actually inhibit cholesterol production in the liver.

Maintain a healthy cholesterol level. It is best to keep your total cholesterol level below 220.

Prostatitis

Prostatitis is inflammation of the prostate gland. The doughnut-shaped, walnut-size prostate gland, which is found only in men, is located behind the pubic bone and in front of the rectum. It produces most of the fluids in semen.

Though rarely discussed, prostatitis is one of the most common medical problems faced by men. Every year, men make about 2 million visits to doctors because of this medical problem.

There are three types of prostatitis: acute bacterial prostatitis, chronic bacterial prostatitis, and nonbacterial prostatitis. Acute bacterial prostatitis develops quickly; you immediately know you are sick. It is not uncommon for this type of prostatitis to require hospitalization. The progression of chronic bacterial prostatitis and nonbacterial prostatitis is slower and more subtle.

Causes and Risk Factors

Many cases of prostatitis are caused by a bacteria-induced infection. Generally, the bacteria travel to the prostate from other parts of the urinary tract, such as the kidneys or bladder. But they may also be transmitted through the urethra during sexual activity. And bacteria found in the large intestine may also be a culprit. Only infrequently are the bacteria spread through the bloodstream. It is well known that the insertion of a catheter into the urethra has the potential to introduce bacteria and trigger an infection. And calcified stones that may form in the prostate gland may attract bacteria.

However, most cases of prostatitis are not a result of bacteria. In these instances, there is no evidence of bacteria in the urine or prostate fluid. Nevertheless, elevated white blood cells in urine specimens will usually indicate inflammation. Though researchers are not certain what causes nonbacterial prostatitis, they have a number of theories. Some think it may be related to inflammation of the urethra or a sexually transmitted disease, such as gonorrhea or chlamydia. There is speculation that it may be connected to a reduction in sexual activity or an undetected infectious agent. Further, it has been theorized that men who start and stop their urination instead of allowing the urine to flow freely may cause a backing up of urine, which irritates the prostate.

Other hypotheses focus on anxiety and stress or lifting heavy objects with a full bladder. Occupations that subject the prostate to a good deal of vibrations—such as riding on heavy equipment—may place men at risk. And recreational bikers and joggers may irritate their prostate glands.

Men who are over 50 who have benign enlargement of the prostate are at increased risk of urinary tract infections, and that increased risk places them at greater risk for prostatitis. Also, men who have suffered a bout of acute bacterial prostatitis are at greater risk for a recurrence, as well as the development of chronic bacterial prostatitis.

Certain behaviors, such as excess alcohol consumption, are believed to cause congestion in the prostate gland. A congested prostate gland is a good environment for bacteria to thrive.

A Quick Guide to Symptoms

Acute bacterial prostatitis
- [ ] **Spiking fever**
- [ ] **Chills**
- [ ] **Sweating**
- [ ] **Cloudy, bloody, or foul-smelling urine**
- [ ] **Pain in the lower back, behind the scrotum, or in the testicles**
- [ ] **Pain with urination or bowel movements**
- [ ] **Inability to urinate and empty the bladder, or the need to urinate frequently**
- [ ] **Painful ejaculation**

Chronic bacterial prostatitis
- [ ] **Pain or burning during urination**
- [ ] **Lower back pain**
- [ ] **Aching sensation in the middle to lower abdomen**
- [ ] **Pain in the penis and scrotum**
- [ ] **Frequent urination**
- [ ] **Blood in the semen**
- [ ] **Low-grade fever**
- [ ] **Painful ejaculation**

Signs and Symptoms

With acute bacterial prostatitis, symptoms may be rather dramatic: a spiking fever, chills, sweating, cloudy urine, and lower back pain. There may be pain behind the scrotum, pain in the testicles, and pain with urination or bowel movements. You may be unable to urinate and empty the bladder, or you may feel the need to urinate frequently. Urine may contain blood or smell bad, and ejaculation may be painful.

The symptoms of chronic bacterial prostatitis and nonbacterial prostatitis tend to develop more slowly. While not as severe as acute bacterial prostatitis, they are definitely worrisome. Among the many possible symptoms are pain or burning during urination, mild lower back pain, aching sensation in the middle to lower abdomen, pain in the penis and scrotum, frequent urination, blood in the semen, low-grade fever, and painful ejaculation. In chronic bacterial prostatitis, there are bacteria in the urine or in the fluid from the prostate. There are no detectable bacteria in nonbacterial prostatitis.

Conventional Treatments

Treatments vary according to the type of prostatitis. Prostatitis does not always respond well to treatments, so a number of different options may be needed.

Medications

Though it may make you quite ill, acute bacterial prostatitis is the easiest form of prostatitis to treat. Depending upon the type of bacteria that is found, your doctor will prescribe an antibiotic. You'll likely also get an antibiotic for chronic bacterial prostatitis, and you will probably take it for a longer period of time.

In general, antibiotics that penetrate the prostate are preferred. Typically, they are prescribed for 4 weeks. These antibiotics include the fluoroquinolones, such as ciprofloxacin and levofloxacin. In addition, trimethoprim-sulfamethoxazole has been found to be effective for treating chronic bacterial prostatitis.

Further, some doctors prescribe antibiotics for their patients with nonbacterial prostatitis. And in certain cases, it does help with the symptoms, although it is not known why this occurs.

If an obstruction in the urinary tract is causing you to have difficulty with urination, your doctor may prescribe an alpha-blocker such as terazosin. This medication relaxes the prostate and bladder neck, which improves the flow of urine. Since the urine will flow more easily, you may not need to urinate as often during the night. If you are experiencing pain during bowel movements, a stool softener such as Colace may be advised.

To help you cope with discomfort and pain, your doctor may recommend a pain reliever. Since you may be taking it over an extended period of time, be sure to review potential side effects.

Physical Therapy

The symptoms of prostatitis may be relieved by learning how to stretch and relax the lower pelvic muscles. A physical therapist may teach you specific exercises as well as ways to heat muscles, thereby making them more limber. In addition, a physical therapist may provide instruction in the use of biofeedback to relax muscles.

Surgery

If you have ongoing pain and complications from chronic bacterial prostatitis, surgery to remove part of the prostate gland may be an option. For the surgery, which is known as a transurethral resection of the prostate (TURP), you will either be under general anesthesia or be anesthetized from the waist down. The surgeon inserts a narrow instrument known as a resectoscope into the urethra. The resectoscope has an electrical loop that may be used to remove prostate tissue and seal blood vessels. Potential complications from TURP include blood in the urine, a sense of urgency to urinate, short-term difficulty controlling urine, and problems with sexual function. Some men develop retrograde or dry ejaculation. In this condition, part of the semen goes backward into the bladder.

If you have an obstruction to the bladder neck, it may be relieved with surgery. The surgery usually is successful in increasing the rate of urine flow.

Warm Baths

Many men find that sitting in a warm tub or sitz bath relieves pain and relaxes muscles. Consider making time for regular warm baths.

Complementary Treatments

Herbal remedies and nutritional supplements may help boost recovery from infection. Therapies and lifestyle changes that strengthen the immune system may be effective in controlling prostatitis.

Aromatherapy

Cedarwood and juniper are essential oils that promote urination and fight infection. Sandalwood also fights infection and stimulates the immune system. All three of these oils are useful for urinary tract infections. As it stimulates the production of infection-fighting white blood cells, lemon is an overall immune system enhancer. Place 8 to 10 drops of any of these oils in a warm bath and soak for 20 minutes. Or use these oils in combination by placing 2 drops of each in the bath.

Diet

Increase your intake of fluids, which will cause you to urinate more often and flush bacteria from the bladder. Studies have shown that zinc deficiency may lead to prostate problems. Zinc may be found in pumpkin and sunflower seeds, so try to include them in your diet.

Avoid foods that tend to irritate the bladder, such as hot or spicy foods and citrus juices. Also, stay away from foods and supplements containing caffeine. Since sugar impairs the ability of white blood cells to kill bacteria and alcohol robs the body of zinc, avoid both sugar and alcohol.

Herbal Medicine

Goldenseal. Goldenseal is an herb with antiseptic and diuretic properties. Although effective in fighting infection, it should be used only for short periods of time. The body may build up an immunity to it, and in higher doses it may be irritating to the throat, mouth, and skin and cause diarrhea and nausea. Goldenseal contains the alkaloid berberine, its most extensively researched constituent. In capsule form, goldenseal may contain 0.5 percent to 6 percent berberine. As dosage may vary depending upon the percentage of berberine in the bottle, take as directed on the label. In tincture form, the daily dose is 4 to 6 milliliters.

Pygeum and stinging nettle. Along with saw palmetto, pygeum and stinging nettle are diuretics, which increase the secretion and flow of urine and reduce irritation of the bladder and urethra. Pygeum, in particular, has been shown to aid males who have trouble initiating urination, and it also supports the complete emptying of the bladder. The typical recommended daily dose for pygeum is 50 milligrams twice a day of extract standardized to 13 percent total sterols. For stinging nettle, the recommended daily dose is 250 milligrams of nettle root twice a day. Both herbs are available in tincture form.

Saw palmetto. Clinical studies have shown saw palmetto to be useful for the relief of symptoms of an inflamed prostate. Saw palmetto is available in capsules containing 160 milligrams of extract standardized to 85 to 95 percent fatty acids and sterols. The typical recommended dose is 320 milligrams. Though you may notice symptom relief within 30 days, you should continue to take the supplement.

Nutritional Supplements

Nutritional supplements are beneficial in shrinking an inflamed prostate.

- Omega-3 fatty acids: 1 tablespoon of flaxseed oil or fish oil capsules as directed on the label. May prevent the prostate from swelling.

- Zinc: 30 milligrams daily. Effective in shrinking an inflamed prostate and enhancing the immune system.

Lifestyle Recommendations

Limit your evening beverage intake. While you should drink a good deal of water during the day, reduce the amount of water you drink in the evening to lessen your need to urinate while you sleep.

Practice yoga. The gentle movement and postures of yoga may increase circulation to the groin area and ease prostate problems.

Preventive Measures

Begin walking. Walking is the most effective exercise for relieving prostatitis. Avoid bicycling, running, rowing, or any other activity that puts pressure on the groin area.

Maintain a healthy cholesterol level. High cholesterol has been linked to prostate problems.

Practice good genital hygiene. Especially if you are uncircumcised, you must keep yourself clean. Also, after a bowel movement, wash your hands before touching your penis. This will reduce the chance of spreading *E. coli* organisms from the rectal area to the genitourinary tract, lessening the likelihood of developing prostatitis.

Engage in safer sex. If you are not in a committed long-term relationship, use a condom during sexual intercourse. This will decrease the risk for sexually transmitted diseases and prostatitis.

Treat urinary infections. Do not delay treatment for a potential urinary infection. And be sure to take the full course of medication recommended by your doctor.

Rashes

Also known as dermatitis, *rash* is a broad term used to describe a number of different inflammations of the skin. Depending upon the type of rash, the skin may scale, itch, flake, crust, ooze, swell, thicken, or redden.

Rashes are extremely common. It has been estimated that every year there are about 13.3 million visits to physicians for skin rashes. Of course, most people probably don't visit a doctor for every rash. During the midlife years, rashes are even more likely to occur.

Causes and Risk Factors

Atopic dermatitis. Atopic dermatitis (eczema) tends to run in families whose members have asthma or allergies. It may begin when exposure to an irritant or allergen causes an itchy rash. Scratching soon follows. The skin becomes extremely itchy and inflamed. Emotional and environmental factors may also play a role. While it often starts in early childhood, by adulthood it is typically limited to one area of the body, such as the hands.

Contact dermatitis. Probably the most common type of rash, contact dermatitis is caused by physical contact with a substance. The skin reaction may be irritant-induced or allergic. The types of irritants vary widely. Some substances are natural irritants, including soaps, detergents, and solvents. Other substances, such as hair dyes, poison ivy, rubber, latex, and nickel, may trigger an allergic reaction in susceptible people. While a larger amount of a natural irritant might be required to trigger a reaction, if you are sensitized to a particular allergen, only a small amount of it is needed before you break out in a rash.

Neurodermatitis. With neurodermatitis (also known as lichen simplex chronicus), a disorder more often seen in women than men, you keep rubbing or scratching a single area of skin or a small number of patches that are thickened, dry, and scaly. The continuous rubbing and scratching produce more lesions and, as a result, more scratching. Over time, the area of skin thickens and becomes leathery. The condition has a definite psychological component and is exacerbated by stress and tension. Neurodermatitis most often appears on the lower legs, wrists, ankles, back, neck, and vulva.

Seborrheic dermatitis. Seborrheic dermatitis is characterized by scales over pink-red patches, believed to be caused by the overproduction of oil by the sebaceous glands. The excess oil dries into flakes and obstructs ducts. While pink-red patches usually appear on the scalp, they may be seen on other parts of the head and face (nose, eyebrows, eyelids, and the skin behind the ears) and on other parts of the body, such as the middle of the chest. In the worst form of the disorder, the scales may thicken, ooze, and crust, becoming yellow to orange in color. About 5 percent of the US population is affected by seborrheic dermatitis, and it is more common in men than women. Seborrheic dermatitis tends to recur throughout life. Dry climate, nutritional deficiencies, scratching, and immune dysfunctions worsen the condition. People with neurological conditions, such as Parkinson's disease, are at increased risk.

Stasis dermatitis. Though less well known than the other forms of dermatitis, stasis dermatitis may appear on the calves, ankles, and feet of people with varicose veins, circulatory problems, and chronic swelling of the feet. The rash may be red and swollen, and there will be some itching. Untreated, the rash will become redder, and it may crust and leak fluid, leading to an infection or ulceration.

Signs and Symptoms

Rash symptoms vary according to the type of rash.

Atopic dermatitis. The skin is itchy, thickened, and fissured. There may be patches of red, dry, flaking skin that are inflamed and oozing, and there is a strong urge to scratch. Affected skin may be located on the upper chest, hands and feet, and the skin over joints, such as the elbows and knees.

Contact dermatitis. The skin will be itchy and swell. It may be red, and there may be blisters that may break open and ooze, crust, or scale, potentially causing an infection.

Neurodermatitis. There is chronic itching and scratching at the nape of the neck, the arms, legs, or ankles. In time, the skin thickens and takes on a leatherlike appearance.

Seborrheic dermatitis. There may be dry, itchy, pink-red, or greasy scales on the scalp and face, including eyebrows, eyelids, and areas behind the ears. There will be flaking

> **Rashes** may be a symptom of a specific disease such as systemic lupus erythematosus. About half of those who suffer from this disorder have a rash over the cheeks and bridge of the nose.

dandruff, itching, scaling, and redness of the scalp and/or facial skin. But other areas of the body, such as the front of the chest, the groin, and underarms, may also be affected.

A Quick Guide to Symptoms

☐ **Atopic dermatitis**—itchy, thickened, and fissured skin; patches of red, dry flaking skin that are inflamed and oozing; strong urge to scratch; rashes located on the upper chest, hands and feet, and the skin over joints

☐ **Contact dermatitis**—itchy, red, and swollen skin; blisters that may break open and ooze, crust, or scale

☐ **Neurodermatitis**—chronic itching and scratching at the nape of the neck, arms, legs, or ankles; skin thickens and takes on a leatherlike appearance

☐ **Seborrheic dermatitis**—dry, itchy, pink-red, or greasy scales on the scalp and face (eyebrows, eyelids, and areas behind the ears); flaking dandruff, itching, scaling, and redness of the scalp and/or face; may also affect the front of the chest, the groin, and the underarms

☐ **Stasis dermatitis**—area around the ankles is swollen; skin is red, thick, scaly, and itchy

Stasis dermatitis. The area around the ankles will be swollen, and the skin will be red, thick, scaly, and itchy.

Conventional Treatments

Recommended treatments vary according to the type of rash.

Atopic Dermatitis

First, you need to determine the cause of the irritation. Once identified, the offending substance should then be avoided. An over-the-counter hydrocortisone cream or lotion and a cool compress may help with the discomfort. If symptoms persist, your doctor may give you a prescription for a stronger medication such as tacrolimus (Protopic), which is a nonsteroidal ointment, or any number of steroid preparations. If you have cracks in the skin, your doctor might suggest applying dressings moistened with a mild astringent to reduce secretions and lessen the chances of infection. If the itching does not stop, you might want to take an over-the-counter antihistamine, but it may make you feel tired.

In some cases, your doctor may recommend phototherapy, treatment with ultraviolet light waves, under the direction of a dermatologist. Some profoundly resistant cases might benefit from photochemotherapy, which combines ultraviolet light therapy with the medication psoralen, a treatment also known as PUVA. However, this treatment has some potential long-term negative side effects, including premature aging of the skin and an increased risk for melanoma and other types of skin cancer. Further, the treatments are expensive.

If you have severe atopic dermatitis and no medical intervention has been helpful, your doctor might recommend a systemic corticosteroid such as prednisone. But you should be aware that these medications could have unpleasant side effects, such as skin damage, thinned or weakened bones, high blood pressure, high blood sugar, increased susceptibility to infections, and cataracts.

For those with intractable severe atopic dermatitis, immunosuppressive drugs such as cyclosporine are an option. These drugs control the overactive immune system. Still, these drugs have potential toxic side effects, such as high blood pressure, kidney problems, headaches, vomiting, tingling or numbness, and nausea. In addition, they may increase your risk for infections and cancer. People receiving these drugs must be closely monitored.

Contact Dermatitis

With contact dermatitis, the goal is to determine the cause of the irritation. Once it is identified, the offending substance should be avoided. To help relieve the discomfort, you may wish to apply a steroid cream and cool compresses.

Neurodermatitis

You need to stop scratching the rash. To help you stop, your doctor may prescribe antihistamines, sedatives, or tranquilizers. These may be particularly useful at night. Sometimes, doctors may inject corticosteroids into the lesions to reduce itching and redness, or they might advise phototherapy or treatments of ultraviolet light. Steroid creams and lotions as well as cool compresses may also help alleviate some of the itching.

Seborrheic Dermatitis

You will need to shampoo your hair frequently and rinse your scalp with a shampoo containing zinc pyrithione, salicylic acid, selenium sulfide, or ketoconazole as the active ingredient. A coal-tar shampoo is another option, though it will tend to darken lighter hair. Allow the shampoos to remain on the hair and scalp for several minutes. While waiting, you may wish to massage your scalp. Under medical supervision, you may use a mild steroid cream or lotion on your face and other parts of the body. A secondary infection may require an antibacterial ointment or a prescription for antibiotics from your doctor.

Stasis Dermatitis

Adequate treatment requires correcting the condition that caused the accumulation of fluid. You will probably first be asked to wear elastic supportive hose and, to control infection, place wet dressings on the thickened skin. Steroid creams may help reduce the inflammatory components of this rash. If the condition has been brought on by varicose veins, your doctor may advise surgery.

Complementary Treatments

Complementary medicine approaches, consisting of internal and external treatments, have been shown to be very effective in the treatment of rashes. Strengthening and improving skin health through diet, finding the underlying cause of the rash, relieving the discomfort, and learning how to reduce stress are the focus of treating the various forms of dermatitis.

Acupuncture

By focusing on blood and energy deficiencies and counteracting the detrimental effects of heat, dampness, and wind, acupuncture is effective for treating rashes. Acupuncture points that have a calming effect on the central nervous system are also used to reduce stress. Stress may be a trigger for conditions such as eczema.

Aromatherapy

Bergamot, chamomile, geranium, lavender, and thyme all decrease inflammation and soothe itchy, irritated skin. They also work on a cellular level to speed up the healing process and promote the regeneration of skin cells. Seek an experienced aromatherapist for advice on the correct oil to use. Using the wrong oil or too much oil may further irritate the skin. Also note that essential oils should never be applied to the skin in undiluted form. Rather, place several drops of the oil in a carrier oil, such as jojoba, olive, or canola oil, before using.

Diet

Some individuals with dermatitis are lacking in B vitamins, which play an important role in how cells grow and are essential for healthy skin. B vitamins are found in dark green, leafy vegetables; whole grains; oranges; avocados; beets; bananas; potatoes; dairy products; nuts; beans; fish; and chicken. In fact, the best thing you can do for your skin is to avoid fried foods, sugar, and other processed food products, and eat a balanced and healthy diet that includes lots of vegetables, fruits, whole grains, nuts, and seeds.

Essential fatty acids found in flaxseed oil and fish (canned salmon, pink salmon, mackerel, and sardines) also support the skin. Taking a tablespoon of flaxseed oil each day is an easy and cost-effective way to get these essential fatty acids.

Deficiencies in vitamins A, B-complex, C, or E may lead to dry skin, which can further irritate dermatitis. In fact, dry skin is a symptom of a deficiency in these vitamins. Vitamin A is derived from animal sources such as eggs and dairy products, including cheese, yogurt, ice cream, and butter. Large amounts are found in beef and chicken liver. Your body

If you decide to eliminate gluten from your diet, be sure to look for hidden sources. Gluten may be found in a host of different products such as salad dressings, soups, and prepared foods. Read labels carefully.

also converts beta-carotene into vitamin A. Beta-carotene is found in almost all fruits and vegetables. It is the substance that gives them their color. It may be healthier to obtain the necessary amount of vitamin A by eating lots of fruits and vegetables, including dark green, leafy vegetables.

By regulating sebaceous glands, which secrete lubricating substances in the skin,

vitamin C helps to prevent dry skin. Vitamin C is found in almost all fruits and green vegetables. Good sources are strawberries, cranberries, melons, oranges, mangoes, papayas, peppers, spinach, kale, broccoli, tomatoes, and potatoes.

Vitamin E, which helps to relieve itching and dryness, may be found in vegetable oils, nuts, seeds, and wheat germ. You may also obtain small amounts of vitamin E by eating leafy vegetables and whole grains.

You might want to check for food allergies and intolerances. For example, it has been shown that people with dermatitis benefit from removing gluten (wheat, oats, barley, and rye) from their diet. Making dietary changes may provide a good deal of relief.

Herbal Medicine

Many herbs are helpful for people with dermatitis. These may be taken internally or used topically.

Burdock root. Burdock root boosts the immune system and reduces inflammation. To prepare a tea, simmer 1 tablespoon of dried herb for 8 to 10 minutes. Burdock is also sold as a tincture; drops may be added to warm water.

Calendula. With its antiseptic and anti-inflammatory properties, calendula is an excellent herb for treating skin abrasions, infections, and rashes. You can buy topical creams made with calendula, often in combination with goldenseal, as discussed on page 467. Use according to the label directions.

Chamomile. Chamomile, which is sold as a tea and as an ingredient in moisturizing products, speeds healing and calms the central nervous system. This is most useful for those whose dermatitis is related to stress.

Chickweed. Another consideration for skin rashes is chickweed, which is sold as a salve. It is most effective when it is left on the skin for a longer period of time. Try applying it after a nighttime bath. It should remain on your skin while you sleep.

Echinacea. Taken orally, echinacea has an antibiotic effect and bolsters the immune system. When applied topically, it is a very effective treatment for eczema. Available in a number of forms such as gel, liquid, and powder, echinacea may be applied directly on a rash. The liquid form can be added to a bath.

Evening primrose oil. Evening primrose oil, which contains gamma-linolenic acid, an omega-6 fatty acid, is good for mild cases of eczema and dry skin–related rashes. It helps relieve the itching and strengthens skin cells, enabling them to hold more moisture. Evening primrose oil is sold in capsules; the typical recommended dose is 500 milligrams, twice a day.

Goldenseal. Goldenseal fights infections, reduces inflammation, and dries rashes that are oozing. It works best for eczema and contact dermatitis.

Licorice. In liquid form, licorice may be applied directly to the skin to relieve the inflammation and itching of an eczema flare-up. Use according to the label directions.

Homeopathy

Homeopathy may be useful for treating rashes. However, since the remedies are specific for each individual's rash symptoms, it is best to seek out a homeopathic physician. For example, a homeopath may prescribe one remedy for skin eruptions that are dry and scaly and another for eruptions that are moist. And remedies are different depending on the time of the year. Remedies for eruptions that are worse in the winter vary from those that are worse in the spring. To find a practitioner trained in homeopathy, visit the Web site of the National Center for Homeopathy at www.homeopathic.org.

Hydrotherapy

Soaking in a bath with Dead Sea salts may provide short-term relief from itching and reduce long-term skin sensitivity. These salts are available at many health food stores and online.

Nutritional Supplements

The following nutrients are necessary for healthy skin and are especially useful for those who have allergies or intolerances and need to avoid certain foods.

- Vitamin A: 10,000 IU daily. Antioxidant that protects skin tissue.

- B-complex vitamins: Take as directed on the label. Antistress vitamins that help reduce anxiety, which can aggravate flare-ups.

- Vitamin C: 1,000 milligrams daily in divided doses of 500 milligrams. Regulates sebaceous glands (which secrete lubricating substances) and increases circulation to the skin.

- Vitamin E: 400 IU daily. Antioxidant that protects against free radical damage to the skin. Deficiency may lead to dry skin.

- Omega-3 fatty acids such as flaxseed oil or fish oil: 1 tablespoon of flaxseed oil daily or 4,000 milligrams daily of fish oil capsules. Help maintain healthy skin.

Lifestyle Recommendations

Keep your environment clean and healthful. Dry skin may be aggravated by the heat that warms our homes. Be sure to have a humidifier or other means to add moisture to the air in your home. Check the filters on your heating vents regularly to see if they are clean. As air conditioners and open windows may bring lots of irritants into the home, central air is best. Regularly clean curtains and carpets, as they may hold quite a bit of dust. Try to avoid pet dander and cigarette smoke.

Stop scratching. Continuous scratching will only make your rash worse, and it may lead to an infection. As a precaution, keep your fingernails short.

Preventive Measures

The skin is the largest organ in the body and subject to the most environmental stresses.

Avoid dry skin. You will reduce your risk for rashes if you avoid dry skin. This may be accomplished in a few easy-to-follow ways. Take shorter showers or baths and use tepid rather than hot water. Oatmeal baths are very soothing to irritated skin. Pat skin dry, don't rub. If possible, liberally moisturize your skin while still damp. Avoid moisturizers and creams that are not specifically formulated for your type of dermatitis; otherwise, you may further irritate your skin. Use superfatted soaps or a cleansing product specifically made for sensitive skin, such as Cetaphil.

Avoid perfumes and dyes. Many people react to products containing perfumes and dyes. You will probably be more comfortable using products that do not contain perfumes and dyes.

Elevate legs. For those suffering from stasis dermatitis, it is extremely important to elevate the legs as often as possible. This reduces the buildup of fluids. Also, be careful not to injure your lower legs, as cuts or open sores may lead to infection.

Identify and avoid irritants and allergens. If your doctor believes that your dermatitis is caused by an irritant or allergen, patch tests may be ordered. If specific irritants and/or allergens are identified, you will need to avoid those substances. If contact is made, wash the exposed area immediately.

Pay attention to clothing. Try to wear 100 percent cotton clothing, because it is less irritating to the skin. If possible, keep clothes loose-fitting. New clothes should be washed before they are worn, preferably with an unscented detergent. Don't hang clothes outdoors to dry, which exposes them to pollen and other allergens.

Rheumatoid Arthritis

If you have rheumatoid arthritis (RA), you may experience a great deal of pain and sometimes the loss of function. In RA, joints throughout the body are inflamed, swollen, and stiff.

There are two types of rheumatoid arthritis. Type 1, which is less common, lasts for a few months and causes no permanent disability. The far more widespread type 2 is chronic and lasts for years or a lifetime. People who have type 2 RA may have periods in which their symptoms are worse, known as flares, and periods when they improve, known as remissions. Others may remain symptomatic all the time. They are at very high risk for serious joint damage and disability.

It has been estimated that more than 2 million Americans have rheumatoid arthritis, around 1 to 2 percent of the US population. While it may affect anyone of any age, it occurs most commonly in people between the ages of 25 and 55.

Causes and Risk Factors

Although researchers are still uncertain of an exact cause for rheumatoid arthritis, they consider it an autoimmune disorder in which the body attacks itself. For an unknown reason, white blood cells cause the synovial membranes (which surround the joints and protect them with a lubricant-filled sac) to become inflamed. This inflammation is known as synovitis. It results in the swelling, redness, and warmth that are characteristic of RA. The inflamed synovial membranes thicken and release chemicals that digest cartilage, bone, tendons, and ligaments. In time, joints lose their shape and alignment, and muscle, bone, and ligaments grow weaker and loosen. Sometimes, joints are eventually destroyed.

Heredity is believed to play a role in rheumatoid arthritis, but other factors may place people who are already susceptible at greater risk. These include heavy smoking, shorter reproductive life, history of blood transfusions, and obesity. Women are $2\frac{1}{2}$ times more likely than men to have this disease.

Signs and Symptoms

If you have RA, you are probably experiencing a number of different symptoms, such as joint stiffness in the morning that continues for at least an hour and swelling and pain in your joints that has lasted for at least 6 weeks. Though joints in the wrists, knuckles, knees, and the ball of the foot are almost always affected, the disease may also affect joints in the hips, shoulders, elbows, neck, and jaw. Typically, both sides of the body are affected, so if the knuckles on one hand show evidence of RA, the knuckles on the other hand probably do too. On occasion, the spine may be misaligned. During the early stages of RA, you may have flulike symptoms, such as fatigue, weight loss, and fever.

In about one out of every four cases of RA, inflamed blood vessels may cause nodules or lumps under the skin. These are called rheumatoid subcutaneous nodules. They tend to be the size of millet (a small grain), but they may be as large as a walnut. While they are frequently located near the elbow, they may appear in other pressure locations in the body, such as the hand, back of the head, and bottom of the spine. On rare occasions, they may become sore and infected, especially if they are located in a part of the body that experiences more stress, such as the ankles.

Rheumatoid arthritis may also cause problems in nonjoint areas of the body, such as muscles, bones, heart, blood vessels, lungs, and eyes. If you have RA, you are at higher risk for peripheral neuropathy, osteoporosis, anemia, periodontal disease, and infections.

A Quick Guide to Symptoms

☐ **Joint stiffness in the morning that continues for at least an hour**
☐ **Swelling and pain in your joints that has lasted for at least 6 weeks**
☐ **Flulike symptoms such as fatigue, weight loss, and fever**
☐ **Nodules or lumps under the skin**

In a small number of cases, you may develop neck pain and dry eyes and mouth. Inflammation of the blood vessels, the lining of the lungs, or the sac enclosing the heart is, on rare occasions, part of this disorder.

Conventional Treatments

Depending upon the degree of illness and disability, doctors use a variety of treatments to address the symptoms of RA. The goals are always to relieve pain, reduce inflammation, decrease joint damage, and improve the overall sense of well-being.

Lifestyle Changes

Reduce stress. Rheumatoid arthritis has a strong emotional component. If you have the disease, you may feel anger, fear, and frustration in addition to your ongoing pain. But stress in your life will only enhance the symptoms, such as increasing the pain. Ask your doctor for suggestions for reducing stress.

Take care of your joints. Ask your doctor if you should be using a splint on your hands, wrists, or ankles. Sometimes, the support from the splint helps reduce swelling. You might also want to consult with an occupational therapist, who can teach you about the many self-help and adaptive devices available for people with disabilities.

Medications

Biological response modifiers. Biological response modifiers are genetically engineered medications that impede certain parts of the autoimmune response in rheumatoid arthritis. They interfere with tumor necrosis factor cytokine, a substance that supports the inflammation process. Initially used for Crohn's disease, infliximab (Remicade) is given by intravenous infusion at 0, 2, 6, and then every 8 weeks. Etanercept (Enbrel) is given by subcutaneous injection one or two times each week. Both of these medications are effective for the symptoms of RA, but, like other medications, they do not cure RA. Since they are newer, the consequences of the long-term use of these drugs are unknown. Moreover, they are quite expensive, and some insurers refuse to cover them. They also have side effects, most frequently at the injection site. More worrisome is their potential to make people more susceptible to severe infections such as tuberculosis, and there are reports of aplastic anemia.

Corticosteroids. Corticosteroids are also used to control the inflammation and pain of RA. When they are combined with disease-modifying antirheumatic drugs (DMARDs), they appear to enhance the effectiveness of the DMARDs. Examples are prednisolone and prednisone (Deltasone, Orasone). Corticosteroids may also be injected directly into the joints for relief. No more than two or three injections should be administered each year. The long-term use of oral corticosteroids has a number of serious side effects, including osteoporosis, diabetes, fluid retention, cataracts, glaucoma, weight gain, susceptibility to infection, high blood pressure, acne, excess hair growth, irritability, loss of muscle mass, insomnia, and psychosis. If you get a prescription for corticosteroids, have a discussion with your doctor about how to mitigate some of the side effects.

COX-2 inhibitors. COX-2 inhibitors are also used effectively to treat rheumatoid arthritis. Examples are celecoxib (Celebrex) and meloxicam (Mobic). They suppress the enzyme cyclooxygenase-2 (COX-2) that causes joint inflammation and pain, while

> **Never stop taking corticosteroids** without the assistance of your doctor. The long-term use of oral corticosteroids suppresses the natural secretion of steroid hormones from your adrenal glands, so your body may need up to a year to begin producing its own steroids. You should be monitored closely by your doctor as you discontinue use.

preserving the COX-1 enzyme, which protects the stomach lining. Patients taking COX-2 inhibitors tend to have fewer gastrointestinal concerns than those taking nonsteroidal anti-inflammatory drugs (NSAIDs). Nevertheless, many of those who take these medications do have gastrointestinal problems. They may also experience other potential side effects, such as headache, dizziness, and kidney problems. Those on anticoagulant drugs may be at greater risk for bleeding. And, in a small number of cases, higher doses of celecoxib have been related to hallucinations, a buildup of fluid, high blood pressure, and excess potassium in the blood.

Disease-modifying antirheumatic drugs (DMARDs). There are medications that actually slow the course of rheumatoid arthritis, called disease-modifying antirheumatic drugs (DMARDs). It is believed that early treatment with DMARDs improves the long-term outcome and quality of life of people with RA. Further, there is some evidence that the early use of DMARDs protects against a variety of heart problems, a serious complication of RA. These are very slow-acting medications. You may be on them for several weeks or months before you notice any changes. They are typically prescribed in conjunction with another medication. Commonly, at least two are prescribed at the same time.

Some of the most well-known DMARDs are hydroxychloroquine (Plaquenil), gold (Myochrysine, Solganal, Ridaura), penicillamine (Cuprimine, Depen), leflunomide (Arava), cyclosporine (Sandimmune, Neoral), and methotrexate (Rheumatrex). All DMARDs tend to have unpleasant side effects, including stomach and intestinal problems (diarrhea, loss of appetite, and vomiting), liver problems, mouth sores, mild hair loss, headaches, muscle aches, rashes, and blood disorders. And, over time, they lose their effectiveness.

Immunosuppressants. If you have not responded to any other medication, your doctor may recommend immunosuppressants. Examples are azathioprine (Imuran), cyclophosphamide (Cytoxan), and chlorambucil (Leukeran). These medicines are extremely toxic and may cause liver damage, increased infections, decreased production of blood cells, and lung inflammation. If you are on any of these medications, your doctor needs to watch you very carefully.

Nonsteroidal anti-inflammatory drugs (NSAIDs). Treatment for RA generally begins with nonsteroidal anti-inflammatory drugs (NSAIDs), such as aspirin, ibuprofen, naproxen, and ketoprofen. These medications block prostaglandins, which dilate blood vessels, causing inflammation and pain. However, they frequently cause gastrointestinal problems, such as ulcers, upset stomach, and internal bleeding. This occurs even when these medications are injected intravenously. NSAIDs may also raise blood pressure. Other potential side effects include headaches, skin rashes, ringing in the ears, dizziness, and depression. There is some evidence that NSAIDs may damage cartilage and/or cause kidney damage. These medications should be used with caution. The longer they are used, the more likely they are to cause side effects.

Surgery

Arthrodesis (joint fusion). If a joint needs to be stabilized but cannot be replaced, arthrodesis

If you have high blood pressure, a severe circulation disorder, or kidney or liver problems, or if you are taking diuretics or oral hypoglycemics, and your doctor places you on an NSAID for an extended period of time, then you need to be monitored carefully. Also, since NSAIDs reduce blood clotting, stop taking them a week before surgery.

may be advised. During the procedure, bones are fused together. When the surgery heals, the joint may bear weight, but it is inflexible. The most common sites for this surgery are the wrist and ankle.

Arthroplasty (joint replacement). In arthroplasty, a surgeon reconstructs the joint with artificial or prosthetic implants. It may be advised when pain and immobility from an osteoarthritic joint have made normal functioning impossible. The most commonly replaced joints are the hip and knee. They account for about 80 percent of such surgeries in the United States. But joints in the ankles, shoulders, elbows, and knuckles are also successfully replaced.

During the surgery, which is done under general anesthesia, the surgeon will open the joint and separate the tendons and ligaments. The surgeon removes the diseased portions of the joint and replaces them with plastic and/or metal prostheses. Sometimes, these are cemented into place. Then, the remainder of the joint parts, as well as the ligaments and tendons, are reattached.

Depending upon the type of surgery, expect to spend 3 to 7 days in the hospital. Then, you will probably be transferred to a rehabilitation facility for a week or two, followed by outpatient therapy. Since some blood loss is associated with arthroplasty, a month or two before your surgery, you may wish to donate one to three units of your own blood. If you require a transfusion, your blood may then be used.

While the majority of people who have

Treating NSAID-Induced Ulcers

If your doctor determines that you are at risk for developing an NSAID-induced ulcer or if you actually develop an ulcer, it may be treated with a number of medications. Generally, proton-pump inhibitors are useful in preventing ulcers in those who are at high risk. Examples are omeprazole (Prilosec), lansoprazole (Prevacid), rabeprazole (Aciphex), and pantoprazole (Protonix). When compared to no treatment, these medications reduce the rate of ulcers by up to 80 percent. Misoprostol has been found valuable in preventing, but not treating, NSAID-induced ulcers. The medication Arthrotec is a combination of misoprostol and the NSAID diclofenac. In one study, people who took Arthrotec reported having 60 percent fewer ulcers than those who took diclofenac alone.

undergone joint replacements are thrilled with the pain relief and newfound independence, as with all surgeries, individuals are at risk for complications. Infections, which occur in about 1 percent of all joint replacements, may require the removal of the implant. You may experience blood clots and damage to the nerves near the joint. A prosthesis may loosen or a joint may dislocate. And the replacements of the weight-bearing joints may wear out and fail. Hips tend to last between 10 and 15 years, while you may have as many as 20 years with new knees.

Arthroscopic debridement. In general,

arthroscopic surgery is performed to remove the bone and cartilage fragments in the hip and knee that are causing pain and inflammation. The surgeon begins by making a small incision into which a sterile solution is injected. Since that makes the joint swell, it is easier to see. A lighted tube called an arthroscope is inserted into a second small incision. Entering through a third incision, the surgeon trims or stitches the damaged tissue. Typically, this procedure is done under local anesthetic. Recovery rarely takes more than a few weeks.

Osteotomy. If the arthritis has caused a deformity in your knee or hip joints, your doctor may recommend an osteotomy. In this surgery, a physician opens your knee or hip and reshapes a wedge of bone, thereby correcting the weight-bearing problems you have been experiencing. This procedure is recommended for heavier adults who are under the age of 60. It may provide pain relief, increased joint stability, and better range of motion.

Synovectomy. During synovectomy, a surgeon removes an inflamed, overgrown joint lining, which reduces joint injury. The surgeon is able to complete this procedure with a large incision or an arthroscope. However it is done, some joint lining is cut away and only enough lining to produce lubricating fluid remains. Allow several weeks to recover. It is important to note that the synovium eventually grows back, but you should have some relief for a few years.

Tendon reconstruction. Rheumatoid arthritis may damage tendons, the tissues that attach muscles to bones. Most often used on the hands, this surgery repairs a damaged tendon by attaching it to another tendon. The function of the hand may be restored.

Complementary Treatments

Complementary medicine treats rheumatoid arthritis by addressing many of the underlying causes, including digestive disorders and food allergies. Dietary changes play a key role in the treatment of this condition. Approaches that help to decrease pain and increase mobility have proven beneficial to people who have RA.

Diet

A diet rich in fruits and vegetables, whole grains, and fiber and low in meats, refined sugar, and other simple carbohydrates, and saturated fats has shown promise in the treatment of rheumatoid arthritis. Among other antioxidant properties, fruits and vegetables contain beta-carotene, flavonoids, and vitamin C. Foods rich in vitamin E and selenium are also recommended. Vitamin E may be found in vegetable oils, nuts, seeds, and wheat germ. Small amounts are also found in leafy vegetables and whole grains. Selenium is available in whole grains, broccoli, asparagus, and onions. Vitamin C and beta-carotene are found in almost all fruits and vegetables, including dark green, leafy vegetables. Anthocyanosides have antioxidant properties that promote healing. Fruits rich in flavonoids that contain anthocyanosides are cherries, cranberries, blackberries, black currants, red grapes, and blueberries.

The high amounts of fat in dairy products and meat are converted into a chemical that stimulates the inflammatory process.

Food allergies and digestive problems also appear to play a major role in RA. Therefore, it is highly recommended that you seek a health care professional who can help in determining foods that may be causing or aggravating this condition. The most common problem foods are wheat, corn, milk, and dairy products. It should be noted that approximately one-third of all people suffering from RA are sensitive to vegetables in the nightshade family, which includes tomatoes, potatoes, eggplant, and peppers.

Herbal Medicine

Bromelain. The enzyme bromelain, which is found in pineapple, has anti-inflammatory properties. The typical recommended daily dose is 400 to 600 milligrams, three times a day between meals. However, drinking fresh pineapple juice may produce similar results.

Curcumin. Curcumin is the yellow pigment found in turmeric. It has powerful antioxidant and anti-inflammatory properties and may be taken in a dose of 400 to 600 milligrams, three times a day between meals. To enhance absorption, it may be taken with bromelain.

Ginger. An excellent anti-inflammatory, ginger is most effective when used fresh. Consuming approximately a $1/4$-inch slice of fresh ginger every day is recommended. It may be grated over a salad or added to a stir-fry or any other meal where the flavor would work well.

Hydrotherapy

Many health clubs are equipped with a heated pool (92° to 99°F) as well as an additional pool that contains cooler water. The warm water stimulates and then relaxes tired, aching joints and muscles. People with non-weight-bearing injuries and those who cannot tolerate traditional exercise programs find the buoyancy of water to be the perfect medium in which to decrease pain and increase mobility.

Movement Therapy

Tai chi, qigong, and yoga are gentle movement therapies that increase joint mobility, range of motion, flexibility, coordination, and balance and help to reduce pain.

Nutritional Supplements

Many nutritional supplements have anti-inflammatory properties and provide healthy cellular structure.

• Multivitamin/mineral: Take as directed on the label. Should include vitamins A, C, and E, beta-carotene, calcium, copper, magnesium, selenium, and zinc to aid in healthy cell structure and to provide anti-inflammatory properties.

• B-complex vitamins: Take as directed on the label. B_5 levels may be low in people who have rheumatoid arthritis. B-complex vitamins work best when taken together.

• Boron: 3 milligrams twice a day. Required for healthy bones and aids in the regulation of calcium.

• Vitamin C: 2,000 milligrams daily in divided doses of 1,000 milligrams. People with rheumatoid arthritis have lower levels of vitamin C.

• Vitamin D: 400 IU daily. Essential for cartilage health; needed for absorption of calcium.

• DLPA (DL-phenylalanine): 750 milligrams daily. Enhances body's ability to deal with pain. Requires 1 to 2 weeks to become effective. May raise blood pressure.

• Vitamin E: 400 IU daily. Increases joint range of motion. Protects against free radical damage.

• Essential fatty acids—omega-3 (flaxseed and fish oil) and omega-6 (borage, evening primrose, and black currant seed oils): Available in oil and capsule form. Take as directed on the labels. Very effective in the treatment of rheumatoid arthritis. Increase anti-inflammatory agents in the body and help to reduce pain.

• Glucosamine sulfate: 500 milligrams daily. Slows the breakdown, aids in the repair, and stimulates the growth of new cartilage. Also important for the formation of synovial fluid. Pain relief may be initially slow, but results are extremely promising.

• MSM (methylsulfonylmethane): 1,000 milligrams daily. Effective against arthritis pain and inflammation.

• SAMe (S-adenosyl-methionine): Dosing varies depending on symptoms. See your doctor for a starting point. Amino acid that helps lubricate joints and relieve pain and stiffness.

• Zinc: 30 milligrams daily. People with rheumatoid arthritis have lower levels of zinc.

Therapeutic Massage

Massage is recommended for those who want to prevent the loss of mobility. It provides a natural way to relax tired, aching muscles and joints and helps to remove waste products that have built up around the joints from the body. Gentle touch also has a nurturing and calming effect, and it relaxes the mind and body.

Trager Approach

The Trager Approach has been shown to be useful for people with rheumatoid arthritis. It is a passive and noninvasive treatment in which the practitioner puts joints through a series of gentle, rhythmic movements. This helps to retrain the nervous system to send new messages of light and free movement to the nerves that control muscle movement and pain messages. To locate a Trager therapist, visit www.trager-us.org (the Web site of the United States Trager Association) or www.

ncbtmb.org (the Web site for the National Certification Board for Therapeutic Massage and Bodywork).

Lifestyle Recommendations

Apply heat. Electric heating pads and dry heat applications are not recommended for RA. Moist heat packs applied over or near the affected area for 20 minutes will penetrate deeper and lessen stiffness and pain much better than dry heat.

Balance rest and exercise. If you have rheumatoid arthritis, you need to find a way to incorporate adequate amounts of rest into your life. However, when you are feeling better, you should make the time to exercise. Exercise will strengthen your muscles and help keep your joints as flexible and mobile as possible. It will also help you to control weight and maintain a positive outlook on life, and people who exercise tend to sleep better.

Consider magnet therapy. Preliminary studies have shown a reduction in pain when magnets are applied directly over the affected area for several hours. It is also thought that low-energy AC and DC fields may help stimulate the production of cartilage-building cells.

Keep a journal. People with rheumatoid arthritis who spend time writing in a personal journal a few times a week improve more readily. There is a definite emotional

Starting an Exercise Program

Begin your exercise program with a short warmup. A brief 3-minute walk will do. After your body is warmed up, begin with slow stretching exercises that will lengthen your muscles and take pressure off your joints. Remember to hold each stretch 30 to 45 seconds and perform each stretch two or three times.

When that is comfortable, progress to mild strength training. Then, try aerobic exercises such as walking, dancing, or swimming. Swimming in a heated pool should make your joints feel better. Tai chi, which uses slow, sweeping movements, is also good for RA. Stay away from exercises that put too much impact on your joints, such as running and jumping.

component to RA, and writing about pain and stress may help relieve anxiety and depression.

Preventive Measures

Lose weight. Excess weight places added strain on the joints.

Stop smoking. Heavy smoking over a long period of time increases your risk for rheumatoid arthritis, especially if you don't have a family history of the disease.

Rosacea

With rosacea, the facial skin becomes inflamed and tends to redden and flush. The facial blood vessels remain dilated, and your face may have small, red, pus-filled bumps or pustules. Though rosacea is often referred to as adult acne or acne rosacea, it actually has little in common with the acne that affects teens.

Rosacea is not infectious. There is no evidence that it spreads from one person to another. Still, when untreated, rosacea tends to worsen over time. In most people, it is cyclic. It appears for a period of time and then goes away until there is a flare-up.

Rosacea is quite common. An estimated 13 million Americans have this skin condition.

Causes and Risk Factors

While the exact cause of rosacea is unknown, there are a few theories. One view is that rosacea is related to a blood vessel disorder. Another hypothesis is that it is associated with an infection of the stomach caused by *Helicobacter pylori*. Other possible causes include microscopic skin mites (demodex), a malfunction of connective tissue under the skin, and a fungus. Some believe that it has a psychological derivation. The cause may be a combination of factors.

Since there is a strong hereditary component to rosacea, individuals who have a relative with this disorder are at greater risk. In addition, in the United States, those who are of Irish, English, Scandinavian, Scottish, Welsh, or Eastern European descent have an increased risk. Rosacea tends to affect those with fair skin who are between the ages of 30 and 60, and it is usually more severe in men.

Signs and Symptoms

Normally, rosacea appears in different phases. During the earliest stages, you may blush more easily. Then, there may be redness in the center of the face, especially the nose. The redness is caused by the dilation of blood vessels that are close to the surface of the skin. This phase of the disorder is called prerosacea.

As the disorder progresses, you may develop vascular rosacea. With this, small blood vessels on your cheeks and nose become visible. In some instances, the skin may be dry and sensitive. In other cases, it may be oily, and you may have dandruff. With time, you may have red bumps or pustules across the nose, cheeks, forehead, and chin. This condition is called inflammatory rosacea. In the worst cases, the oil or sebaceous glands in your nose and/or cheeks may enlarge and result in a buildup of tissue on and around the nose. This complication, which is called rhinophyma, occurs far more often in men than it does in women.

About half of those with rosacea experience a burning and gritty feeling in the eyes, known as ocular rosacea. And rosacea may cause an inflammation or scaling of the inner skin of the eyelids, which is called conjunctivitis.

Conventional Treatments

There is no cure for rosacea. Nevertheless, there are a number of helpful treatments. Generally, more than one treatment is required.

Antibiotics

For mild cases of rosacea, your doctor may prescribe a topical antibiotic cream, such as metronidazole. It is applied directly to the skin. If you appear to have a more difficult case of rosacea, you may get a prescription for an oral antibiotic, such as tetracycline, minocycline, doxycycline, or erythromycin. Antibiotics are quite useful for treating the papules and pustules, but less useful for the redness and flushing. In some cases, both topical and oral antibiotics are called for. Frequently, after you have completed taking the oral antibiotics, you will be asked to use a topical antibiotic once each day, which may prevent future flare-ups.

Glycolic Acid Peel

To accelerate the rate of healing, you may receive a glycolic acid peel along with antibiotics. Peels, which take only 3 to 5 minutes,

A Quick Guide to Symptoms

- ☐ Redness in the center of the face, especially the nose
- ☐ Dry, sensitive skin or oily skin with dandruff
- ☐ Red bumps or pustules across the nose, cheeks, forehead, and chin
- ☐ Rhinophyma (a buildup of tissue on and around the nose)
- ☐ Burning and gritty feeling in the eyes
- ☐ Conjunctivitis

may be performed every 2 to 4 weeks. After the procedure, your skin will be red for several hours. During this time, you should not use makeup. The peels may be combined with glycolic acid washes and topical creams.

Laser Therapy

Laser therapy, which reduces redness and removes visible blood vessels, may be a valuable tool in the treatment of rosacea. Normally, you will require at least three treatments. Though the removed vessels do not reappear, after treatment new vessels may emerge. Laser therapy may also be used to slow the buildup of excess tissue or to remove unwanted tissue.

Other Treatments

If you have a severe case of rosacea, you may receive a prescription for isotretinoin (Accutane), which inhibits the production of oil by the sebaceous glands. However, there may be serious side effects from isotretinoin, so you will need to be carefully monitored. Eye problems from rosacea are treated with oral antibiotics, especially tetracycline and doxycycline. You may be asked to practice eyelid hygiene with an over-the-counter eyelid cleaner and warm compresses. When the eyes are severely affected, steroid eye drops may be used.

Complementary Treatments

In order to find the best treatment, people with rosacea should be individually assessed. However, dietary changes, supplementation with certain vitamins and minerals, strengthening of the immune system, and herbal remedies taken internally and/or used topically may be helpful in eliminating or reducing the symptoms and flare-ups of rosacea.

Acupuncture

By toning the meridian of the liver and eliminating waste material from the body, acupuncture is effective in the treatment of certain skin conditions such as rosacea. The accumulation of waste material in the body may irritate the skin, causing inflammation and flare-ups of rosacea.

Diet

The diet plays an important role in the condition of the skin. It is essential to eat a diet high in nutrients, consisting of fruits, vegetables, and whole grains. Try to include a minimum of five servings of vegetables, four servings of fruit, and six servings of whole grains each day. Since it may reduce the inflammation, the magnesium found in dark green, leafy vegetables is especially useful for this condition. These vegetables also contain other nutrients beneficial to the health of the skin. Juicing is an easy way to obtain a substantial amount of these vegetables in your system every day. Since less digestive breakdown is required, juices allow the body to begin absorbing the nutrients immediately.

Food allergies, low stomach acid, and a low level of digestive enzymes, particularly pancreatic enzymes, may contribute to rosacea flare-ups. In the area of food, an allergy or intolerance to yeast is a likely culprit. See a doctor who can evaluate your particular situation. People with low stomach acid have trouble absorbing nutrients. Your body will better absorb nutrients if your diet is healthier. It's possible that low stomach acid allows more toxins into the body, which may cause a rosacea flare-up.

As saturated fat causes inflammation, saturated fats such as fried and processed foods should be eliminated. Saturated fats and trans fatty acids are also difficult to digest. People with rosacea who also have digestive problems should be particularly vigilant in avoiding saturated fat. If you eat meat, consume only the leanest cuts.

Because it supplies the essential fatty acids necessary for healthy skin, flaxseed oil is useful for people with rosacea. Take 1 teaspoon daily.

Naturopathy

By identifying food intolerances through an elimination diet, strengthening the immune system, assessing nutritional deficiencies, and making dietary and nutritional supplementation recommendations, naturopathic physicians have been successful in treating rosacea. Lifestyle factors may also be addressed.

A naturopath may prescribe azelaic acid cream, which should be applied topically. Azelaic acid is a natural substance found in barley, rye, and wheat. Preliminary studies have shown it to be useful in mild to moderate cases of rosacea. Since studies have shown that people with rosacea produce less of the digestive enzyme lipase, naturopathic physicians may further address the need for lipase.

Nutritional Supplements

The following nutrients protect against free radicals, support the immune system, and are beneficial for maintaining healthy skin.

• Vitamin A: 10,000 IU daily. Beneficial for healing and the development of new skin tissue.

• B-complex vitamins: Take as directed on the label. Antistress vitamins that help reduce anxiety, which can aggravate rosacea flare-ups.

• Vitamin C: 1,000 milligrams daily in divided doses of 500 milligrams. Supports the immune system as well as the capillaries.

• Vitamin E: 400 IU daily. Antioxidant that protects against free radicals and helps strengthen the immune system.

• Essential fatty acids—omega-3 (flaxseed and fish oil) and omega-6 (borage, evening primrose, and black currant seed oils): Available in oil and capsule form. Take as directed on the labels. Help maintain healthy skin.

• Evening primrose oil: 3,000 milligrams daily in divided doses of 1,000 milligrams each to provide 240 milligrams of GLA (gamma-linolenic acid). Helps heal skin tissue.

Other Supplements to Consider

When low stomach acid is addressed, rosacea symptoms and flare-ups may greatly improve. Hydrochloric acid capsules are the recommended treatment for people with low stomach acid. Before taking these capsules, you will need a gastric analysis. The unsupervised dosing and use of hydrochloric acid supplementation could cause an ulcer. It has been found that taking acidophilus (healthy bacteria) capsules along with the hydrochloric acid is especially effective.

Pancreatic digestive enzymes have also been found to be useful in reducing symptoms and rosacea flare-ups. Some studies have shown that individuals with rosacea produce less pancreatic lipase, a digestive enzyme. In order to determine if you are, in fact, low in pancreatic lipase, consult with your doctor before taking digestive enzyme supplementation.

Lifestyle Recommendations

Avoid triggers. Trigger factors vary from person to person. While avoiding trigger factors will not prevent rosacea, if you are able to identify your trigger factors, you may help mitigate the symptoms and reduce the probability of a flare-up. The following are some of the reported trigger factors: heated beverages, hot baths, alcohol, spicy foods, heavy exercise, corticosteroids, drugs that dilate the blood vessels, caffeine withdrawal, emotional stress, sun exposure, hot or cold weather, wind, and some skin care products.

Be gentle with your skin. Use a mild soap or cleanser to wash your skin and stay away from grainy or abrasive products. Ask your doctor for suggestions. While you can use a soft pad or washcloth, you should not use rough products such as sponges or brushes. After you wash your skin, dry it with a soft towel. Before applying topical medication, allow your skin several minutes to dry. Further, give your skin 5 to 10 minutes to absorb the antibiotic ointment before applying other skin care products or makeup.

Don't be discouraged. Rosacea responds slowly to treatment. It may take a few months before you see significant improvement.

Drink water. Drinking plenty of purified water helps remove excess waste products from the body and reduces the buildup of toxins. Drink at least 8 glasses of water per day.

Keep a food journal. To determine which foods may be triggering a rosacea flare-up, keep a food diary. Eliminating the offending foods may greatly improve your condition.

Limit your alcohol consumption. While alcohol may not be the cause of rosacea, since it causes the blood vessels to dilate, it may definitely have an effect on the reddening of the skin.

Stop smoking. Because nicotine constricts blood vessels and deprives the skin of necessary nutrients and oxygen, smoking can irritate this condition.

Use sunscreen. If you have rosacea, it is particularly important for you to use a sunscreen that protects against ultraviolet rays (both UVA and UVB). It should have an SPF of 15 or higher. Remember to use it every day and in all types of weather.

Preventive Measures

There is no proven method to prevent rosacea. If rosacea runs in your family, you may want to be periodically checked. Your treatments will be most effective if they begin early in the progression of the disease.

Excess stress and worry may lead to digestive imbalance, which may be a cause of rosacea. It is important to find some way to reduce the stress in your life. Regular exercise in moderation and the practice of yoga, tai chi, and qigong are all beneficial. Deep breathing exercises, meditation, or simply finding the time to be alone and quiet are all good ways to unwind and reduce stress.

Shingles

If you had chickenpox as a kid, the virus that caused that itchy, unpleasant disease could revisit you in your later years. Only this time, what happens is a lot worse than chickenpox. The virus (varicella zoster) causes shingles, also known as herpes zoster, which begins with pain and tingling in the trunk area of the body. This early period, which is known as prodrome, may be accompanied by flulike symptoms. Though it may sometimes take longer, normally within a few days there will be blisters. The disorder is then called active shingles.

Shingles are very common. At some point, about 20 percent of the population who previously had chickenpox is affected. In those who live until the age of 80, about 50 percent will deal with a bout of shingles. It is estimated that each year about 1 million Americans become ill with this disorder.

In some people, shingles may involve the nerves in the face and ears. This is called Ramsey Hunt syndrome or herpes zoster oticus. There may be severe pain, facial paralysis, loss of taste, dizziness, hearing loss, and mild inflammation of the brain. While most of the symptoms pass, the facial paralysis may be permanent. If shingles affects the eye, the cornea may become infected, which may cause temporary or permanent blindness.

Shingles may lead to a complication, known as postherpetic neuralgia (PHN), which is pain that continues for more than a month. It is most likely to occur in those who had shingles with many blisters and severe pain. If you have PHN, you no longer have shingles. However, shingles damaged your nervous system, which is now sending exaggerated pain messages to the brain. When PHN occurs, it tends to take one of three forms. It may result in continuous burning or aching pain, you may have periodic intense pain, or you may have pain from very light stimulation, such as the touch of clothing.

PHN is usually worse at night, and it may be affected by temperature changes. The pain may even extend beyond the area in which you had blisters. About 200,000 Americans have PHN, and approximately 25 percent of people over the age of 50 who have shingles will develop it. The older you are, the longer the PHN will tend to last, but most cases resolve within a year.

Doctors sometimes refer to the three syndromes associated with shingles (prodrome, active shingles, and PHN) with a single term, *zoster-associated pain (ZAP)*.

Causes and Risk Factors

If you never had chickenpox, you cannot develop shingles. But anyone who has had

fatigue, rash, tremor, and (in rare instances) seizure.

Pain medications. To deal with the pain, you may wish to try capsaicin ointment (Zostrix), which contains an active ingredient from hot chili peppers. But this ointment may not be used until the blisters have dried and fallen off. Apply with a gloved hand three or four times each day. Initially, you will feel a burning sensation, but it will subside. You may also want to take acetaminophen (Tylenol) or ibuprofen (Motrin).

If pain fails to respond to these medications, your doctor my prescribe opioids, such as oxycodone. Since there is the potential for addiction, oxycodone should be carefully monitored. Or, you may be given an injection of an anesthetic or steroid to block the nerves. Other pain-relieving options include a patch that contains the anesthetic lidocaine (Lidoderm) and a spray that has a combination of ethyl chloride (Chloroethane) and Fluorimethane, which cools the blood vessels in the skin.

Procedures

Some people with PHN obtain relief from transcutaneous electrical nerve stimulation (TENS) treatments, which suppress pain with low-level electrical pulses. Generally, individuals are given 80 to 100 pulses per second for 45 minutes, three times a day. Another procedure known as iontophoresis uses direct electrical current to deliver ions of medication through the skin. Laser therapy has also been used for PHN. Because it carries a high risk for permanent damage, surgery on the brain or spinal cord to reduce pain is used only as a last resort and only for intolerable pain.

Complementary Treatments

Complementary medicine approaches are effective in reducing the symptoms of shingles while the disease runs its course. They can also be helpful in aiding the recovery process.

Acupuncture

Acupuncture may accelerate the healing process, cool the body, and aid in the reduction of pain. To locate an acupuncturist in your area, visit the Web site of the National Certification Commission for Acupuncture and Oriental Medicine (NCCAOM) at www.nccaom.org.

Diet

Eating a diet full of whole grains, legumes, and fresh fruits and vegetables is beneficial in recovering from shingles. Try to include a minimum of five servings of vegetables, four servings of fruit, and six servings of whole grains each day. Whole grains, legumes, eggs, and fish contain B vitamins that help protect nerve endings. Fruits and vegetables contain vitamins A and C, which aid in the healing of skin lesions. Foods high in vitamin A are apricots, cantaloupes, carrots, mangoes, pumpkin, romaine lettuce, spinach, and sweet potatoes. Vitamin C may be found in apricots, broccoli, cabbage, cantaloupes, kiwifruit, oranges, pineapple, plums, spinach, tomatoes, and watermelon.

Calcium and magnesium are also beneficial to nerve health. They may be found in green, leafy vegetables. Lysine is an amino acid that may actually prevent the virus from replicating. It is also useful in reducing the severity of a shingles outbreak and speeds the recovery process. Lysine may be found in nonfat dairy products such as yogurt.

Flower Essences

Rescue Remedy, a Bach flower essence, is widely used to treat emotional trauma. It is useful both for a stressful acute disturbance and a condition that requires long-term support, such as shingles. It is available in tincture form. Place 4 drops in a glass of water or juice and sip. Take one dose in the morning, two doses during the day, and one dose before bed. Rescue Remedy is also available as a cream that can be applied directly to the affected area. Rescue Remedy is available at natural and organic health food stores.

Herbal Medicine

A number of herbal remedies may be valuable in treating shingles.

Chamomile and valerian root. When taken as a tea at bedtime, chamomile and valerian root may promote a restful night of sleep. These teas are available at health food stores. Follow the directions on the package.

Lemon balm. Lemon balm may have an antiviral effect. It should be applied to the affected area several times a day with a cotton ball. Steep 2 teaspoons of the dried leaf of lemon balm per cup of boiling water.

Licorice. Licorice is an immune-booster as well as an antiviral herb. If you do not have high blood pressure, you may drink it as a tea up to three times a day. (Those with high blood pressure should avoid it.) There is also a licorice gel that may be applied to the affected area to fight the infection.

Homeopathy

Homeopathy has been shown to be effective for the pain associated with shingles, and it aids in the recovery process. While homeopathic remedies are not harmful and may be used for self-treatment, to ensure that you are using the remedy and dose best suited for your symptoms, you may wish to seek the advice of a homeopathic practitioner. The remedy chosen should most closely match your symptoms, and dosing may range from taking a remedy several times an hour to a couple of times each day. With the appropriate homeopathic remedy, your recovery may progress faster. To find a practitioner trained in homeopathy, visit the Web site of the National Center for Homeopathy at www.homeopathic.org.

Hydrotherapy

In the early stages of a shingles outbreak, cool down the area with ice. Apply ice for 5 minutes and then remove it for 5 minutes. Repeat this procedure two more times and then again every few hours. The cold from the ice confuses the nerves and helps break the pain cycle. If you are unable to tolerate the ice, try a cold compress. Soak a washcloth in very cold water, squeeze out the excess water, and apply directly to the affected area until the washcloth feels warm. Repeat this throughout the day. Soaking in a lukewarm bath for 20 to 30 minutes is also a way to calm the nervous system.

Naturopathy

Since they provide dietary, nutritional supplement, herbal, and homeopathic recommendations, naturopathic physicians may be a valuable resource when dealing with shingles. To find a naturopathic practitioner in your area, contact the American Association of Naturopathic Physicians at www.naturopathic.org.

Nutritional Supplements

Complications of shingles generally occur in people with weakened immune systems, so supplements that boost the immune system and protect the nerves are essential in combating a shingles outbreak.

- Multivitamin/mineral: Take as directed on the label. Should include calcium, magnesium, and vitamin D.

- B-complex vitamins: Take as directed on the label. Essential for nerve function.

- Vitamin B_{12}: Injections or 1,000-microgram sublingual tablet daily. Useful in preventing nerve damage. Injections

are recommended. If not, sublingual tablets.

- Vitamin C: 2,000 milligrams daily in divided doses of 500 milligrams each. Acts as an antiviral agent, destroying the herpes virus.

- Vitamin E: 400 IU daily. Helps prevent scar tissue from forming.

- Beta-carotene: 25,000 IU daily. Protects against infection.

- Lysine: 1,000 milligrams daily in divided doses of 500 milligrams. Symptoms, severity, and duration of outbreak may be greatly reduced when taken at onset.

- Zinc: 30 milligrams daily. Antioxidant that boosts the immune system.

Lifestyle Recommendations

Avoid heat. Because they become more irritated with heat, keep blisters cool. Keep your baths lukewarm.

Consider visiting several doctors. If you have a debilitating case of shingles or if you are left with PHN, you are facing serious physical and psychological challenges. In addition to your primary care physician, you may benefit from visits with a pain specialist and/or a psychiatrist.

Reduce stress. Excess stress has been known to trigger an outbreak of shingles as well as increase the severity of an outbreak. Stress impairs the immune system and prevents it from fighting off illness. Try a number of stress-reduction techniques, such as deep breathing exercises, meditation, guided imagery, or visualization. Yoga, tai chi, and qigong are movement exercises that may calm the mind and reduce stress.

Take an oatmeal bath. Taking a lukewarm bath with colloidal oatmeal right before bedtime may enable you to feel more comfortable and help you to get a good night's sleep. Colloidal oatmeal is available at your local pharmacy.

Wear loose clothing. You will feel more comfortable if you wear loose clothing that does not rub against the area of pain and blisters.

Preventive Measures

Get a vaccine. In 2006, the FDA approved the shingles vaccine known as Zostavax for people 60 years and older. Studies have shown that the vaccine can prevent shingles in about half the people vaccinated. About 20 percent of individuals who have had chickenpox will develop shingles during their lifetime. Speak to your physician to see if you are able to receive the vaccine.

Practice tai chi. Recent studies have shown that individuals who practiced tai chi had stronger immune systems against the shingles virus.

Sleep Apnea

In sleep apnea, there are brief breathing interruptions, usually greater than 10 seconds, during sleep. In some instances, these interruptions (called involuntary breathing pauses or apneic events) may occur 20 to 30 times per hour. Though it is possible to have sleep apnea without snoring, usually there is snoring between the breathing interruptions. There may also be choking. Because the sleep pattern is so interrupted, people with sleep apnea are unable to obtain sufficient amounts of deep, restorative sleep. They tend to have morning headaches and excessive daytime sleepiness.

Sleep apnea is very common. It may affect as many as 12 to 25 million Americans, but only about 1 million are aware that they have this disorder.

Because there are sudden drops in blood oxygen levels, sleep apnea is viewed as a serious medical problem. It strains the cardio-

Because of their breathing disorder, people with sleep apnea have increased risks when undergoing major surgery. If you have sleep apnea, be sure to share this information with your surgeon.

vascular system. About half of those with this disorder develop high blood pressure, which increases the risk for heart failure and stroke.

Sleep apnea has also been associated with diabetes, gastroesophageal reflux disease (GERD), kidney failure, peripheral nerve damage, and eye disorders. And people dealing with sleep apnea are often depressed.

According to a study completed at Yale University and published in the *New England Journal of Medicine*, sleep apnea may lead to stroke. The study found that in participants over the age of 50, obstructive sleep apnea more than doubles the risk of stroke or death. Further, severe cases of sleep apnea may triple the risk for stroke or death.

Causes and Risk Factors

There are two types of sleep apnea, each with a different cause. With obstructive sleep apnea, the more common form, while you are sleeping, the muscles in the walls of the throat (pharynx) relax and impede the flow of air. As seconds pass and there is no exchange of air, you enter a lighter level of sleep. The muscles regain their muscle tone, and then you breathe. Many people with this form of sleep apnea are unaware that they have a problem.

With central sleep apnea, the brain sends improper signals to the throat muscles that are involved with breathing. When breathing is interrupted, the amount of carbon dioxide in your blood rises, which may cause you to awaken. If you have central sleep apnea, you are more likely to be aware that you have a problem.

A number of factors place you at greater risk for sleep apnea. Most cases occur in people between the ages of 40 and 70. Men have a greater risk than women. Other factors that increase risk include excess weight, especially around the neck; enlarged tonsils or adenoids; physical abnormality in the nose; a narrow throat; use of alcohol, sedatives, or tranquilizers; an overbite; receding chin; larger tongue; long lower part of the face; narrow upper jaw; soft palate in the throat; and a family history of the disorder. Smokers and alcohol users have higher rates, and African Americans appear to have the highest risk of any ethnic group.

Signs and Symptoms

Though many people with sleep apnea are unaware they have a problem, the disorder is associated with a number of symptoms. These include severe daytime sleepiness, episodes of breathing stoppage during the night, awakening with a dry mouth or throat, irritability, problems with concentration and memory, depression, frequent nighttime urination, heartburn, impotence, and morning headaches. Sleep apnea may be present with or without snoring.

Conventional Treatments

Your doctor will recommend that you stop sleeping on your back. If you are overweight,

A Quick Guide to Symptoms

- ☐ **Episodes of stopped breathing during the night**
- ☐ **Severe daytime sleepiness**
- ☐ **Awakening with a dry mouth or throat**
- ☐ **Irritability**
- ☐ **Problems with concentration and memory**
- ☐ **Depression**
- ☐ **Frequent nighttime urination**
- ☐ **Heartburn**
- ☐ **Impotence**
- ☐ **Morning headaches**
- ☐ **Snoring**

you should also lose excess weight. In some instances, the change in position and weight loss will be sufficient to correct the sleep apnea. You will also be told to avoid alcohol, tobacco, and sleep medications. However, you may need to consider additional options.

Devices and Machines

Your dentist can fit you with a device that brings your jaw forward. Called a mandibular advancement device (MAD), it opens your throat and may relieve mild cases of apnea. Potential MAD side effects include pain, dry lips, tooth discomfort, and excessive salivation.

For moderate or severe cases of sleep apnea, you might use a nasal continuous positive airway pressure (nCPAP) system. With an nCPAP, a machine delivers air through a mask that is

Self-Testing

If you suspect that you have sleep apnea, you should evaluate yourself with the following Epworth Sleepiness Scale. Rate the following eight activities from 0 to 3. A "0" means that you would never doze; "1" means that there is a slight chance you would doze; "2" indicates that there is a moderate chance you would doze; and a "3" means that there is a high chance you may doze. If you score 9 or more, you should visit your doctor.

1. Sitting and reading

2. Watching TV

3. Sitting inactive in a public place

4. Sitting as a passenger in a car for an hour without a break

5. Lying down to rest in the afternoon

6. Sitting and talking to someone

7. Sitting quietly after a lunch without alcohol

8. Sitting in a car while stopped for a few minutes in traffic

Also, consider keeping a sleep journal. Every morning, record how you slept and how you are feeling. Share the journal with your doctor.

placed over your nose. The pressure keeps your airway passages open. In some instances, you will be asked to use a humidifier with your nCPAP. While some people find the systems to be cumbersome and the mask claustrophobic, they often bring dramatic improvements in symptoms. Potential side effects include irritation in the nose and throat and over the bridge of the nose, upper respiratory infections, eye irritation or conjunctivitis, and mild chest muscle discomfort. Rare side effects include heart rhythm disorders, severe nosebleeds, and air pockets in the skull.

Clinical studies have demonstrated that nCPAP may improve sleep quality and reduce both daytime sleepiness and cognitive impairment (caused by obstructive sleep apnea). In a few studies, nCPAP has also reduced blood pressure in people with both normal and high blood pressure who have obstructive sleep apnea.

If you are having trouble tolerating an nCPAP, your doctor may recommend a bilevel positive airway pressure (BiPAP) device. It reduces the air pressure when a person exhales and appears to be more comfortable than the nCPAP. However, it tends to be significantly more expensive than nCPAP.

Surgery

Uvulopalatopharyngoplasty (UPPP) is the most common surgical procedure used to treat sleep apnea and snoring. During UPPP, tissue is removed from the top of the throat and the rear of the mouth. Normally, the tonsils and adenoids are also removed. However, tissue that is farther down the throat may continue to block your air passage. This surgical procedure requires a general anesthetic. After surgery, expect a severe sore throat, and you will only be able to eat soft foods until you heal. Allow yourself about a month to recover fully. Frequent complications include impaired sense of smell, swallowing problems, mucus in the throat, infection, reduced functioning of the soft palate and throat muscles, and regurgitation of fluids through the mouth or nose.

Depending upon what your doctor finds,

you may have surgery to remove nasal polyps or to align the partition between your nostrils (a condition known as a deviated nasal septum). You may have surgery to move your tongue and jaw forward or surgery that removes only the tonsils and/or adenoids.

If all previous treatments have failed and if you are experiencing life-threatening sleep apnea, your doctor may advise a tracheostomy. During this procedure, a surgeon creates an opening in your neck and inserts a tube that enables you to breathe. When you are awake, the opening is covered. When you sleep, it is uncovered, thereby allowing air to pass in and out of the lungs.

Complementary Treatments

To reduce and eliminate sleep apnea and its associated symptoms, practitioners of complementary medicine recommend lifestyle and dietary changes.

Acupuncture

Acupuncture has been found to increase serotonin levels in the body. Low levels of serotonin have been linked to sleep apnea. To find a practitioner in your area, contact the National Certification Commission for Acupuncture and Oriental Medicine (NCCAOM) at www.nccaom.org.

Diet

Eating a well-balanced diet that limits the amount of sugar, caffeine, and processed foods may help you maintain a healthy weight, which reduces your risk of developing sleep apnea.

Also, calcium, magnesium, and vitamins B_6 and B_{12} are all useful nutrients for their ability to calm the nervous system, which may aid in getting a restful night's sleep. Foods high in calcium and magnesium are tofu, shrimp, almonds, black beans, potatoes, and green leafy vegetables, such as spinach, kale, or broccoli. Meat, fish, and eggs are foods that naturally contain vitamin B_{12}. B_{12} is often added to breakfast cereals as well. Poultry and fish are the best natural sources for vitamin B_6.

Flower Essences

Flower essence remedies may be valuable in dealing with the emotional component of sleep apnea, such as depression. Vervain is one remedy that is calming. Flower essences are available in prepared tinctures and may be found in natural health food stores. Take as directed on the label.

Naturopathy

To detect potential food allergies, it may be useful to see a naturopathic physician who may start you on a food elimination diet. These allergies have been linked to blockages in the air passageway. A naturopath may also use other techniques such as homeopathy and nutritional supplementation to treat sleep apnea.

Nutritional Supplements

5-HTP is a precursor to serotonin. To release serotonin and produce a more restful night's sleep, it may be useful to take 100 milligrams of 5-HTP at bedtime. Studies have found it to be useful for sleep apnea and the associated symptoms, such as daytime sleepiness and depression. Serotonin receptors are also responsible for controlling the hormone cortisol, which regulates the muscles needed for breathing.

Lifestyle Recommendations

Avoid alcohol. In addition to relaxing the muscles in the back of the throat, alcohol consumption, especially within 4 to 6 hours of bedtime, may increase the frequency and severity of sleep apnea. It has been found that alcohol is a trigger for sleep apnea, even in individuals who might otherwise only snore.

Avoid tranquilizers and sleeping medications. Since these drugs may relax the muscles in the back of the throat, they can interfere with breathing.

Exhale. When people are awakened from their sleep because they momentarily stop breathing, the initial response is to gasp and inhale quickly. This will only make the condition worse. Instead, try to remember to first sharply exhale and then inhale slowly. Repeat until breathing becomes natural and relaxed.

Gargle before bed. Gargle before bed with warm water and salt. This can help shrink your tonsils.

Keep your nasal passages open when you sleep. Experiment with nasal decongestants, which may help keep nasal passages clear.

Lose excess weight. If you have been carrying excess weight, you may improve your sleep apnea by dropping some pounds. Losing weight tends to relieve the constriction in your throat. Even a small loss may make a big difference.

Raise the head of the bed or mattress. To raise the entire top half of your body, elevate the head of the bed with 4- to 6-inch blocks or a wedge support. Don't attempt to accomplish this goal with pillows, as this will only further interrupt your breathing.

Relax before bed. Before getting into bed, try some relaxation techniques. One way to relax is to lie on your bed without pillows and with your legs and arms spread wide apart. Tilt your head slightly back. Take a long, deep breath through the nose and exhale slowly through the mouth for as long as you can. The exhale should be longer than the inhale. Get into a rhythm and continue until you feel the muscles of your body relax. When you are ready to get under the blankets and use a pillow, turn on your side. Try to maintain this long and relaxed way of breathing as you drift off to sleep.

Try sleeping on your side. When you sleep on your back, your tongue and soft palate lie against the back of your throat, thereby blocking the airway. If you are a back sleeper and need some assistance training yourself to sleep on your side, try placing a thick pillow behind your back after you get into bed and lie on your side. This may prevent you from rolling over onto your back.

Preventive Measures

Live a healthier lifestyle. People who maintain a healthier weight and don't smoke are less likely to develop sleep apnea.

Stop smoking. Smoking may swell the throat tissue and increase mucus buildup, interfering with the ability of air to pass through without obstruction.

Snoring

Snoring is the noisy breathing sounds that you may make while you sleep. It occurs when air does not flow smoothly through your air passages or when structures in your air passages vibrate. Snoring is extremely common. About half of men and 25 percent of women snore. Most are 40 years old or older.

Causes and Risk Factors

A number of factors are believed to cause snoring. Your risk for snoring increases as you age. When you sleep on your back, your tongue may fall backward into your throat. When that happens, the tongue blocks your throat and makes the passageway smaller. As air passes over your tongue, it may vibrate, creating the snoring sounds.

Snoring may also be caused by a blockage in your nose, resulting from allergies, a cold, or a sinus infection. If your adenoids, which are located in the back of your nose, are enlarged, they may cause snoring. Snoring may also be caused by an injury to the nose or an obstruction, such as a polyp.

When people gain a lot of weight, there is more accumulation of fat tissue, and air passages may become smaller. So, weight gain may trigger snoring. Also, by relaxing the muscles in the throat, some relaxation or sedation medications are known to cause snoring, including sleeping pills, antihistamines, and pain medications. Alcohol may have a similar effect. Smokers are far more likely to snore than people who have never smoked.

Signs and Symptoms

People who snore have noisy breaths while they sleep. These may occur when they are breathing in or breathing out or both.

Conventional Treatments

In many instances, the treatments for snoring are fairly direct. For example, if your doctor believes that your snoring is related to excess weight, you will be told to lose weight. Similarly, your doctor will tell you to avoid sleeping on your back. Your doctor may

Snoring and Sleep Apnea

Sometimes snoring is a symptom of a serious condition known as sleep apnea. If you have this disorder, your sleep is being interrupted by frequent periods of breathing stoppages. During these episodes, you take in less oxygen. Sleep apnea is associated with a number of additional medical problems. If you suspect that you have sleep apnea, be sure to talk with your doctor about it.

suggest medication for nasal congestion, or advise against drinking alcoholic beverages or taking sedating medications. If you have an obstruction in your nasal passages, you will be referred to a physician who will surgically correct the problem.

However, if none of these treatments is appropriate for your snoring and if it continues to bother you and your sleeping partner, additional treatments may be offered.

Dental Devices

A variety of dental devices are available to reposition your mouth, stabilize your lower jaw and tongue, or increase the muscle tone of the tongue. The goal is to improve the passage of air and decrease snoring.

Nasal Strips

You may wish to try over-the-counter nasal strips. Since they increase the area of the nasal passages, they improve breathing. But nasal strips tend to be effective for only mild cases of snoring.

Surgery

Laser surgery. With laser surgery, known as laser-assisted uvulopalatoplasty (LAUP), your doctor uses a laser to remove excess tissue in your throat and enlarge the airway. Depending upon the severity of your snoring, you may require two to five sessions, each lasting for about 30 minutes. Your doctor will probably recommend a period of 4 to 6 weeks between treatments.

Somnoplasty. With somnoplasty, also known as radiofrequency tissue volume reduction, your doctor uses a low-intensity radiofrequency to remove part of the soft palate. Performed under local anesthesia, the procedure results in slight scarring of the soft palate, which is thought to reduce snoring.

Traditional surgery. While you are under general anesthesia, a surgeon will trim and tighten the excess tissues in the throat. Normally, this will reduce the amount of snoring. Still, you should be aware that there will be a good deal of postoperative pain. Allow yourself at least 2 weeks to recover.

Complementary Treatments

To reduce or eliminate snoring, practitioners of complementary medicine recommend a number of lifestyle and dietary changes.

Aromatherapy

The essential oils of eucalyptus and menthol have been shown to be effective in reducing nasal congestion, which may cause snoring. To clear your nasal passages, try placing a few drops of these oils on a handkerchief and breathing in before bed. You may want to place a few drops on a lamp in your bedroom and let the heat of the lightbulb disperse the essential oils into the air.

Nutritional Supplements

Preliminary studies on chondroitin sulfate nasal spray have shown promise in reducing snoring. The chondroitin spray coats the nasal passages.

Lifestyle Recommendations

Keep a clean room. Be sure that your room is free of dust and any other pollutants or irritants that could be causing nasal congestion. Feather pillows or blankets, fresh flowers, and dust trapped in curtains may be potential irritants.

Raise the head of the bed or mattress. To raise the entire top half of your body, elevate the head of the bed with 4- to 6-inch blocks or a wedge support. Don't attempt to accomplish this goal with pillows, as this will only further interrupt your breathing.

Stop smoking. Smoking may swell the throat tissue and increase mucus buildup, interfering with the ability of air to pass through without obstruction.

Preventive Measures

Avoid alcohol and sedatives before bed. Alcohol and sedatives cause the throat muscles to relax and the tongue to pull back into the airway. If you drink alcoholic beverages or take a sedative before bed, you are at increased risk for snoring.

Lose weight. If you have been carrying excess weight, you may improve your snoring by dropping some pounds. Losing weight tends to relieve the constriction in your throat. Even a small loss may make a big difference.

Sleep on your side. When you sleep on your back, your tongue and soft palate lie against the back of your throat, thereby blocking your airway and possibly leading to snoring. If you sleep on your back and need to train yourself to sleep on your side, after lying on your side in bed, try placing a thick pillow behind your back. This may prevent you from rolling onto your back.

Unclog your nasal passages. If your nasal passages are clogged, you are more likely to snore. Take the medication you require to unclog them.

Tinnitus

Tinnitus is noise that you hear inside your head, in the absence of real sounds. For obvious reasons, tinnitus is also known as head noise. The noise may be evident in one or both ears, and while it may be quite soft, in some instances it is so loud that you are unable to hear properly or concentrate. Tinnitus may occur for a relatively brief time and then disappear. It may begin quickly or slowly over an extended period of time. Tinnitus may also be intermittent or persistent, and it seems to be more apparent when the environment is quiet. About 40 percent of those who have tinnitus also have hyperacusis, a heightened sensitivity to normal sounds. And about 90 percent of those who have severe tinnitus have hearing loss.

If you are the only one who can hear your tinnitus, it is referred to as "subjective tinnitus." If it is audible to your doctor when listening with a stethoscope, your tinnitus is known as "objective tinnitus."

Tinnitus is extremely common. Though statistics vary, it has been estimated that it may affect as many as 50 million Americans. About 10 million are so disturbed by the condition that they seek medical care. Of these, about 2.5 million people are seriously disabled.

Causes and Risk Factors

There are a number of causes of tinnitus. Most often, tinnitus seems to be the result of some form of damage to the sensory (hair) cells in the inner ear (cochlea) or in the cells along the auditory nerve that connects the inner ear to the brain. Tinnitus appears to be related to exposure to loud noises and/or age-related hearing loss (presbycusis). But it has also been associated with ear injuries, Ménière's syndrome, infections, head trauma, hypothyroidism, diabetes, allergies, psychological disorders, and diseases of the circulatory system, such as atherosclerosis (pulsatile tinnitus), high or low blood pressure, A-V malformation (malformation of capillaries), and the narrowing of the carotid artery.

More than 200 medications have been linked with tinnitus. These include aspirin and other nonsteroidal anti-inflammatories, quinine, antibiotics, chemotherapy, beta-blockers, anti-inflammatory drugs, and antidepressants. And tinnitus has been related to caffeine, alcohol, and illegal drugs such as marijuana.

Tinnitus may also be the result of jaw joint (temporomandibular) disorders, the stiffening of the bones in the middle ear (otosclerosis), and (rarely) head and neck tumors. Because of the abrupt change in atmospheric pressure, people who scuba dive may experience tinnitus. If you already have tinnitus, your symptoms may worsen if you have earwax buildup, an ear infection, or a rupture of your eardrum.

People between the ages of 40 and 70 are at most risk for tinnitus. It may appear in about one-third of those over the age of 55. It affects men more often than women.

Signs and Symptoms

With tinnitus, you hear noises in one or both of your ears. This occurs despite the fact that there is no external sound. The noise may sound like buzzing, ringing, humming, escaping air, running water, sizzling, or chirping. In some instances, the noise may be so loud and persistent that you have trouble concentrating.

Conventional Treatments

Though you may be experiencing tinnitus, your medical tests may find no cause. In most cases, the results of all the tests are normal. If a specific cause of your tinnitus is determined, then treating the medical problem should help correct the tinnitus. Thus, if your doctor concludes that the tinnitus is caused by high blood pressure, you will probably be advised to take measures to lower your blood pressure, such as medication. Similarly, if your tinnitus is caused by a medication, after a drug or dosage adjustment is made, the noise should stop.

However, for the vast majority of those who have tinnitus, especially from age-related hearing loss and exposure to loud noises, there is no cure. But there are a number of treatments that have proven to be effective.

A Quick Guide to Symptoms

☐ Noises in one or both ears when there is no external sound
☐ Sounds like buzzing, ringing, humming, escaping air, running water, sizzling, or chirping
☐ Trouble concentrating due to noise

Cochlear Implant

Though cochlear implants are generally used for people who have little or no hearing, in some instances they are also being offered to people with tinnitus. With a cochlear implant, a surgeon inserts electrodes into the cochlea and implants a receiver in the skull behind the ear. Combined with a microphone, speech processor, and transmitter, these pick up sounds and send signals to the brain.

Self-Testing

Though there are no self-tests for tinnitus, if you are hearing continuous sounds, you probably have it. Since tinnitus may be related to something you are ingesting, keep a diary of everything you consume, and also record your bouts of tinnitus. You may be able to note associations.

Counseling

People who are coping with tinnitus often become depressed. Talking about your situation with a therapist or with members of a support group may be useful.

Hearing Aids

The vast majority of people with serious tinnitus also have hearing loss. By amplifying the sounds around you, a hearing aid may make the tinnitus less noticeable. Hearing aids will probably not be a solution if your hearing loss is in the same frequency range as the tinnitus.

Medication

The short-term use of antidepressants and anti-anxiety medications may help people with severe forms of tinnitus deal with their stress.

Sound-Generating Devices

Sound-generating devices, which look like hearing aids, are able to reduce or block the sounds from tinnitus. You will need to be fitted by a tinnitus professional (otolaryngologist, audiologist, or neuroscientist). If your tinnitus is making it difficult for you to sleep, consider purchasing a pillow that has small speakers. These may be plugged into a tape or CD player. You can accomplish a similar goal by using a tabletop machine that creates external white noise or by setting a radio between stations so that it produces static.

Tinnitus Retraining Therapy (TRT)

With tinnitus retraining therapy (TRT), education and counseling are used to teach the brain to view the sounds from tinnitus as nonthreatening and to retrain the brain not to hear them. A team of physicians, audiologists, and psychologists combine counseling and the use of low-level broadband noise generators. People wear small devices behind their ears that deliver pleasant sounds. This reduces the effect of the tinnitus sounds. After 12 to 18 months of this treatment, your brain learns to ignore both kinds of sounds. It is reported that TRT is effective in about 75 to 80 percent of cases.

Complementary Treatments

The symptoms of tinnitus may be controlled and possibly eliminated by various complementary medicine approaches. Practitioners work to address the underlying cause of the tinnitus and create a specific treatment plan. Positive outcomes may also be achieved in relieving the symptoms of tinnitus through general lifestyle changes, nutritional recommendations, bodywork, and relaxation/meditation techniques.

Acupuncture

Acupuncture may decrease the sound level of tinnitus and remove blockages to the middle ear. To locate an acupuncturist in your area, visit the Web site of the National Certification Commission for Acupuncture and Oriental Medicine (NCCAOM) at www. nccaom.org.

Alexander Technique

By correcting the position of the head on the spine, the Alexander Technique may improve circulation to the inner ear, helping to alleviate tinnitus. It also may ease other symptoms of Meniere's disease, such as dizziness and nausea. To locate a teacher of the Alexander Technique, visit the Web site of the American Society for the Alexander Technique at www. alexandertech.org.

Biofeedback

With biofeedback, you are able to learn how to control your physiological response to stress, thereby preventing stress from exacerbating your condition.

Chiropractic

Chiropractic adjustment and manipulation of the neck and spine may increase circulation to the inner ear and relieve blockages of the nerves that supply the inner ear.

Craniosacral Therapy

Imbalances and discrepancies in the rhythm of the cerebrospinal fluid lead to impaired body functions, which may result in tinnitus. The craniosacral practitioner works to reestablish a balanced rhythm and normal function of the cerebrospinal fluid. To search for a qualified therapist in your area, visit the Web site of the International Associa-

tion of Healthcare Practitioners at www. iahp.com.

Diet

Eating plenty of raw fruits and vegetables may clear mucus that is clogging the ears and improve circulation. If you have tinnitus due to high blood pressure, you should avoid foods that are high in fat and cholesterol. These foods impede circulation. You should also take brewer's yeast, which contains choline, an important nutrient in preventing or eliminating tinnitus.

Apricots, baked potatoes, bananas, green leafy vegetables, and nuts are good sources of magnesium and potassium, which are essential nutrients for treating tinnitus. Vitamin A is important for the membranes of the ear and overall ear health. The body converts beta-carotene into vitamin A. Beta-carotene is found in many fruits and vegetables, especially those that are red, yellow, and orange. If you follow a diet high in fresh fruits and vegetables, you should be getting enough vitamin A.

Make sure you eat lots of garlic, which dilates tiny capillaries, including those that supply the inner ear. Zinc is valuable for reducing some of the symptoms associated with tinnitus. Good food sources of zinc are oysters, whole grains, nuts, cereals, fish, spinach, papaya, brussels sprouts, string beans, asparagus, and prunes.

Avoid sodium or greatly reduce your intake. Sodium fosters the retention of water in the middle ear, which may cause tinnitus and hearing loss. Foods high in saturated fats and trans fatty acids place stress on the body and constrict the arteries. Sugar narrows the blood vessels of the inner ear and impairs the immune system. As a result, these foods should be avoided.

Herbal Medicine

If your tinnitus is caused by a circulation problem or an allergy, the following herbs may be helpful.

Black cohosh. Black cohosh has been shown to decrease the symptoms of tinnitus. It may be purchased as a capsule or in a tincture. It works best when taken in conjunction with ginkgo. The recommended daily dose is 20 milligrams twice a day of standardized extract of 2.5 percent triterpene glycosides.

Ginger. Ginger improves circulation and bloodflow to the ear and aids in reducing nausea from tinnitus. It is available in capsule and tincture form as well as a tea.

Ginkgo biloba. Ginkgo increases bloodflow to the inner ear and relieves dizziness. The typical recommended daily dose is 120 milligrams of standardized extract containing 24 percent flavone glycosides and 6 percent terpene lactones. (As mentioned above, ginkgo works best when taken with black cohosh, as medical trials have shown it to be no better than a placebo when taken alone.)

Nutritional Supplements

Nutritional supplements play a role in the function of the inner ear and alleviate deficiencies that may cause ear problems.

- Multivitamin/mineral: Take as directed on the label. Should include calcium, magnesium, and potassium, which are essential nutrients for treating tinnitus.

- Vitamin A: 10,000 IU daily. Stimulates auditory nerve and aids in proper functioning of the cochlea.

- B-complex vitamins: Take as directed on the label. Deficiency linked to ear problems; relaxes and widens blood vessels, increasing circulation to inner ear; reduces tinnitus; and stabilizes fluid in inner ear.

- Vitamin B_{12}: Injections or 1,000-microgram sublingual tablet daily. Deficiency found in many individuals with tinnitus. Injections of B_{12} have been more effective with this condition.

- Vitamin D: 400 IU daily. Supports the cochlea, prevents damage to bones of the middle ear, and may restore some hearing loss.

- Melatonin: 3 milligrams daily. May improve the symptoms of tinnitus.

- Zinc: 30 milligrams daily. May control symptoms of tinnitus.

Relaxation/Meditation

Relaxation/meditation techniques may decrease stress and increase circulation. Deep breathing exercises, tai chi, guided imagery, biofeedback, and visualization techniques decrease the stress associated with tinnitus. Stress only makes tinnitus worse, so it is important to find an outlet that helps you relax.

Lifestyle Recommendations

Having low-level background noise such as music will usually make you much less aware of tinnitus.

Be tested for food allergies. Tinnitus has been linked to food allergies. If you do not have any of the other conditions associated with tinnitus, you may wish to be tested for allergies.

Consult your dentist. TMJ (temporomandibular joint) dysfunction has been associated with tinnitus. See your dentist to determine if TMJ may be causing your tinnitus.

Exercise. If you do not already exercise, begin a program of regular exercise. It will improve circulation. Your exercise program should include some form of aerobic activity (brisk walking, bicycling, or swimming) at least 5 days each week, strength training (weight lifting) at least two or three times per week, and everyday stretching.

Try hypnosis. Hypnosis is helpful in eliminating the unwanted sounds of tinnitus. To bring immediate relief for tinnitus and its associated symptoms, a practitioner may also recommend self-hypnosis techniques.

Limit exposure to tinnitus irritants. It is well known that tinnitus may be aggravated by loud noises, nicotine, caffeine, and certain medications, such as aspirin. If you are exposed to loud noises, use earplugs or wear earmuffs, and be careful about ingesting potential irritants.

Try massage. To increase circulation and bring relief from tinnitus, gently massage the hollows and the top of the jawbone directly behind both earlobes. To further increase circulation to the ears, you may want to apply a hot compress to the neck area.

Preventive Measures

Avoid loud noises. Since exposure to loud noises may trigger tinnitus, whenever possible, protect your ears from excessive noise.

Chew to increase circulation. Chewing gum or eating dried fruits may increase circulation to the ears.

Ulcerative Colitis

Ulcerative colitis is a form of recurring inflammatory bowel disease. Ulcers form in the inner lining (mucosa) of the large intestine and/or rectum. Most often, the left side of the colon (sigmoid colon) and rectum are affected. However, ulcerative colitis may occur throughout the colon (extensive colitis or pancolitis). Generally, the larger the area of the intestine that is affected, the greater the severity of the symptoms. Still, sometimes much of the intestines is affected but the symptoms remain mild.

Ulcerative colitis is more common than most people realize. It has been estimated that out of every 100,000 Americans, 10 to 15 have this disorder.

People with ulcerative colitis may be forced to deal with several complications. With the most serious one, toxic megacolon, the colon dilates and shuts down, and the person is unable to have a bowel movement or pass gas. This causes abdominal pain, swelling, fever, and weakness. This is a condition requiring emergency attention. Without such care, the colon may rupture.

Other complications associated with ulcerative colitis are liver disease and skin, joint, and eye inflammation. And there is an increased risk for colon cancer. Your degree of risk is a function of the amount of the large intestine affected—the larger the area of intestine affected, the greater the risk for cancer.

Causes and Risk Factors

Though the exact cause of ulcerative colitis is unknown, there are a number of strong possibilities. Some researchers suggest that it is the result of an unknown virus or bacterium. The large intestine and rectum may become inflamed in an attempt to combat the virus or bacterium, or the inflammation may be a direct result of the invaders.

Since about 20 percent of those with ulcerative colitis have a parent, sibling, or child who also has the disease, there is probably a genetic component. Still, another potential culprit is the environment and/or the diet. Ulcerative colitis is more common among those who live in cities and industrialized

Ulcerative Colitis or Crohn's Disease?

Since they are both inflammatory bowel diseases, ulcerative colitis is often confused with Crohn's disease. However, ulcerative colitis is confined to the large intestine or rectum and affects the innermost layer of the colon and rectum. Crohn's disease, which is less common than ulcerative colitis, may occur anywhere in the gastrointestinal tract.

nations. And a diet higher in fat or refined foods may play a role.

Most people with ulcerative colitis are diagnosed between the ages of 15 and 35, but it may appear at any age. It affects men and women about equally. Whites have the highest risk, especially people who are of Jewish and European descent, who are four to five times more likely to have this disorder than whites of other ethnicities.

Signs and Symptoms

A number of symptoms are associated with ulcerative colitis, which may develop slowly or appear quite quickly. The symptoms include chronic diarrhea, abdominal pain and cramping, blood in the stool, diminished appetite, weight loss, and fever.

If you have a mild case of ulcerative colitis, you may have an urgent need to move your bowels, even when you are sleeping. You may have frequent stools, loose or liquid stools, and blood and mucus in bowel movements. With more severe cases, you may also experience weight loss, anemia, fever, and poor energy level. While some people suffer continuously, others have years or even decades in which they are symptom-free.

Conventional Treatments

The treatments for ulcerative colitis attempt to reduce the inflammation in the large intestine and rectum. The goal is to attain symptom relief and extended periods of remission.

A Quick Guide to Symptoms

- ☐ **Chronic diarrhea**
- ☐ **Frequent stools**
- ☐ **Abdominal pain and cramping**
- ☐ **Blood and mucus in the stool**
- ☐ **Diminished appetite**
- ☐ **Weight loss**
- ☐ **Fever**
- ☐ **Urgent need to move the bowels**

Dietary Modifications

Though dietary intake does not cause ulcerative colitis, it may affect the symptoms of the disorder. Many people with ulcerative colitis are lactose intolerant, so you may wish to restrict your intake of dairy products, or consume dairy products that are naturally lower in lactose, such as Swiss and Cheddar cheeses. You may also try using Lactaid, an enzyme that breaks down lactose.

Carefully scrutinize the fibrous foods that you eat, especially if you have abdominal cramps. Raw fruits and vegetables may bother you. You may need to steam, bake, or stew them. In addition, you may find that you tolerate certain fruits and vegetables better than others. People with ulcerative colitis tend to have more trouble with crunchy foods (raw apples and carrots) and foods in the cabbage family (cauliflower and broccoli).

Other foods that tend to bother those with ulcerative colitis are citrus fruits, fruits with simple sugars (such as grapes, pineapples, and watermelon), carbonated beverages, products containing sorbitol, spicy foods, dried fruit, popcorn, alcohol, and caffeine-containing foods and drinks. "Gassy foods," such as beans, may also cause problems. Many people with ulcerative colitis find that their symptoms worsen when they eat foods containing corn, gluten (wheat, oats, barley, and rye), soy, eggs, peanuts, and tomatoes.

Try increasing your intake of lean protein foods, especially oily fish such as salmon. And you may find that your symptoms improve if you consume five or six smaller meals throughout the day instead of two or three larger meals. Be sure to drink lots of water.

To reduce the risk of kidney stones—a common complication for people with ulcerative colitis, particularly those who have had intestinal surgery—you should consider additional dietary modifications. Be sure to limit your intake of salt and increase your consumption of potassium-rich foods, such as bananas, papayas, sweet potatoes, and canned salmon. Since many kidney stones are formed from calcium oxalate, you should limit or avoid oxalate-rich foods such as beets, black tea, chocolate, parsley, spinach, and rhubarb.

Medications

Many medications are used to treat ulcerative colitis, including anti-inflammatory drugs, immune system suppressors, antibiotics, antidiarrheals, laxatives, pain relievers, iron supplements, and vitamin B_{12} injections. Don't become discouraged if it takes a while to find the right combination for you.

Anti-inflammatory drugs. Your doctor will probably begin by prescribing an anti-inflammatory drug. Though sulfasalazine (Azulfidine) has been used for many years, it has potential side effects such as nausea, vomiting, heartburn, and headache. Mesalamine (Asacol, Rowasa) and olsalazine (Dipentum) have fewer side effects than sulfasalazine. The chemical structure of mesalamine is similar to aspirin, so if you are allergic to aspirin, do not take mesalamine.

Corticosteroids have also been used successfully, but they have potential side effects such as puffy face, excessive facial hair, night sweats, insomnia, hyperactivity, high blood pressure, diabetes, osteoporosis, cataracts, and increased susceptibility to infection. Budesonide (Entocort EC) is a newer type of corticosteroid that seems to have fewer side effects.

Immune system suppressors. Other drugs reduce inflammation by suppressing the immune system. Azathioprine (Imuran) and mercaptopurine (Purinethol) are widely used for ulcerative colitis. Still, you should be aware that they work very slowly. It may take 3 months before you see significant improvement.

If you have not responded to other medications, your doctor may recommend cyclosporine (Neoral, Sandimmune). Cyclosporine may be effective in those who are hospitalized with severe ulcerative colitis. High doses may be able to achieve short-term control of the disease. Unfortunately, after the short-term control of the disease is achieved, a significant percentage of individuals will still need surgery. Potential side effects include kidney damage, high blood pressure, and an increased risk for infection.

Infliximab, an antibody that has been shown to be useful in the treatment of Crohn's disease, was studied in people who had active ulcerative colitis despite traditional medical therapy. One group of people with moderate to severe ulcerative colitis received infliximab over a period of up to 1 year. The other group received a placebo for the same period of time. When compared to those who received a placebo, the ones who received infliximab were more likely to show improvement.

Medications for symptom relief. Other medications address the signs and symptoms of ulcerative colitis. For mild to moderate diarrhea, your doctor may suggest a fiber supplement, such as psyllium powder (Metamucil) or methylcellulose (Citrucel). If diarrhea is more severe, consider loperamide (Imodium). If the inflammation in the intestines has caused constipation, you may require a laxative. Over-the-counter laxatives are likely to be too strong for your system, so ask your doctor to suggest a laxative.

For mild pain relief, your doctor may advise acetaminophen (Tylenol). Do not take any nonsteroidal anti-inflammatory drugs such as aspirin, naproxen sodium (Aleve), or ibuprofen (Advil), as they will probably exacerbate your symptoms. If you have experienced any intestinal bleeding, you may be anemic and your health care provider may recommend iron supplements.

Surgery

For people with ulcerative colitis, the surgical removal of the colon (a proctocolectomy) generally cures the disease. After the colon is removed, the surgeon may create an opening (known as a stoma) in the right lower portion of the abdomen; this procedure is called an ileostomy. Waste will leave the body from the stoma and be collected in a pouch. Instead of a stoma, whenever possible, surgeons construct a pouch from the end of the small intestine and attach it to the anus. This procedure, an ileoanal anastomosis, permits the normal expulsion of waste. But without a colon, excess water is not absorbed, so waste will be watery. It is estimated that between 25 and 40 percent of people with ulcerative colitis ultimately require surgery.

Complementary Treatments

Changes in lifestyle and diet may be effective in providing relief from ulcerative colitis as well as in helping to relieve the pain associated with its symptoms.

Naturopathy

Naturopathy is a system of holistic therapy that relies on natural remedies, such as homeopathy, hydrotherapy, diet, herbs, massage, acupuncture, and exercise. Naturopathic medicine has proven very effective in the treatment of digestive disorders. To find a naturopathic practitioner in your area, contact the American Association of Naturopathic Physicians at www.naturopathic.org.

Nutritional Counseling

Once ulcerative colitis has been established as a diagnosis, it is beneficial to consider nutritional counseling. Nutritional counselors help individuals determine food hypersensitivities, allergies, or food intolerances through elimination diets. Nutritional counseling can help individuals design specific diets that provide both variety and proper nutrition.

Nutritional Supplements

Due to their inability to absorb vitamins and minerals, individuals with ulcerative colitis often have difficulty maintaining proper nutrition levels in the body. Taking a daily multivitamin/mineral supplement can ensure the body maintains the proper level of these nutrients.

- Multivitamin/mineral: Take as directed on the label. Supplement should contain vitamins A, D, E, folic acid, iron, magnesium, and zinc.
- Vitamin B_{12}: 1,000-microgram sublingual tablet daily. Necessary due to inability to absorb adequate amounts of B_{12}.
- Omega-3 fatty acids such as flaxseed oil or fish oil: 1 tablespoon of flaxseed oil daily or 4,000 milligrams daily of fish oil cap-

sules. Prostaglandins formed from omega-3 fatty acids aid in the regulation of inflammation, pain, and swelling. Particularly effective in the digestive tract.

Lifestyle Recommendations

Address related psychological issues. Dealing with ulcerative colitis exacts a strong psychological toll. People with severe symptoms may fear leaving their homes, worried about the accessibility of bathrooms. Even those with milder symptoms may be reluctant to leave their homes. It is very easy for those with ulcerative colitis to become isolated. Anxiety and depression go hand in hand with this disorder.

Consider joining a support group. Participating in a support group may enable you to cope better with the disease. You may benefit from the advice and suggestions offered by others with the same condition.

Manage the stress in your life. While stress does not cause ulcerative colitis, it may trigger flare-ups and increase the severity of symptoms. When you are experiencing stress, the digestive area often becomes a holding place for tension-causing emotions, resulting in additional digestive difficulties. Try to include stress-reducing techniques in your everyday life. These may include exercise, biofeedback, yoga, meditation, massage, progressive relaxation exercises, deep breathing, and hypnosis.

Practice deep breathing. Deep breathing

can help relax abdominal muscles, which can promote regular bowel movements. While flat on your back, place both hands on your abdomen. Slowly inhale through the nose, pushing your abdomen up as if blowing up a balloon. Then, exhale slowly through the mouth, and feel your abdomen deflate. Practice this breathing process as often as possible.

Watch what you eat. Studies show that a diet high in saturated fat, trans fatty acids, and sugar and low in fruits, vegetables, and other whole grains may increase the risk of ulcerative colitis. Fruits, vegetables, and other fiber may also be useful during an acute attack.

Preventive Measures

Though there is no known way to prevent ulcerative colitis, by making a few changes in your lifestyle, you may reduce the chances for a flare-up.

Consider an elimination diet. In order to determine which foods trigger your condition, try an elimination diet. For the first 10 days, eliminate all citrus fruits and foods containing corn, dairy, eggs, and gluten. After 7 to 10 days, if your symptoms remain unchanged, you most likely do not have a sensitivity to these foods. On the other hand, if your symptoms improve and you have more energy and a better mood, then you need to add these food groups back into your diet one at a time, every 3 or 4 days. That will enable you to determine the culprit or culprits. During this time, a food journal may help you track symptoms.

Exercise. Regular exercise reduces the pressure inside the colon, moves food along faster, and promotes normal bowel function. For improved bowel health, try to exercise at least 30 minutes a day as often as possible. One of the best exercises is a daily walk of 20 to 30 minutes. By including exercise in your daily lifestyle, you will help maintain your strength and reduce stress.

Uterine Fibroids

Uterine fibroids are growths either inside the wall of the uterus or attached to the wall of the uterus. Though in rare instances they may be cancerous, uterine fibroids (also known as leiomyoma, leiomyomata, myoma, or fibromyoma) are generally benign tumors made of smooth muscle and connective tissue. Uterine fibroids that grow in the uterine lining are called submucosal. Those in between the muscles of the uterus are intramural. And those on the outside surface of the uterus are subserosal.

Uterine fibroids may be as small as a pea or as large as a cantaloupe. Often, there are several fibroids. When uterine fibroids grow large, they may deform the uterus and put pressure on the nearby bladder or intestine, resulting in increased urination, constipation, and pain.

Uterine fibroids are quite common: 20 to 40 percent of women over the age of 35 have them. They are the most frequently seen tumors of the genital tract.

Causes and Risk Factors

While the exact cause of uterine fibroids is not known, it has been speculated that they are related to the levels of the hormones estrogen and progesterone and levels of proteins called growth factors. Further, there also seems to be a genetic component.

African American women have the highest risk for uterine fibroids. They are three to five times more likely than white women to have them. Asian women have the lowest risk of them all. Obesity as well as the consumption of beef, other red meat, and ham have been associated with uterine fibroids, while the consumption of green vegetables has been related to a decreased risk of uterine fibroids. Women who have given birth seem to be at lower risk for uterine fibroids. And women who have taken oral contraceptive pills may have some protection against fibroids. After menopause, uterine fibroids have a tendency to shrink.

Signs and Symptoms

Though many women who have uterine fibroids have no related symptoms, fibroids have been associated with a number of symptoms. These include heavy menstrual bleeding, painful menstrual periods, periods that last longer than usual, pelvic pain or pressure, constipation, backache, bloating, more frequent or uncomfortable urination, incontinence, and miscarriage. Uterine fibroids do not affect ovulation, but since the uterine cavity may be distorted by a submucosal fibroid, they may lead to infertility.

Conventional Treatments

Most uterine fibroids do not require treatment. If you are not experiencing symptoms from the fibroids, your doctor will probably evaluate them at each annual physical examination, and ask you to watch for symptoms. Factors that are important to the management of uterine fibroids include their size, location, symptoms, and a woman's age and reproductive plans.

However, if you are losing a great deal of blood or the uterine fibroid is growing quickly or causing severe symptoms, treatment may be advised. Of course, if the uterine fibroids are determined to be cancerous, you need to be treated.

Medications

For pain from uterine fibroids, your doctor will probably recommend the use of a nonsteroidal anti-inflammatory drug such as ibuprofen (Motrin) or naproxen sodium (Naprosyn). Oral contraceptives or the hormone danazol (Danocrine) may be prescribed to control bleeding. Another group of medications, known as gonadotropin-releasing hormone analogues (Lupron), shrink fibroids by reducing the amount of estrogen in the body. They are administered by injection. However, these drugs cause the symptoms associated with menopause, such as bone loss, mood swings, hot flashes, headaches, and vaginal dryness. Generally, they are used for a relatively short period of time, such as to shrink fibroids before surgery.

A Quick Guide to Symptoms

- ☐ Heavy menstrual bleeding
- ☐ Painful menstrual periods
- ☐ Periods that last longer than usual
- ☐ Pelvic pain or pressure
- ☐ Constipation
- ☐ Backache
- ☐ Bloating
- ☐ More frequent or uncomfortable urination
- ☐ Incontinence
- ☐ Miscarriage

Surgery

Cryomyolysis. In a cryomyolysis, which is an outpatient procedure, your doctor begins by making three or four incisions in the abdomen. Then, using a laparoscope to view the inside of the abdomen, your doctor will insert a cryoprobe into the fibroids and freeze them with liquid nitrogen at minus 180°C. The freezing process is monitored with an ultrasound. Cryomyolysis reduces the size of fibroids by 20 to 50 percent.

Hysterectomy. In the United States every year, more than half a million women have a hysterectomy (the surgical removal of the uterus), and about a third of these procedures are for treatment of uterine fibroids. The uterus may be removed either through the vagina with a laparoscope or with an abdominal incision. The type of procedure is a function of the size of the uterus, any previous surgeries, and any other medical problems the woman is experiencing. All types of hysterectomies are performed under general anesthesia. Expect to spend a few days in the hospital and to recover at home for several weeks. There is a 2 percent risk of postoperative bleeding and a 15 to 38 percent risk of postoperative fever.

Myomectomy. In a myomectomy, the uterine fibroids are removed surgically, usually by a gynecologist. There are three main types of this procedure: hysteroscopic myomectomy, laparoscopic myomectomy, and abdominal myomectomy. A hysteroscopic myomectomy may be used only for fibroids that are submucosal (on the inside of the uterus), just below the lining and projecting into the uterine cavity. While you are under general anesthesia, your doctor inserts a hysteroscope (flexible fiber-optic scope) into the uterus via the vagina and cervix. Using a special surgical tube that is attached to the hysteroscope, your doctor removes the fibroids. About 10 to 20 percent of all fibroids may be removed in this way.

If the fibroids are on the outside of the uterus (subserosal), your doctor may advise a laparoscopic myomectomy. While you are under general anesthesia, your doctor makes a few small incisions in the abdomen. Then, your doctor inserts a probe with a tiny camera into one of the incisions and a probe with surgical instruments into a second incision. The fibroids are then removed.

An abdominal myomectomy is a more extensive procedure that requires a recovery of 4 to 6 weeks. While you are under general anesthesia, your doctor makes an incision in the abdomen and a second incision into the uterus. After the fibroids are removed, the uterus and the abdomen are stitched closed. You will probably remain in the hospital for several days of recovery.

Uterine Fibroid Embolization

Uterine fibroids have a large blood supply that enables them to grow. In a uterine fibroid embolization, this blood supply is stopped or blocked. As a result, the uterine fibroids shrink, or even shrivel up and die. This procedure may be of interest to those women who want to keep their uteruses or who are high-risk surgical candidates. Before the procedure, which is done in a hospital, you will be given medication to help you relax and make you sleepy. Your doctor, who should be an interventional radiologist (a radiologist who has received extensive specialized training in these procedures), will make a small cut in the skin of the groin area. Then, a tiny tube will be passed via an artery to the uterus. Through this tube, tiny particles of plastic or gelatin sponge will be sent to the arteries supplying blood to the fibroids, thereby stopping the blood supply. Without a supply of blood, the fibroids shrink. In about 85 percent of cases, the surgery brings a good deal of symptom relief.

The procedure, which is not considered surgery, is usually followed by several hours of moderate to severe cramps. Nausea and fever are not uncommon. Some women develop an infection, which is treated with antibiotics. In about 1 percent of cases, the uterus is injured, and a hysterectomy may be needed. Allow yourself at least 1 to 2 weeks to recover.

Researchers studied women with symptomatic uterine fibroids. One group of 106 women had uterine fibroid embolization; a second group of 51 women had surgery, including 43 hysterectomies and eight myomectomies. Women who had embolization recovered faster. However, within a year after the procedure, because of continuing symptoms, 10 of the women who received the embolization required a second embolization or a hysterectomy. After the first year, another 11 women who had the embolization were hospitalized for recurrent symptoms.

Complementary Treatments

Complementary medicine treatments may be very effective in lessening or eliminating the symptoms generally related to uterine fibroids. Approaches that decrease pain and control excessive bleeding, as well as those that include dietary changes, have been found to be beneficial. Relief from the associated symptoms, such as constipation, incontinence, bloating, and backache, may also be addressed.

Effectiveness of Complementary Medicine for Uterine Fibroids

A study was conducted on the effectiveness of complementary medicine for the treatment of uterine fibroids. The study, which lasted 6 months, included 37 women who used complementary medicine and 37 women who used the standard treatments offered by conventional medicine. The treatments used in the complementary medicine group included traditional Chinese medicine (acupuncture, herbal therapy, and nutritional therapy), guided visual imagery, self-hypnosis, and deep-tissue massage. The results were as follows:

	Complementary	Conventional
Completely cured	3	0
Reduced fibroid size	11	1
Fibroids stopped growing	8	2
Rate of growth decreased	10	9
No change in growth	3	20
Rate of growth increased	2	4

Diet

Eating a well-balanced diet that includes lots of fresh fruits, vegetables, whole grains, seeds, and nuts may help reduce the chances of getting uterine fibroids or prevent them from growing. These foods contain antioxidant nutrients such as vitamins C and E, the B vitamins, and bioflavonoids, which are essential for the body to fight against the damaging free radicals that foster the growth of uterine fibroids. Try to include a minimum of five servings of vegetables, four servings of fruit, and six servings of whole grains each day.

Red meat and pork have been associated with an increased risk of uterine fibroids and should be eaten rarely or eliminated from the diet. On the other hand, soy products, which are a good source of protein, contain phytoestrogens known as isoflavones (genistein, daidzein, and glycitein). These act like antioxidants, helping to prevent the development of blood vessels that supply oxygen to the fibroids. Without this oxygen supply, the fibroids are reduced in size and, in some cases, eliminated completely. Isoflavones also act as weak estrogen, which blocks stronger estrogen from binding and stimulating fibroid growth. Soy, with its protective health benefits, is a major component in the traditional Asian diet, whose population is at the lowest risk for uterine fibroids. Soy is found in soybeans, soy milk, tofu, tempeh, and miso.

Because they decrease the excessive production of estrogen, flaxseeds may be beneficial. The seeds may be used whole or as a flour. Another option is flaxseed oil. Take 1 tablespoon daily; to reduce the oily residue, follow with the juice of a freshly squeezed lemon.

If you are losing a good deal of blood, which may cause anemia, you should increase your consumption of iron-containing foods. Green leafy vegetables, especially parsley and spinach, are rich in iron. Other sources are shellfish, brewer's yeast, dried fruits, and wheat bran.

Nutritional Supplements

Antioxidant nutrients mentioned in the Diet section may also be taken in supplement form.

- Vitamin A: 10,000 IU daily. Inhibits the development of fibroids.

- B-complex vitamins: Take as directed on the label. Builds red blood cells, improves circulation, and aids in tissue repair.

- Vitamin C: 2,000 milligrams daily in divided doses of 1,000 milligrams. Antioxidant and anti-inflammatory properties.

- Vitamin E: 400 IU daily. Regulates hormone production and may shrink existing fibroids.

- Iron: Check with your doctor. If you are losing significant amounts of blood each month, you may want to check to see if you need iron supplementation. However, if constipation is a symptom, you may want to avoid iron supplements and concentrate on iron-rich foods.

Traditional Chinese Medicine

The treatment of uterine fibroids using traditional Chinese medicine dates back thousands of years. The combination of acupuncture and Chinese herbs has been very useful in eliminating fibroids and decreasing their symptoms. Studies have shown that the combination of Chinese herbs known as KBG (keishi-buku-ryo-gan) is very effective in shrinking fibroids and reducing menstrual bleeding and pain. This herbal formula may help inhibit the production of estrogen and is considered a safe alternative for the treatment of uterine fibroids. To locate a practitioner trained in traditional Chinese medicine, visit the Web site of the National Certification Commission for Acupuncture and Oriental Medicine (NCCAOM) at www.nccaom.org or the American Association of Acupuncture and Oriental Medicine at www.aaaomonline.org.

Uterine Prolapse

With uterine prolapse, the uterus drops from its normal position at the top of the vagina in the pelvis. This condition is also known as pelvic relaxation, pelvic floor hernia, and prolapsed uterus. The uterus may drop to the lower part of the vagina or even outside the vagina. When the uterus has dropped only partway into the vagina, it is called an incomplete prolapse. When the uterus and cervix protrude out of the vagina and the vagina is inverted, it is a complete prolapse. A uterine prolapse may result in the extension of part of the bladder or rectum into the vagina.

Uterine prolapse is graded on a 4-point scale. A scale reading of 0 means that there is no prolapse and the uterus is well supported. A scale reading of 4 means that the degree of prolapse is severe, and the uterus is protruding from the vagina.

Uterine prolapse is believed to be somewhat common. The National Center for Health Statistics lists genital prolapse as one of the three most common reasons for hysterectomy.

Causes and Risk Factors

Most often, uterine prolapse is believed to be caused either by the loss of muscle tone and the relaxation of muscles that occurs with normal aging or by the reduction of the hormone estrogen that takes place during menopause. With declines in the level of estrogen comes a lowering in the amount of the protein collagen. Lowered amounts of collagen reduce the ability of the connective tissue in the pelvis to stretch.

However, other conditions have also been associated with the development of uterine prolapse, including obesity, chronic coughing, and straining. Generally, this is caused by a genetic tendency for weak muscles. Collagen defects, such as Marfan syndrome, are believed to be linked to uterine prolapse. And medical problems that affect the spinal cord, such as multiple sclerosis and muscular dystrophy, may result in a paralysis of pelvic muscles. In rare instances, uterine prolapse is caused by a pelvic tumor.

White and Hispanic women and those who have had one or more vaginal births are at increased risk for uterine prolapse. (On occasion, however, women who have never given birth may have this disorder.) The risk is also greater if you had a difficult birth that required the use of instruments, such as forceps, or if you delivered babies who were 9 pounds in size or larger. Further, those who have a "tipped uterus" are at increased risk. Uterine prolapse is most often seen in postmenopausal women.

Signs and Symptoms

With mild uterine prolapse, you may not have any noticeable symptoms. However, when the protrusion progresses, you may experience a number of uncomfortable symptoms, including lower backache, a sensation of heaviness or pulling in the pelvis, the feeling that you are sitting on an egg, lower abdominal discomfort, increased vaginal discharge, urinary tract infections, painful or frequent urination, stress incontinence, feeling of not completely emptying the bladder, constipation, painful bowel movements, protrusion from the vaginal opening, and painful intercourse. Symptoms tend to be exacerbated by prolonged standing and relieved when lying down. Sometimes, women with this disorder feel better in the morning and worse as the day progresses.

A Quick Guide to Symptoms

☐ Lower backache
☐ Sensation of heaviness or pulling in the pelvis
☐ Feeling that you are sitting on an egg
☐ Lower abdominal discomfort
☐ Increased vaginal discharge
☐ Urinary tract infections
☐ Painful or frequent urination
☐ Stress incontinence
☐ Feeling of not completely emptying the bladder
☐ Constipation
☐ Painful bowel movements
☐ Protrusion from the vaginal opening
☐ Painful intercourse

Conventional Treatments

Unless you are dealing with profoundly uncomfortable symptoms from a severe case of uterine prolapse, take time to try the more conservative, nonsurgical options. In many instances, improvement may be sufficient to avoid surgery.

Estrogen Replacement Therapy

If you are experiencing menopausal symptoms and are not already taking estrogen replacement therapy, you may be asked to begin a course of therapy. Estrogen replacement strengthens the muscles around the bladder and vagina.

Pelvic Floor Muscle (Kegel) Exercises

Kegel exercises, which reinforce the muscles of the pelvic floor that support the bladder and close the sphincter, were originally designed to assist women before and after childbirth. However, they have been found useful for uterine prolapse.

Begin by identifying your pelvic muscles—this may be done by slowing or stopping the urine flow while you are urinating. These are the muscles you need to make stronger. Try to perform 5 to 15 contractions, three to five times daily. Hold each Kegel for a count of 5 to start, and gradually work your way to a count of 10. However, don't do too many, as

women who overexercise these muscles may make them too tight. Once you learn to do Kegel exercises, try to avoid them when you are urinating. This practice has the tendency to weaken the muscles.

You will need to commit to Kegel exercises for your lifetime. If you discontinue, any benefits you have achieved will disappear. Also, it may take several months of Kegel exercises before you see any improvements.

Pessary

In some instances, your doctor may recommend a pessary, a plastic device that fits in the vagina. When properly inserted, a pessary returns the pelvic organs to the correct position. It my be combined with vaginal estrogen, which can help strengthen the muscles that support the bladder and vagina. Pessaries are effective in about 80 percent of women. However, a pessary may cause complications such as open sores in the vaginal wall and bleeding. If the pessary fits well, the chance for complications is reduced. Follow your doctor's instructions on how and when to clean and reinsert the pessary.

Surgery

Surgery is the only permanent solution for uterine prolapse. The goal of surgery is to repair each defect of pelvic support leading to uterine prolapse. Most patients with prolapse have defects in more than one location.

If you wish to keep your uterus intact, there are a few options that restore the uterus to its proper place. With a Manchester procedure, the cervix is removed through the vagina and the remaining ligaments are attached to the lower portion of the uterus. With respect to fertility and pelvic support, the long-term results of this procedure are generally satisfactory. However, in women who have had this procedure, delivery by cesarean section is mandatory.

For the majority of midlife women who have completed their biological families, a vaginal hysterectomy is a more realistic and preferred surgical option for uterine prolapse. During this procedure, which is considered major surgery, the uterus is removed via the vagina, and the vagina is resuspended. If there has also been prolapse of the bladder or rectum, then additional surgery of the front (anterior repair) and back (posterior repair) may be completed. In some instances, part of the procedure is completed with a laparoscope, a surgery known as a laparoscope-assisted vaginal hysterectomy (LAVH). When this occurs, a portion of the surgery is done through tiny incisions in the abdomen. Expect to remain in the hospital for at least 2 or 3 days and allow yourself 2 to 6 weeks to recuperate at home. Potential complications include bleeding and infection.

Complementary Treatments

Complementary medicine incorporates various techniques to help stimulate and strengthen uterine muscles.

Biofeedback

Biofeedback is useful in the treatment of mild uterine prolapse. While you do Kegel exercises, a small, pressure-sensitive balloon is placed in the vagina. The feedback helps to ensure that you are squeezing the correct muscles. This leads to strengthening the pelvic floor muscles.

Diet

To compensate for the body's low estrogen production, it may be helpful to eat certain foods that are high in plant phytoestrogens, such as soybeans, flaxseeds, lentils, beans, and whole grains. These foods also contain fiber that is useful in the prevention of constipation, which worsens this condition.

Herbal Medicine

Because of the lack of estrogen after menopause, the ligaments in the pelvic area tend to atrophy. Herbal medicine has been effective in helping to replace estrogen naturally.

Black cohosh. Black cohosh, which is a natural alternative to hormone replacement therapy, may be taken in capsule form. The minimum recommended daily dose is 20 milligrams in the morning and 20 milligrams at night of standardized extract of 2.5 percent triterpene glycosides. However, your doctor may recommend a higher dose.

Dong quai and Asian ginseng. Dong quai and Asian ginseng are herbs with estrogenic properties that may be helpful for those with low estrogen levels. Dong quai promotes relaxation and strengthens blood vessels. The recommended daily dose is 200 milligrams three times a day of extract standardized to 0.8 to 1.1 percent ligustilide. However, if you are taking a prescription blood-thinning medication, be sure to consult your doctor before taking dong quai supplements. The recommended daily dose of Asian ginseng is 100 to 200 milligrams, standardized to 4 to 7 percent ginsenosides. However, do not use ginseng if you have high blood pressure, heart disorders, or hypoglycemia.

Hydrotherapy

Alternating between 3 minutes sitting in hot water and 1 minute sitting in cold water has been effective in toning the pelvic muscles.

Preventive Measures

Avoid constipation. If you are frequently constipated, you are straining. People who strain are more likely to develop uterine prolapse.

Don't wear tight clothing. Try not to wear clothing that places excess pressure on your abdomen.

Maintain a healthy weight. Overweight women are at increased risk for uterine prolapse.

Stop smoking. Many people who smoke develop a chronic cough, which is associated with uterine prolapse.

Try to avoid heavy lifting. Lifting heavy objects is associated with uterine prolapse.

Vaginal Atrophy

Vaginal atrophy is the drying of vaginal tissue. The tissues in and near the vagina have less lubricant and produce fewer secretions. When the tissues become inflamed, dry, and rough, the disorder is called atrophic vaginitis or urogenital atrophy. The skin in the vagina as well as the urethra and bladder becomes thinner, more easily injured, and vulnerable to infection. In some women, vaginal atrophy is the first sign of menopause.

Until menopause, the ovaries produce estrogen, and one of the functions of this hormone is to keep the vaginal tissues adequately lubricated. However, after menopause, the ovaries cease production of estrogen. Without estrogen, bloodflow to the vagina decreases, and the vaginal tissues dry.

Among postmenopausal women, vaginal atrophy is believed to be quite common. Some have estimated that up to 40 percent of post-menopausal women have symptoms of this disorder.

Causes and Risk Factors

Going through menopause places women at risk for vaginal atrophy. Menopausal and postmenopausal women who are not on hormone replacement therapy (HRT) have a higher risk for vaginal atrophy than those who are on HRT.

Signs and Symptoms

A number of symptoms are associated with vaginal atrophy. These include vaginal itching and/or burning of the vulva (area around the vaginal opening), problems with urination (frequency, urgency, pain, loss of urine), bleeding or spotting, and pain or bleeding with intercourse.

A Quick Guide to Symptoms

- ☐ Vaginal itching and/or burning of the vulva
- ☐ Problems with urination (frequency, urgency, pain, loss of urine)
- ☐ Bleeding or spotting
- ☐ Pain or bleeding with intercourse

Conventional Treatments
Hormone Replacement

You may be advised to go on hormone replacement therapy. This may be in the form of estrogen alone or estrogen and progesterone. HRT is available in a variety of forms, such as tablets, capsules, creams, rings, and skin patches. As long as you remain on HRT, your symptoms should improve. If you discontinue the medication, your symptoms will most likely return.

Kegel Exercises

You may wish to try pelvic floor muscle (Kegel) exercises. Start by identifying your pelvic muscles—this may be done by slowing or stopping the urine flow while you are urinating. These are the muscles you need to make stronger. Try to perform 5 to 15 contractions, three to five times daily. Hold each Kegel for a count of 5 to start, and gradually work your way to a count of 10. But don't do too many, as women who overexercise these muscles may make them too tight. Once you learn to do Kegel exercises, try to avoid them when you are urinating. This practice has the tendency to weaken the muscles.

You will need to commit to Kegel exercises for your lifetime. If you discontinue, any benefits you have achieved will disappear. Also, it may take several months of Kegel exercises before you see any improvements.

Complementary Treatments

To help relieve the pain associated with vaginal atrophy, practitioners of complementary medicine attempt to assist the woman's body to regulate itself naturally through dietary and lifestyle changes, nutritional and herbal supplementation, and therapies such as acupuncture. The primary focus is to reduce the

Potential Risks of HRT

HRT is not without risks. It has been linked to a number of medical problems such as cancer of the uterus, endometrial cancer, gallbladder disease, and abnormal blood clotting. Further, it has been associated with many potential side effects, such as abnormal bleeding from the vagina, dizziness, increased blood pressure, anxiety, and bloating. Share your complete medical history with your doctor. Working together, you can determine if you are a good candidate for HRT.

More likely, your doctor may prescribe estrogen in the form of vaginal creams (Premarin or Estrace), a vaginal pill (Vagifem), or vaginal rings (Estring). Improvement or relief of vaginal symptoms has been reported by 80 to 100 percent of women who use these preparations. Since they have little impact on the estrogen levels in the bloodstream, women who use these products properly do not need to take progesterone. You should notice improvement in 2 to 4 weeks.

dosage of HRT and potentially eliminate it altogether.

Diet

To compensate for the body's low estrogen production, it may be useful to eat certain foods that are high in phytoestrogens, such as soybeans (tofu and soy milk are the best sources), flaxseeds (the oil is also available in liquid form), cashews, peanuts, almonds, lentils, beans, and whole grains. In addition, maintaining a low-fat, high-fiber diet that includes lots of fresh vegetables, fruits, and grains helps the body to adjust to hormonal changes. Try to include a minimum of five servings of vegetables, four servings of fruit, and six servings of whole grains each day.

Herbal Medicine

Herbal medicine may be useful in naturally replacing estrogen, which helps to relieve vaginal atrophy. A number of herbs have been shown to be effective for the symptoms associated with menopause. These include burdock root, licorice root, raspberry leaf, black cohosh, and dong quai. In order to assure proper dosing of herbs specific to your body and symptoms, seek the assistance of an herbal medicine practitioner or a naturopath.

Black cohosh and dong quai. Black cohosh and dong quai have long been used for vaginal atrophy. Black cohosh is a phytoestrogen (plant-based estrogen) and a natural alternative to hormone replacement therapy. Dong quai is a precursor to estrogen.

Nutritional Supplements

Certain nutritional supplements may help reduce the symptoms of vaginal atrophy.

- Multivitamin/mineral: Take as directed on the label. Although a multivitamin may not specifically reduce vaginal atrophy, maintaining a healthy level of nutrients helps to retain overall body strength.

- Vitamin A: 10,000 IU daily. Strengthens mucous membranes and reduces vaginal dryness and atrophy. Take with vitamin E.

- Vitamin E: 400 IU daily. Assists the body in maintaining synthetic or natural estrogen.

- Omega-3 fatty acids: 1 tablespoon flaxseed oil or a 2,000-milligram fish oil capsule twice a day. Reduces vaginal dryness.

Traditional Chinese Medicine

By increasing the elasticity of tissue and strengthening the overall health of the female body, traditional Chinese medicine has successfully treated vaginal atrophy through dietary changes, acupuncture, herbal remedies, qigong, and tai chi. Traditional Chinese medicine is particularly useful in treating symptoms such as urinary problems, vaginal dryness, and itching.

Lifestyle Recommendations

Avoid chemical irritants. Avoid douches, bubble bath, and vaginal sprays, as these will only aggravate your condition.

Don't use tampons. If you have bleeding or spotting, use unscented sanitary pads.

Don't wear underwear at night. By not wearing underwear at night, you allow your vaginal area to have more contact with the air, which will help it heal.

Drink plenty of water or herbal tea. This is very important for preventing vaginal dryness. Try to drink at least 2 quarts each day.

Use a lubricant. If you have pain during sexual intercourse, try using a vaginal lubricant such as Astroglide. However, don't use petroleum jelly.

Use a vaginal moisturizer. Vaginal moisturizers are nonhormonal products that you insert into the vagina on a regular basis. (Replens is an example.)

Wear cotton underwear. Cotton underwear enables air to better circulate.

Wipe front to back. After a bowel movement, wipe from front to back—you will be less likely to have feces touch the irritated areas.

Preventive Measures

Don't smoke. Smokers are at greater risk for developing vaginal atrophy. Smoking deprives the body of oxygen, which contributes to weakening of the vaginal muscles. Smokers also have earlier menopause than nonsmokers.

Remain sexually active. Regular sexual activity with or without a partner improves blood circulation in the vagina, thus decreasing the risk for vaginal atrophy. To have greater protection from sexually transmitted diseases, women who are not in monogamous relationships should insist on condoms.

Varicose Veins

Varicose veins are enlarged blood vessels close to the surface of the skin. While many veins have the potential to become varicose, varicose veins are more likely to be found in the thighs, legs, and feet. When they appear in and around the anus, they are called hemorrhoids.

Varicose veins occur when the valves in the veins (which return blood to the heart) lose elasticity and malfunction. As a result, blood flows backward and the veins enlarge. Because they contain de-oxygenated blood, the veins may appear dark purple or blue. In addition, the veins may be twisted or bulging. On occasion, they may rupture or form open sores (ulcers). When left untreated, varicose veins are almost certain to worsen.

In the United States, varicose veins are considered quite common. About 6 to 7 million people have some evidence of varicose veins. In a Scottish study of 1,566 adults between the ages of 18 and 65, varicose veins were present in 40 percent of the men and 32 percent of the women. The first signs of venous problems—very small dilated veins—were found in 80 percent of the men and 85 percent of the women. These venous problems frequently lead to varicose veins.

While most cases of varicose veins are uncomfortable, they are not serious. However, in some instances, there is reason for significant concern. If the area around the varicose veins does not receive adequate nourishment, sores or skin ulcers may develop. Further, if there is severe clogging of the blood in the vein and blood is prevented from returning to the heart, you may have a condition called venous insufficiency. This may cause a bleeding infection or deep vein thrombosis (blood clot). Since blood clots may travel from the veins to the lungs and heart, where they may be deadly, this is a serious situation.

Causes and Risk Factors

Most cases of varicose veins first appear between the ages of 30 and 70. In women, they may be associated with hormonal changes that take place during pregnancy and menopause.

Being overweight adds to the risk, as does standing for prolonged periods of time. Hemorrhoids are associated with constipation. And genetics plays a very strong role. It is the main contributing factor to this disorder. If members of your family have varicose veins, there is a good chance that you will too.

Signs and Symptoms

Several symptoms are associated with varicose veins, including an aching, "heavy" feeling in the legs, muscle cramping, swelling, throbbing, and burning in the lower legs.

These symptoms may be present even before the enlarged varicose veins actually appear under the skin. Other symptoms include a brownish-gray discoloration of your ankles and skin ulcers near the ankles, as well as restless legs.

Conventional Treatments

A number of conventional treatments may offer you some relief, including special stockings and several surgical procedures. Your doctor will probably recommend that you wear compression stockings throughout the day. By squeezing your legs, they help move blood along. Also, a simple elevation of the legs above heart level for 30 minutes, three times a day, may be helpful. If these fail to achieve the desired result, your doctor may suggest other treatments.

Surgery

Ambulatory phlebectomy. In this procedure, used for treating smaller veins, a vein is removed through a series of tiny skin punctures. During this outpatient procedure, local anesthesia will be used. The most common side effect is slight bruising.

Catheter-assisted procedure. In this procedure, a small tube (catheter) is inserted into an enlarged vein. After the tip of the catheter is heated, it is removed, and the heated vein is destroyed. Radio waves may also be used to destroy the vein (radiofrequency ablation). There may be some slight bruising.

Electrodesiccation. With electrodesicca-

A Quick Guide to Symptoms

☐ Aching, "heavy" feeling in the legs
☐ Muscle cramping, swelling, throbbing, and burning in the lower legs
☐ Enlarged veins under the skin
☐ Brownish-gray discoloration of the ankles
☐ Skin ulcers near the ankles
☐ Restless legs

tion, veins are treated with electrical current. Scarring is common.

Endoscopic vein surgery. This procedure is reserved for more serious forms of varicose veins, particularly those cases in which there may be leg ulcers. During the procedure, a thin video camera is inserted in your leg and the surgery is performed after small incisions are made.

Laser surgery. Smaller varicose veins may respond to laser surgery, in which strong bursts of light are sent into the vein. When the laser hits the skin, there is a small pinch, and the vein gradually fades and disappears. There are no incisions and no needles. Treatments last for 15 to 20 minutes, and you may

You should be aware that while treatments may correct your varicose veins, it is likely that you will develop new ones in the future. Once you have varicose veins, you are a good candidate for more.

require two to five treatments. Potential side effects include redness or swelling that resolves in a few days. Any discoloration should fade in a few weeks.

Sclerotherapy. With sclerotherapy, your doctor injects small- or medium-size varicose veins with a solution that closes the vein. Blood is thus forced to travel through other, healthier veins. While evidence of the varicose veins should fade in a few weeks, sometimes veins may need to be injected more than once. No anesthesia is required, and your doctor will perform the procedure in his or her office.

Potential side effects at the site of the injection include stinging; red, raised patches of skin; cramping; bruises; and small skin ulcers. It is not uncommon for spots, fine red vessels, and brown lines to appear around the treated vein. On occasion, the vein may become inflamed or develop lumps of coagulated or congested blood. Though they are not dangerous, if you experience this last group of side effects, contact your doctor.

Vein stripping. With vein stripping, a long vein is removed through a number of small incisions. Though vein stripping is usually an outpatient procedure, allow yourself at least 2 weeks to recover. Other veins will assume the work of the removed vein.

Potential side effects of the surgery include bleeding, blood congestion, infection, inflammation, swelling, redness, nerve tissue damage around the vein, and permanent scarring. In rare cases, the surgery creates a deep vein blood clot that travels to the lungs and heart. To reduce the chances that a clot will be created, your doctor may order injections of heparin before surgery. Heparin reduces blood coagulation, but increases the risk of bleeding and bruising after the surgery.

Complementary Treatments

For the prevention and treatment of varicose veins, complementary medicine offers many options. In addition to specific treatments, a combination of lifestyle and dietary changes as well as herbal medicine can usually help relieve symptoms and prevent further progression of the condition.

Acupuncture

Acupuncture has been found effective in relieving pain and in stopping the progression of varicose veins. Treatments focus on moving the stagnant blood. However, it should be noted that acupuncture does not alter the appearance of varicose veins.

Aromatherapy

The essential oils of cypress, geranium, and rosemary all help to improve circulation in areas affected with varicose veins. To create a healing massage oil, they may be combined with soy or sunflower oil. Add 3 drops of each essential oil to 1 ounce of carrier oil. Or the essential oils may be used in a warm bath, where they will be absorbed though the skin. Add 3 drops of each oil to the tub and soak for 20 minutes.

Chiropractic

To improve bloodflow throughout the body, chiropractors focus on adjustments to the skeletal system. In order to promote bloodflow to the lower limbs, the proper alignment of the pelvic area is of significant importance. As part of their overall plan, chiropractors may also incorporate diet and lifestyle changes.

Diet

In order to prevent and reduce the effects of varicose veins, it is important that the body be properly nourished. Bioflavonoids, which have been shown to aid blood circulation, are found in many fruits and vegetables. More specifically, studies have shown that rutin, a bioflavonoid found in citrus fruits, apricots, blueberries, cherries, and blackberries, is particularly important for vein health. In fact, for strengthening the walls of the veins, drinking a fresh juice of cherries, blackberries, blueberries, and other dark berries may be even more effective than eating them. Quercetin, a flavonoid found in apples, onions, and black tea, reduces inflammation.

Many fruits and vegetables also contain vitamin C. A deficiency in vitamin C may make small capillaries fragile and more prone to breaking. B-complex vitamins, found in brewer's yeast, help to keep blood vessels strong. Brewer's yeast may be added to cereal or to a fresh juice drink.

Fiber is another crucial component for vein health. Be sure to add lots of whole grains to your fruit and vegetable regimen.

Further, fiber reduces constipation, which may exacerbate existing varicose veins. Found in pineapples, the enzyme bromelain may reduce swelling and soreness and help prevent blood clots in people who have varicose veins.

Though not commonly mentioned, liver deficiency may contribute to varicose veins by placing pressure on the vascular system. So, you should eat foods that support the liver, including dark green, leafy vegetables; carrots; onions; beets; and artichoke hearts. Try to avoid foods that are high in sugar and reduce your intake of foods with white flour and animal fats. Since they prevent healthy circulation and do not nourish the body, eliminate processed foods and foods high in saturated fat and trans fatty acids.

Herbal Medicine

Butcher's broom. Butcher's broom tones the veins and reduces inflammation. It is available as a capsule, tea, tincture, or ointment. The recommended daily dose is 150 milligrams three times a day of extract standardized to 9 to 11 percent ruscogenins.

Ginkgo biloba. Ginkgo supports blood vessels and increases the flow of blood to the lower limbs. Ginkgo is rich in quercetin, a powerful flavonoid. The typical recommended daily dose is 40 milligrams of extract standardized to 24 percent of flavone glycosides and 6 percent terpene lactones three times per day.

Gotu kola. Gotu kola (centella) improves circulation to the limbs, provides nutritional support, and strengthens blood vessels. Recommended doses vary widely, but it may be best to start with a low dose, such as 30 milligrams twice daily of extract standardized to 10 percent asiaticosides. Then, you may slowly increase the amount. Gotu kola is also available as a tea and tincture. People who suffer from liver disease should not take gotu kola.

Grape seed or pine bark extract. Both of these extracts stimulate circulation and support vein health. Take 80 milligrams daily, in divided doses of 40 milligrams each.

Horse chestnut. Horse chestnut, which contains aescin, a compound known to increase vein wall strength and promote circulation, has been found to be useful in reducing pain and swelling associated with varicose veins. The recommended daily dose for the treatment of varicose veins is 300 milligrams, two times a day, of extract standardized to 16 to 21 percent aescin content. The dosage can be reduced to a maintenance dose of 50 milligrams per day once beneficial results are noticeable. It is also available in a tincture and as a topical cream. Since the leaves and nuts of horse chestnut are toxic, be sure to avoid those. People who suffer from liver or kidney problems should not use horse chestnut.

Witch hazel. Witch hazel, which is used primarily for hemorrhoids, may be applied externally to the affected areas three or more times per day.

Homeopathy

Homeopathic remedies are available for specific varicose vein symptoms, such as weak, restless, heavy legs and red, swollen, tender varicose veins. Remedies are specific to each individual. Though these remedies are available over-the-counter in pellet or ointment form, it may be useful to seek a homeopathic practitioner or naturopath who has experience selecting the correct remedy and proper dose. To find a practitioner trained in homeopathy, visit the Web site of the National Center for Homeopathy at www.homeopathic.org.

Hydrotherapy

Alternating between hot and cold baths may stimulate circulation in the legs and slow the progression of varicose veins. Use two wastebaskets or buckets that are sufficiently large to submerge your legs up to the knees. Fill one with warmer water and the other with colder water. Soak your legs in the warm water for 3 to 4 minutes and then immediately soak them in the cold water for 30 seconds. Every day, repeat this procedure three times.

Nutritional Supplements

Certain nutritional supplements support vein health and improve circulation.

- Vitamin C: 2,000 milligrams daily in divided doses of 1,000 milligrams. Improves circulation and strengthens vein walls. Deficiency can lead to varicose veins.

- Vitamin E: 400 IU daily. Improves circulation, reduces the risk of having varicose veins.

- Quercetin: 400 milligrams daily in divided doses of 200 milligrams. Powerful bioflavonoid routinely prescribed in the treatment of this disorder.

Therapeutic Massage

Because they reduce swelling in the veins and may alleviate pain, daily leg massages may be beneficial. Sit up with your legs raised on a pillow and begin massaging the ankle area. Work your way up toward the thigh. Don't massage directly over the varicose veins. Do this daily on each leg for 3 to 5 minutes. You may wish to use an essential oil mixture as discussed in the Aromatherapy section on page 526.

Yoga

Because the stretches promote circulation and the deep breathing helps bring oxygen into the bloodstream, yoga is very beneficial for people who have varicose veins.

Lifestyle Recommendations

Avoid tight garments. Pantyhose and other garments that are tight around the groin may keep blood pooled in the legs.

Beware of bogus treatments. Many ads offer quick-fix solutions for varicose veins. Treat them with an enormous amount of caution.

Drink lots of water. Drinking at least eight 8-ounce glasses of water each day may help rid the body of unwanted toxins, relieve constipation, and maintain skin elasticity.

Elevate your legs. Try sleeping on your back with a small pillow under your legs. Elevating the legs to just above heart level helps the pooled blood drain. If you can, during the day, elevate your legs for 10 minutes every 3 hours.

Preventive Measures

Change positions. Try not to stand or sit for extended periods of time. If you are sitting, stand up every 30 minutes or so. If you are standing, periodically shift your weight from one leg to the other.

Consider making lifestyle changes. Many poor lifestyle habits contribute to the development of varicose veins and may aggravate existing ones. Smoking, consuming large amounts of processed foods and saturated fats, and consuming excess alcohol and coffee may all contribute to free radical damage and the weakening of vein walls. They may also cause elevated blood pressure and an increase in circulation problems.

Don't cross your legs. When you are sitting, avoid crossing your legs. Crossing your legs impairs the flow of blood. If this is a habit that is difficult to stop, try crossing your legs at the ankles and not the knees.

Eat high-fiber foods. Including high-fiber foods in your diet lowers the risk for constipation, which is associated with varicose veins.

Exercise. Regular exercise will improve circulation as well as leg and vein strength. It will also tone the muscles and help you to maintain a healthy weight. A daily walk may keep blood from settling in your legs. Swimming is another gentle way to improve circulation. However, varicose veins may be exacerbated by high-impact aerobic activity.

Watch your weight. If you are overweight, you are placing more pressure on your legs.

Wrinkles

Lines that radiate from the corners of the eyes are known as crow's feet, while the lines between the eyebrows are called frown lines. But skin may lose its elasticity on any part of the face, thereby resulting in wrinkles. Gravity only further aggravates the situation, contributing to jowls and drooping eyelids.

As we age, we are quite likely to develop facial wrinkles. Just about every midlife person has at least a few wrinkles, and some people have many.

Causes and Risk Factors

A wide variety of factors contribute to wrinkles. Probably the four most significant are excessive exposure to sun, smoking, the aging process, and genetics. But other elements may play a role, including the overuse of astringents, dry skin, excessive scrubbing of the skin, and air pollution.

Signs and Symptoms

Wrinkles are the lines on the face. You are easily able to see them when you look in the mirror.

Conventional Treatments

The appropriate conventional treatment varies from person to person, according to the individual's specific needs, level of sun damage, the amount he or she is willing to spend, and age. In many instances, it is wise to begin with the mildest treatments. Frequently, it is best to consult with your doctor.

Botulinum (Botox)

Botulinum is a deadly toxin that may be found in spoiled, uncooked foods. But in its purified form, called Botox, it is also a muscle relaxant and may be injected into wrinkles to relax the surrounding muscles. Botox has been found useful for treating wrinkles in lower eyelids, lines on the side of the nose, frown lines on the forehead, crow's feet, expression lines, and the area between the upper lip and nose. Unfortunately, the benefits of Botox last only a few months. So, if you decide you like how Botox has improved your appearance, you will need to have shots several times each year. Botox injections do decrease your ability to frown and squint, and they have caused the sides of the mouth to turn down. You may also have temporary muscle weakness near the site of the injection.

Chemical Peels

In a chemical peel, the top layers of skin are stripped away and new, younger skin appears in its place. While especially useful for the upper lip and chin and sun-induced skin damage, it may not be used for the eye area. During the procedure, a dermatologist applies chemicals to the skin. These may include trichloroacetic acid or high concentrations of alpha-hydroxy or beta-hydroxy acids. Sometimes, a combination of acids is used. To improve the results, the dermatologist may recommend that you begin using tretinoin or alpha-hydroxy acid 4 to 6 weeks before the peel. Then, you should start using it again the day after the peel.

Within 24 hours of the peel, expect a crust or scab to form on the skin. It may be removed with gentle cleansing. Though your skin will look a deep red, as the days pass, it will lighten. Your skin will need about a week to heal.

Even with a skilled dermatologist, there is the possibility of complications, such as scarring, numbness, infection, whiteheads, cold sores, and permanent discoloration of the skin, especially in those with darker skin.

Dermabrasion

Dermabrasion removes deeper layers of skin than a chemical peel, so it may remove deeper wrinkles and scarring. It is most useful for wrinkles on the upper lip and chin and may not be used for those around the eyes. In a typical dermabrasion, a dermatologist will use a rotating brush to remove the top layers of skin, thereby exposing the lower layers of skin. As with a chemical peel, the skin will ooze and form a scab. The postoperative care and complications are the same as for the chemical peel.

There is a milder form of dermabrasion known as microdermabrasion in which the skin is polished with tiny crystals. The skin does not become nearly as red afterward. For best results, microdermabrasion should be repeated every week or two for a total of five or six times.

Home Exfoliation and Alpha-Hydroxy Acid

Exfoliation or removal of the top layer of skin is a good method for removing small wrinkles. This may be accomplished in a variety of ways. Probably the easiest method is to wash your face with a mildly abrasive material, such as cleansing grains with microbeads, and a soap that contains salicylic acid. Wash using a motion that is perpendicular to the wrinkles. Stay away from loofahs and sea sponges, which often foster the growth of bacteria. Do not use scrubs. They may have crushed walnut or apricot seeds, which can cause tiny cuts in the skin.

Alpha-hydroxy acid products trigger the removal of dead skin cells, and they may facilitate the production of collagen and elastin. After months of daily applications, you should note a subtle improvement of wrinkling. Alpha-hydroxy acid is found naturally in the following products.

- Lactic acid: in milk
- Citric acid: in oranges and lemons
- Tartaric acids: in grapes
- Malic acid: in apples and pears
- Glycolic acid: in sugarcane

Lactic and glycolic acids are frequently found in commercial preparations. Some contend that products with lactic acid are a little more effective than those with glycolic acid. And there are preparations such as poly-alpha-hydroxy acid and beta-hydroxy acid. Over-the-counter alpha-hydroxy acid products have acid concentrations between 2 and 10 percent. Prescription creams have at least 12 percent glycolic acid. Even stronger concentrations of glycolic acid (between 30 and 70 percent) may be administered by a physician in a procedure known as a glycolic peel.

While low concentrations of alpha-hydroxy acid are generally safe, some people experience side effects, especially when using the higher concentrations. These potential side effects include burning, pain, itching, and the potential for scarring. If you have any of these side effects, you should stop using the product. Alpha-hydroxy acid also seems to increase the risk of damage from the sun, so you should be extra vigilant with your sunscreen.

Implants

A number of different implant substances may be injected into wrinkles. In microlipoinjection, fat tissue is taken from an individual's own thighs, buttocks, knees, or abdomen and injected into wrinkles around the nose and mouth and folds in the forehead. It has also been used for wrinkles in the hands. Since the body will reabsorb the fat, the wrinkle will probably eventually reappear. However, there is some evidence that a good amount of the fat remains for at least a year.

In collagen implants, bovine (cow) collagen is injected into wrinkles around the eyes and mouth. A repeat treatment is usually needed within 4 to 12 months. People with autoimmune diseases are advised against this procedure.

During a surgical procedure, Gore-Tex, a highly porous and inert synthetic material, may be inserted under the skin to fill out a wrinkle. While Gore-Tex does not degrade, there may be a small scar and, though rare, allergic reactions are possible. Artecoll, another highly porous and inert synthetic material that is enclosed in tiny droplets of natural collagen, may be injected into deep wrinkles. It does not degrade as quickly as collagen, but repeat treatments may be required and there is at least the potential for an allergic reaction.

Laser Resurfacing

This is the most effective method for treating wrinkles. During laser resurfacing, which involves laser pulses penetrating the skin, the skin is actually tightened. It is most useful for the areas around the mouth and eyes.

Though the actual procedure is relatively painless, the recovery period may be quite difficult. For at least a week, you will be quite uncomfortable. The skin will become very red and irritated, and your face will be swollen and require constant moisturizing. It is not uncommon for the skin to be sensitive and red for several months. During this time, you will need to stay out of the sun. In about 1 percent of cases, individuals will experience scarring and/or infections. Those with a history of herpes simplex may have a flare-up, including flu symptoms and facial pain for 5 or 6 days. Since it may cause a dramatic lightening of the skin, it is often not advised for people with darker skin.

Surgery

Blepharoplasty (eye lift). This procedure involves the removal of excess skin, muscle, and fat from the upper and lower eyelids. Normally, results will last for between 5 and 10 years. Increasingly, this surgery is being done with lasers rather than scalpels. A related procedure, transconjunctival upper blepharoplasty, removes fat from the membrane lining the eyelids.

Rhytidectomy (face-lift). If you are seriously bothered by wrinkles, you may decide to have a rhytidectomy or face-lift. Relatively simple face-lifts generally take about 2 hours and are often done under local anesthesia in a physician's office. More complicated procedures are usually scheduled in the hospital under general anesthesia and may take up to 6 hours.

There are two main types of face-lifts. In a superficial musculoaponeurotic system (SMAS), the most common type, a surgeon makes an incision at the hairline and separates the skin from underlying tissue and muscle. Excess fat and tissue are removed, and the muscles are tightened. In the less common endoscopic subperiosteal or subgaleal face-lift, the surgeon raises facial structures instead of cutting flaps of skin. As a result, there is minimal scarring.

Neither type of face-lift is useful for the wrinkles in the middle of the face. And recovery times vary considerably, from weeks to months. Expect swelling and discoloration. Some people have temporary tingling or numbing sensations. A small percentage of individuals develop postsurgical hematomas or collections of blood that need to be drained. Less common complications are infection, asymmetrical facial muscles, scarring, delayed healing, excessive bleeding, and permanent injury to the nerves that control movement in the face.

Topical Products

Topical products that contain a natural form of vitamin A (retinol) or vitamin A derivatives known as retinoic acids (tretinoin) are effective in reducing wrinkles. Skin preparations containing retinol are available over-the-counter. However, the actual amount of retinol that they contain may vary widely. Tretinoin, which is better known as Retin-A, is available by prescription only. You should apply it at least twice each week at night. Within 2 to 6 months, you should notice a reduction in some large wrinkles. Since Retin-A will make the skin quite sensitive to the sun, you need to be extra vigilant about using sunscreen and avoiding the sun as much as possible. Frequent side effects include itching, burning, scaling, and redness.

Complementary Treatments

Complementary medicine works toward strengthening the body through proper nutrition, exercise, and a change in lifestyle in order to help protect the skin from further damage.

Acupuncture

Acupuncture has been shown to be very effective in treating wrinkles. It is a well-known and highly used treatment. Needles are placed at specific points on the face to increase circulation, tone the facial muscles, and rebalance the body's natural energy, improving the health and appearance of facial skin.

Aromatherapy

Frankincense, palmarosa, and rose are three essential oils that restore moisture to dry skin, smooth out lines and wrinkles, and stimulate new cell growth. Use them as facial moisturizers or masks. Find a natural, unscented facial moisturizer and add 10 drops of each oil for every 3 ounces of moisturizer. Blend together and use daily, morning and night. For a facial mask, mix 1 tablespoon of cold-pressed olive oil, 2 teaspoons of honey, and 1 drop of each oil, or 3 drops if you use just one oil. Spread the mixture over your face, but be careful of the eye area. Let it sit for 20 minutes, and then rinse. You may repeat this twice a week.

Diet

To help prevent and manage wrinkles, your diet should be rich in the antioxidant nutrients, such as vitamins A, C, and E, the B vitamins, and zinc. Vitamin A stimulates bloodflow and encourages new cell formation. Vitamin C helps the sebaceous glands lubricate the skin and is a nutrient necessary for collagen production, as is zinc. Vitamin E has been shown to slow the aging process and prevent premature wrinkles.

The B vitamins are essential for healthy skin. By eating lots of whole grains, fruits, and vegetables, you consume a good amount of these nutrients. In addition, the B vitamins are found in dark green, leafy vegetables; whole grains; oranges; avocados; beets; bananas; potatoes; dairy products; nuts; beans; fish; and chicken. Brewer's yeast is another good way to get B vitamins into your system. Stir 1 tablespoon of brewer's yeast in a glass of juice or water, two times a day, for improved skin texture and a healthy glow.

Vitamin E may be found in vegetable oils, nuts, seeds, and wheat germ. Small amounts are also found in leafy vegetables and whole grains. High amounts of zinc are found in oysters (canned, raw, or smoked). Smaller amounts are found in whole grains, eggs, sunflower seeds, peanuts, walnuts, cashews, and meats such as ground beef, chicken, and turkey. Zinc works with vitamin A. Low levels of zinc may appear as a vitamin A deficiency. Symptoms include dry skin and premature wrinkling.

Protein is one more factor that is key to maintaining healthy skin. The following protein foods contain collagen, which is beneficial in preventing and smoothing out wrinkles: whole-grain cereals, sunflower seeds, nuts, sesame seeds, dried legumes, and avocados. The protein found in fish, meats, dairy products, and poultry helps your body balance between new and dying skin cells.

Selenium, which is available in whole grains, tomatoes, red meat, chicken, broccoli, asparagus, egg yolks, milk, and onions, supports your skin's elasticity. Iodine, iron, and potassium are useful for promoting healthy skin. Good sources of iodine are iodized salt, kelp, onions, vegetable oils, and seafood. Iron is found in lean red meat; dark green, leafy vegetables; blackstrap molasses; whole wheat; and dried fruits and legumes. Potassium is found in dried apricots, bananas, peanuts, lean meats, potatoes, and fresh vegetables.

It should be apparent that many of these nutrients are in the same foods. By eating them, you are well on your way to reducing wrinkles and having healthier skin. Whenever possible, avoid fried, processed foods, foods containing trans fatty acids, and products made with refined white flour and sugar.

Herbal Medicine

With its antioxidant properties, green tea has been shown to be very beneficial to holding back the aging process. It is available without caffeine. Drink 3 cups per day, allowing the tea bag or loose leaves to steep for 2 to 3 minutes.

Nutritional Supplements

The following nutrients are necessary to slow wrinkle formation and soften those that have already appeared.

- Vitamin A: 10,000 IU daily. Antioxidant that protects skin tissue, encourages new cell formation, and helps prevent aging of the skin.

- B-complex vitamins: Take as directed on the label. Prevent aging of the skin.

- Vitamin C: 1,000 milligrams daily in divided doses of 500 milligrams. Regulates the sebaceous glands (which secrete lubricating substances) and increases circulation to the skin. Necessary for collagen production.

- Vitamin E: 400 milligrams daily. Antioxidant that protects against free radical damage to the skin and prevents premature wrinkles.

- Essential fatty acids—omega-3 (flaxseed and fish oils) and omega-6 (borage, evening primrose, and black currant seed oils): Available in oil and capsule form. Take as directed on the labels. Help maintain healthy skin.

- Selenium: 200 micrograms daily. Helps maintain healthy skin and protect against ultraviolet damage. Take with vitamin E.

- Zinc: 30 milligrams daily. Necessary for collagen production and tissue repair.

Therapeutic Massage

Facial massage is easy to do and should be practiced in the morning when applying moisturizer or after shaving and each night after washing your face. This aids in the removal of damaging waste products that build up on the skin and increases circulation with fresh blood that nourishes the skin.

Begin at the center of the chin. Make small circular motions around the outside of the face all the way up to the top of the forehead. Do this three times. Then apply gentle pressure in an upsweeping motion along the same area, and lightly brush down the sides of your face with your fingertips. Next, using your index and middle fingers, start under your nose and glide along the base of your cheekbones outward toward the ears. Repeat along the cheekbones.

Using your fingers, press on each side of the nose between the eyes. Apply comfortable pressure and sweep down and along the top of the cheekbones under the eyes. Sweep all the way out to the temples, ending at the temples with slow, circular motions. Repeat this five times.

When you are done, bring your fingers back to the top of your nose between your eyebrows. Apply comfortable pressure and hold for 6 seconds. Trace up and along the top of the eyebrows out to the temples, again ending in slow, circular motions. Repeat five times.

Return to the top of your nose between the eyebrows and, using the fingertips, sweep up the forehead toward the hairline. Do this until the entire forehead area has been massaged. End by sweeping up the front and sides of the neck to the chin and along the jaw. Tap the skin underneath the chin gently with the back of your hand. To stimulate the skin cells, gently tap your entire face with your fingertips, including around your mouth, nose, and under and above your eyes.

Lifestyle Recommendations

Exercise. Daily exercise will aid circulation, including circulation in your face and skin, which may reduce wrinkles. Exercise also stimulates the formation of new skin cells in the base layer of the skin. If you frequently exercise outdoors, remember to protect yourself from the sun, or the damaging rays will counteract all the hard work of stimulating new cell growth.

Preventive Measures

Preventive measures should begin as early as possible. There are a number of ways to reduce the number of wrinkles on your face and their degree of severity.

Avoid gaining and losing weight. The process of gaining and losing weight stretches the skin, resulting in a loss of elasticity. Becoming too thin may cause wrinkles to become more apparent, as the face loses some of its plumpness. Try to reach a target weight range and maintain that through healthy eating and regular exercise, including strength training.

Drink lots of water. Drinking eight glasses of water a day supports healthy skin by removing toxins and keeping you hydrated.

Give your eyes a rest. To soothe puffy eyes,

place two slices of fresh cucumber that have been in the freezer for 3 minutes on each eye and cover with a cold washcloth. Cucumbers, used as a cold compress, have been shown to be useful in treating the eye area. It is also a good way to relax for 10 to 15 minutes.

Keep the air moist. In the colder months, heating systems, particularly forced hot air, and hotter showers may cause skin to become much drier and accentuate wrinkles. Humidifiers in the home, at least in the bedroom at night, may help. Keeping the door open during a hot shower allows the steam to escape and lets moisture into other areas of the house. Houseplants may also put moisture back into the air.

Practice daily preventive care. Wash your face daily with a mild moisturizing soap. Stay away from alkaline soaps, which are drying. After patting your skin dry, apply a moisturizer and a sunscreen.

Reduce alcohol consumption. Regular alcohol consumption may cause your face to become puffy, stretching your skin and creating new wrinkles.

Reduce stress. People who have excess amounts of stress in their lives often find that they go about their day holding their face in a constant frown or strained position, where the forehead is filled with lines. Reducing stress and clearing the mind may allow the muscles of the face to relax and circulation to the skin to flow more freely.

Reduce your sun exposure. The sun will shrivel your skin. A plum becomes a prune, a grape becomes a raisin, and smooth skin becomes wrinkled, all due to sun exposure. Try to limit your exposure to the sun, especially during the hours between 10:00 a.m. and 4:00 p.m., when sunlight is most direct. Be especially careful when you are in an area with reflective surfaces, such as water, sand, concrete, and areas that are painted white. Remember that the sun is stronger at higher elevations. Avoid tanning booths as well, because they have the same effect as sun exposure.

Sleep on your back. Pressing your face against a pillow while sleeping on your stomach may create squint-pressure wrinkles. Getting enough sleep is also important, as the lack of sleep is immediately evident on the face.

Stop smoking. Smokers tend to have skin that is leathery and wrinkled, and they have far more wrinkles than nonsmokers. This is because smoking decreases the blood supply to the skin, depleting it of oxygen and other nutrients. It also damages collagen and elastin, which causes premature wrinkling and sagging of the skin. Wrinkles are particularly noticeable around the mouth and eyes due to the repetitive expressions used when smoking, such as pursing the lips and squinting the eyes.

Wear a hat and sunglasses. Stop squinting, which deepens existing wrinkles or creates new ones. It is a good idea to wear a protective hat and sunglasses that block out 100 percent of ultraviolet (UVA and UVB) rays and filter out at least 85 percent of blue-violet sunrays. Some contend that brown to yellow lenses are better alternatives. Be aware that some medications make the skin and the eyes more sensitive to light. Ask your doctor if any of your medications has this potential. If you are taking such a medicine, you need to be extra vigilant with protecting yourself.

Wear sunscreen. Apply a sunscreen with an SPF of at least 15 every morning, 30 to 45 minutes before going outside. If you spend a good deal of time outside, reapply every few hours.

Part 3

References

Resources for Specific Disorders

AGE SPOTS

American Academy of Dermatology
P.O. Box 4014
Schaumburg, IL 60618-4014
Phone: 866-503-SKIN (7546)
Web site: www.aad.org

American Society for Dermatologic Surgery
5550 Meadowbrook Drive, Suite 120
Rolling Meadows, IL 60008
Phone: 847-956-0900
Web site: www.asds-net.org

National Institute on Aging
Building 31, Room 5C27
31 Center Drive, MSC 2292
Bethesda, MD 20892
Phone: 301-496-1752 or 800-222-4225 (TTY)
Web site: www.nia.nih.gov

ALZHEIMER'S DISEASE

Alzheimer's Association
225 North Michigan Avenue, 17th Floor
Chicago, IL 60601-7633
Phone: 800-272-3900 (Helpline) or 312-335-8700
Web site: www.alz.org

Alzheimer's Foundation of America
322 Eighth Avenue, 7th Floor
New York, NY 10001
Phone: 866-232-8484
Web site: www.alzfdn.org

ARCH National Respite Network
800 Eastowne Drive, Suite 105
Chapel Hill, NC 27514
Phone: 919-490-5577
Web site: www.archrespite.org

National Family Caregivers Association
10400 Connecticut Avenue, Suite 500
Kensington, MD 20895-3944
Phone: 800-896-3650 or 301-942-6430
Web site: www.nfcacares.org

ANEMIA

American Academy of Family Physicians
Mailing Address:
P.O. Box 11210
Shawnee Mission, KS 66207-1210
Street Address:
11400 Tomahawk Creek Parkway
Leawood, KS 66211-2672
Phone: 800-274-2237 or 913-906-6000
Web site: aafp.org

Division of Nutrition, Physical Activity and Obesity
National Center for Chronic Disease Prevention and Health Promotion
Centers for Disease Control and Prevention
1600 Clifton Road
Atlanta, GA 30333
Phone: 800-CDC-INFO (232-4636) or 404-639-3311 or 888-232-6348 (TTY)
Web site: www.cdc.gov/nccdphp/dnpa

Iron Disorders Institute
Mailing Address:
P.O. Box 675
Taylors, SC 29687
Street Address:
2722 Wade Hampton Boulevard, Suite A
Greenville, SC 29615
Phone: 888-565-IRON (4766) or 864-292-1175
Web site: www.irondisorders.org

ANGINA

American College of Cardiology
Heart House
2400 N Street NW
Washington, DC 20037
Phone: 202-375-6000
Web site: www.acc.org

American Heart Association
7272 Greenville Avenue
Dallas, TX 75231
Phone: 800-AHA-USA-1 (242-8721)
Web site: www.americanheart.org

Heart Information Center
Texas Heart Institute
Mailing Address:
P.O. Box 20345
Houston, TX 77225-0345
Street Address:
6770 Bertner Avenue
Houston, TX 77030
Phone: 800-292-2221 or 832-355-4011
Web site: www.texasheartinstitute.org

National Heart, Lung, and Blood Institute Health
  Information Center
P.O. Box 30105
Bethesda, MD 20824-0105
Phone: 301-592-8573
Web site: www.nhlbi.nih.gov

ANXIETY DISORDERS

American Psychiatric Association
1000 Wilson Boulevard, Suite 1825
Arlington, VA 22209-3901
Phone: 703-907-7300
Web site: www.psych.org

American Psychological Association
750 First Street NE
Washington, DC 20002-4242
Phone: 800-374-2721 or 202-336-5500
Web site: www.apa.org

Anxiety Disorders Association of America
8730 Georgia Avenue, Suite 600
Silver Spring, MD 20910
Phone: 240-485-1001
Web site: www.adaa.org

Mental Health America
2000 North Beauregard Street, 6th Floor
Alexandria, VA 22311
Phone: 800-969-6642 or 703-684-7722
Web site: www.nmha.org

National Institute of Mental Health
Science Writing, Press, and Dissemination
  Branch
6001 Executive Boulevard, Room 8184,
  MSC 9663
Bethesda, MD 20892-9663
Phone: 866-615-6464 or 301-443-4513
Web site: www.nimh.nih.gov

Obsessive-Compulsive Foundation
P.O. Box 961029
Boston, MA 02196
Phone: 617-973-5801
Web site: www.ocfoundation.org

ATHEROSCLEROSIS

American College of Cardiology
Heart House
2400 N Street NW
Washington, DC 20037
Phone: 202-375-6000
Web site: www.acc.org

American Heart Association
7272 Greenville Avenue
Dallas, TX 75231
Phone: 800-AHA-USA-1 (242-8721)
Web site: www.americanheart.org

Heart Information Center
Texas Heart Institute
Mailing Address:
P.O. Box 20345
Houston, TX 77225-0345
Street Address:
6770 Bertner Avenue
Houston, TX 77030
Phone: 800-292-2221 or 832-355-4011
Web site: www.texasheartinstitute.org

National Heart, Lung, and Blood Institute Health
  Information Center
P.O. Box 30105
Bethesda, MD 20824-0105
Phone: 301-592-8573
Web site: www.nhlbi.nih.gov

BACK PAIN

American Academy of Orthopaedic Surgeons
6300 North River Road
Rosemont, IL 60018-4262
Phone: 847-823-7186
Web site: www.aaos.org

American Chronic Pain Association
P.O. Box 850
Rocklin, CA 95677
Phone: 800-533-3231
Web site: www.theacpa.org

American Pain Society
4700 West Lake Avenue
Glenview, IL 60025
Phone: 847-375-4715
Web site: www.ampainsoc.org

CATARACTS

American Academy of Ophthalmology
P.O. Box 7424
San Francisco, CA 94120-7424
Phone: 415-561-8500
Web site: www.aao.org

American Optometric Association
243 North Lindbergh Boulevard
St. Louis, MO 63141
Phone: 800-365-2219
Web site: www.aoa.org

Foundation Fighting Blindness
11435 Cronhill Drive
Owings Mills, MD 21117
Phone: 800-683-5555 or 800-683-5551 (TDD)
Web site: www.blindness.org

National Eye Institute
2020 Vision Place
Bethesda, MD 20892-3655
Phone: 301-496-5248
Web site: www.nei.nih.gov

Prevent Blindness America
211 West Wacker Drive, Suite 1700
Chicago, IL 60606
Phone: 800-331-2020
Web site: www.preventblindness.org

CELIAC DISEASE

American Dietetic Association
120 South Riverside Plaza, Suite 2000
Chicago, IL 60606-6995
Phone: 800-877-1600
Web site: www.eatright.org

Celiac Disease Foundation
13251 Ventura Boulevard, #1
Studio City, CA 91604
Phone: 818-990-2354
Web site: www.celiac.org

Celiac Sprue Association
P.O. Box 31700
Omaha, NE 68131-0700
Phone: 877-CSA-4CSA (272-4272)
Web site: www.csaceliacs.org

Gluten Intolerance Group (GIG)
31214 124th Avenue SE
Auburn, WA 98092-3667
Phone: 253-833-6655
Web site: www.gluten.net

CHRONIC FATIGUE SYNDROME

American Chronic Pain Association
P.O. Box 850
Rocklin, CA 95677
Phone: 800-533-3231
Web site: www.theacpa.org

American Pain Society
4700 West Lake Avenue
Glenview, IL 60025
Phone: 847-375-4715
Web site: www.ampainsoc.org

CFIDS Association of America
P.O. Box 220398
Charlotte, NC 28222-0398
Phone: 704-365-2343
Web site: www.cfids.org

International Association for CFS/ME
27 North Wacker Drive, Suite 416
Chicago, IL 60606
Phone: 847-258-7248
Web site: www.iacfsme.org

International Association for the Study of Pain
111 Queen Anne Avenue North, Suite 501
Seattle, WA 98109-4955
Phone: 206-283-0311
Web site: www.iasp-pain.org

National Institute of Allergy and Infectious Diseases
NIAID Office of Communications and Public Liaison
6610 Rockledge Drive, MSC 6612
Bethesda, MD 20892-6612
Phone: 866-284-4107 or 800-877-8339 (TDD)
Web site: www.niaid.nih.gov

COLON POLYPS

American College of Gastroenterology
P.O. Box 342260
Bethesda, MD 20827-2260
Phone: 301-263-9000
Web site: www.acg.gi.org

American Gastroenterological Association
4930 Del Ray Avenue
Bethesda, MD 20814
Phone: 301-654-2055
Web site: www.gastro.org

American Society for Gastrointestinal Endoscopy
1520 Kensington Road, Suite 202
Oak Brook, IL 60523
Phone: 630-573-0600
Web site: www.asge.org

American Society of Colon and Rectal Surgeons
85 West Algonquin Road, Suite 550
Arlington Heights, IL 60005
Phone: 847-290-9184
Web site: www.fascrs.org

CONSTIPATION

American College of Gastroenterology
P.O. Box 342260
Bethesda, MD 20827-2260
Phone: 301-263-9000
Web site: www.acg.gi.org

American Gastroenterological Association
4930 Del Ray Avenue
Bethesda, MD 20814
Phone: 301-654-2055
Web site: www.gastro.org

American Society for Gastrointestinal Endoscopy
1520 Kensington Road, Suite 202
Oak Brook, IL 60523
Phone: 630-573-0600
Web site: www.asge.org

American Society of Colon and Rectal Surgeons
85 West Algonquin Road, Suite 550
Arlington Heights, IL 60005
Phone: 847-290-9184
Web site: www.fascrs.org

International Foundation for Functional
Gastrointestinal Disorders (IFFGD)
P.O. Box 170864
Milwaukee, WI 53217-8076
Phone: 888-964-2001 or 414-964-1799
Web site: www.iffgd.org

CORONARY ARTERY DISEASE

American College of Cardiology
Heart House
2400 N Street NW
Washington, DC 20037
Phone: 202-375-6000
Web site: www.acc.org

American Heart Association
7272 Greenville Avenue
Dallas, TX 75231
Phone: 800-AHA-USA-1 (242-8721)
Web site: www.americanheart.org

Heart Information Center
Texas Heart Institute
Mailing Address:
P.O. Box 20345
Houston, TX 77225-0345
Street Address:
6770 Bertner Avenue
Houston, TX 77030
Phone: 800-292-2221 or 832-355-4011
Web site: www.texasheartinstitute.org

National Heart, Lung, and Blood Institute Health
Information Center
P.O. Box 30105
Bethesda, MD 20824-0105
Phone: 301-592-8573
Web site: www.nhlbi.nih.gov

CROHN'S DISEASE

American College of Gastroenterology
P.O. Box 342260
Bethesda, MD 20827-2260
Phone: 301-263-9000
Web site: www.acg.gi.org

American Gastroenterological Association
4930 Del Ray Avenue
Bethesda, MD 20814
Phone: 301-654-2055
Web site: www.gastro.org

American Society of Colon and Rectal Surgeons
85 West Algonquin Road, Suite 550
Arlington Heights, IL 60005
Phone: 847-290-9184
Web site: www.fascrs.org

Crohn's and Colitis Foundation of America
386 Park Avenue South, 17th Floor
New York, NY 10016
Phone: 800-932-2423
Web site: www.ccfa.org

DEEP VEIN THROMBOSIS

American Academy of Orthopaedic Surgeons
6300 North River Road
Rosemont, IL 60018-4262
Phone: 847-823-7186
Web site: www.aaos.org

American Heart Association
7272 Greenville Avenue
Dallas, TX 75231
Phone: 800-AHA-USA-1 (242-8721)
Web site: www.americanheart.org

American Public Health Association
800 I Street NW
Washington, DC 20001-3710
Phone: 202-777-APHA (2742)
Web site: www.apha.org

Society of Interventional Radiology
3975 Fair Ridge Drive, Suite 400 North
Fairfax, VA 22033
Phone: 800-488-7284 or 703-691-1805
Web site: www.sirweb.org

DEGENERATIVE DISK DISEASE

American Academy of Orthopaedic Surgeons
6300 North River Road
Rosemont, IL 60018-4262
Phone: 847-823-7186
Web site: www.aaos.org

American Chronic Pain Association
P.O. Box 850
Rocklin, CA 95677
Phone: 800-533-3231
Web site: www.theacpa.org

American Pain Society
4700 West Lake Avenue
Glenview, IL 60025
Phone: 847-375-4715
Web site: www.ampainsoc.org

North American Spine Society
7075 Veterans Boulevard
Burr Ridge, IL 60527
Phone: 866-960-6277 or 630-230-3600
Web site: www.spine.org

DEPRESSION

American Psychiatric Association
1000 Wilson Boulevard, Suite 1825
Arlington, VA 22209-3901
Phone: 703-907-7300
Web site: www.psych.org

American Psychological Association
750 First Street NE
Washington, DC 20002-4242
Phone: 800-374-2721 or 202-336-5500
Web site: www.apa.org

Anxiety Disorders Association of America
8730 Georgia Avenue, Suite 600
Silver Spring, MD 20910
Phone: 240-485-1001
Web site: www.adaa.org

Depression and Bipolar Support Alliance
730 North Franklin Street, Suite 501
Chicago, IL 60610-7224
Phone: 800-826-3632
Web site: www.dbsalliance.org

International Foundation for Research and
Education on Depression (iFred)
2017-D Renard Court
Annapolis, MD 21401
Phone: 410-268-0044
Web site: www.ifred.org

Mental Health America
2000 North Beauregard Street, 6th Floor
Alexandria, VA 22311
Phone: 800-969-6642 or 703-684-7722
Web site: www.nmha.org

National Institute of Mental Health
Science Writing, Press, and Dissemination
Branch
6001 Executive Boulevard, Room 8184,
MSC 9663
Bethesda, MD 20892-9663
Phone: 866-615-6464 or 301-443-4513
Web site: www.nimh.nih.gov

DIABETES

American Diabetes Association
1701 North Beauregard Street
Alexandria, VA 22311
Phone: 800-DIABETES (342-2383)
Web site: www.diabetes.org

American Dietetic Association
120 South Riverside Plaza, Suite 2000
Chicago, IL 60606-6995
Phone: 800-877-1600
Web site: www.eatright.org

National Diabetes Information Clearinghouse
1 Information Way
Bethesda, MD 20892-3560
Phone: 800-860-8747
Web site: www.diabetes.niddk.nih.gov

National Eye Institute
2020 Vision Place
Bethesda, MD 20892-3655
Phone: 301-496-5248
Web site: www.nei.nih.gov

DIVERTICULOSIS/DIVERTICULITIS

American College of Gastroenterology
P.O. Box 342260
Bethesda, MD 20827-2260
Phone: 301-263-9000
Web site: www.acg.gi.org

American Gastroenterological Association
4930 Del Ray Avenue
Bethesda, MD 20814
Phone: 301-654-2055
Web site: www.gastro.org

American Society for Gastrointestinal Endoscopy
1520 Kensington Road, Suite 202
Oak Brook, IL 60523
Phone: 630-573-0600
Web site: www.asge.org

American Society of Colon and Rectal Surgeons
85 West Algonquin Road, Suite 550
Arlington Heights, IL 60005
Phone: 847-290-9184
Web site: www.fascrs.org

International Foundation for Functional
   Gastrointestinal Disorders (IFFGD)
P.O. Box 170864
Milwaukee, WI 53217-8076
Phone: 888-964-2001 or 414-964-1799
Web site: www.iffgd.org

National Institute of Diabetes and Digestive and
   Kidney Diseases
Building 31, Room 9A06
31 Center Drive, MSC 2560
Bethesda, MD 20892-2560
Phone: 301-496-3583
Web site: www.niddk.nih.gov

DRY SKIN

American Academy of Dermatology
P.O. Box 4014
Schaumburg, IL 60618-4014
Phone: 866-503-SKIN (7546)
Web site: www.aad.org

American Society for Dermatologic Surgery
5550 Meadowbrook Drive, Suite 120
Rolling Meadows, IL 60008
Phone: 847-956-0900
Web site: www.asds-net.org

National Institute on Aging
Building 31, Room 5C27
31 Center Drive, MSC 2292
Bethesda, MD 20892
Phone: 301-496-1752 or 800-222-4225 (TTY)
Web site: www.nia.nih.gov

EMPHYSEMA

American Association for Respiratory Care
9425 North MacArthur Boulevard, Suite 100
Irving, TX 75063-4706
Phone: 972-243-2272
Web site: www.aarc.org

American Lung Association
61 Broadway, 6th Floor
New York, NY 10006
Phone: 800-548-8252 or 212-315-8700
Web site: www.lungusa.org

National Heart, Lung, and Blood Institute Health
   Information Center
P.O. Box 30105
Bethesda, MD 20824-0105
Phone: 301-592-8573
Web site: www.nhlbi.nih.gov

National Jewish Medical and Research Center
1400 Jackson Street
Denver, CO 80206
Phone: 800-222-LUNG (5864)
Web site: www.njc.org

ERECTILE DYSFUNCTION

American Diabetes Association
1701 North Beauregard Street
Alexandria, VA 22311
Phone: 800-DIABETES (342-2383)
Web site: www.diabetes.org

American Urological Association
1000 Corporate Boulevard
Linthicum, MD 21090
Phone: 866-746-4282 (United States only) or
   410-689-3700
Web site: www.auanet.org

Endocrine Society
8401 Connecticut Avenue, Suite 900
Chevy Chase, MD 20815
Phone: 301-941-0200
Web site: www.endo-society.org

Hormone Foundation
8401 Connecticut Avenue, Suite 900
Chevy Chase, MD 20815
Phone: 800-HORMONE (467-6663)
Web site: www.hormone.org

ESSENTIAL TREMOR

American Neurological Association
5841 Cedar Lake Road, Suite 204
Minneapolis, MN 55416
Phone: 952-545-6284
Web site: www.aneuroa.org

International Essential Tremor Foundation
P.O. Box 14005
Lenexa, KS 66285-4005
Phone: 888-387-3667 or 913-341-3880
Web site: www.essentialtremor.org

National Institute of Neurological Disorders and
Stroke
P.O. Box 5801
Bethesda, MD 20824
Phone: 800-352-9424 or 301-496-5751 or
301-468-5981 (TTY)
Web site: www.ninds.nih.gov

WE MOVE
204 West 84th Street
New York, NY 10024
Phone: 212-875-8312
Web site: www.wemove.org

FALLEN BLADDER

American Urogynecologic Society
2025 M Street NW, Suite 800
Washington, DC 20036
Phone: 202-367-1167
Web site: www.augs.org

American Urological Association
1000 Corporate Boulevard
Linthicum, MD 21090
Phone: 866-746-4282 (United States only) or
410-689-3700
Web site: www.auanet.org

National Association for Continence
P.O. Box 1019
Charleston, SC 29402-1019
Phone: 800-BLADDER (252-3337) or
843-377-0900
Web site: www.nafc.org

FATIGUE

If you have a medical condition that is causing your
fatigue, be sure to see the resources for that condition,
in addition to those below.

American Geriatrics Society
The Empire State Building
350 Fifth Avenue, Suite 801
New York, NY 10118
Phone: 212-308-1414
Web site: www.americangeriatrics.org

National Institute on Aging
Building 31, Room 5C27
31 Center Drive, MSC 2292
Bethesda, MD 20892
Phone: 301-496-1752 or 800-222-4225 (TTY)
Web site: www.nia.nih.gov

US Department of Health and Human Services
Office of Disease Prevention and Health
Promotion
Office of Public Health and Science, Office of the
Secretary
1101 Wootton Parkway, Suite LL100
Rockville, MD 20852
Phone: 240-453-8280
Web site: www.odphp.osophs.dhhs.gov

FEMALE SEXUAL DYSFUNCTION

American Association for Marriage and Family
Therapy
112 South Alfred Street
Alexandria, VA 22314-3061
Phone: 703-838-9808
Web site: www.aamft.org

American College of Obstetricians and
Gynecologists
409 12th Street SW, P.O. Box 96920
Washington, DC 20090-6920
Phone: 202-638-5577
Web site: www.acog.org

American Diabetes Association
1701 North Beauregard Street
Alexandria, VA 22311
Phone: 800-DIABETES (342-2383)
Web site: www.diabetes.org

American Urological Association
1000 Corporate Boulevard
Linthicum, MD 21090
Phone: 866-746-4282 (United States only) or
410-689-3700
Web site: www.auanet.org

Endocrine Society
8401 Connecticut Avenue, Suite 900
Chevy Chase, MD 20815
Phone: 301-941-0200
Web site: www.endo-society.org

Hormone Foundation
8401 Connecticut Avenue, Suite 900
Chevy Chase, MD 20815
Phone: 800-HORMONE (467-6663)
Web site: www.hormone.org

FIBROMYALGIA

American Chronic Pain Association
P.O. Box 850
Rocklin, CA 95677
Phone: 800-533-3231
Web site: www.theacpa.org

American College of Rheumatology
1800 Century Place, Suite 250
Atlanta, GA 30345-4300
Phone: 404-633-3777
Web site: www.rheumatology.org

American Fibromyalgia Syndrome Association
Mailing Address:
P.O. Box 32698
Tucson, AZ 85751
Street Address:
7371 East Tanque Verde Road
Tucson, AZ 85715
Phone: 520-733-1570
Web site: www.afsafund.org

American Pain Society
4700 West Lake Avenue
Glenview, IL 60025
Phone: 847-375-4715
Web site: www.ampainsoc.org

Arthritis Foundation
P.O. Box 7669
Atlanta, GA 30357-0669
Phone: 800-283-7800
Web site: www.arthritis.org

National Chronic Fatigue Syndrome and
Fibromyalgia Association
P.O. Box 18426
Kansas City, MO 64133
Phone: 816-737-1343
Web site: www.ncfsfa.org

National Fibromyalgia Partnership
P.O. Box 160
Linden, VA 22642-0160
Web site: www.fmpartnership.org

FLATULENCE

American College of Gastroenterology
P.O. Box 342260
Bethesda, MD 20827-2260
Phone: 301-263-9000
Web site: www.acg.gi.org

American Gastroenterological Association
4930 Del Ray Avenue
Bethesda, MD 20814
Phone: 301-654-2055
Web site: www.gastro.org

International Foundation for Functional
Gastrointestinal Disorders (IFFGD)
P.O. Box 170864
Milwaukee, WI 53217-8076
Phone: 888-964-2001 or 414-964-1799
Web site: www.iffgd.org

FLOATERS

American Optometric Association
243 North Lindbergh Boulelvard
St. Louis, MO 63141
Phone: 800-365-2219
Web site: www.aoa.org

National Eye Institute
2020 Vision Place
Bethesda, MD 20892-3655
Phone: 301-496-5248
Web site: www.nei.nih.gov

Saint Luke's Cataract and Laser Institute
Retina Center
43309 U.S. Highway 19 North
Tarpon Springs, FL 34689
Phone: 888-648-4393
Web site: www.theretinasource.com

GALLSTONES

American College of Gastroenterology
P.O. Box 342260
Bethesda, MD 20827-2260
Phone: 301-263-9000
Web site: www.acg.gi.org

American Gastroenterological Association
4930 Del Ray Avenue
Bethesda, MD 20814
Phone: 301-654-2055
Web site: www.gastro.org

American Society for Gastrointestinal Endoscopy
1520 Kensington Road, Suite 202
Oak Brook, IL 60523
Phone: 630-573-0600
Web site: www.asge.org

GASTROESOPHAGEAL REFLUX DISEASE (GERD)

American College of Gastroenterology
P.O. Box 342260
Bethesda, MD 20827-2260
Phone: 301-263-9000
Web site: www.acg.gi.org

American Gastroenterological Association
4930 Del Ray Avenue
Bethesda, MD 20814
Phone: 301-654-2055
Web site: www.gastro.org

American Society for Gastrointestinal Endoscopy
1520 Kensington Road, Suite 202
Oak Brook, IL 60523
Phone: 630-573-0600
Web site: www.asge.org

GLAUCOMA

American Academy of Ophthalmology
P.O. Box 7424
San Francisco, CA 94120-7424
Phone: 415-561-8500
Web site: www.aao.org

American Optometric Association
243 North Lindbergh Boulevard
St. Louis, MO 63141
Phone: 800-365-2219
Web site: www.aoa.org

Foundation Fighting Blindness
11435 Cronhill Drive
Owings Mills, MD 21117
Phone: 800-683-5555 or 800-683-5551 (TDD)
Web site: www. blindness.org

Glaucoma Research Foundation
251 Post Street, Suite 600
San Francisco, CA 94108
Phone: 800-826-6693 or 415-986-3162
Web site: www.glaucoma.org

National Eye Institute
2020 Vision Place
Bethesda, MD 20892-3655
Phone: 301-496-5248
Web site: www.nei.nih.gov

Prevent Blindness America
211 West Wacker Drive, Suite 1700
Chicago, IL 60606
Phone: 800-331-2020
Web site: www.preventblindness.org

GOUT

American College of Rheumatology
1800 Century Place, Suite 250
Atlanta, GA 30345-4300
Phone: 404-633-3777
Web site: www.rheumatology.org

American Pain Society
4700 West Lake Avenue
Glenview, IL 60025
Phone: 847-375-4715
Web site: www.ampainsoc.org

Arthritis Foundation
P.O. Box 7669
Atlanta, GA 30357-0669
Phone: 800-283-7800
Web site: www.arthritis.org

GUM DISEASE

Academy of General Dentistry
211 East Chicago Avenue, Suite 900
Chicago, IL 60611-1999
Phone: 888-243-3368
Web site: www.agd.org

American Academy of Periodontology
737 North Michigan Avenue, Suite 800
Chicago, IL 60611-6660
Phone: 312-787-5518
Web site: www.perio.org

American Board of Cosmetic Surgery
18525 Torrence Avenue
Lansing, IL 60438
Phone: 866-907-3100 or 708-474-7200
Web site: www.americanboardcosmeticsurgery.org

American Dental Association
211 East Chicago Avenue
Chicago, IL 60611-2678
Phone: 312-440-2500
Web site: www.ada.org

HAIR LOSS

American Academy of Dermatology
P.O. Box 4014
Schaumburg, IL 60618-4014
Phone: 866-503-SKIN (7546)
Web site: www.aad.org

American Society for Dermatologic Surgery
5550 Meadowbrook Drive, Suite 120
Rolling Meadows, IL 60008
Phone: 847-956-0900
Web site: www.asds-net.org

National Institute on Aging
Building 31, Room 5C27
31 Center Drive, MSC 2292
Bethesda, MD 20892
Phone: 301-496-1752 or 800-222-4225 (TTY)
Web site: www.nia.nih.gov

HEARING LOSS

Alexander Graham Bell Association for the Deaf
and Hard of Hearing
3417 Volta Place NW
Washington, DC 20007
Phone: 202-337-5220 or 202-337-5221 (TTY)
Web site: www.agbell.org

American Academy of Otolaryngology–Head and
Neck Surgery
One Prince Street
Alexandria, VA 22314-3357
Phone: 703-836-4444
Web site: www.entnet.org

American Speech-Language-Hearing Association
2200 Research Boulevard
Rockville, MD 20850-3289
Phone: 800-498-2071 (member) or 800-638-
8255 (nonmember); 301-296-5650 (TTY)
Web site: www.asha.org

American Tinnitus Association
Mailing Address:
P.O. Box 5
Portland, OR 97207-0005
Street Address:
65 SW Yamhill Street, Suite 200
Portland, OR 97204
Phone: 800-634-8978 (United States only) or
503-248-9985
Web site: www.ata.org

Hearing Loss Association of America
7910 Woodmont Avenue, Suite 1200
Bethesda, MD 20814
Phone: 301-657-2248
Web site: www.shhh.org

HEART PALPITATIONS

American College of Cardiology
Heart House
2400 N Street NW
Washington, DC 20037
Phone: 202-375-6000
Web site: www.acc.org

American Heart Association
7272 Greenville Avenue
Dallas, TX 75231
Phone: 800-AHA-USA-1 (242-8721)
Web site: www.americanheart.org

National Heart, Lung, and Blood Institute Health
Information Center
P.O. Box 30105
Bethesda, MD 20824-0105
Phone: 301-592-8573
Web site: www.nhlbi.nih.gov

HEMORRHOIDS

American College of Gastroenterology
P.O. Box 342260
Bethesda, MD 20827-2260
Phone: 301-263-9000
Web site: www.acg.gi.org

American Gastroenterological Association
4930 Del Ray Avenue
Bethesda, MD 20814
Phone: 301-654-2055
Web site: www.gastro.org

American Society of Colon and Rectal Surgeons
85 West Algonquin Road, Suite 550
Arlington Heights, IL 60005
Phone: 847-290-9184
Web site: www.fascrs.org

HIGH BLOOD PRESSURE

American Heart Association
7272 Greenville Avenue
Dallas, TX 75231
Phone: 800-AHA-USA-1 (242-8721)
Web site: www.americanheart.org

American Society of Hypertension
148 Madison Avenue, Fifth Floor
New York, NY 10016
Phone: 212-696-9099
Web site: www.ash-us.org

National Heart, Lung, and Blood Institute Health
   Information Center
P.O. Box 30105
Bethesda, MD 20824-0105
Phone: 301-592-8573
Web site: www.nhlbi.nih.gov

National Hypertension Association, Inc.
324 East 30th Street
New York, NY 10016
Phone: 212-889-3557
Web site: www.nathypertension.org

US Food and Drug Administration
5600 Fishers Lane
Rockville, MD 20857-0001
Phone: 888-INFO-FDA (463-6332)
Web site: www.fda.gov

HIGH CHOLESTEROL

American College of Cardiology
Heart House
2400 N Street NW
Washington, DC 20037
Phone: 202-375-6000
Web site: www.acc.org

American Heart Association
7272 Greenville Avenue
Dallas, TX 75231
Phone: 800-AHA-USA-1 (242-8721)
Web site: www.americanheart.org

National Heart, Lung, and Blood Institute Health
   Information Center
P.O. Box 30105
Bethesda, MD 20824-0105
Phone: 301-592-8573
Web site: www.nhlbi.nih.gov

HIP FRACTURE

American Academy of Orthopaedic Surgeons
6300 North River Road
Rosemont, IL 60018-4262
Phone: 847-823-7186
Web site: www.aaos.org

American Pain Society
4700 West Lake Avenue
Glenview, IL 60025
Phone: 847-375-4715
Web site: www.ampainsoc.org

American Physical Therapy Association
1111 North Fairfax Street
Alexandria, VA 22314-1488
Phone: 800-999-APTA (2782) or
   703-684-APTA (2782) or 703-683-6748 (TDD)
Web site: www.apta.org

Hip Society
951 Old County Road, #182
Belmont, CA 94002
Phone: 650-525-1074
Web site: www.hipsoc.org

National Osteoporosis Foundation
1232 22nd Street NW
Washington, DC 20037-1202
Phone: 800-231-4222 or 202-223-2226
Web site: www.nof.org

HYPERTHYROIDISM

American Association of Clinical Endocrinologists
245 Riverside Avenue, Suite 200
Jacksonville, FL 32202
Phone: 904-353-7878
Web site: www.aace.com

American Thyroid Association
6066 Leesburg Pike, Suite 550
Falls Church, VA 22041
Phone: 703-998-8890
Web site: www.thyroid.org

Endocrine Society
8401 Connecticut Avenue, Suite 900
Chevy Chase, MD 20815
Phone: 301-941-0200
Web site: www.endo-society.org

The Thyroid Foundation of America
One Longfellow Place, Suite 1518
Boston, MA 02114
Phone: 800-832-8321
Web site: www.tsh.org

HYPOTHYROIDISM

American Association of Clinical Endocrinologists
245 Riverside Avenue, Suite 200
Jacksonville, FL 32202
Phone: 904-353-7878
Web site: www.aace.com

American Thyroid Association
6066 Leesburg Pike, Suite 550
Falls Church, VA 22041
Phone: 703-998-8890
Web site: www.thyroid.org

Endocrine Society
8401 Connecticut Avenue, Suite 900
Chevy Chase, MD 20815
Phone: 301-941-0200
Web site: www.endo-society.org

The Thyroid Foundation of America
One Longfellow Place, Suite 1518
Boston, MA 02114
Phone: 800-832-8321
Web site: www.tsh.org

INCONTINENCE

American Urogynecologic Society
2025 M Street NW, Suite 800
Washington, DC 20036
Phone: 202-367-1167
Web site: www.augs.org

American Urological Association
1000 Corporate Boulevard
Linthicum, MD 21090
Phone: 866-746-4282 (United States only) or
  410-689-3700
Web site: www.auanet.org

National Association for Continence
P.O. Box 1019
Charleston, SC 29402-1019
Phone: 800-BLADDER (252-3337) or
  843-377-0900
Web site: www.nafc.org

National Kidney and Urologic Diseases
  Information Clearinghouse
3 Information Way
Bethesda, MD 20892-3580
Phone: 800-891-5390
Web site: www.kidney.niddk.nih.gov

National Kidney Foundation
30 East 33rd Street
New York, NY 10016
Phone: 800-622-9010
Web site: www.kidney.org

The Simon Foundation for Continence
P.O. Box 815
Wilmette, IL 60091
Phone: 800-23-SIMON (237-4666)
Web site: www.simonfoundation.org

INDIGESTION

American College of Gastroenterology
P.O. Box 342260
Bethesda, MD 20827-2260
Phone: 301-263-9000
Web site: www.acg.gi.org

American Gastroenterological Association
4930 Del Ray Avenue
Bethesda, MD 20814
Phone: 301-654-2055
Web site: www.gastro.org

International Foundation for Functional
  Gastrointestinal Disorders (IFFGD)
P.O. Box 170864
Milwaukee, WI 53217-8076
Phone: 888-964-2001 or 414-964-1799
Web site: www.iffgd.org

INFLUENZA

American Lung Association
61 Broadway, 6th Floor
New York, NY 10006
Phone: 800-548-8252 or 212-315-8700
Web site: www.lungusa.org

Centers for Disease Control and Prevention
1600 Clifton Road
Atlanta, GA 30333
Phone: 800-311-3435 or 404-498-1515
Web site: www.cdc.gov

Infectious Diseases Society of America
1300 Wilson Boulevard, Suite 300
Arlington, VA 22209
Phone: 703-299-0200
Web site: www.idsociety.org

National Foundation for Infectious Diseases
4733 Bethesda Avenue, Suite 750
Bethesda, MD 20814
Phone: 301-656-0003
Web site: www.nfid.org

US Food and Drug Administration
5600 Fishers Lane
Rockville, MD 20857-0001
Phone: 888-INFO-FDA (463-6332)
Web site: www.fda.gov

INSOMNIA

American Academy of Family Physicians
Mailing Address:
P.O. Box 11210
Shawnee Mission, KS 66207-1210
Street Address:
11400 Tomahawk Creek Parkway
Leawood, KS 66211-2672
Phone: 800-274-2237 or 913-906-6000
Web site: aafp.org

American Academy of Sleep Medicine
One Westbrook Corporate Center, Suite 920
Westchester, IL 60154
Phone: 708-492-0930
Web site: www.aasmnet.org

National Center on Sleep Disorders Research
National Heart, Lung, and Blood Institute, NIH
6701 Rockledge Drive
Bethesda, MD 20892
Phone: 301-435-0199
Web site: www.nhlbi.nih.gov/about/ncsdr

National Sleep Foundation
1522 K Street NW, Suite 500
Washington, DC 20005
Phone: 202-347-3471
Web site: www.sleepfoundation.org

IRRITABLE BOWEL SYNDROME

American College of Gastroenterology
P.O. Box 342260
Bethesda, MD 20827-2260
Phone: 301-263-9000
Web site: www.acg.gi.org

American Gastroenterological Association
4930 Del Ray Avenue
Bethesda, MD 20814
Phone: 301-654-2055
Web site: www.gastro.org

International Foundation for Functional
Gastrointestinal Disorders (IFFGD)
P.O. Box 170864
Milwaukee, WI 53217-8076
Phone: 888-964-2001 or 414-964-1799
Web site: www.iffgd.org

KIDNEY STONES

American Urological Association
1000 Corporate Boulevard
Linthicum, MD 21090
Phone: 866-746-4282 (United States only) or
410-689-3700
Web site: www.auanet.org

National Kidney and Urologic Diseases
Information Clearinghouse
3 Information Way
Bethesda, MD 20892-3580
Phone: 800-891-5390
Web site: www.kidney.niddk.nih.gov

National Kidney Foundation
30 East 33rd Street
New York, NY 10016
Phone: 800-622-9010
Web site: www.kidney.org

MACULAR DEGENERATION

American Academy of Ophthalmology
P.O. Box 7424
San Francisco, CA 94120-7424
Phone: 415-561-8500
Web site: www.aao.org

American Optometric Association
243 North Lindbergh Boulevard
St. Louis, MO 63141
Phone: 800-365-2219
Web site: www.aoa.org

Association for Macular Diseases, Inc.
210 East 64th Street, 8th Floor
New York, NY 10021
Phone: 212-605-3719
Web site: www.macula.org

Foundation Fighting Blindness
11435 Cronhill Drive
Owings Mills, MD 21117
Phone: 800-683-5555 or 800-683-5551 (TDD)
Web site: www.blindness.org

Macular Degeneration Foundation
P.O. Box 531313
Henderson, NV 89053
Phone: 888-633-3937
Web site: www.eyesight.org

National Eye Institute
2020 Vision Place
Bethesda, MD 20892-3655
Phone: 301-496-5248
Web site: www.nei.nih.gov

MALE MENOPAUSE

American Association of Clinical Endocrinologists
245 Riverside Avenue, Suite 200
Jacksonville, FL 32202
Phone: 904-353-7878
Web site: www.aace.com

American Geriatrics Society
The Empire State Building
350 Fifth Avenue, Suite 801
New York, NY 10118
Phone: 212-308-1414
Web site: www.americangeriatrics.org

Hormone Foundation
8401 Connecticut Avenue, Suite 900
Chevy Chase, MD 20815
Phone: 800-HORMONE (467-6663)
Web site: www.hormone.org

National Institute on Aging
Building 31, Room 5C27
31 Center Drive, MSC 2292
Bethesda, MD 20892
Phone: 301-496-1752 or 800-222-4225 (TTY)
Web site: www.nia.nih.gov

MEMORY LOSS

Alzheimer's Association
225 North Michigan Avenue, 17th Floor
Chicago, IL 60601-7633
Phone: 800-272-3900 (Helpline) or
   312-335-8700
Web site: www.alz.org

American Geriatrics Society
The Empire State Building
350 Fifth Avenue, Suite 801
New York, NY 10118
Phone: 212-308-1414
Web site: www.americangeriatrics.org

National Institute on Aging
Building 31, Room 5C27
31 Center Drive, MSC 2292
Bethesda, MD 20892
Phone: 301-496-1752 or 800-222-4225 (TTY)
Web site: www.nia.nih.gov

MENOPAUSE

American College of Obstetricians and
   Gynecologists
409 12th Street SW, P.O. Box 96920
Washington, DC 20090-6920
Phone: 202-638-5577
Web site: www.acog.org

American Geriatrics Society
The Empire State Building
350 Fifth Avenue, Suite 801
New York, NY 10118
Phone: 212-308-1414
Web site: www.americangeriatrics.org

National Institute on Aging
Building 31, Room 5C27
31 Center Drive, MSC 2292
Bethesda, MD 20892
Phone: 301-496-1752 or 800-222-4225 (TTY)
Web site: www.nia.nih.gov

National Women's Health Network
514 10th Street NW, Suite 400
Washington, DC 20004
Phone: 202-347-1140
Web site: www.nwhn.org

The North American Menopause Society
P.O. Box 94527
Cleveland, OH 44101
Phone: 440-442-7550
Web site: www.menopause.org

METABOLIC SYNDROME

American Association of Clinical Endocrinologists
245 Riverside Avenue, Suite 200
Jacksonville, FL 32202
Phone: 904-353-7878
Web site: www.aace.com

American Heart Association
7272 Greenville Avenue
Dallas, TX 75231
Phone: 800-AHA-USA-1 (242-8721)
Web site: www.americanheart.org

Endocrine Society
8401 Connecticut Avenue, Suite 900
Chevy Chase, MD 20815
Phone: 301-941-0200
Web site: www.endo-society.org

National Center for Chronic Disease Prevention and Health Promotion
Centers for Disease Control and Prevention
4770 Buford Highway NE, MS K-40
Atlanta, GA 30341-3717
Phone: 800-CDC-INFO (232-4636) or
    404-639-3311 or 888-232-6348 (TTY)
Web site: www.cdc.gov/nccdphp

National Heart, Lung, and Blood Institute Health Information Center
P.O. Box 30105
Bethesda, MD 20824-0105
Phone: 301-592-8573
Web site: www.nhlbi.nih.gov

MUSCLE CRAMPS

American Academy of Orthopaedic Surgeons
6300 North River Road
Rosemont, IL 60018-4262
Phone: 847-823-7186
Web site: www.aaos.org

American Physical Therapy Association
1111 North Fairfax Street
Alexandria, VA 22314-1488
Phone: 800-999-APTA (2782) or 703-684-APTA (2782) or 703-683-6748 (TDD)
Web site: www.apta.org

NAIL FUNGUS

American Academy of Dermatology
P.O. Box 4014
Schaumburg, IL 60618-4014
Phone: 866-503-SKIN (7546)
Web site: www.aad.org

American Podiatric Medical Association
9312 Old Georgetown Road
Bethesda, MD 20814-1621
Phone: 301-581-9200
Web site: www.apma.org

National Institute on Aging
Building 31, Room 5C27
31 Center Drive, MSC 2292
Bethesda, MD 20892
Phone: 301-496-1752 or 800-222-4225 (TTY)
Web site: www.nia.nih.gov

NIGHT VISION PROBLEMS

American Society of Cataract and Refractive Surgery
4000 Legato Road, Suite 700
Fairfax, VA 22033
Phone: 703-591-2220
Web site: www.ascrs.org

US National Library of Medicine
8600 Rockville Pike
Bethesda, MD 20894
Phone: 888-FIND-NLM (346-3656) or
    301-594-5983
Web site: www.nlm.nih.gov

Vision Surgery Rehab Network
1643 North Alpine Road, Suite 104, PMB 180
Rockford, IL 61107
Phone: 877-666-VSRN (8776)
Web site: www.visionsurgeryrehab.org

OBESITY

American Dietetic Association
120 South Riverside Plaza, Suite 2000
Chicago, IL 60606-6995
Phone: 800-877-1600
Web site: www.eatright.org

American Society of Bariatric Physicians
2821 South Parker Road, Suite 625
Aurora, CO 80014
Phone: 303-770-2526
Web site: www.asbp.org

Association for Behavioral and Cognitive Therapies
305 7th Avenue, 16th Floor
New York, NY 10001
Phone: 212-647-1890
Web site: www.aabt.org

Council on Size & Weight Discrimination
P.O. Box 305
Mount Marion, NY 12456
Phone: 845-679-1209
Web site: www.cswd.org

The Obesity Society
8630 Fenton Street, Suite 814
Silver Spring, MD 20910
Phone: 301-563-6526
Web site: www.obesity.org

Overeaters Anonymous
Wood Service Office
P.O. Box 44020
Rio Rancho, NM 87174-4020
Phone: 505-891-2664
Web site: www.oa.org

President's Council on Physical Fitness and
    Sports
Department W
200 Independence Avenue SW, Room 738-H
Washington, DC 20201-0004
Phone: 202-690-9000
Web site: www.fitness.gov

Shape Up America!
6707 Democracy Boulevard, Suite 306
Bethesda, MD 20817
Web site: www.shapeup.org

The Society for Surgery of the Alimentary Tract
900 Cummings Center, #221-U
Beverly, MA 01915
Phone: 978-927-8330
Web site: www.ssat.com

OSTEOARTHRITIS

American Academy of Orthopaedic Surgeons
6300 North River Road
Rosemont, IL 60018-4262
Phone: 847-823-7186
Web site: www.aaos.org

American Chronic Pain Association
P.O. Box 850
Rocklin, CA 95677
Phone: 800-533-3231
Web site: www.theacpa.org

American College of Rheumatology
1800 Century Place, Suite 250
Atlanta, GA 30345-4300
Phone: 404-633-3777
Web site: www.rheumatology.org

American Pain Society
4700 West Lake Avenue
Glenview, IL 60025
Phone: 847-375-4715
Web site: www.ampainsoc.org

Arthritis Foundation
P.O. Box 7669
Atlanta, GA 30357-0669
Phone: 800-283-7800
Web site: www.arthritis.org

OSTEOPOROSIS

American Society for Bone and Mineral Research
2025 M Street NW, Suite 800
Washington, DC 20036-3309
Phone: 202-367-1161
Web site: www.asbmr.org

National Osteoporosis Foundation
1232 22nd Street NW
Washington, DC 20037-1202
Phone: 800-231-4222 or 202-223-2226
Web site: www.nof.org

NIH Osteoporosis and Related Bone Diseases
    National Resource Center
2 AMS Circle
Bethesda, MD 20892-3676
Phone: 800-624-BONE (2663) or
    202-223-0344 or 202-466-4315 (TTY)
Web site: www.niams.nih.gov/bone

The North American Menopause Society
P.O. Box 94527
Cleveland, OH 44101
Phone: 440-442-7550
Web site: www.menopause.org

OVERACTIVE BLADDER

American Urogynecologic Society
2025 M Street NW, Suite 800
Washington, DC 20036
Phone: 202-367-1167
Web site: www.augs.org

American Urological Association
1000 Corporate Boulevard
Linthicum, MD 21090
Phone: 866-746-4282 (United States only) or
    410-689-3700
Web site: www.auanet.org

National Association for Continence
P.O. Box 1019
Charleston, SC 29402-1019
Phone: 800-BLADDER (252-3337) or
    843-377-0900
Web site: www.nafc.org

The Simon Foundation for Continence
P.O. Box 815
Wilmette, IL 60091
Phone: 800-23-SIMON (237-4666)
Web site: www.simonfoundation.org

PAGET'S DISEASE

American Society for Bone and Mineral Research
2025 M Street NW, Suite 800
Washington, DC 20036-3309
Phone: 202-367-1161
Web site: www.asbmr.org

NIH Osteoporosis and Related Bone Diseases
    National Resource Center
2 AMS Circle
Bethesda, MD 20892-3676
Phone: 800-624-BONE (2663) or
    202-223-0344 or 202-466-4315 (TTY)
Web site: www.niams.nih.gov/bone

Paget Foundation
120 Wall Street, Suite 1602
New York, NY 10005-4001
Phone: 800-23-PAGET (237-2438) or
    212-509-5335
Web site: www.paget.org

PARKINSON'S DISEASE

American Association of Neurological Surgeons
5550 Meadowbrook Drive
Rolling Meadows, IL 60008
Phone: 888-566-AANS (2267) or 847-378-
    0500
Web site: www.aans.org

American Neurological Association
5841 Cedar Lake Road, Suite 204
Minneapolis, MN 55416
Phone: 952-545-6284
Web site: www.aneuroa.org

The Michael J. Fox Foundation for Parkinson's
    Research
Church Street Station
P.O. Box 780
New York, NY 10008-0780
Phone: 800-708-7644
Web site: www.michaeljfox.org

National Parkinson Foundation
1501 NW 9th Avenue/Bob Hope Road
Miami, FL 33136-1494
Phone: 800-327-4545 or 305-243-6666
Web site: www.parkinson.org

Parkinson's Disease Foundation
1359 Broadway, Suite 1509
New York, NY 10018
Phone: 800-457-6676 or 212-923-4700
Web site: www.pdf.org

WE MOVE
204 West 84th Street
New York, NY 10024
Phone: 212-875-8312
Web site: www.wemove.org

PERIPHERAL NEUROPATHY

American Chronic Pain Association
P.O. Box 850
Rocklin, CA 95677
Phone: 800-533-3231
Web site: www.theacpa.org

American Pain Society
4700 West Lake Avenue
Glenview, IL 60025
Phone: 847-375-4715
Web site: www.ampainsoc.org

The National Foundation for the
    Treatment of Pain
P.O. Box 70045
Houston, TX 77270-0045
Phone: 713-862-9332
Web site: www.paincare.org

The Neuropathy Association
60 East 42nd Street, Suite 942
New York, NY 10165
Phone: 212-692-0662
Web site: www.neuropathy.org

PERIPHERAL VASCULAR DISEASE

American College of Cardiology
Heart House
2400 N Street NW
Washington, DC 20037
Phone: 202-375-6000
Web site: www.acc.org

American Heart Association
7272 Greenville Avenue
Dallas, TX 75231
Phone: 800-AHA-USA-1 (242-8721)
Web site: www.americanheart.org

National Heart, Lung, and Blood Institute Health
    Information Center
P.O. Box 30105
Bethesda, MD 20824-0105
Phone: 301-592-8573
Web site: www.nhlbi.nih.gov

PICK'S DISEASE

Alzheimer's Association
225 North Michigan Avenue, 17th Floor
Chicago, IL 60601-7633
Phone: 800-272-3900 (Helpline) or
    312-335-8700
Web site: www.alz.org

American Geriatrics Society
The Empire State Building
350 Fifth Avenue, Suite 801
New York, NY 10118
Phone: 212-308-1414
Web site: www.americangeriatrics.org

National Institute on Aging
Building 31, Room 5C27
31 Center Drive, MSC 2292
Bethesda, MD 20892
Phone: 301-496-1752 or 800-222-4225 (TTY)
Web site: www.nia.nih.gov

Office of Rare Diseases
National Institutes of Health
6100 Executive Boulevard, Room 3B01,
    MSC 7518
Bethesda, MD 20892-7518
Phone: 301-402-4336
Web site: http://rarediseases.info.nih.gov

PROSTATE ENLARGEMENT

American Urological Association
1000 Corporate Boulevard
Linthicum, MD 21090
Phone: 866-746-4282 (United States only) or
    410-689-3700
Web site: www.auanet.org

SeniorNet
900 Lafayette Street, Suite 604
Santa Clara, CA 95050
Phone: 408-615-0699
Web site: www.seniornet.org

PROSTATITIS

American Urological Association
1000 Corporate Boulevard
Linthicum, MD 21090
Phone: 866-746-4282 (United States only) or
    410-689-3700
Web site: www.auanet.org

Prostatitis Foundation
1063 30th Street, Box 8
Smithshire, IL 61478
Voice mail: 888-891-4200
Web site: www.prostatitis.org

RASHES

American Academy of Dermatology
P.O. Box 4014
Schaumburg, IL 60618-4014
Phone: 866-503-SKIN (7546)
Web site: www.aad.org

American Society for Dermatologic Surgery
5550 Meadowbrook Drive, Suite 120
Rolling Meadows, IL 60008
Phone: 847-956-0900
Web site: www.asds-net.org

National Eczema Association
4460 Redwood Highway, Suite 16-D
San Rafael, CA 94903-1953
Phone: 800-818-7546 or 415-499-3474
Web site: www.nationaleczema.org

**National Institute of Arthritis and Musculoskeletal
    and Skin Diseases**
Information Clearinghouse
National Institutes of Health
1 AMS Circle
Bethesda, MD 20892-3675
Phone: 877-22-NIAMS (226-4267) or
    301-495-4484 or 301-565-2966 (TTY)
Web site: www.niams.nih.gov

National Institute on Aging
Building 31, Room 5C27
31 Center Drive, MSC 2292
Bethesda, MD 20892
Phone: 301-496-1752 or 800-222-4225 (TTY)
Web site: www.nia.nih.gov

RHEUMATOID ARTHRITIS

American Academy of Orthopaedic Surgeons
6300 North River Road
Rosemont, IL 60018-4262
Phone: 847-823-7186
Web site: www.aaos.org

American Chronic Pain Association
P.O. Box 850
Rocklin, CA 95677
Phone: 800-533-3231
Web site: www.theacpa.org

American College of Rheumatology
1800 Century Place, Suite 250
Atlanta, GA 30345-4300
Phone: 404-633-3777
Web site: www.rheumatology.org

American Pain Society
4700 West Lake Avenue
Glenview, IL 60025
Phone: 847-375-4715
Web site: www.ampainsoc.org

Arthritis Foundation
P.O. Box 7669
Atlanta, GA 30357-0669
Phone: 800-283-7800
Web site: www.arthritis.org

ROSACEA

American Academy of Dermatology
P.O. Box 4014
Schaumburg, IL 60618-4014
Phone: 866-503-SKIN (7546)
Web site: www.aad.org

American Society for Dermatologic Surgery
5550 Meadowbrook Drive, Suite 120
Rolling Meadows, IL 60008
Phone: 847-956-0900
Web site: www.asds-net.org

National Institute of Arthritis and Musculoskeletal
and Skin Diseases
Information Clearinghouse
National Institutes of Health
1 AMS Circle
Bethesda, MD 20892-3675
Phone: 877-22-NIAMS (226-4267) or
301-495-4484 or 301-565-2966 (TTY)
Web site: www.niams.nih.gov

National Rosacea Society
800 South Northwest Highway, Suite 200
Barrington, IL 60010
Phone: 888-NO-BLUSH (662-5874)
Web site: www.rosacea.org

SHINGLES

American Chronic Pain Association
P.O. Box 850
Rocklin, CA 95677
Phone: 800-533-3231
Web site: www.theacpa.org

American Pain Society
4700 West Lake Avenue
Glenview, IL 60025
Phone: 847-375-4715
Web site: www.ampainsoc.org

National Institute of Neurological Disorders and
Stroke
P.O. Box 5801
Bethesda, MD 20824
Phone: 800-352-9424 or 301-496-5751 or
301-468-5981 (TTY)
Web site: www.ninds.nih.gov

SLEEP APNEA

American Academy of Dental Sleep Medicine
One Westbrook Corporate Center, Suite 920
Westchester, IL 60154
Phone: 708-273-9366
Web site: www.dentalsleepmed.org

American Academy of Sleep Medicine
One Westbrook Corporate Center, Suite 920
Westchester, IL 60154
Phone: 708-492-0930
Web site: www.aasmnet.org

American Sleep Apnea Association
1424 K Street NW, Suite 302
Washington, DC 20005
Phone: 202-293-3650
Web site: www.sleepapnea.org

National Center on Sleep Disorders Research
National Heart, Lung, and Blood Institute, NIH
6701 Rockledge Drive
Bethesda, MD 20892
Phone: 301-435-0199
Web site: www.nhlbi.nih.gov/about/ncsdr

National Sleep Foundation
1522 K Street NW, Suite 500
Washington, DC 20005
Phone: 202-347-3471
Web site: www.sleepfoundation.org

SNORING

American Academy of Dental Sleep Medicine
One Westbrook Corporate Center, Suite 920
Westchester, IL 60154
Phone: 708-273-9366
Web site: www.dentalsleepmed.org

American Academy of Sleep Medicine
One Westbrook Corporate Center, Suite 920
Westchester, IL 60154
Phone: 708-492-0930
Web site: www.aasmnet.org

National Center on Sleep Disorders Research
National Heart, Lung, and Blood Institute, NIH
6701 Rockledge Drive
Bethesda, MD 20892
Phone: 301-435-0199
Web site: www.nhlbi.nih.gov/about/ncsdr

National Sleep Foundation
1522 K Street NW, Suite 500
Washington, DC 20005
Phone: 202-347-3471
Web site: www.sleepfoundation.org

TINNITUS

Alexander Graham Bell Association for the Deaf
and Hard of Hearing
3417 Volta Place NW
Washington, DC 20007
Phone: 202-337-5220 or 202-337-5221 (TTY)
Web site: www.agbell.org

American Academy of Audiology
11730 Plaza America Drive, Suite 300
Reston, VA 20190
Phone: 800-AAA-2336 (222-2336) or
    703-790-8466
Web site: www.audiology.org

American Speech-Language-Hearing Association
2200 Research Boulevard
Rockville, MD 20850-3289
Phone: 800-498-2071 (member) or
    800-638-8255 (nonmember)
Web site: www.asha.org

American Tinnitus Association
Mailing Address:
P.O. Box 5
Portland, OR 97207-0005
Street Address:
65 SW Yamhill Street, Suite 200
Portland, OR 97204
Phone: 800-634-8978 (United States only) or
    503-248-9985
Web site: www.ata.org

Hearing Loss Association of America
7910 Woodmont Avenue, Suite 1200
Bethesda, MD 20814
Phone: 301-657-2248
Web site: www.shhh.org

National Institute on Aging
Building 31, Room 5C27
31 Center Drive, MSC 2292
Bethesda, MD 20892
Phone: 301-496-1752 or 800-222-4225 (TTY)
Web site: www.nia.nih.gov

National Institute on Deafness and Other
    Communication Disorders
National Institutes of Health
31 Center Drive, MSC 2320
Bethesda, MD 20892-2320
Phone: 800-241-1044 or 800-241-1055 (TTY)
Web site: www.nidcd.nih.gov

ULCERATIVE COLITIS

American College of Gastroenterology
P.O. Box 342260
Bethesda, MD 20827-2260
Phone: 301-263-9000
Web site: www.acg.gi.org

American Gastroenterological Association
4930 Del Ray Avenue
Bethesda, MD 20814
Phone: 301-654-2055
Web site: www.gastro.org

American Society of Colon and Rectal Surgeons
85 West Algonquin Road, Suite 550
Arlington Heights, IL 60005
Phone: 847-290-9184
Web site: www.fascrs.org

Crohn's and Colitis Foundation of America
386 Park Avenue South, 17th Floor
New York, NY 10016
Phone: 800-932-2423
Web site: www.ccfa.org

UTERINE FIBROIDS

American College of Obstetricians and
    Gynecologists
409 12th Street SW, P.O. Box 96920
Washington, DC 20090-6920
Phone: 202-638-5577
Web site: www.acog.org

National Uterine Fibroids Foundation
P.O. Box 9688
Colorado Springs, CO 80932-0688
Phone: 800-874-7247 or 719-633-3454
Web site: www.nuff.org

Society of Interventional Radiology
3975 Fair Ridge Drive, Suite 400 North
Fairfax, VA 22033
Phone: 800-488-7284 or 703-691-1805
Web site: www.sirweb.org

UTERINE PROLAPSE

American College of Obstetricians and
Gynecologists
409 12th Street SW, P.O. Box 96920
Washington, DC 20090-6920
Phone: 202-638-5577
Web site: www.acog.org

American Urogynecologic Society
2025 M Street NW, Suite 800
Washington, DC 20036
Phone: 202-367-1167
Web site: www.augs.org

National Women's Health Network
514 10th Street NW, Suite 400
Washington, DC 20004
Phone: 202-347-1140
Web site: www.nwhn.org

The North American Menopause Society
P.O. Box 94527
Cleveland, OH 44101
Phone: 440-442-7550
Web site: www.menopause.org

VAGINAL ATROPHY

American Geriatrics Society
The Empire State Building
350 Fifth Avenue, Suite 801
New York, NY 10118
Phone: 212-308-1414
Web site: www.americangeriatrics.org

National Institute on Aging
Building 31, Room 5C27
31 Center Drive, MSC 2292
Bethesda, MD 20892
Phone: 301-496-1752 or 800-222-4225 (TTY)
Web site: www.nia.nih.gov

The North American Menopause Society
P.O. Box 94527
Cleveland, OH 44101
Phone: 440-442-7550
Web site: www.menopause.org

VARICOSE VEINS

American Academy of Dermatology
P.O. Box 4014
Schaumburg, IL 60618-4014
Phone: 866-503-SKIN (7546)
Web site: www.aad.org

American College of Phlebology
100 Webster Street, Suite 101
Oakland, CA 94607-3724
Phone: 510-834-6500
Web site: www.phlebology.org

American Society for Dermatologic Surgery
5550 Meadowbrook Drive, Suite 120
Rolling Meadows, IL 60008
Phone: 847-956-0900
Web site: www.asds-net.org

American Venous Forum
203 Washington Street, PMB 311
Salem, MA 01970
Phone: 978-744-5005
Web site: www.venous-info.com

National Heart, Lung, and Blood Institute Health
Information Center
P.O. Box 30105
Bethesda, MD 20824-0105
Phone: 301-592-8573
Web site: www.nhlbi.nih.gov

WRINKLES

American Academy of Dermatology
P.O. Box 4014
Schaumburg, IL 60618-4014
Phone: 866-503-SKIN (7546)
Web site: www.aad.org

American Society for Aesthetic Plastic Surgery
11081 Winners Circle
Los Alamitos, CA 90720-2813
Phone: 888-ASAPS-11 (272-7711)
Web site: www.surgery.org

American Society for Dermatologic Surgery
5550 Meadowbrook Drive, Suite 120
Rolling Meadows, IL 60008
Phone: 847-956-0900
Web site: www.asds-net.org

American Society for Laser Medicine and Surgery
2100 Stewart Avenue, Suite 240
Wausau, WI 54401
Phone: 715-845-9283
Web site: www.aslms.org

American Society of Plastic Surgeons
444 East Algonquin Road
Arlington Heights, IL 60005
Phone: 888-4-PLASTIC or 888-475-2784
Web site: www.plasticsurgery.org

National Institute on Aging
Building 31, Room 5C27
31 Center Drive, MSC 2292
Bethesda, MD 20892
Phone: 301-496-1752 or 800-222-4225 (TTY)
Web site: www.nia.nih.gov

Professional Organizations for Complementary Therapies

The following professional organizations and teaching institutions can provide further information and/or a referral to a practitioner in your area.

ACUPRESSURE

American Organization for Bodywork Therapies of Asia (AOBTA)
Web site: www.aobta.org

National Certification Board for Therapeutic Massage and Bodywork
Web site: www.ncbtmb.org

National Certification Commission for Acupuncture and Oriental Medicine (NCCAOM)
Web site: www.nccaom.org

ACUPUNCTURE

American Association of Acupuncture and Oriental Medicine (AAAOM)
Web site: www.aaaomonline.org

National Certification Commission for Acupuncture and Oriental Medicine (NCCAOM)
Web site: www.nccaom.org

ALEXANDER TECHNIQUE

American Society for the Alexander Technique
Web site: www.alexandertech.org

AQUATIC THERAPY

Aquatic Exercise Association
Web site: www.aeawave.com

Red Cross
(Local chapters can be found in the Yellow Pages.)

AROMATHERAPY

Aromatherapy Registration Council (ARC)
Web site: www.aromatherapycouncil.org

National Association for Holistic Aromatherapy (NAHA)
Web site: www.naha.org

AYURVEDA

Ayurvedic Institute
Web site: www.ayurveda.com

BIOFEEDBACK

Biofeedback Certification Institute of America (BCIA)
Web site: www.bcia.org

CHIROPRACTIC

American Chiropractic Association (ACA)
Web site: www.amerchiro.org

CRANIOSACRAL THERAPY

International Association of Healthcare Practitioners (IAHP)
Web site: www.iahp.com

FELDENKRAIS METHOD

Feldenkrais Educational Foundation of North America (FEFNA)
Web site: www.feldenkrais.com

FLOWER ESSENCES

Flower Essence Society (FES)
Web site: www.flowersociety.org

HERBAL MEDICINE

American Association of Acupuncture and Oriental Medicine (AAAOM)
Web site: www.aaaomonline.org

American Holistic Medical Association (AHMA)
Web site: www.holisticmedicine.org

National Certification Commission for
Acupuncture and Oriental Medicine (NCCAOM)
Web site: www.nccaom.org

HOMEOPATHY

National Center for Homeopathy
Web site: www.homeopathic.org

HYPNOTHERAPY

American Society of Clinical Hypnosis
Web site: www.asch.net

National Guild of Hypnotists, Inc.
Web site: www.ngh.net

NATUROPATHY

American Association of Naturopathic Physicians
Web site: www.naturopathic.org

NUTRITIONAL COUNSELING

American Association of Nutritional Consultants
Web site: www.aanc.net

POLARITY THERAPY

National Certification Board for Therapeutic
Massage and Bodywork
Web site: www.ncbtmb.org

PSYCHOTHERAPY

American Psychiatric Association
Web site: www.psych.org

American Psychological Association
Web site: www.apa.org

National Association of Social Workers
Web site: www.naswdc.org

QIGONG

American Organization for Bodywork Therapies
of Asia (AOBTA)
Web site: www.aobta.org

REFLEXOLOGY

International Institute of Reflexology
Web site: www.reflexology-usa.net

REIKI

International Center for Reiki Training
Web site: www.reiki.org

Reiki Alliance
Web site: www.reikialliance.org

RELAXATION/MEDITATION

American Organization for Bodywork Therapies
of Asia (AOBTA)
Web site: www.aobta.org
(For tai chi and qigong)

International Association of Yoga Therapists (IAYT)
Web site: www.iayt.org

Transcendental Meditation Program
Web site: www.tm.org

ROLFING

National Certification Board for Therapeutic
Massage and Bodywork
Web site: www.ncbtmb.org

Rolf Institute of Structural Integration
Web site: www.rolf.org

SHIATSU

American Organization for Bodywork Therapies
of Asia (AOBTA)
Web site: www.aobta.org

National Certification Board for Therapeutic
Massage and Bodywork
Web site: www.ncbtmb.org

National Certification Commission for
Acupuncture and Oriental Medicine (NCCAOM)
Web site: www.nccaom.org

TAI CHI

American Organization for Bodywork Therapies
of Asia (AOBTA)
Web site: www.aobta.org

THERAPEUTIC MASSAGE

American Massage Therapy Association
Web site: www.massagetherapy.org

National Certification Board for Therapeutic
Massage and Bodywork
Web site: www.ncbtmb.org

THERAPEUTIC TOUCH

Nurse Healers–Professional Associates
 International
Web site: www.therapeutic-touch.org

TRADITIONAL CHINESE MEDICINE

American Association of Acupuncture and
 Oriental Medicine (AAAOM)
Web site: www.aaaomonline.org

American Association of Oriental Medicine
 (AAOM)
Web site: www.aaom.org

National Certification Commission for
 Acupuncture and Oriental Medicine (NCCAOM)
Web site: www.nccaom.org

TRAGER APPROACH

National Certification Board for Therapeutic
 Massage and Bodywork
Web site: www.ncbtmb.org

Trager International
Web site: www.trager.com

TRIGGER POINT THERAPY

International Myotherapy Association
Web site: www.myotherapy.org

YOGA

International Association of Yoga Therapists (IAYT)
Web site: www.iayt.org

Practitioners' Credentials for Complementary Therapies

When you're looking for a practitioner of a specific therapeutic approach, it is important to familiarize yourself with the degrees, certifications, licenses, and other credentials that are necessary or at least recommended for that discipline. The list below identifies appropriate credentials for the various complementary therapies that we discuss in this book. If a particular therapy doesn't appear here, it means that there are no formal educational or training requirements or relevant state licensing guidelines.

Please be aware that there is a difference between licensure and certification. For example, a person who uses the designation CMT (for certified massage therapist) or CMP (certified massage practitioner) is "certified" by virtue of having graduated from an accredited school of therapeutic massage. The designation LMT (licensed massage therapist) or LMP (licensed massage practitioner) indicates that in addition to having graduated from an accredited school of therapeutic massage, the person has met the licensing requirements of a particular state.

Note that licensing is not available in all states. For example, in Massachusetts, massage therapists are certified, since the state does not offer licensure at the present time.

ACUPRESSURE

AOBTA: American Organization for Bodywork Therapies of Asia
DiplABT: diplomate in Asian bodywork therapy
NCBTMB: National Certification Board for Therapeutic Massage and Bodywork

ACUPUNCTURE

CA: certified acupuncturist
DiplAc: diplomate in acupuncture
LAc, LicAc: licensed acupuncturist
MAc: master of acupuncture
RAc: registered acupuncturist

ALEXANDER TECHNIQUE

AmSAT: American Society for the Alexander Technique

AQUATIC THERAPY

WSI: water safety instructor (American Red Cross certification)

AROMATHERAPY

NAHA: National Association for Holistic Aromatherapy
RA: registered aromatherapist

AYURVEDA

BAMS: bachelor of Ayurveda medical studies

BIOFEEDBACK

BCIAC: Biofeedback Certification Institute of America certified

CHIROPRACTIC

DC: doctor of chiropractic

CRANIOSACRAL THERAPY

CST: craniosacral therapist
IAHP: International Association of Healthcare Practitioners

FELDENKRAIS METHOD

GCFP: guild certified Feldenkrais practitioner
Practitioners certified by the Feldenkrais Guild of North America (FGNA) also may use the following service marks:
Guild Certified Feldenkrais Practitioner
Guild Certified Feldenkrais Teacher

HOMEOPATHY

CCH: certified in classical homeopathy
DHANP: diplomate in Homeopathic Academy of Naturopathic Physicians
DHt: diplomate in homeotherapeutics

HYPNOTHERAPY

CH: certified hypnotherapist

LYMPHATIC MASSAGE

CMLDT: certified manual lymph drainage therapist
IAHP: International Association of Healthcare Practitioners

NATUROPATHY

ND: naturopathic doctor

NUTRITIONAL COUNSELING

CNC: certified nutritional consultant
LD: licensed dietitian
RD: registered dietitian

POLARITY THERAPY

NCBTMB: National Certification Board for Therapeutic Massage and Bodywork
RPP: registered polarity practitioner

PSYCHIATRIST

MD: medical doctor

PSYCHOLOGIST

EdD: doctor of education
MA: master of arts
PhD: doctor of philosophy
PsyD: doctor of psychology

PSYCHOTHERAPY

MA: master of arts
MEd: master of education

REFLEXOLOGY

NCBTMB: National Certification Board for Therapeutic Massage and Bodywork

REIKI

RM: Reiki Master

ROLFING

ACR, CAR: advanced certified Rolfer; certified advanced Rolfer
CR: certified Rolfer
NCBTMB: National Certification Board for Therapeutic Massage and Bodywork

SHIATSU

AOBTA: American Organization for Bodywork Therapies of Asia
DiplABT: diplomate in Asian Bodywork Therapy
NCBTMB: National Certification Board for Therapeutic Massage and Bodywork

SOCIAL WORKER

ACSW: Academy of Certified Social Workers
BCD: board-certified diplomate in clinical social work
CSW: certified social worker
DSW: doctor of social work
LCSW: licensed clinical social worker
LICSW: licensed independent clinical social worker
MSW: master of social work
PhD: doctor of philosophy

SPORTS MASSAGE

CSMT: certified sports massage therapist
NCBTMB: National Certification Board for
Therapeutic Massage and Bodywork

THERAPEUTIC MASSAGE (GENERAL)

CMP, CMT: certified massage practitioner,
certified massage therapist
LMP, LMT: licensed massage practitioner,
licensed massage therapist
MT/MsT: massage therapist (does not necessarily
indicate certification or licensure)
NCBTMB: National Certification Board for
Therapeutic Massage and Bodywork

TRADITIONAL CHINESE MEDICINE

DOM or OMD: doctor of oriental medicine
MOM: master of oriental medicine

TRAGER APPROACH

CTP: certified Trager practitioner
NCBTMB: National Certification Board for
Therapeutic Massage and Bodywork

TRIGGER POINT THERAPY

CBPM: certified Bonnie Prudden myotherapist

Source Notes

INTEGRATIVE MEDICINE: THE BEST OF ALL WORLDS

Kim DH, et al. CT colonography versus colonoscopy for the detection of advanced neoplasia. *New England Journal of Medicine*, October 4, 2007: 1403-1412.

SIGNS AND SYMPTOMS OF LIFE-THREATENING CONDITIONS

SOS-KANTO Study Group. Cardiopulmonary resuscitation by bystanders with chest compression only (SOS-KANTO): an observational study. *Lancet*, March 17, 2007: 920-926.

ALZHEIMER'S DISEASE

Cummings JL. Alzheimer's disease. *New England Journal of Medicine*, July 1, 2004: 56-67.

ANGINA

Yeghiazarians Y, et al. Unstable angina pectoris. *New England Journal of Medicine*, January 13, 2000: 101-114.

ANXIETY DISORDERS

Fricchione G. Clinical practice. Generalized anxiety disorder. *New England Journal of Medicine*, August 12, 2004: 675-682.

Morris N. The effects of lavender (Lavendula angustifolium) baths on psychological well-being: two exploratory randomised control trials. *Complementary Therapies in Medicine*, December 2002: 223-228.

ARTHRITIS (OSTEO- AND RHEUMATOID)

Berman BM, et al. Effectiveness of acupuncture as adjunctive therapy in osteoarthritis of the knee: a randomized, controlled trial. *Annals of Internal Medicine*, December 21, 2004: 901-910.

Geis GS. Arthrotec: a therapeutic option in the management of arthritis. *European Journal of Rheumatology and Inflammation*, January 1993: 25-32.

Han A, et al. Tai chi for treating rheumatoid arthritis. *Cochrane Database of Systematic Reviews*, 2004: CD004849.

Kulkarni B, et al. Arthritic pain is processed in brain areas concerned with emotions and fear. *Arthritis and Rheumatism*, April 2007: 1345-1354.

NCCAM, National Institutes of Health. Acupuncture found to be of benefit in knee osteoarthritis. *CAM at the NIH—Focus on Complementary and Alternative Medicine,* Winter 2005, Volume XII, Number 1.

Nicklas BJ, et al. Diet-induced weight loss, exercise, and chronic inflammation in older, obese adults: a randomized controlled clinical trial. *American Journal of Clinical Nutrition*, April 2004: 544-551.

Olsen NJ, Stein CM. New drugs for rheumatoid arthritis. *New England Journal of Medicine,* May 20, 2004: 2167-2179.

Sharma L, et al. Quadriceps strength and osteoarthritis progression in malaligned and lax knees. *Annals of Internal Medicine,* April 15, 2003: 613-619.

Towheed TE, Anastassiades TP. Glucosamine and chondroitin for treating symptoms of osteoarthritis: evidence is widely touted but incomplete. *JAMA,* March 15, 2000: 1483-1484.

Trock DH. Electromagnetic fields and magnets. Investigational treatment for musculoskeletal disorders. *Rheumatic Disease Clinic of North America,* February 2000: 51-62, viii.

van Baar ME, et al. Effectiveness of exercise therapy in patients with osteoarthritis of the hip or knee: a systematic review of randomized clinical trials. *Arthritis and Rheumatism,* July 1999: 1361-1369.

Witt C, et al. Acupuncture in patients with osteoarthritis of the knee: a randomised trial. *Lancet,* July 9-15, 2005: 136-143.

ATHEROSCLEROSIS

Howard G, et al. Cigarette smoking and progression of atherosclerosis: The Atherosclerosis Risk in Communities (ARIC) Study. *JAMA,* January 14, 1998: 119-124.

BACK PAIN

Brinkhaus B, et al. Acupuncture in patients with chronic low back pain: a randomized controlled trial. *Archives of Internal Medicine*, February 27, 2006: 450-457.

Carragee EJ. Clinical practice. Persistent low back pain. *New England Journal of Medicine,* May 5, 2005: 1891-1898.

Hayden JA, et al. Meta-analysis: exercise therapy for nonspecific low back pain. *Annals of Internal Medicine*, May 3, 2005: 765-775.

CARDIOVASCULAR CONDITIONS

Andersen LF, et al. Consumption of coffee is associated with reduced risk of death attributed to inflammatory and cardiovascular diseases in the Iowa Women's Health Study. *American Journal of Clinical Nutrition*, May 2006: 1039-1046.

Greenberg JA, et al. Caffeinated beverage intake and the risk of heart disease mortality in the elderly: a prospective analysis. *American Journal of Clinical Nutrition*, February 2007: 392-398.

Hansson GK. Inflammation, atherosclerosis, and coronary artery disease. *New England Journal of Medicine*, April 21, 2005: 1685-1695.

Jayadevappa R, et al. Effectiveness of transcendental meditation on functional capacity and quality of life of African Americans with congestive heart failure: a randomized control study. *Ethnicity & Disease,* Winter 2007: 72-77.

Johnsen SP, et al. Intake of fruit and vegetables and the risk of ischemic stroke in a cohort of Danish men and women. *American Journal of Clinical Nutrition*, July 2003: 57-64.

Joshipura KJ, et al. Fruit and vegetable intake in relation to risk of ischemic stroke. *JAMA*, October 6, 1999: 1233-1239.

Joshipura KJ, et al. The effect of fruit and vegetable intake on risk for coronary heart disease. *Annals of Internal Medicine,* June 19, 2001: 1106-1114.

Khatta M, et al. The effect of coenzyme Q_{10} in patients with congestive heart failure. *Annals of Internal Medicine,* April 18, 2000: 636-640.

Lee IM, et al. Relative intensity of physical activity and risk of coronary heart disease. *Circulation*, March 4, 2003: 1110-1116.

Manson JE, et al. Walking compared with vigorous exercise for the prevention of cardiovascular events in women. *New England Journal of Medicine,* September 5, 2002: 716-725.

Mink PJ, et al. Flavonoid intake and cardiovascular disease mortality: a prospective study in postmenopausal women. *American Journal of Clinical Nutrition*, March 2007: 895-909.

Whooley MA. Depression and cardiovascular disease: healing the broken-hearted. *JAMA,* June 28, 2006: 2874-2881.

Wilkinson IB, et al. Oral vitamin C reduces arterial stiffness and platelet aggregation in humans. *Journal of Cardiovascular Pharmacology,* November 1999: 690-693.

Yochum LA, et al. Intake of antioxidant vitamins and risk of death from stroke in postmenopausal women. *American Journal of Clinical Nutrition*, August 2000: 476-483.

CATARACTS

Chasan-Taber L, et al. A prospective study of carotenoid and vitamin A intakes and risk of cataract extraction in US women. *American Journal of Clinical Nutrition*, October 1999: 509-516.

Christen WG, et al. Fruit and vegetable intake and the risk of cataract in women. *American Journal of Clinical Nutrition*, June 2005: 1417-1422.

Hankinson SE, et al. A prospective study of cigarette smoking and risk of cataract surgery in women. *JAMA*, August 26, 1992: 994-998.

Schaumberg DA, et al. Relations of body fat distribution and height with cataract in men. *American Journal of Clinical Nutrition*, December 2000: 1495-1502.

Taylor A, et al. Long-term intake of vitamins and carotenoids and odds of early age-related cortical and posterior subcapsular lens opacities. *American Journal of Clinical Nutrition*, March 2002: 540-549.

Taylor A, et al. Relations among aging, antioxidant status, and cataract. *American Journal of Clinical Nutrition*, December 1995: 1439S-1447S.

Valero MP, et al. Vitamin C is associated with reduced risk of cataract in a Mediterranean population. *Journal of Nutrition,* June 2002: 1299-1306.

CELIAC DISEASE

Catassi C, et al. Risk of non-Hodgkin lymphoma in celiac disease. *JAMA,* March 20, 2002: 1413-1419.

Dahele A, Ghosh S. Vitamin B_{12} deficiency in untreated celiac disease. *American Journal of Gastroenterology,* March 2001: 745-750.

Murray JA, et al. Effect of a gluten-free diet on gastrointestinal symptoms in celiac disease. *American Journal of Clinical Nutrition*, April 2004: 669-673.

CHRONIC FATIGUE SYNDROME

Prins JB, et al. Chronic fatigue syndrome. *Lancet*, January 28, 2006: 346-355.

Wang O, Xiong JX. Clinical observation on effect of electro-acupuncture on back-shu points in treating chronic fatigue syndrome. *Zhongguo Zhong Xi Yi Jie He Za Zhi,* September 2005: 834-836.

Whiting P, et al. Interventions for the treatment and management of chronic fatigue syndrome: a systematic review. *JAMA,* September 19, 2001: 1360-1368.

COLON POLYPS

Chan AT, et al. Aspirin and the risk of colorectal cancer in relation to the expression of COX-2. *New England Journal of Medicine,* May 24, 2007: 2131-2142.

Lieberman DA, et al. Risk factors for advanced colonic neoplasia and hyperplastic polyps in asymptomatic individuals. *JAMA,* December 10, 2003: 2959-2967.

CROHN'S DISEASE

Joos S, et al. Acupuncture and moxibustion in the treatment of active Crohn's disease: a randomized controlled study. *Digestion,* 2004;69: 131-139.

Korzenik JR, et al. Sargramostim for active Crohn's disease. *New England Journal of Medicine,* May 26, 2005: 2193-2201.

DEEP VEIN THROMBOSIS

Bates SM, Ginsberg JS. Clinical practice. Treatment of deep-vein thrombosis. *New England Journal of Medicine*, July 15, 2004: 268-277.

Pittler MH, Ernst E. Horse-chestnut seed extract for chronic venous insufficiency: a criteria-based systematic review. *Archives of Dermatology,* November 1998: 1356-1360.

Steffen LM, et al. Greater fish, fruit, and vegetable intakes are related to lower incidence of venous thromboembolism: the Longitudinal Investigation of Thromboembolism Etiology. *Circulation,* January 16, 2007: 188-195.

DEPRESSION

Eich H, et al. Acupuncture in patients with minor depressive episodes and generalized anxiety. Results of an experimental study. *Fortschritte der Neurologie–Psychiatrie,* March 2000: 137-144.

Rush AJ, et al. Bupropion-SR, sertraline, or venlafaxine-XR after failure of SSRIs for depression. *New England Journal of Medicine,* March 23, 2006: 1231-1242.

DIABETES

Belcaro G, et al. Diabetic ulcers: microcirculatory improvement and faster healing with pycnogenol. *Clinical and Applied Thrombosis/Hemostasis,* July 2006: 318-323.

Hu FB, et al. Walking compared with vigorous physical activity and risk of type 2 diabetes in women: a prospective study. *JAMA,* October 20, 1999: 1433-1439.

Jenkins DJ, et al. Type 2 diabetes and the vegetarian diet. *American Journal of Clinical Nutrition*, September 2003: 610S-616S.

McGinnis RA, et al. Biofeedback-assisted relaxation in type 2 diabetes. *Diabetes Care,* September 2005: 2145-2149.

Meisinger C, et al. Body fat distribution and risk of type 2 diabetes in the general population: are there differences between men and women? The MONICA/KORA Augsburg cohort study. *American Journal of Clinical Nutrition,* September 2006: 483-489.

Meyer KA, et al. Carbohydrates, dietary fiber, and incident type 2 diabetes in older women. *American Journal of Clinical Nutrition*, April 2000: 921-930.

Nathan DM, et al. Intensive diabetes treatment and cardiovascular disease in patients with type 1 diabetes. *New England Journal of Medicine*, December 22, 2005: 2643-2653.

Nissen SE, Wolski K. Effect of rosiglitazone on the risk of myocardial infarction and death from cardiovascular causes. *New England Journal of Medicine,* June 14, 2007: 2457-2471.

Pham AQ, et al. Cinnamon supplementation in patients with type 2 diabetes mellitus. *Pharmacotherapy,* April 2007: 595-599.

Pittas AG, et al. Vitamin D and calcium intake in relation to type 2 diabetes in women. *Diabetes Care,* March 2006: 650-656.

Salmerón J, et al. Dietary fat intake and risk of type 2 diabetes in women. *American Journal of Clinical Nutrition,* June 2001: 1019-1026.

Vuksan V, et al. American ginseng (Panax quinquefolius L) reduces postprandial glycemia in nondiabetic subjects and subjects with type 2 diabetes mellitus. *Archives of Internal Medicine,* April 10, 2000: 1009-1013.

EMPHYSEMA

Fishman A., et al. A randomized trial comparing lung-volume-reduction surgery with medical therapy for severe emphysema. *New England Journal of Medicine,* May 22, 2003: 2059-2073.

Gigliotti F, et al. Breathing retraining and exercise conditioning in patients with chronic obstructive pulmonary disease (COPD): a physiological approach. *Respiratory Medicine,* March 2003: 197-204.

ERECTILE DYSFUNCTION

Aydin S, et al. Acupuncture and hypnotic suggestions in the treatment of non-organic male sexual dysfunction. *Scandinavian Journal of Urology and Nephrology,* June 1997: 271-274.

Bacon CG, et al. Sexual function in men older than 50 years of age: results from the Health Professionals Follow-up Study. *Annals of Internal Medicine,* August 5, 2003: 161-168.

Chen J, et al. Effect of oral administration of high-dose nitric oxide donor L-arginine in men with organic erectile dysfunction: results of a double-blind, randomized, placebo-controlled study. *BJU International,* February 1999: 269-273.

Dorey G, et al. Pelvic floor exercises for erectile dysfunction. *BJU International,* September 2005: 595-597.

Esposito K, et al. Effect of lifestyle changes on erectile dysfunction in obese men: a randomized controlled trial. *JAMA,* June 23, 2004: 2978-2984.

Hong B, et al. A double-blind crossover study evaluating the efficacy of Korean red ginseng in patients with erectile dysfunction: a preliminary report. *Journal of Urology,* November 2002: 2070-2073.

Kho HG, et al. The use of acupuncture in the treatment of erectile dysfunction. *International Journal of Impotence Research,* February 1999: 41-46.

Thompson IM, et al. Erectile dysfunction and subsequent cardiovascular disease. *JAMA,* December 21, 2005: 2996-3002.

ESSENTIAL TREMOR

Louis ED. Clinical practice. Essential tremor. *New England Journal of Medicine,* September 20, 2001: 887-891.

FEMALE SEXUAL DYSFUNCTION

Clayton AH, et al. Prevalence of sexual dysfunction among newer antidepressants. *Journal of Clinical Psychiatry,* April 2002: 357-366.

Kennedy SH, et al. Sexual dysfunction before antidepressant therapy in major depression. *Journal of Affective Disorders,* December 1999: 201-208.

Laumann EO, et al. Sexual dysfunction in the United States: prevalence and predictors. *JAMA,* February 10, 1999: 537-544.

Lindau ST, et al. A study of sexuality and health among older adults in the United States. *New England Journal of Medicine,* August 23, 2007: 762-774.

FIBROMYALGIA

Field T, et al. Fibromyalgia pain and substance P decrease and sleep improves after massage therapy. *Journal of Clinical Rheumatology,* April 2002: 72-76.

Goldenberg DL, et al. Management of fibromyalgia syndrome. *JAMA,* November 17, 2004: 2388-2395.

Leventhal LJ. Management of fibromyalgia. *Annals of Internal Medicine,* December 7, 1999: 850-858.

Meyer BB, Lemley KJ. Utilizing exercise to affect the symptomology of fibromyalgia: a pilot study. *Medicine and Science in Sports and Exercise,* October 2000: 1691-1697.

Rossy LA, et al. A meta-analysis of fibromyalgia treatment interventions. *Annals of Behavioral Medicine,* Spring 1999: 180-191.

FLATULENCE

Tomlin J, et al. Investigation of normal flatus production in healthy volunteers. *Gut,* June 1991: 665-669.

GALLSTONES

Cabrera C, et al. Beneficial effects of green tea—a review. *Journal of the American College of Nutrition*, April 2006: 79-99.

Leitzmann MF, et al. A prospective study of coffee consumption and the risk of symptomatic gallstone disease in men. *JAMA,* June 9, 1999: 2106-2112.

Misciagna G, et al. Diet, physical activity, and gallstones—a population-based, case-control study in southern Italy. *American Journal of Clinical Nutrition*, January 1999, 120-126.

Tsai CJ, et al. Long-term intake of *trans*-fatty acids and risk of gallstone disease in men. *Archives of Internal Medicine,* May 9, 2005: 1011-1015.

Tsai CJ, et al. Prospective study of abdominal adiposity and gallstone disease in US men. *American Journal of Clinical Nutrition*, July 2004: 38-44.

Tsai CJ, et al. Weight cycling and risk of gallstone disease in men. *Archives of Internal Medicine.* November 27, 2006: 2369-2374.

GASTROESOPHAGEAL REFLUX DISEASE (GERD)

Jacobson BC, et al. Body-mass index and symptoms of gastroesophageal reflux in women. *New England Journal of Medicine,* June 1, 2006: 2340-2348.

Lagergren J. Body measures in relation to gastroesophageal reflux. *Gut,* June 2007: 741-742.

Spechler SJ, et al. Long-term outcome of medical and surgical therapies for gastroesophageal reflux disease: follow-up of a randomized, controlled trial. *JAMA,* May 9, 2001: 2331-2338.

GLAUCOMA

Alward WL. Medical management of glaucoma. *New England Journal of Medicine*, October 29, 1998: 1298-1307.

GOUT

Choi HK, et al. Pathogenesis of gout. *Annals of Internal Medicine*, October 4, 2005: 499-516.

GUM DISEASE

Staudte H, et al. Grapefruit consumption improves vitamin C status in periodontitis patients. *British Dental Journal*, August 27, 2005: 213-217.

Tomar SL, Asma S. Smoking-attributable periodontitis in the United States: findings from NHANES III. National Health and Nutrition Examination Survey. *Journal of Periodontology,* May 2000: 743-751.

Vandana KL, Reddy MS. Assessment of periodontal status in dental fluorosis subjects using community periodontal index of treatment needs. *Indian Journal of Dental Research,* April-June 2007: 67-71.

HAIR LOSS

Price VH. Treatment of hair loss. *New England Journal of Medicine,* September 23, 1999: 964-973.

HEARING LOSS

Dobie RA. Folate supplementation and age-related hearing loss. *Annals of Internal Medicine,* January 2, 2007: 63-64.

Durga J, et al. Effects of folic acid supplementation on hearing in older adults: a randomized, controlled trial. *Annals of Internal Medicine,* January 2, 2007: 1-9.

Houston DK, et al. Age-related hearing loss, vitamin B_{12}, and folate in elderly women. *American Journal of Clinical Nutrition*, March 1999: 564-571.

Mizoue T, et al. Combined effect of smoking and occupational exposure to noise on hearing loss in steel factory workers. *Occupational and Environmental Medicine,* January 2003: 56-59.

Rueter A. Nutrients might prevent hearing loss in war zones, concert halls and workplaces, new animal study suggests. www.med.umich.edu/opm/newspage/2007/hearingloss.htm. March 28, 2007.

HEART PALPITATIONS

Zimetbaum P, Josephson ME. Evaluation of patients with palpitations. *New England Journal of Medicine,* May 7, 1998: 1369-1373.

HIGH BLOOD PRESSURE

Beulens JW, et al. Alcohol consumption and risk for coronary heart disease among men with hypertension. *Annals of Internal Medicine,* January 2, 2007: 10-19.

Burgess E, et al. Lifestyle recommendations to prevent and control hypertension. 6. Recommendations on potassium, magnesium and calcium. Canadian Hypertension Society, Canadian Coalition for High Blood Pressure Prevention and Control, Laboratory Centre for Disease Control at Health Canada, Heart and Stroke Foundation of Canada. *Canadian Medical Association Journal,* May 4, 1999: S35-S45.

Cabrera C, et al. Beneficial effects of green tea— a review. *Journal of the American College of Nutrition,* April 2006: 79-99.

Chiu YJ, et al. Cardiovascular and endocrine effects of acupuncture in hypertensive patients. *Clinical and Experimental Hypertension,* October 1997: 1047-1063.

Choudhury A, Lip GY. Exercise and hypertension. *Journal of Human Hypertension,* August 2005: 585-587.

Hagberg JM, et al. The role of exercise training in the treatment of hypertension: an update. *Sports Medicine,* September 2000: 193-206.

Hulsman CA, et al. Blood pressure, arterial stiffness, and open-angle glaucoma: the Rotterdam study. *Archives of Ophthalmology,* June 2007: 805-812.

Kaushik RM, et al. Effects of mental relaxation and slow breathing in essential hypertension. *Complementary Therapies in Medicine,* June 2006: 120-126.

Laterza MC, et al. Exercise training restores baroreflex sensitivity in never-treated hypertensive patients. *Hypertension,* June 2007: 1298-1306.

Messerli FH, et al. Essential hypertension. *Lancet,* August 18, 2007: 591-603.

Peluso MR. Flavonoids attenuate cardiovascular disease, inhibit phosphodiesterase, and modulate lipid homeostasis in adipose tissue and liver. *Experimental Biology and Medicine,* September 2006: 1287-1299.

Peppard PE, et al. Prospective study of the association between sleep-disordered breathing and hypertension. *New England Journal of Medicine,* May 11, 2000: 1378-1384.

Welty FK, et al. Effect of soy nuts on blood pressure and lipid levels in hypertensive, prehypertensive, and normotensive postmenopausal women. *Archives of Internal Medicine,* May 28, 2007: 1060-1067.

HIGH CHOLESTEROL

Kodama S, et al. Effect of aerobic exercise training on serum levels of high-density lipoprotein cholesterol: a meta-analysis. *Archives of Internal Medicine,* May 28, 2007: 999-1008.

Nissen SE, et al. Statin therapy, LDL cholesterol, C-reactive protein, and coronary artery disease. *New England Journal of Medicine,* January 6, 2005: 29-38.

Welty FK, et al. Effect of soy nuts on blood pressure and lipid levels in hypertensive, prehypertensive, and normotensive postmenopausal women. *Archives of Internal Medicine,* May 28, 2007: 1060-1067.

HIP FRACTURE

Baron JA, et al. Cigarette smoking, alcohol consumption, and risk of hip fracture in women. *Archives of Internal Medicine,* April 9, 2001: 983-988.

Feskanich D, et al. Vitamin K intake and hip fractures in women: a prospective study. *American Journal of Clinical Nutrition,* January 1999: 74-79.

Kujala UM, et al. Physical activity and osteoporotic hip fracture risk in men. *Archives of Internal Medicine,* March 13, 2000: 705-708.

Langlois JA, et al. Hip fracture risk in older white men is associated with change in body weight from age 50 years to old age. *Archives of Internal Medicine,* May 11, 1998: 990-996.

Sellmeyer DE, et al. A high ratio of dietary animal to vegetable protein increases the rate of bone loss and the risk of fracture in postmenopausal women. Study of Osteoporotic Fractures Research Group. *American Journal of Clinical Nutrition*, January 2001: 118-122.

HYPERTHYROIDISM

Cooper DS. Antithyroid drugs. *New England Journal of Medicine,* March 3, 2005: 905-917.

HYPOTHYROIDISM

Pearce EN, et al. Thyroiditis. *New England Journal of Medicine,* June 26, 2003: 2646-2655.

INCONTINENCE

Albo ME, et al. Burch colposuspension versus fascial sling to reduce urinary stress incontinence. *New England Journal of Medicine,* May 24, 2007: 2143-2155.

Ouslander JG. Management of overactive bladder. *New England Journal of Medicine,* February 19, 2004: 786-799.

INDIGESTION

Holtmann G, et al. A placebo-controlled trial of itopride in functional dyspepsia. *New England Journal of Medicine,* February 23, 2006: 832-840.

INFLUENZA

Barak V, et al. The effect of Sambucol, a black elderberry-based, natural product, on the production of human cytokines: I. Inflammatory cytokines. *European Cytokine Network,* April-June 2001: 290-296.

Barrett BP, et al. Treatment of the common cold with unrefined echinacea. A randomized, double-blind, placebo-controlled trial. *Annals of Internal Medicine,* December 17, 2002: 936-946.

Cabrera C, et al. Beneficial effects of green tea—a review. *Journal of the American College of Nutrition*, April 2006: 79-99.

Fortes C, et al. The effect of zinc and vitamin A supplementation on immune response in an older population. *Journal of the American Geriatrics Society*, January 1998: 19-26.

Moscona A. Neuraminidase inhibitors for influenza. *New England Journal of Medicine,* September 29, 2005: 1363-1373.

INSOMNIA

Cerny A, Schmid K. Tolerability and efficacy of valerian/lemon balm in healthy volunteers (a double-blind, placebo-controlled, multicentre study). *Fitoterapia,* June 1, 1999: 221-228.

Lin Y. Acupuncture treatment for insomnia and acupuncture analgesia. *Psychiatry and Clinical Neurosciences,* May 1995: 119-120.

Silber MH. Clinical practice. Chronic insomnia. *New England Journal of Medicine,* August 25, 2005: 803-810.

IRRITABLE BOWEL SYNDROME

Chan J, et al. The role of acupuncture in the treatment of irritable bowel syndrome: a pilot study. *Hepatogastroenterology,* September-October 1997: 1328-1330.

Hayee B, Forgacs I. Psychological approach to managing irritable bowel syndrome. *BMJ,* May 26, 2007: 1105-1109.

Horwitz BJ, Fisher S. The irritable bowel syndrome. *New England Journal of Medicine,* June 14, 2001: 1846-1850.

Li Y, et al. The effect of acupuncture on gastrointestinal function and disorders. *American Journal of Gastroenterology,* October 1992: 1372-1381.

KIDNEY STONES

Hollingsworth JM, et al. Medical therapy to facilitate urinary stone passage: a meta-analysis. *Lancet,* September 30, 2006: 1171-79.

MACULAR DEGENERATION

de Jong PT. Age-related macular degeneration. *New England Journal of Medicine*, October 5, 2006: 1474-1485.

Krinsky NI, et al. Biologic mechanisms of the protective role of lutein and zeaxanthin in the eye. *Annual Review of Nutrition,* 2003;23: 171-201.

Mares JA, Moeller SM. Diet and age-related macular degeneration: expanding our view. *American Journal of Clinical Nutrition*, April 2006: 733-734.

Seddon JM. Multivitamin-multimineral supplements and eye disease: age-related macular degeneration and cataract. *American Journal of Clinical Nutrition*, January 2007: 304S-307S.

MALE MENOPAUSE

Federman DD. The biology of human sex differences. *New England Journal of Medicine,* April 6, 2006: 1507-1514.

MEMORY LOSS

Wilson RS, et al. Chronic distress and incidence of mild cognitive impairment. *Neurology,* June 12, 2007: 2085-2092.

MENOPAUSE

Albertazzi P, et al. The effect of dietary soy supplementation on hot flushes. *Obstetrics and Gynecology,* January 1998: 6-11.

Elavsky S, McAuley E. Physical activity and mental health outcomes during menopause: a randomized controlled trial. *Annals of Behavioral Medicine*, April 2007: 132-142.

Kronenberg F, Fugh-Berman A. Complementary and alternative medicine for menopausal symptoms: a review of randomized, controlled trials. *Annals of Internal Medicine,* November 19, 2002: 805-813.

Messina MJ. Soy foods and soybean isoflavones and menopausal health. *Nutrition in Clinical Care,* November-December 2002: 272-282.

Miszko TA, Cress ME. A lifetime of fitness. Exercise in the perimenopausal and postmenopausal woman. *Clinics in Sports Medicine,* April 2000: 215-232.

METABOLIC SYNDROME

Ford ES, et al. Prevalence of the metabolic syndrome among US adults: findings from the third National Health and Nutrition Examination Survey. *JAMA,* January 16, 2002: 356-359.

Lakka HM, et al. The metabolic syndrome and total and cardiovascular disease mortality in middle-aged men, *JAMA,* December 4, 2002: 2709-2716.

Wannamethee SG, et al. Metabolic syndrome vs Framingham Risk Score for prediction of coronary heart disease, stroke, and type 2 diabetes mellitus. *Archives of Internal Medicine,* December 12-26, 2005: 2644-2650.

MUSCLE CRAMPS

Thompson PD, et al. Statin-associated myopathy. *JAMA,* April 2, 2003: 1681-1690.

NAIL FUNGUS

Buck DS, et al. Comparison of two topical preparations for the treatment of onychomycosis: Melaleuca alternifolia (tea tree) oil and clotrimazole. *Journal of Family Practice,* June 1994: 601-605.

Gupta AK, et al. Ciclopirox nail lacquer topical solution 8% in the treatment of toenail onychomycosis. *Journal of the American Academy of Dermatology,* October 2000: S70-S80.

OBESITY

Jakicic JM, et al. Effect of exercise duration and intensity on weight loss in overweight, sedentary women: a randomized trial. *JAMA,* September 10, 2003: 1323-1330.

Sjöström L, et al. Effects of bariatric surgery on mortality in Swedish obese subjects. *New England Journal of Medicine*, August 23, 2007: 741-752.

Stenlöf K, et al. Topiramate in the treatment of obese subjects with drug-naive type 2 diabetes. *Diabetes, Obesity and Metabolism,* May 2007: 360-368.

Wansink B, Chandon P. Meal size, not body size, explains errors in estimating the calorie content of meals. *Annals of Internal Medicine,* September 5, 2006: 326-332.

Wing RR, Hill JO. Successful weight loss maintenance. *Annual Review of Nutrition,* 2001;21: 323-341.

OSTEOPOROSIS

Bone HG, et al. Ten years' experience with alendronate for osteoporosis in postmenopausal women. *New England Journal of Medicine,* March 18, 2004: 1189-1199.

Marini H, et al. Effects of the phytoestrogen genistein on bone metabolism in osteopenic post-menopausal women: a randomized trial. *Annals of Internal Medicine,* June 19, 2007: 839-847.

Meunier PJ, et al. The effects of strontium ranelate on the risk of vertebral fracture in women with postmenopausal osteoporosis. *New England Journal of Medicine,* January 29, 2004: 459-68.

Orwoll E, et al. Alendronate for the treatment of osteoporosis in men. *New England Journal of Medicine,* August 31, 2000: 604-610.

Tang BM, et al. Use of calcium or calcium in combination with vitamin D supplementation to prevent fractures and bone loss in people aged 50 years and older: a meta-analysis. *Lancet,* August 25, 2007: 657-666.

OVERACTIVE BLADDER

Ouslander JG. Management of overactive bladder. *New England Journal of Medicine,* February 19, 2004: 786-799.

PAGET'S DISEASE

Whyte MP. Clinical practice. Paget's disease of bone. *New England Journal of Medicine,* August 10, 2006: 593-600.

PARKINSON'S DISEASE

Deuschl G, et al. A randomized trial of deep-brain stimulation for Parkinson's disease. *New England Journal of Medicine,* August 31, 2006: 896-908.

Dick FD, et al. Environmental risk factors for Parkinson's disease and parkinsonism: the Geoparkinson study. *Occupational and Environmental Medicine,* October 2007: 666-672.

PERIPHERAL NEUROPATHY

Mendell JR, Sahenk Z. Clinical practice. Painful sensory neuropathy. *New England Journal of Medicine,* March 27, 2003: 1243-1255.

PICK'S DISEASE

McKhann GM, et al. Clinical and pathological diagnosis of frontotemporal dementia: report of the Work Group on Frontotemporal Dementia and Pick's Disease. *Archives of Neurology,* November 2001: 1803-1809.

PROSTATE ENLARGEMENT

Wilt TJ, et al. Saw palmetto extracts for treatment of benign prostatic hyperplasia: a systematic review. *JAMA,* November 11, 1998: 1604-1609.

PROSTATITIS

Schaeffer AJ. Clinical practice. Chronic prostatitis and the chronic pelvic pain syndrome. *New England Journal of Medicine,* October 19, 2006: 1690-1698.

ROSACEA

Chiu AE, et al. Double-blinded, placebo-controlled trial of green tea extracts in the clinical and histologic appearance of photoaging skin. *Dermatologic Surgery,* July 2005: 855-860.

Hsu S. Green tea and the skin. *Journal of the American Academy of Dermatology,* June 2005: 1049-1059.

SHINGLES

Irwin MR, et al. Augmenting immune responses to varicella zoster virus in older adults: a randomized, controlled trial of Tai Chi. *Journal of the American Geriatrics Society,* April 2007: 511-517.

SLEEP APNEA

Basner RC. Continuous positive airway pressure for obstructive sleep apnea. *New England Journal of Medicine,* April 26, 2007: 1751-1758.

Wang XH, et al. Clinical observation on effect of auricular acupoint pressing in treating sleep apnea syndrome. *Zhongguo Zhong Xi Yi Jie He Za Zhi,* October 2003: 747-749.

Yaggi HK, et al. Obstructive sleep apnea as a risk factor for stroke and death. *New England Journal of Medicine,* November 10, 2005: 2034-2041.

SNORING

Lenclud C, et al. Effects of chondroitin sulfate on snoring characteristics: a pilot study. *Current Therapeutic Research,* April 1998: 234-243.

Nieto FJ, et al. Association of sleep-disordered breathing, sleep apnea, and hypertension in a large community-based study. Sleep Heart Health Study. *JAMA,* April 12, 2000: 1829-1836.

TINNITUS

Lockwood AH, et al. Tinnitus. *New England Journal of Medicine,* September 19, 2002: 904-910.

ULCERATIVE COLITIS

Podolsky DK. Inflammatory bowel disease. *New England Journal of Medicine,* August 8, 2002: 417-429.

Rutgeerts P, et al. Infliximab for induction and maintenance therapy for ulcerative colitis. *New England Journal of Medicine,* December 8, 2005: 2462-2476.

UTERINE FIBROIDS

Edwards RD, et al. Uterine-artery embolization versus surgery for symptomatic uterine fibroids. *New England Journal of Medicine,* January 25, 2007: 360-370.

VAGINAL ATROPHY

Grady D. Clinical practice. Management of menopausal symptoms. *New England Journal of Medicine,* November 30, 2006: 2338-2347.

VARICOSE VEINS

Bergan JJ, et al. Chronic venous disease. *New England Journal of Medicine,* August 3, 2006: 488-498.

Lee AJ, et al. Lifestyle factors and the risk of varicose veins: Edinburgh Vein Study. *Journal of Clinical Epidemiology,* February 2003: 171-179.

WRINKLES

Helfrich YR, et al. Effect of smoking on aging of photoprotected skin: evidence gathered using a new photonumeric scale. *Archives of Dermatology,* March 2007: 397-402.

Reading List
for Complementary Therapies

Aihara, Cornelia, and Aihara, Herman, with Carl Ferré. *Natural Healing from Head to Toe: Traditional Macrobiotic Remedies.* Garden City Park, NY: Avery Publishing Group, 1994.

Ain, Kenneth B., M.D., and Rosenthal, M. Sara, Ph.D. *The Complete Thyroid Book.* New York: McGraw-Hill, 2005.

Alexander, Ivy M., and Knight, Karla A., R.N., M.S.N. *100 Questions and Answers about Osteoporosis and Osteopenia.* Sudbury, MA: Jones and Bartlett, 2006.

Alon, Ruthy. *Mindful Spontaneity: Lessons in the Feldenkrais Method.* Berkeley, CA: North Atlantic Books, 1996.

Altman, Nathaniel. *Everybody's Guide to Chiropractic Health Care.* Los Angeles: J.P. Tarcher, 1990.

Anson, Briah. *Rolfing: Stories of Personal Empowerment.* Kansas City, MO: Heartland Personal Growth Press, 1992.

Antol, Marie Nadine. *Healing Teas: How to Prepare and Use Teas to Maximize Your Health.* Garden City Park, NY: Avery Publishing Group, 1996.

Ash, Richard N., M.D., with Conkling, Winifred. *What Your Doctor May Not Tell You about IBS.* New York: Warner Books, 2004.

Astor, Stephen. *Hidden Food Allergies.* Garden City Park, NY: Avery Publishing Group, 1997.

Aubin, Michel, and Picard, Philippe. *Homeopathy and Your Health.* Garden City Park, NY: Avery Publishing Group, 1996.

Bach, Edward, M.D., and Wheeler, F.J. *The Bach Flower Remedies.* New Canaan, CT: Keats Publishing, 1979.

Baginski, Bodo J., and Sharamon, Shalila. *Universal Life Energy.* Mendocino, CA: LifeRhythm, 1988.

Baker, Jan. *Yoga for Real People.* Boston: Weiser Books, 2002.

Balch, James F., M.D., and Balch, Phyllis A., C.N.C. *Prescription for Nutritional Healing.* Garden City Park, NY: Avery Publishing Group, 1997.

Bandler, Richard, and Grinder, John. *Reframing: Neuro-Linguistic Programming and the Transformation of Meaning.* Moab, UT: Real People Press, 1982.

Barksy, Arthur J., M.D., and Deans, Emily C., M.D. *Stop Being Your Symptoms and Start Being Yourself: The 6-Week Mind-Body Program to Ease Your Chronic Symptoms.* New York: Collins, 2006.

Barnett, Libby, and Chambers, Maggie, with Davidson, Susan. *Reiki Energy Medicine.* Rochester, VT: Healing Arts Press, 1996.

Beaulieu, John, N.D., Ph.D., R.P.P. *Polarity Therapy Workbook.* New York: BioSonic Enterprises, 1994.

Beck, Mark F. *Milady's Theory and Practice of Therapeutic Massage.* 2nd ed. Albany, NY: Milady Publishing Company, 1994.

Benjamin, Patricia J., and Lamp, Scott P. *Understanding Sports Massage.* Champaign, IL: Human Kinetics, 1996.

Benson, Herbert, M.D., with Klipper, Miriam Z. *The Relaxation Response.* New York: Wings Books, 1992.

Benson, Herbert, M.D., with Proctor, William. *Your Maximum Mind.* New York: Times Books, 1987.

Benson, Herbert, M.D., with Stark, Marg. *Timeless Healing: The Power and Biology of Belief.* New York: Scribner, 1996.

Benson, Herbert, M.D., and Stuart, Eileen M., R.N., M.S. *The Wellness Book.* New York: Simon & Schuster, 1993.

Bentley, Eilean. *The Essential Massage Book: The Complete Guide to the Primary Hands-On Therapy.* London, UK: Gaia Books Limited, 2005.

Beresford-Cooke, Carola, and Albright, Peter. *Acupressure (Naturally Better).* New York: Quarto, 1996.

Berger, Stuart M., M.D. *How to Be Your Own Nutritionist.* New York: Morrow, 1987.

Berry, Linda, D.C., C.C.D. *Internal Cleansing.* 2nd ed. Roseville, CA: Prima Health, 2000.

Biermann, June, and Toohey, Barbara. *The Stroke Book: A Guide to Life after Stroke for Survivors and Those Who Care for Them.* New York: Jeremy P. Tarcher/Penguin, 2005.

Birch, Beryl Bender. *Power Yoga.* New York: Simon & Schuster, 1995.

Blanchard, Kenneth M., M.D., Ph.D. *What Your Doctor May Not Tell You about Hypothyroidism.* New York: Warner Books, 2004.

Blumenfield, Larry (editor). *The Big Book of Relaxation.* Roslyn, NY: The Relaxation Company, 1994.

Blumenthal, Mark (editor). *Herbal Medicine.* Newton, MA: Integrative Medicine Communications, 2000.

Bond, Mary. *Balancing Your Body: A Self-Help Approach to Rolfing Movement.* Rochester, VT: Healing Arts Press, 1996.

Borysenko, Joan, with Rothstein, Larry. *Minding the Body, Mending the Mind.* New York: Bantam Books, 1988, 1987.

Bourne, Edmund J., Ph.D. *The Anxiety and Phobia Workbook.* Oakland, CA: New Harbinger Publications, 1995.

Brody, Jane E. *Jane Brody's Nutrition Book.* New York: Bantam Books, 1987.

Bruckner-Gordon, Fredda, D.S.W., Gangi, Barbara Kuerer, C.S.W., and Wallman, Geraldine Urbach, D.S.W. *Making Therapy Work: Your Guide to Choosing, Using, and Ending Therapy.* New York: Harper & Row, 1988.

Burstall, Dawn, R.D., Vallis, T. Michael, Ph.D., and Turnball, Geoffrey K., M.D. *IBS Relief: A Complete Approach to Managing Irritable Bowel Syndrome.* Hoboken, NJ: John Wiley, 2006.

Carrico, Mara. *Yoga Basics.* New York: Henry Holt, 1997.

Carter, Mildred. *Body Reflexology: Healing at Your Fingertips.* West Nyack, NY: Parker Publishing Company, 1983.

Carter, Mildred, and Weber, Tammy. *Healing Yourself with Foot Reflexology.* Englewood Cliffs, NJ: Prentice Hall, 1997.

Casey, Aggie, R.N., M.S., and Benson, Herbert, M.D., with O'Neill, Brian. *The Harvard Medical School Guide to Lowering Your Blood Pressure.* New York: McGraw Hill, 2006.

Castleman, Michael. *The New Healing Herbs.* Emmaus, PA: Rodale, 2001.

Chilton, Floyd H. "Ski", Ph.D., with Tucker, Laura. *Inflammation Nation: The First Clinically Proven Eating Plan to End Our Nation's Secret Epidemic.* New York: Fireside, 2005.

Chin, Richard, M.D., O.M.D. *The Energy Within: The Science behind Every Oriental Therapy from Acupuncture to Yoga.* New York: Marlowe, 1998.

Chopra, Deepak, M.D. *Perfect Health: The Complete Mind/Body Guide.* New York: Harmony Books, 1991.

Clark, Jan. *Natural Menopause.* London, UK: Hamlyn, 2004.

Clark, Nancy. *Nancy Clark's Sports Nutrition Guidebook.* Champaign, IL: Leisure Press, 1990.

Cohen, Dan. *An Introduction to Craniosacral Therapy: Anatomy, Function and Treatment.* Berkeley, CA: North Atlantic Books, 1995.

Cohen, Ken S. *The Way of Qigong.* New York: Ballantine Books, 1997.

Contreras, Francisco, M.D., and Kennedy, Daniel E. *Fighting Cancer 20 Different Ways.* Lake Mary, FL: Siloam, 2005.

Crayhon, Robert, M.S. *Robert Crayhon's Nutrition Made Simple.* New York: M. Evans, 1996.

Danskin, David G., Ph.D., and Crow, Mark A., Ph.D. *Biofeedback: An Introduction and Guide.* Palo Alto, CA: Mayfield Publishing Company, 1981.

Davies, Clair, NCTMB, with Davies, Amber. *The Trigger Point Therapy Workbook: Your Self-Treatment Guide for Pain Relief.* 2nd ed. Oakland, CA: New Harbinger Publications, 2004.

Davis, Martha, Ph.D., Eshelman, Elizabeth Robbins, M.S.W., and McKay, Matthew, Ph.D. *The Relaxation and Stress Reduction Workbook.* 4th ed. New York: New Harbinger Publications, 1995.

Dilts, Robert, Hallbom, Tim, and Smith, Suzi. *Beliefs: Pathways to Health and Well-Being.* Portland, OR: Metamorphous Press, 1990.

Dossey, Larry, M.D. *Prayer Is Good Medicine.* San Francisco: HarperSanFrancisco, 1996.

Dougans, Inge. *The New Reflexology: A Unique Blend of Traditional Chinese Medicine and Western Reflexology Practice for Better Health and Healing.* New York: Marlowe & Company, 2006.

Dull, Harold. *WATSU: Freeing the Body in Water.* Middletown, CA: Harbin Springs, 1993.

Eckert, Achim. *Chinese Medicine for Beginners.* Rocklin, CA: Prima Publishing, 1996.

Editors of *Prevention* Magazine Health Books. *The Doctors Book of Home Remedies.* New York: Bantam Dell, 2002.

Eisenberg, David, M.D., with Wright, Thomas Lee. *Encounters with Qi: Exploring Chinese Medicine.* 3rd ed. New York: Norton, 1995.

Elinwood, Ellae. *The Everything T'ai Chi and Qigong Book.* Avon, MA: Adams Media, 2002.

Ellyard, Lawrence. *Reiki Q&A: 200 Questions and Answers for Beginners.* UK: O Books, 2006.

Elwart, Harry A., N.D., Ph.D. *Let's Stop the #1 Killer of Americans Today: A Natural Approach to Preventing and Reversing Heart Disease.* Bloomington, IN: AuthorHouse, 2006.

Feldenkrais, Moshé. *Awareness through Movement: Health Exercises for Personal Growth.* San Francisco: HarperSan Francisco, 1990.

Fielding, Deborah, with Fielding, Simon. *The Healthy Back Exercise Book: Achieving and Maintaining a Healthy Back.* New York: Barnes & Noble Books, 2001.

Finando, Donna, L.A.c., L.M.T. *Trigger Point Self-Care Manual for Pain-Free Movement.* Rochester, VT: Healing Arts Press, 2005.

Firebrace, Peter, and Hill, Sandra. *Acupuncture: How It Works, How It Cures.* New Canaan, CT: Keats Publishing, 1994.

Fischer, Harry D., M.D., and Yu, Winnie. *What to Do When the Doctor Says It's Rheumatoid Arthritis: Cure Your Pain, Become More Active, and Take Control of Your Medical Care.* Gloucester, MA: Fair Winds Press, 2005.

Fisher, Stanley, Ph.D., with Ellison, James. *Discovering the Power of Self-Hypnosis.* New York: Newmarket Press, 2001.

Frantzis, Bruce. *Tai Chi: Health for Life.* Berkeley, CA: Blue Snake Books, and Fairfax, CA: Energy Arts, 2006.

Fulghum Bruce, Debra, Ph.D., and McIlwain, Harris H., M.D. *Pain Free Arthritis: A 7-Step Program for Feeling Better Again.* New York: Henry Holt & Co., 2003.

Gandee, William S., D.C. *Triumph Over Illness.* Garden City Park, NY: Avery Publishing Group, 1998.

Gascoigne, Stephen. *The Chinese Way to Health: A Self-Help Guide to Traditional Chinese Medicine.* Boston: Tuttle Publishing, 1997.

Gelb, Michael. *Body Learning: An Introduction to the Alexander Technique.* New York: Holt, 1995.

Gillespie, Larrian, M.D. *You Don't Have to Live with Cystitis.* New York: Quill, 2002.

Goldsmith, Joel S. *The Art of Meditation.* 2nd ed. San Francisco: Harper & Row, 1990.

Goodman, Saul. *The Book of Shiatsu: The Healing Art of Finger Pressure.* Garden City Park, NY: Avery Publishing Group, 1990.

Gordon, James S., M.D. *Stress Management.* New York: Chelsea House Publishers, 1990.

Greene, Robert A., M.D., and Feldon, Leah. *Perfect Balance: Dr. Robert Greene's Breakthrough Program for Finding the Lifelong Hormonal Health You Deserve.* New York: Clarkson Potter Publishers, 2005.

Hallowell, Michael. *Herbal Healing.* Garden City Park, NY: Avery Publishing Group, 1994.

Harrison, Sheila. *Help Your Child with Homeopathy.* Garden City Park, NY: Avery Publishing Group, 1996.

Hatcher, Chris, and Himelstein, Philip (editors). *The Handbook of Gestalt Therapy.* New York: J. Aronson, 1995.

Heussenstamm, Frances K., Ph.D. *Blame It On Freud: A Guide to the Language of Psychology.* Georgetown, MA: North Star Publications, 1993.

Honervogt, Tanmaya. *The Power of Reiki.* New York: Henry Holt, 1998.

Houston, F.M. *The Healing Benefits of Acupressure: Acupuncture without Needles.* 2nd ed. New Canaan, CT: Keats Publishing, 1993.

Houston, Mark C., M.D., with Fox, Barry, Ph.D., and Taylor, Nadine, M.S., R.D. *What Your Doctor May Not Tell You about Hypertension: The Revolutionary Nutrition and Lifestyle Program to Help Fight High Blood Pressure.* New York: Warner Books, 2003.

Huang, Alfred. *Complete Tai Chi.* Rutland, VT: Charles E. Tuttle Company, 1993.

Huey, Lynda, and Forster, Robert, P.T. *The Complete Waterpower Workout Book.* New York: Random House, 1993.

Hunt Christensen, Jackie. *The First Year— Parkinson's Disease: An Essential Guide for the Newly Diagnosed.* New York: Marlowe & Co., 2005.

Ingham, Eunice D. *The Original Works of Eunice D. Ingham: Stories the Feet Can Tell and Stories the Feet Have Told.* St. Petersburg, FL: Ingham Publishing, 1984.

Jahnke, Roger. *The Most Profound Medicine.* Santa Barbara, CA: Health Action Books, 1990.

Jarmey, Chris, and Mojay, Gabriel. *Shiatsu: The Complete Guide.* London: Thorsons, 1991.

Jensen, Bernard. *Foods That Heal: A Guide to Understanding and Using the Healing Powers of Natural Foods.* Garden City Park, NY: Avery Publishing Group, 1993.

Johnson, Joan. *The Healing Art of Sports Massage.* Emmaus, PA: Rodale Press, 1995.

Kabat-Zinn, Jon, Ph.D. *Full Catastrophe Living: Using the Wisdom of Your Body and Mind to Face Stress, Pain and Illness.* New York: Delacorte Press, 1990.

Kalibjian, Cliff. *Straight from the Gut: Living with Crohn's Disease and Ulcerative Colitis.* Sebastopol, CA: O'Reilly, 2003.

Kaptchuk, Ted J. *The Web That Has No Weaver: Understanding Chinese Medicine.* New York: Congdon & Weed, 1983.

Kaslof, Leslie J. *The Bach Remedies: A Self Help Guide.* New Canaan, CT: Keats Publishing, 1988.

Katz, Aaron E., M.D. *Dr. Katz's Guide to Prostate Health: From Conventional to Holistic Therapies.* Topanga, CA: Freedom Press, 2006.

Kean, Frances, and Voorhees, Susan. *A Simple Guide to Yoga.* White Plains, NY: Peter Pauper Press, 2002.

Kenyon, J.N. *Acupressure Techniques: A Self-Help Guide.* Rochester, VT: Healing Arts Press, 1998.

Kloss, Jethro. *Back to Eden.* 2nd ed. Twin Lakes, WI: Lotus Press, 2005.

Kogler, Aladar, Ph.D. *Yoga for Every Athlete.* St. Paul, MN: Llewwellyn Publications, 1995.

Koury, Joanne M., M.Ed. *Aquatic Therapy Programming.* Champaign, IL: Human Kinetics, 1996.

Krasner, A.M., Ph.D. *The Wizard Within: The Krasner Method of Hypnotherapy.* Santa Ana, CA: American Board of Hypnotherapy Press, 1990.

Krieger, Dolores, Ph.D., R.N. *Accepting Your Power to Heal: The Personal Practice of Therapeutic Touch.* Santa Fe, NM: Bear & Co., 1993.

Krieger, Dolores, Ph.D., R.N. *Therapeutic Touch Inner Workbook: Ventures in Transpersonal Healing.* Santa Fe, NM: Bear & Co., 1997.

Kushi, Michio. *The Macrobiotic Way.* Garden City Park, NY: Avery Publishing Group, 1993.

Lad, Vasant, B.A.M.S. *The Complete Book of Ayurvedic Home Remedies.* New York: Harmony Books, 1998.

Lange, Vladimir, M.D. *Be a Survivor: Your Guide to Breast Cancer Treatment.* Los Angeles, CA: Lange Publications, 2005.

Lawless, Julia. *The Encyclopedia of Essential Oils.* Rockport, MA: Element, 1992.

Leibowitz, Judith, and Connington, Bill. *The Alexander Technique.* New York: HarperCollins Publishers, 1991.

Lenarz, Michael, D.C., with St. George, Victoria. *The Chiropractic Way: How Chiropractic Care Can Stop Your Pain and Help You Regain Your Health without Drugs or Surgery.* New York: Bantam Books, 2003.

Lipski, Elizabeth, Ph.D., C.C.N. *Digestive Wellness.* 3rd ed. New York: McGraw-Hill, 2005.

Lockie, Andrew, M.D. *Encyclopedia of Homeopathy.* New York: D. Kindersley Publishing, 2006.

Lowen, Alexander, M.D. *Bioenergetics.* New York: Penguin/Arkana, 1994.

Lowen, Alexander, M.D. *Joy: The Surrender to the Body and to Life.* New York: Arkana, 1995.

Lu, Henry C. *Chinese Natural Cures: Traditional Methods for Remedy and Prevention.* New York: Black Dog and Leventhal Publishers, Inc., 2006.

Lu, Henry C. *Traditional Chinese Medicine: An Authoritative and Comprehensive Guide.* Laguna Beach, CA: Basic Health Publications, Inc., 2005.

Lukas, Christopher. *The First Year—Prostate Cancer: An Essential Guide for the Newly Diagnosed.* New York: Marlowe & Co., 2005.

MacDonald, Glynn. *Illustrated Elements of Alexander Technique.* Hammersmith, London: Element, 2002.

Macrae, Janet. *Therapeutic Touch: A Practical Guide.* New York: Knopf, 1988.

Magee, Elaine, M.P.H., R.D. *Tell Me What to Eat If I Have Irritable Bowel Syndrome.* Franklin Lakes, NJ: Career Press, 2000.

maranGraphics Development Group. *Maran Illustrated Weight Training.* Boston: Thomson Course Technology PTR, 2005.

Mark, Bow-Sim. *Combined Tai Chi Chuan.* Boston: Chinese Wushu Research Institute, 1979.

Maxwell-Hudson, Clare. *Aromatherapy Massage.* New York: DK Publishing, 1997.

McCarty, Meredith. *American Macrobiotic Cuisine.* Garden City Park, NY: Avery Publishing Group, 1996.

McCarty, Patrick. *A Beginner's Guide to Shiatsu.* Garden City Park, NY: Avery Publishing Group, 1995.

McDermott, Ian, and O'Connor, Joseph. *Neuro-Linguistic Programming and Health.* San Francisco: Thorsons, 1996.

McGee, Charles T., M.D., with Poy Yew Chow, Effie. *Miracle Healing from China—Qigong.* Coeur d'Alene, ID: Medipress, 1994.

McGill, Leonard. *The Chiropractor's Health Book: Simple, Natural Exercises for Relieving Headaches, Tension, and Back Pain.* New York: Crown Trade Paperbacks, 1997.

McLaughlin, Chris, and Hall, Nicola. *Secrets of Reflexology.* New York: Dorling Kindersley, 2001.

Meagher, Jack, and Boughton, Pat. *Sportsmassage.* Barrytown, NY: Station Hill Press, 1990.

Miles, Pamela. *Reiki: A Comprehensive Guide.* New York: Jeremy P. Tarcher/Penguin, 2006.

Miller, Lyle H., Ph.D., Smith, Alma Dell, Ph.D., with Rothstein, Larry, Ed.D. *The Stress Solution.* New York: Pocket Books, 1993.

Morrison, Judith H. *The Book of Ayurveda: A Holistic Approach to Health and Longevity.* New York: Simon & Schuster, 1995.

Müller, Brigitte, and Gunther, Horst H. (Gerken, Teja, translator.) *A Complete Book of Reiki Healing.* Mendocino, CA: LifeRhythm, 1995.

Mumford, Susan. *The Complete Guide to Massage.* New York: Plume, 1996.

Murray, Michael T., and Pizzorno, Joseph E. *Encyclopedia of Natural Medicine.* Rocklin, CA: Prima Publishing, 1991.

Murray, Michael T., and Pizzorno, Joseph E., with Pizzorno, Lara. *The Encyclopedia of Healing Foods.* New York: Atria Books, 2005.

Naparstek, Belleruth. *Staying Well with Guided Imagery.* New York: Warner Books, 1994.

Nelson, Miriam E., Ph.D. *Strong Women and Men Beat Arthritis.* New York: Perigee Books, 2003.

Neustaedter, Randall, O.M.D. *Flu: Alternative Treatments and Prevention.* Berkeley, CA: North Atlantic Books, 2004.

Nevis, Edwin C. (editor). *Gestalt Therapy: Perspectives and Applications.* New York: Gardner Press, 1992.

O'Connor, John, and Bensky, Dan (translators and editors). *Acupuncture: A Comprehensive Text.* Chicago: Eastland Press, 1981.

Ody, Penelope. *The Holistic Herbal Directory.* Edison, NJ: Chartwell Books, 2001.

Page, Phil, and Ellenbecker, Todd. *Strength Band Training.* Champaign, IL: Human Kinetics, 2005.

Parfitt, Andrew. *Seated Acupressure Bodywork: A Practical Handbook for Therapists.* Berkeley, CA: North Atlantic Books, 2006.

Paris, Bob. *Natural Fitness.* New York: Warner Books, 1996.

Parsa-Stay, Flora, D.D.S. *The Complete Book of Dental Remedies.* Garden City Park, NY: Avery Publishing Group, 1996.

Patterson Wildemann, Ann. *Sessions: A SelfHelp Guide through Psychotherapy.* New York: Crossroad Publishing, 1996.

Peeke, Pamela, M.D., M.P.H. *Fight Fat after Forty: The Revolutionary Three-Pronged Approach That Will Break Your Stress-Fat Cycle and Make You Healthy, Fit, and Trim for Life.* New York: Penguin, 2001.

Peper, Erik, and Holt, Catherine F. *Creating Wholeness: A Self-Healing Workbook Using Dynamic Relaxation, Images and Thoughts.* New York: Plenum Press, 1993.

Perricone, Nicholas, M.D. *The Clear Skin Prescription: The Perricone Program to Eliminate Problem Skin.* New York: Harper Resources, 2004.

Phaneuf, Holly, Ph.D. *Herbs Demystified: A Scientist Explains How the Most Common Herbal Remedies Really Work.* New York: Marlowe & Co., 2005.

Pierrakos, John C., M.D. *Core Energetics: Developing the Capacity to Love and Heal.* Mendocino, CA: LifeRhythm Publications, 1987.

Piscatella, Joseph C., and Franklin, Barry A., Ph.D. *Take a Load Off Your Heart: 109 Things You Can Actually Do to Prevent, Halt, or Reverse Heart Disease.* New York: Workman Publishing, 2003.

Pratt, Steven, M.D., and Matthews, Kathy. *SuperFoods Rx: Fourteen Foods That Will Change Your Life.* New York: Harper Paperbacks, 2005.

Prudden, Bonnie. *Myotherapy: Bonnie Prudden's Complete Guide to Pain Free Living.* 2nd ed. New York: Dial Press, 1984.

Prudden, Bonnie. *Pain Erasure: The Bonnie Prudden Way.* New York: Ballantine Books, 1985.

Reader's Digest Association. *Magic and Medicine of Plants.* Pleasantville, NY: Reader's Digest Association, 1986.

Rimmerman, Curtis. *Heart Attack.* Cleveland, OH: Cleveland Clinic Press, 2006.

Robinson, Ronnie. *Total Tai Chi: The Step-by-Step Guide to Tai Chi at Home for Everybody.* London, UK: Duncan Baird Publishers, 2006.

Roizen, Michael F., M.D. *The realAge Makeover: Take Years Off Your Looks and Add Them to Your Life.* New York: HarperCollins, 2004.

Rolf, Ida P. (Feitis, Rosemary, editor.) *Rolfing and Physical Reality.* Rochester, VT: Healing Arts Press, 1990.

Rolf, Ida P. *Rolfing: Re-establishing the Natural Alignment and Structural Integration of the Human Body for Vitality and Well-Being.* Rochester, VT: Healing Arts Press, 1989.

Rosenthal, M. Sara. *The Hypothyroid Sourcebook.* Chicago: Contemporary Books, 2002.

Ross, Gary, and Bieling, Peter J. *Depression and Your Thyroid: What You Need to Know.* Oakland, CA: New Harbinger Publications, 2006.

Rossman, Martin L., M.D. *Guided Imagery for Self-Healing.* Tiburon, CA: H.J. Kramer, 2000.

Rubin, Jordan S., N.M.D., Ph.D. *Patient Heal Thyself.* Topanga, CA: Freedom Press, 2003.

Runowicz, Carolyn D., M.D., and Cherry, Sheldon H., M.D., with Lange, Dianne Partie. *The Answer to Cancer.* Emmaus, PA: Rodale, 2004.

Ruoti, Richard G., Morris, David M., and Cole, Andrew J. *Aquatic Rehabilitation.* Philadelphia: Lippincott, 1997.

Samskrti and Veda. *Hatha Yoga. Manual I.* 2nd ed. Honesdale, PA: Himalayan International Institute of Yoga Science and Philosophy, 1985.

Saputo, Len, M.D. *Boosting Immunity: Creating Wellness Naturally.* Novato, CA: New World Library, 2002.

Schneider, Jennifer P., M.D., Ph.D. *Living with Chronic Pain.* Long Island City, NY: Healthy Living Books, 2004.

Schneider, Robert H., M.D., F.A.C.C., and Fields, Jeremy Z., Ph.D. *Total Heart Health.* Laguna Beach, CA: Basic Health Publications, 2006.

Seidman, Maruti. *A Guide to Polarity Therapy: The Gentle Art of Hands-On Healing.* Boulder, CO: Elan Press, 1991.

Shafarman, Steven. *Awareness Heals: The Feldenkrais Method for Dynamic Health.* Reading, MA: Addison-Wesley, 1997.

Sharon, Michael. *Complete Nutrition.* Garden City Park, NY: Avery Publishing Group, 1989.

Shomon, Mary J. *Living Well with Chronic Fatigue Syndrome and Fibromyalgia: What Your Doctor Doesn't Tell You—That You Need to Know.* New York: HarperCollins, 2004.

Sibley, Veronica. *Aromatherapy Solutions: Essential Oils to Lift the Mind, Body and Spirit.* London, UK: Hamlyn, 2003.

Sinatra, Stephen T., M.D., F.A.C.C. *The Sinatra Solution: New Hope for Preventing and Treating Heart Disease.* North Bergen, NJ: Basic Health Publications, Inc., 2005.

Singh, Rajinder. *Inner and Outer Peace through Meditation.* Rockport, MA: Element Books, 1996.

Sklar, Jill. *The First Year—Crohn's Disease and Ulcerative Colitis: An Essential Guide for the Newly Diagnosed.* New York: Marlowe and Co., 2002.

So, James Tin Yau. *The Book of Acupuncture Points.* Brookline, MA: Paradigm Publications, 1985.

Stone, Randolph. Dr. Randolph Stone's *Polarity Therapy: The Complete Collected Works, Volume I and II.* Reno, NV: CRCS Publications, 1986.

Tagliaferri, Mary, M.D., L.A.c., Cohen, Isaac, O.M.D., L.A.c., and Tripathy, Debu, M.D. (editors). *The New Menopause Book.* New York: Avery, 2006.

Tappan, Frances M., Ed.D., M.A. *Tappan's Handbook of Healing Massage Techniques.* 3rd ed. Stanford, CT: Appleton & Lange, 1998.

Thompson, Rob, M.D. *The Glycemic Load Diet.* New York: McGraw-Hill, 2006.

Tousley, Dirk. *The Chiropractic Handbook for Patients.* Independence, MO: White Dove Publishing Company, 1985.

Trager, Milton, M.D., and Hammond, Cathy. *Movement as a Way to Agelessness: A Guide to Trager Mentastics.* Barrytown, NY: Station Hill Press, 1995.

Trivieri, Larry Jr., and Anderson, John W. (editors). *Alternative Medicine: The Definitive Guide.* 2nd ed. Berkeley, CA: Celestial Arts, 2002.

Tweed, Vera. (Challem, Jack, editor.) *Basic Health Publications User's Guide to Carnitine and Acetyl-L-Carnitine.* Laguna Beach, CA: Basic Health Publications, Inc., 2006.

Ullman, Dana. *The Consumer's Guide to Homeopathy.* New York: Jeremy P. Tarcher, 1996.

Ullman, Dana. *Homeopathy A–Z.* Carlsbad, CA: Hay House, 1999.

Upledger, John E., D.O., F.A.A.O. *Your Inner Physician and You: Craniosacral Therapy* and *Somatoemotional Release.* Berkeley, CA: North Atlantic Books, 1997.

Varona, Verne. *Nature's Cancer Fighting Foods.* Paramus, NJ: Rewards Books, 2001.

Vishnudevananda, Swami. *The Complete Illustrated Book of Yoga.* New York: Harmony Books, 1988.

Voner, Valerie, C.R.T., C.T.M., R.M.T. *The Everything Reflexology Book.* Avon, MA: Adams Media Corporation, 2003.

Vukovic, Laurel, M.S.W. *Overcoming Sleep Disorders Naturally.* Laguna Beach, CA: Basic Health Publications, 2005.

Walser, Mackenzie, M.D., with Thorpe, Betsy. *Coping with Kidney Disease: A 12-Step Treatment Program to Help You Avoid Dialysis.* Hoboken, NJ: John Wiley & Sons, 2004.

Walsh, William, M.D., F.A.C.A. *The Food Allergy Book.* Garden City Park, NY: Avery Publishing Group, 1995.

Weil, Andrew, M.D. *Natural Health, Natural Medicine.* Boston: Houghton Mifflin, 2004.

Weiner, Michael. *The Complete Book of Homeopathy.* New York: MJF Books, 1997.

Whichello Brown, Denise. *Reflexology Basics.* New York: Sterling Publishing, 2001.

Wilde, Christian. *Hidden Causes of Heart Attack and Stroke: Inflammation, Cardiology's New Frontier.* Valley Village, CA: Abigon Press, 2003.

Wildwood, Chrissie. *The Encyclopedia of Aromatherapy.* Rochester, VT: Healing Arts Press, 1996.

Wildwood, Christine. *Flower Remedies: Natural Healing with Flower Essences.* Rockport, MA: Element, 1995.

Wilk, Chester A., D.C. *Medicine, Monopolies and Malice.* Garden City Park, NY: Avery Publishing Group, 1996.

Williams, Tom. *Chinese Medicine.* Rockport, MA: Element Books, 1997.

Williamson, Vivien. *Bach Remedies and Other Flower Essences.* New York: Lorenz Books, Anness Publishing, 2000.

Wilson, James L., N.D., D.C., Ph.D. *Adrenal Fatigue: 21st Century Stress Syndrome.* Petaluma, CA: Smart Publications, 2001.

Wilson, Roberta. *Aromatherapy for Vibrant Health and Beauty.* Garden City Park, NY: Avery Publishing Group, 1995.

Wise, Anna. *The High-Performance Mind: Mastering Brainwaves for Insight, Healing and Creativity.* New York: Putnam, 1995.

Wolberg, Lewis R. *Hypnosis: Is It for You?* New York: Dembner Books, 1982.

Yamamoto, Shizuko, and McCarty, Patrick. *The Shiatsu Handbook: A Guide to the Traditional Art of Shiatsu Acupressure.* Garden City Park, NY: Avery Publishing Group, 1996.

Index

Underscored page references indicate boxed text.